Atlas of Film-Screen Mammography

Second Edition

Atlas of Film-Screen Mammography

Second Edition

Ellen Shaw de Paredes, M.D.

Department of Radiology
University of Virginia School of Medicine
Charlottesville, Virginia

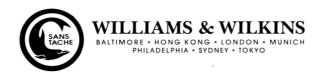

WILLIAMS & WILKINS
BALTIMORE · HONG KONG · LONDON · MUNICH
PHILADELPHIA · SYDNEY · TOKYO

Editor: Timothy H. Grayson
Managing Editor: Victoria M. Vaughn
Copy Editor: Bill Cady
Designer: Norman W. Och
Illustration Planner: Lorraine Wrzosek
Production Coordinator: Kathleen C. Millet

Accurate indications, adverse reactions, and dosage schedules for drugs are provided in this book, but it is possible that they may change. The reader is urged to review the package information data of the manufacturers of the medications mentioned.

Printed in the United States of America

First Edition 1989

Library of Congress Cataloging-in-Publication Data

De Paredes, Ellen Shaw.
    Atlas of film-screen mammography / Ellen Shaw de Paredes.—2nd
ed.
       p. cm.
    Includes bibliographical references and index.
    ISBN 0-683-06758-3
    1. Breast—Cancer—Diagnosis—Atlases. 2. Breast—Radiography—
Atlases. I. Title. II. Title: Atlas of film-screen mammography.
    [DNLM: 1. Breast Neoplasms—radiography—atlases. WO 17 D419a]
RC280.B8D38   1992
616.99′44907572—dc20
DNLM/DLC
for Library of Congress   91-21627
                                        CIP

92 93 94 95
2 3 4 5 6 7 8 9 10

To Victor

For his idea to write this book
and for his tremendous encouragement,
support, and advice,
I am always grateful.

Foreword

Although many years of effort have been spent in improving surgical and radiotherapeutic techniques, the mortality rate from breast cancer remains appalling. It is commonly conceded that early detection is the best means of reducing this mortality. Fortunately, mammography has finally evolved as a means of achieving this purpose. At last we have an opportunity to improve significantly the cure rate for patients with breast cancer.

Mammography today is far different from what it was when I became involved with it more than 25 years ago. Progress has resulted from the dedicated efforts of the pioneers in this field, such as Egan and Wolfe and their associates. Today, this progress continues with further improvement in image quality, techniques for localizing lesions, and biopsy procedures. These advances have led to greatly improved detection rates. They have also made it necessary for the radiologist constantly to modify his or her patterns of practice and to become a perennial student in the field.

Dr. Ellen Shaw de Paredes has been tireless in the pursuit of excellence in her mammographic program at the University of Virginia. Her work exemplifies the enlightened state of modern mammography. This book reflects her clinical experience and contains a wealth of teaching axioms gleaned from working with many residents, fellows, and surgical colleagues. Her new edition includes additional case material to amplify her teaching points. Also included are discussions of interventional procedures and a valuable chapter on the postoperative breast. These additions should further enhance the scope of this valuable work.

Theodore E. Keats, M.D.
Professor and Chairman
Department of Radiology
University of Virginia School of Medicine
Charlottesville, Virginia

Preface to the Second Edition

In the past 5 years there has been a rapid burst in mammography utilization, and increasing numbers of asymptomatic women are undergoing screening procedures. A well-thought-out quality assurance program for mammography is necessary to optimize the benefits of early detection of breast cancer through screening. Such a quality assurance program includes not only the quality control of equipment and processing, but also the training and monitoring of performance of physicians and technologists.

The accuracy of the diagnostic skills of the radiologist greatly affects the rate of detection of early breast cancer as well as the recognition of lesions that are benign and do not need to be biopsied. New accreditation programs for mammography facilities and board examinations for radiologists and technologists assess quality of image production and interpretative and technical skills in mammography.

The goal of this book is to present, through mammographic images, the appearances of the normal breast and spectrum of benign and malignant conditions that affect the breast. This atlas can be a reference source when one is faced with an imaging dilemma, and it can serve as a tool for developing pattern recognition skills in mammography. This book will be useful to practicing radiologists or to radiology residents learning mammography. The second edition expands the chapters with new cases and more radiographic presentations of the various disease processes.

Each chapter is introduced with a review of the various benign and malignant diseases that can be manifested as a certain mammographic pattern (well-defined or ill-defined masses, calcifications, prominent ducts, edema) and is followed with a series of radiographs demonstrating each process. In each case, clinical findings and mammographic and histologic diagnoses are correlated, and in some cases additional sonographic or histopathologic images are presented.

In this second edition, the chapters on foundation of normal anatomy, techniques and positioning, and approach to mammography are followed by the various pattern recognition chapters, the axilla, and the male breast. The chapter on interventional procedures has been expanded to reflect the growing role of the radiologist in evaluation of breast abnormalities. A discussion of stereotaxis for needle localization and fine-needle aspiration biopsy has been incorporated into this chapter. Also, to reflect the increasing numbers of mammograms we read on patients who have undergone a prior surgical procedure, a separate chapter on the postsurgical breast has been added.

All mammographic images are film-screen images produced almost entirely at the University of Virginia Health Sciences Center. The new cases in the second edition were performed on Siemens Mammomat II mammographic units and were produced on Min-R E film (Eastman Kodak Company) and Min-R medium screens with extended cycle processing. Sonographic images were produced with 7.5-MHz linear array transducers using Siemens Sonoline SL-1 or Aloka ultrasound equipment. The presentation of all the radiography is with the patient's left breast toward the reader's left. For film reading, I place the mammograms as mirror images with the patient's left to the reader's left, in order to reduce the surface glare from the nonemulsion side of the film.

I wish to acknowledge the following individuals for their significant contributions to this book. My technologists, Diane Loudermilk, Deborah Smith, Marie Bickers, Mary Baldwin, Edith Pollard, Diane Quinn, and Melissa Spagnuolo, are responsible for the excellent radiographs that serve as the source material for the book. My special thanks go to Deborah Smith for assisting in writing the section on patient positioning. My thanks go to Patsie Cutright for her fine work in the preparation of the manuscript. Additional secretarial and production support was provided by Catherine Payne, Richard Cubbage, and Susan Moss, and editorial assistance was provided by Julia Shaw. Ursula Miller and Norman Carter of the Biomedical Communications Division produced the photographs of the images. Dr. Philip Feldman assisted me with the images and descriptions of histopathologic sections. My postresidency fellow, Dr. Christine Brown, assisted greatly with clinical work, allowing me time to complete the second edition.

Several individuals have been instrumental in directing my interests and area of subspecialization toward mammography. Pat Barnette was important in influencing my career move into mammography. Dr. Theodore Keats, Chairman of the Radiology Department, has provided me with direction, opportunity, and support to develop the breast imaging section. Lastly, special thanks go to my husband, Dr. Victor Paredes, for guiding my career into radiology, for suggesting that I write this atlas, and for encouraging and supporting me throughout this lengthy endeavor.

Ellen Shaw de Paredes, M.D.

Preface to the First Edition

"People see only what they are prepared to see."
(Ralph Waldo Emerson, Journals, 1863)

The early detection of breast cancer depends primarily on mammography. With the increasing emphasis on screening mammography by organizations such as the American Cancer Society, there is a rapidly expanding utilization of mammography services, and there is a concomitant need for increased training of radiologists and radiology residents.

High-quality images are absolutely necessary for the detection of subtle abnormalities. There are tremendous differences in patterns of the breast parenchyma among women. Although the number of diseases that affect the breast is not vast, the perception and analysis of an abnormality can make mammography seem difficult.

The purpose of this book is to present through images the various manifestations of breast diseases, so that the reader may use it not only as a reference source, but also as a tool for developing pattern recognition skills in mammography. The book will be useful to practicing radiologists or to radiology residents in the process of learning mammography.

Each chapter is introduced with a brief review of the various processes that are manifested as a specific pattern, and is followed by a series of radiographs demonstrating the lesions. Correlation of clinical findings, mammographic findings, and histologic diagnosis is made. In some cases, not only mammography but also ultrasound images and histopathologic sections are correlated.

The initial sections discuss the anatomy and physiology of the breast, the proper techniques for performing film-screen mammography, and the analysis of a mammogram. The body of the text deals with chapters divided by patterns—well-defined masses, ill-defined masses, calcifications, prominent ducts, and thickened skin. The remainder of the text covers the axilla, the male breast, and interventional procedures in mammography.

The recent technical trends are towards film-screen mammography. This book covers only film-screen techniques, and all images are film radiographs. The images were produced almost entirely at the University of Virginia on either an Elscint Mam-II unit, which does not utilize a grid, or newer Siemens Mammomat B and the Mammomat-2 units with grids. The higher contrast and improved image quality on the radiographs from the equipment with grids are apparent on the reproductions. Film-screen systems that have been utilized are Kodak Ortho M film and Min-R screens and Kodak T-Mat M film with Min-R Fast screens.

I wish to acknowledge the fine work of my dedicated technologists. Deborah Smith, Diane Loudermilk, Mary Owens, Bonnie Mallan, Marie Bickers, Theresa Breeden, and Lisa Elgin, who are responsible for the radiographs. My special thanks go to Deborah Smith for assisting in writing the section on patient positioning. Manuscript preparation was carried out by Joy Bottomly and Patsie Cutright. Esther Spears, Catherine Payne, Kim Nash, Adair Crawford, Susan Bywaters, Tracy Bowles, and Lisa Crickenberger assisted in the collection of cases and other production work. The line drawings were produced by Craig Harding, and the reproductions of radiographs were done by Ursula Bunch, Connie Gardner, and Patricia Pugh of the Biomedical Communications Division. I wish to thank Dr. Sana Tabbarah for her assistance with the pathology slides and descriptions. My postresidency fellows, Drs. Patricia Abbitt and Thomas Langer, have assisted greatly with clinical work, leaving me time to work on this project. My appreciation also goes to other physicians who have sent me interesting cases: Drs. Luisa Marsteller, George Oliff, Jay Levine, Alexander Girevendulis, A. C. Wagner, Bernard Savage, M. C. Wilhelm, Melvin Vinik, and James Lynde. Lastly, I wish to thank my husband, Dr. Victor Paredes, for his assistance with the production and editing of the book. Without their help, this work would not have been possible.

Ellen Shaw de Paredes, M.D.

Contents

Atlas of Film-Screen Mammography

Second Edition

1

ANATOMY OF THE BREAST

The breast or mammary gland is a modified sweat gland that has the specific function of milk production. An understanding of the basic anatomy, physiology, and histology is important in the interpretation of mammography. With an understanding of the normal breast, one is better able to correlate radiologic-pathologic entities.

Development

The development of the breast begins in the fifth-week embryo with the formation of the primitive milk streak from axilla to groin. The band develops into the mammary ridge in the thoracic area and regresses elsewhere.

If there is incomplete regression or dispersion of the milk streak, there is accessory mammary tissue present in the adult, occurring in 2–6% of women (1). Accessory breast tissue, particularly in the axillary area, that is separate from the bulk of the parenchyma may be identified on mammography in these women (2).

At 7–8 weeks, there is an invagination into the mesenchyma of the chest wall. Mesenchymal cells differentiate into the smooth muscle of the nipple and areola (1, 3). At 16 weeks, epithelial buds develop and branch. Between 20 and 32 weeks, placental sex hormones entering the fetal circulation induce canalization of the epithelial buds to form the mammary ducts. At 32–40 weeks, differentiation of the parenchyma occurs, with the formation of the lobules (3, 4).

The mammary gland mass increases by fourfold, and the nipple-areolar complex develops (1). Developmental anomalies include polymastia (accessory breasts along the milk streak), polythelia (accessory nipples), hypoplasia of the breast, amastia (absence of the breast), and amazia (absence of breast parenchyma) (1).

During puberty in girls, the release of follicle-stimulating hormone and luteinizing hormone by the pituitary causes release of estrogens by the ovary. Hormonal stimulation induces growth and maturation of the breasts. In early adolescence, the estrogen synthesis by the ovary predominates over progesterone synthesis. The physiologic effect of estrogen on the developing breast is to stimulate longitudinal ductal growth and the formation of terminal ductule buds (1). Periductal connective tissue and fat deposition increase (1).

Structure

The adult breast is composed of three basic structures: the skin, the subcutaneous fat, and the breast tissue, which includes the parenchyma and the stroma. Beneath the breast is the pectoralis major muscle, which is also imaged during mammography. The breast parenchyma is enveloped by deep and superficial fascial layers; Cooper's ligaments, the fibrous strands that support the breasts, traverse the parenchyma and attach to the fascial layers. The parenchyma is divided into 15–20 segments, with each drained by a lactiferous duct (Fig. 1.1). The ducts converge beneath the nipple, with about 5–10 major ducts draining into the nipple (Fig. 1.1). Each duct drains a lobe composed of 20–40 lobules (1).

The microanatomy of the breast was described by Parks in 1959 (4). Each lobule is 1–2 mm in diameter and con-

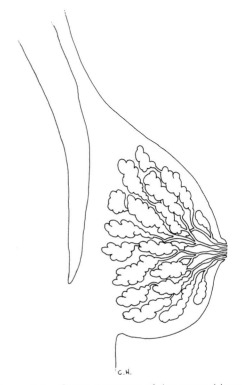

Figure 1.1 Gross anatomy of the normal breast.

tains a complex system of tiny ducts, the ductules, which terminate in blind endings. The ductules can respond to hormonal stimulation of pregnancy by proliferation and formation of alveoli (3). Two types of stroma are present: the perilobular connective tissue, which contains collagen and fat, and the intralobular connective tissue, which does not contain fat (4).

Wellings et al. (5) further classified the microstructure of the normal breast into the terminal duct lobular unit (TDLU) (Fig. 1.2). Small branches of the lactiferous ducts lead into terminal ducts that drain a single lobule. The terminal duct is composed of the extralobular segment and the intralobular segment. The lobule is composed of the intralobular terminal duct and the blindly ending ductules (5). The ductules are lined by a single layer of epithelial cells and a flattened peripheral layer of myoepithelial cells (5). A loose fibrous connective tissue stroma supports the ductules of the lobule.

The TDLU is a hormone-sensitive gland varying from 1 to 8 mm in diameter in the nonpregnant state and having the potential of milk production (6). The lobules normally regress at menopause, leaving blunt terminal ducts (6); but in women over 55 years with breast cancer, Jensen et al. (6) found the TDLUs to remain well developed.

The work of Wellings et al. (5) has suggested that the TDLU is a basic histopathologic unit of the breast from which many benign and malignant lesions arise. Fibroadenomas, sclerosing adenosis, apocrine cysts, epithelial cysts, and lobular carcinoma in situ are thought to develop in the lobule itself; atypical lobules and ductal carcinoma in situ develop in the TDLU, and only intraductal papillomas and epithelial hyperplasias of the larger ducts occur in the main lactiferous ducts (4). Correlative studies between radiographic and histologic appearances of the breast parenchyma suggest that small nodular densities on mammography rep-

resent lesions of the terminal duct lobular units and that linear densities are due to periductal and perilobular fibrosis (7).

Blood Supply and Lymphatic Drainage

The primary arterial supply to the breast is from the perforating branches of the internal mammary and lateral thoracic arteries. Minor contributions to the blood come from the branches of the thoracoacromial, subscapular, and thoracodorsal arteries (1). Venous drainage is primarily via branches of the internal mammary, intercostal, and axillary veins. If there is obstruction of the subclavian vein, collateral drainage produces dilated, tortuous vascular structures, easily visible on mammography (Fig. 1.4).

Lymphatic drainage is via the superficial plexus to the deep plexus to the axillary and internal mammary lymph nodes. The low axillary nodes are often visible on mammography, as are small intramammary nodes. It is unusual to identify on mammography intramammary nodes in a location other than the superficial region of the middle to upper outer quadrant of the breast.

Life Cycle

At birth and in childhood, only rudimentary ducts are present (Fig. 1.3). At puberty, growth and elongation of ducts occur, and buds of the future lobules form at the end of the ducts (4, 8). Periductal collagen is deposited, and mammographically the breast appears very dense and homogeneous. In the adult breast in response to progesterone, the second stage of glandular development occurs, namely, the formation of the lobules (8) (Figs. 1.5 and 1.6). Systemic or iatrogenic influences in childhood may be related to breast hyperplasia or amazia. Iatrogenic causes of amazia include excision of the breast bud during biopsy of the prepubertal breast and the use of radiation therapy to the chest (1) (Figs. 1.7–1.9).

With pregnancy, changes in the parenchyma occur to make milk secretion possible (8). There is a marked increase in numbers of lobules and an increase in their size and complexity (4). In the second and third trimesters of pregnancy, the terminal ductules expand into the secreting alveoli (4). Prolactin, in the presence of insulin, growth hormone, and cortisol, changes the epithelial cells of the alveoli into a secretory state (1). With the onset of lactation, the alveoli become maximally dilated and milk production occurs. On mammography (Figs. 1.10 and 1.11), the lactating breast appears extremely dense and dilated ducts may be imaged. After lactation ceases, the hypertrophied lobules shrink and may disappear. The breasts of parous women tend to appear more fatty and radiolucent than those of nulliparous women (Figs. 1.12–1.14)

With menopause, there is further involution of the paren-

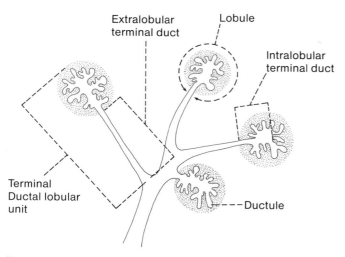

Figure 1.2. Classification of the microstructure of the breast (from Wellings et al. (5)).

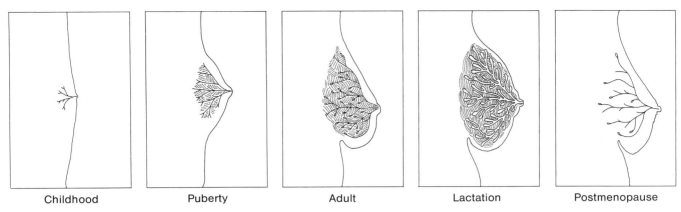

| Childhood | Puberty | Adult | Lactation | Postmenopause |

Figure 1.3. Changes that the normal breast undergoes during the life cycle.

chyma. The terminal lobules disappear and the small ducts eventually atrophy. The main ducts are not greatly affected (4). The postmenopausal breast appears more radiolucent (9), and only minimal glandular elements are generally seen (Figs. 1.15–1.17).

The effects of endogenous hormones related to the menstrual cycle have been observed on the histologic appearance of the normal breast (10). During the first half of the menstrual cycle, the effect of estrogen is to stimulate breast epithelial proliferation. In the second half of the cycle, after ovulation, progesterone causes ductal dilatation and differentiation of the ductural epithelial cells into secretory cells. In the 3–4 days before menses, edema and enhanced ductural acinar proliferation occur (1, 10, 11). Mammography at this time is more difficult because the breasts are tender and may appear more dense (Fig. 1.18). Postmenstrually, the edema is reduced and secretory activity of the epithelium regresses (1, 10).

Exogenous hormones may also have an effect on the mammographic appearance of the breast (Figs. 1.19 and 1.20). In some women placed on estrogen replacement therapy, an overall increase in density of the breasts may be observed (12). Stomper et al. (13) found changes related to hormonal influences in 24% of women placed on estrogen; these changes included diffuse increase in density (14%), multifocal areas of asymmetry (4%), and cyst formation (6%). Trapido et al. (14) found an increased risk of benign breast disease, both fibroadenomas and fibrocystic disease, in women on estrogen replacement therapy in comparison with a control group. The risk of benign breast disease was greater with increasing years of use of estrogen and was also higher in women with bilateral oophorectomy than in other postmenopausal women (14).

Danazol is sometimes used in the treatment of severe fibrocystic and cystic disease of the breast. The effect of danazol on the breast is to decrease pain and tenderness. The density of the breast also may decrease on the mammogram, allowing better visualization of the parenchyma (15).

Another systemic effect on the breast, weight loss, may produce a striking change in the mammogram (Fig. 1.21). The loss of body fat is accompanied by a loss of fat in the breasts, and the density of the parenchyma may appear much greater on mammography.

By keeping in mind the normal structure of the breast (Figs. 1.22–1.24), macroscopically and microscopically, and the effects on the breast of the hormonal changes during the life cycle, one can be better prepared to interpret the normal and the abnormal mammogram.

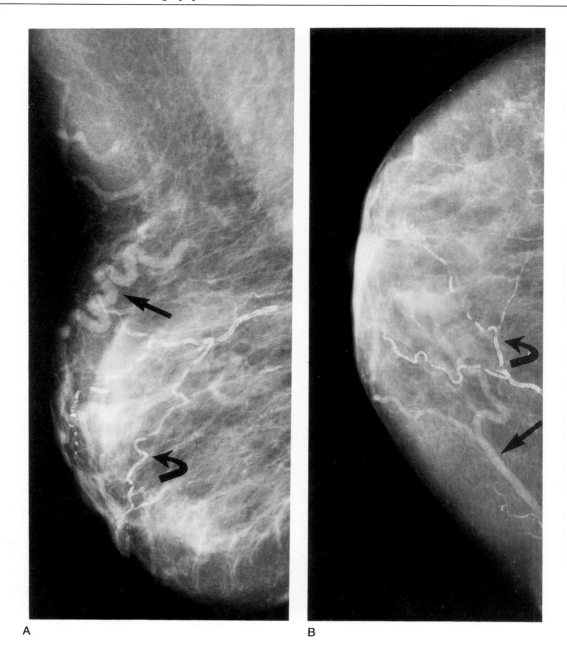

A

B

Figure 1.4.

Clinical: 65-year-old woman with a new thickening in the left upper inner quadrant.

Mammogram: Left oblique (**A**) and craniocaudal (**B**) views. The breast is moderately dense, but no mass is identified in the area of palpable concern. There is, however, a smoothly undulating tubular density *(arrows)* in the upper inner quadrant that has an appearance of a dilated vein. This vascular

structure contrasts with the densely calcified, serpiginous arteries of a smaller diameter *(curved arrows)*. By history it was found that the patient had previously had a left subclavian vein thrombosis.

Impression: Dilated venous collateral secondary to subclavian vein thrombosis.

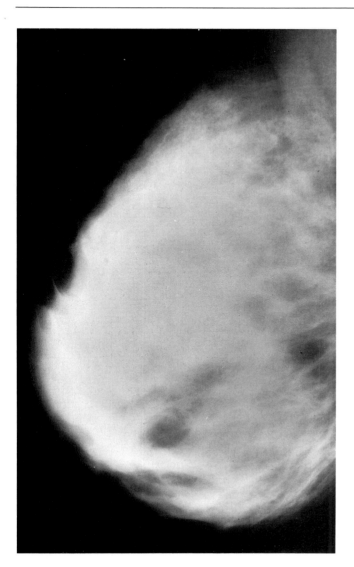

Figure 1.5.

Clinical: 15-year-old nulliparous woman.

Mammogram: The adolescent breast is very dense and glandular, particularly because of a large amount of collagen. A small amount of fat is present in the subcutaneous areas and within the parenchyma.

Figure 1.6.

Clinical: 25-year-old G2, P2 woman with pain in the right breast.

Mammogram: Bilateral oblique (**A**) and craniocaudal (**B**) views. The breasts are very dense and glandular but symmetrical in appearance. The mammographic appearance is normal for the age and parity of the patient.

Impression: Normal breast pattern for a 25-year-old woman.

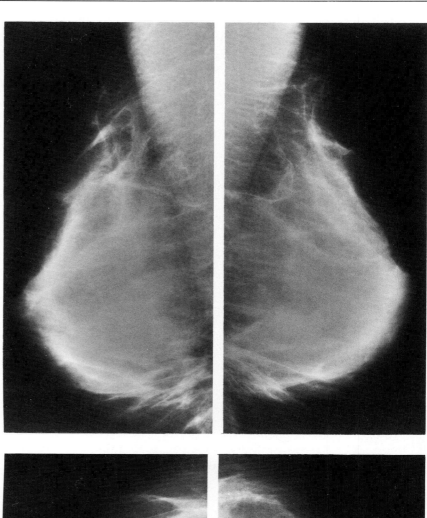

A

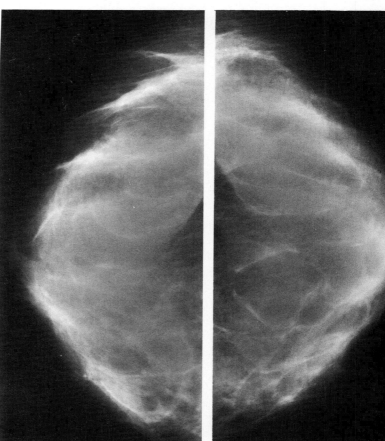

B

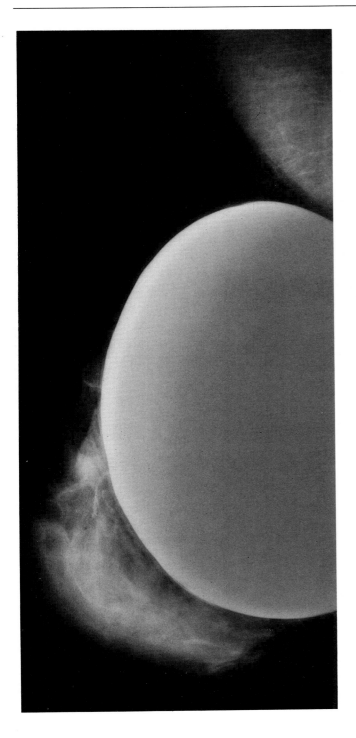
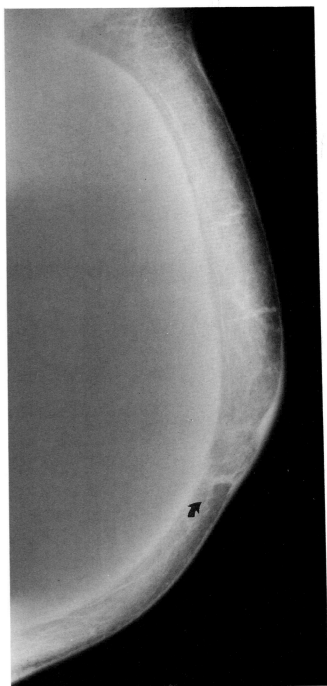

Figure 1.7.

Clinical: 26-year-old G0, P0 woman with a history of ectodermal dysplasia. She had bilateral breast implants placed during adolescence because of the lack of breast development.

Mammogram: Bilateral oblique views. There are bilateral breast implants present. There is some fairly dense glandular tissue in the subareolar area on the left side, but there are only rudimentary ducts on the right *(arrow).* The appearance on the right is similar to a normal male breast or a preado-lescent female breast. In the condition of ectodermal dysplasia, there is a lack of normal development of epithelial structures such as nails, teeth, skin, hair, and sweat glands. Since the breast is a modified sweat gland and is derived from epithelium, the development of the breast can be impaired in this condition.

Impression: Maldevelopment of the breast secondary to ectodermal dysplasia.

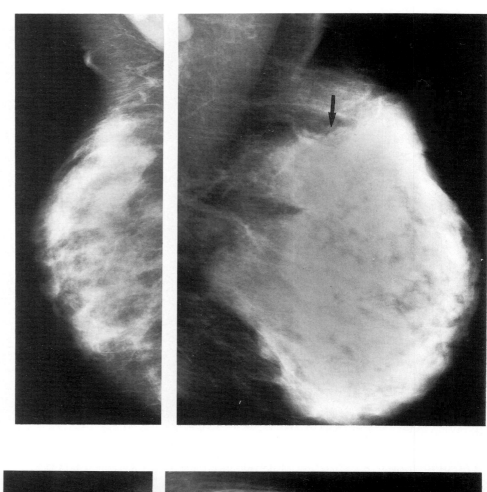

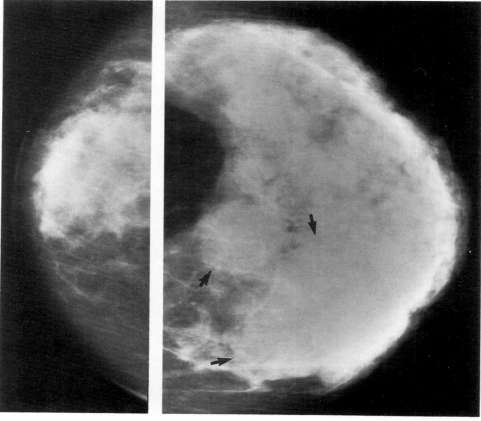

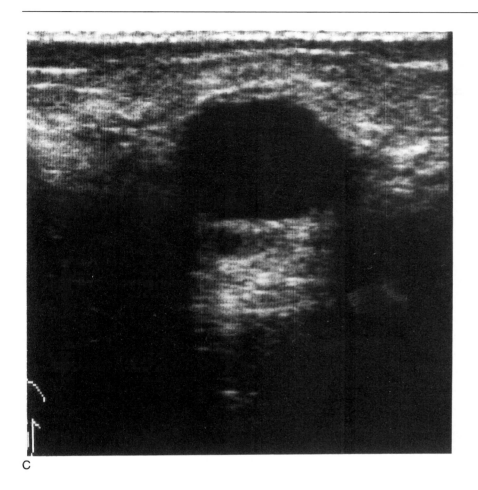

C

Figure 1.8.

Clinical: 48-year-old G1, P1 patient with a right upper inner quadrant mass and no previous history of breast surgery. Her breasts have been asymmetric in size since development.

Mammogram: Bilateral oblique (**A**) and craniocaudal (**B**) views and ultrasound (**C**) of the right breast. The breasts are markedly asymmetric in size, with the right being larger and generally more glandular than the left. Two well-circumscribed medium-density masses *(arrows)* are present on the right (**A**, and **B**), the more medial of which corresponded in location to the palpable finding. Ultrasound (**C**) shows the masses to be simple cysts—anechoic with a well-defined back wall and good through-transmission of sound.

Impression: Hypoplastic left breast with associated fibrocystic changes in larger, more glandular breast.

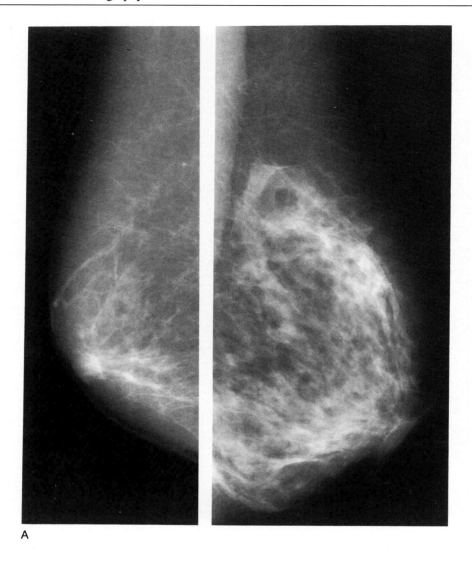

A

Figure 1.9.

Clinical: 49-year-old G2, P2 woman with a history of a plasma cell granuloma tumor of the left lung, treated with pneumonectomy and radiation therapy at age 4 years. At the thoracotomy, a resection of the entire left fifth and sixth ribs was performed. The left breast has been significantly smaller than the right since development. The patient has no history of breast surgery.

Mammogram: Bilateral oblique (**A**) and craniocaudal (**B**) views. Marked asymmetry in the appearance of the breasts is seen. The left breast is significantly smaller, and there is a paucity of glandular tissue in comparison with the right. This striking lack of glandular development is presumably related to the lack of development of the breast bud, either from atrophy secondary to the radiation therapy or from surgery in the left midchest area, which may have involved incidental removal of part of the breast bud.

Impression: Hypoplasia of the left breast, presumably of iatrogenic origin.

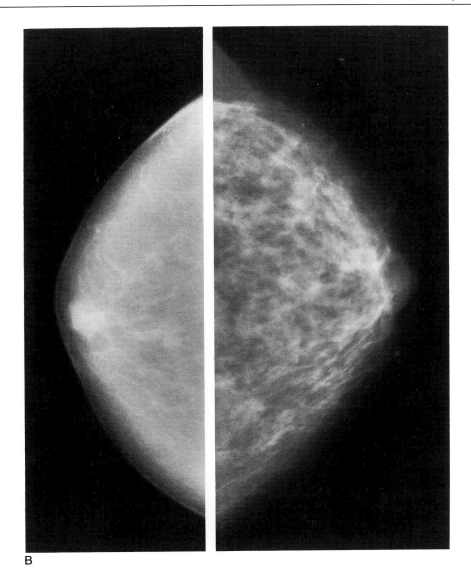

B

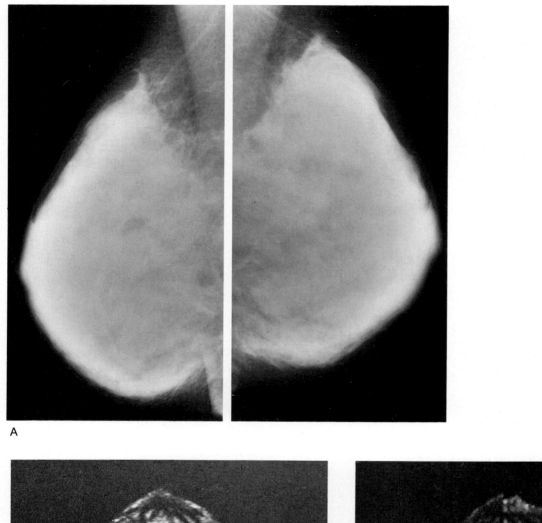

A

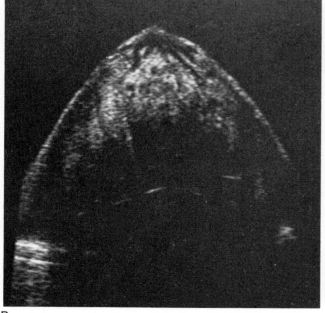

B

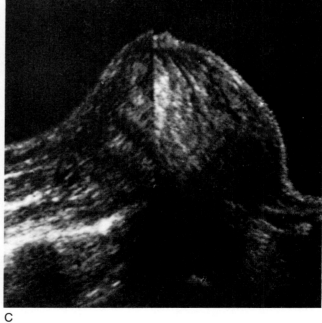

C

Figure 1.10.

Clinical: 29-year-old woman 3 months postpartum who is lactating.

Mammogram: Bilateral oblique views (**A**) and whole-breast sonography of right (**B**) and left (**C**) breasts. The breasts are extremely dense, normal for a lactating state (**A**). On sonography (**B**, and **C**), tubular structures are radiating from the nipples, representing dilated lactiferous ducts.

Impression: Lactating breasts.

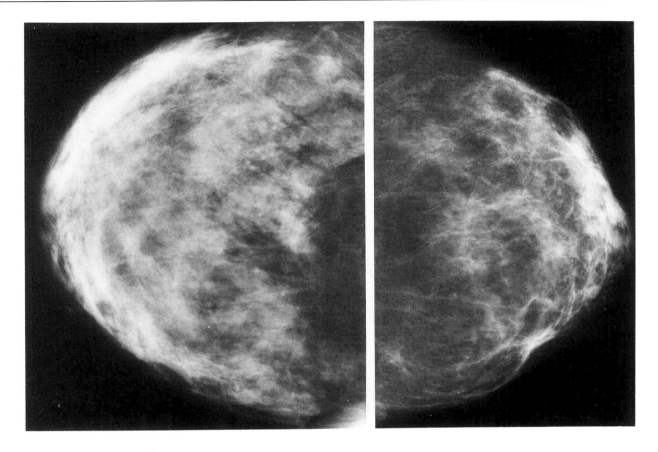

Figure 1.11.

Clinical: 34-year-old G2, P2 woman 6 months postpartum who has been breast-feeding only from the left breast.

Mammogram: Bilateral craniocaudal views. The breasts are asymmetric in size and density. The left breast, from which the patient has been lactating, is significantly larger and more glandular than the right. These changes are related to lactation, where the acini are engorged and the ducts are dilated.

Impression: Asymmetry in the breasts, related to lactation.

Figure 1.12.

Clinical: 35-year-old premenopausal G2, P2 woman.

Mammogram: The breasts are moderately dense, but there are areas of fatty tissue located medially and superficially. This is a normal pattern that one might expect to see in a patient of this age and parity. Note the normal pectoralis muscle shadow (arrow) on the right side. The pectoralis major muscle may appear larger on the ipsilateral side of the patient's handedness.

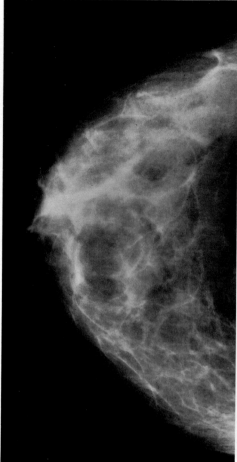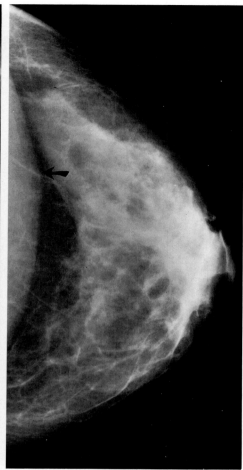

Figure 1.13.

Clinical: 36-year-old obese G4, P3, Ab1 woman.

Mammogram: The breasts show fatty replacement and appear more fatty than those of most young women. This degree of fatty replacement is more commonly seen in multiparous and obese women.

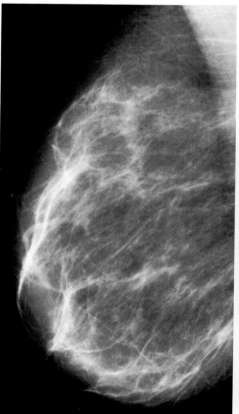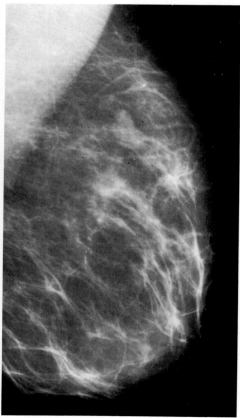

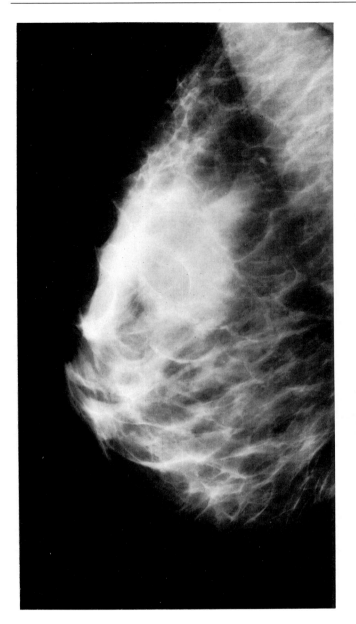
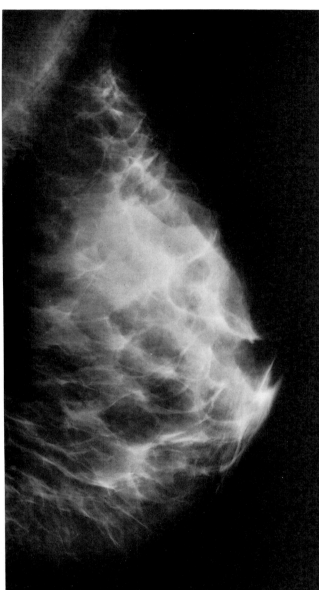

Figure 1.14.
Clinical: 40-year-old G2, P2 woman.
Mammogram: There is moderate glandularity in the upper quadrants with fatty replacement elsewhere.

Figure 1.15.

Clinical: 50-year-old postmeno-pausal G5, P3 woman.

Mammogram: The breasts show fatty replacement, with minimal glandular elements remaining. Partial involution of the paren-chyma is normally seen by age 50 years.

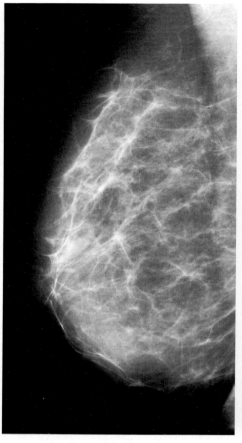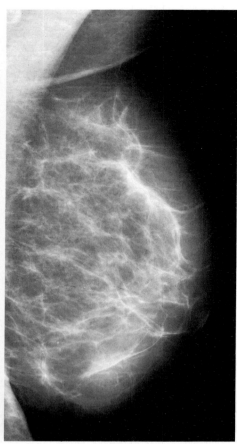

Figure 1.16.

Clinical: 64-year-old G3, P3 woman.

Mammogram: The breasts show fatty replacement. There has been further involution of the pa-renchyma in the postmenopau-sal patient.

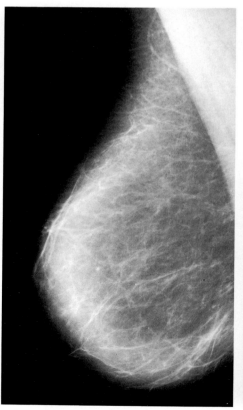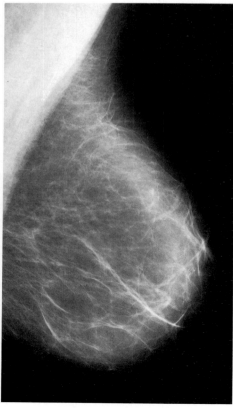

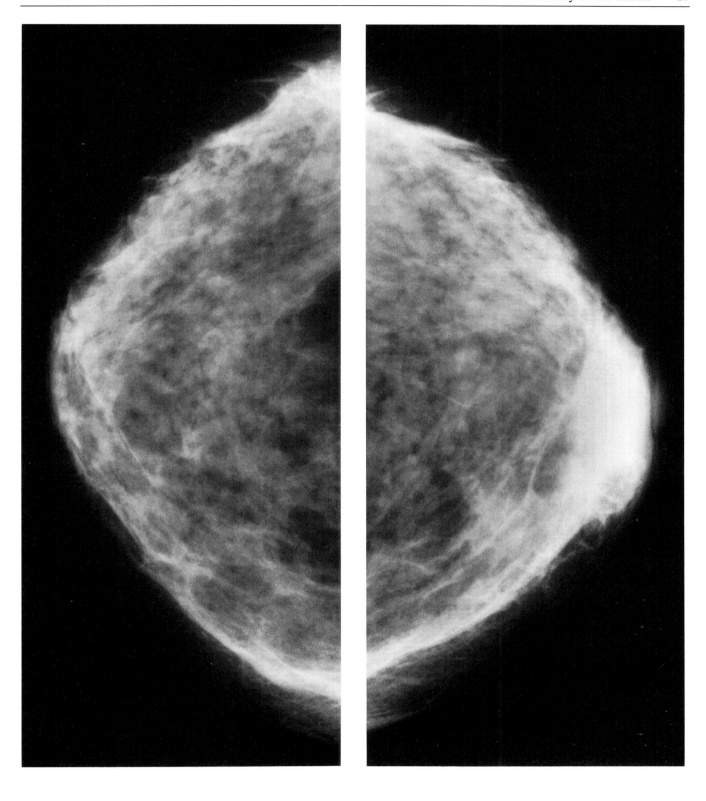

Figure 1.17.

Clinical: 72-year-old nulliparous woman.

Mammogram: The breasts are moderately dense and somewhat nodular. This appearance is more dense than usual for a postmenopausal patient, but this pattern may be seen in a nulliparous woman.

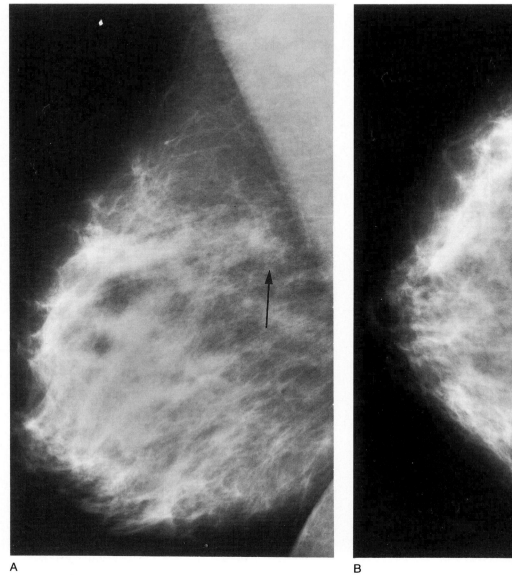

A

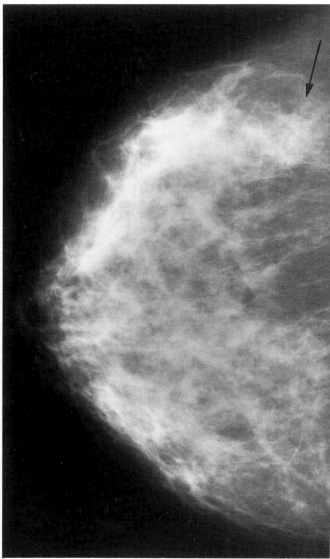

B

Figure 1.18.

Clinical: 47-year-old premenopausal G2, P2 patient with tender breasts.

Mammogram: left oblique (**A**) and craniocaudal (**B**) views on day 21 of her menstrual cycle, and left oblique (**C**) and craniocaudal (**D**) views on day 10 of the following menstrual cycle. On the initial films (**A**, and **B**), the left breast is dense, and there is a focal area of irregular increased density *(ar-*row) in the upper outer quadrant. On the subsequent films (**C** and **D**) in the early phase of the patient's following menstrual cycle, the overall density of the breast and the focal asymmetry have diminished, consistent with the effect of hormonal stimulation on the breast.

Impression: Effect of intrinsic hormonal status on the breast density.

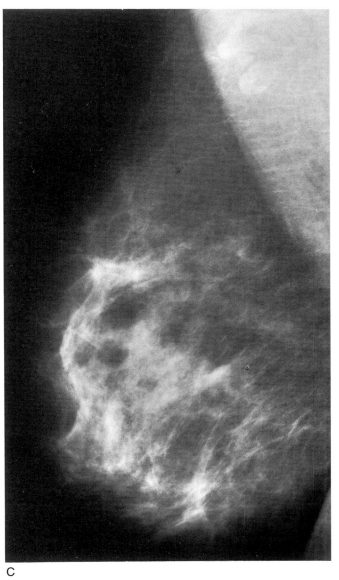

C

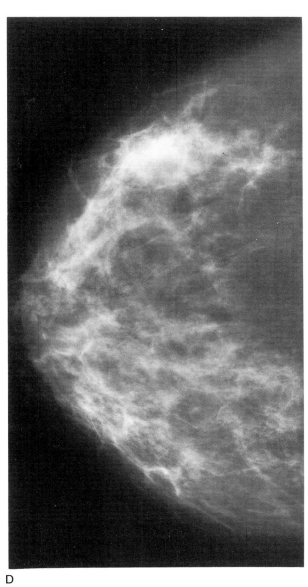

D

Figure 1.19.

Clinical: 56-year-old postmenopausal G2, P2 woman for screening. Initial mammograms were taken prior to the beginning of estrogen replacement therapy.

Mammogram: Bilateral oblique views, October 1988 (**A**), and bilateral oblique views, December 1989 (**B**). On the initial examination (**A**), the breasts are mildly glandular, and no focal abnormalities are seen. On the subsequent examination (**B**), after 1 year of estrogen replacement therapy, there is generalized increased glandularity bilaterally, consistent with the effects of the hormones.

Impression: Increased glandularity consistent with estrogen effects.

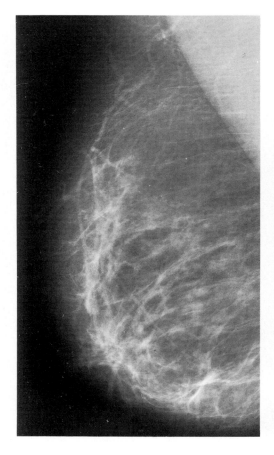
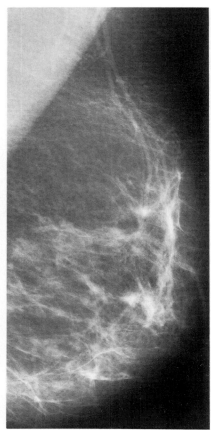

A

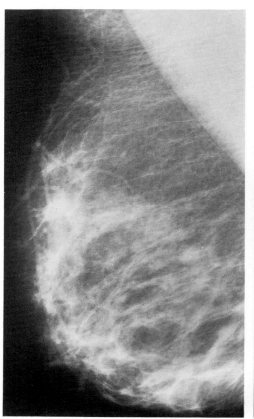
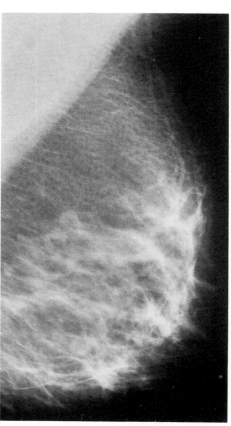

B

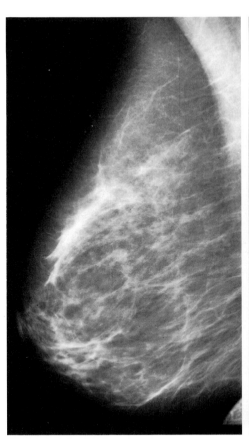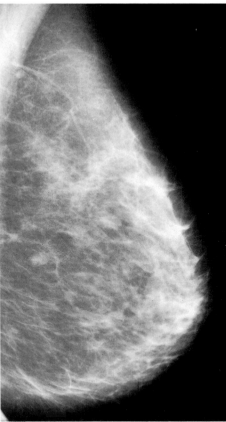

Figure 1.20.

Clinical: 63-year-old G3, P3 woman for screening mammography. (She had been placed on estrogen replacement therapy between the two studies.)

Mammogram: Initial bilateral oblique views (**A**) and bilateral oblique views 1 year later (**B**). Initially (**A**), the breasts were mildly glandular, normal for a postmenopausal patient. After 1 year of estrogen replacement therapy (**B**), the breasts have become diffusely more dense and glandular, having an appearance more like that in a premenopausal state.

Impression: Effect of estrogen therapy.

A

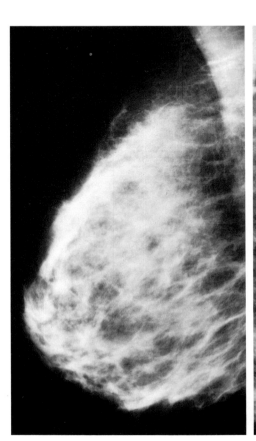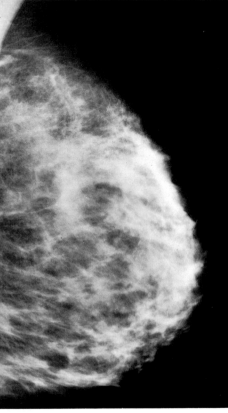

B

Figure 1.21.

Clinical: 44-year-old G0 woman who had a 50-pound weight loss in the previous 2 years.

Mammogram: Bilateral craniocaudal views in 1981 (**A**) and in 1986 (**B**). In 1981 (**A**), the breasts show largely fatty replacement, with mild glandularity present. In 1986 (**B**), the breasts are considerably more dense, presumably related to the weight loss.

Impression: Effects of weight loss on the appearance of the breasts.

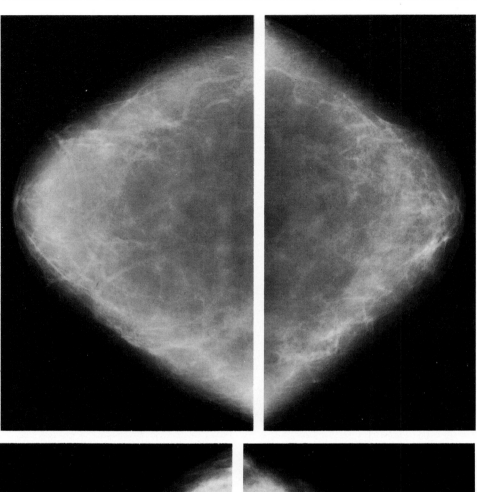

A

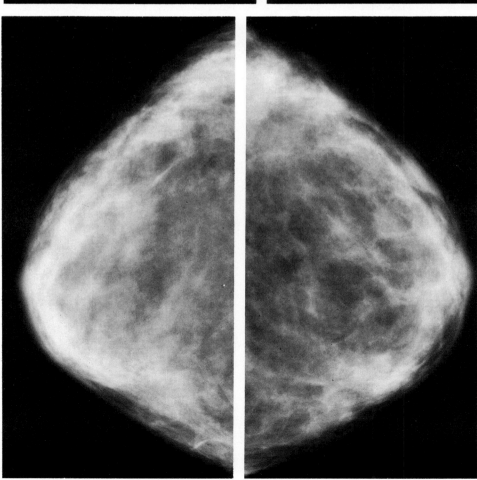

B

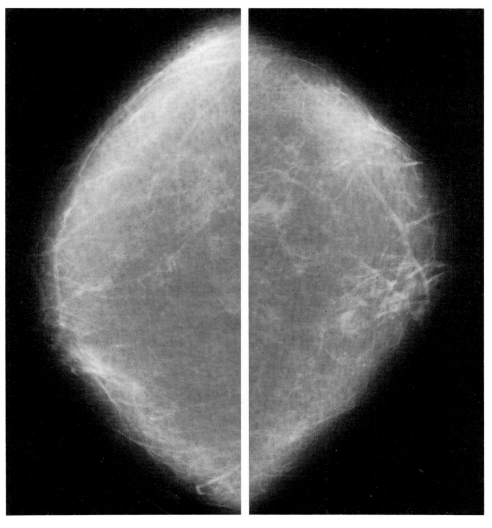

A

Figure 1.22. When the breast is well compressed, the pores in the skin are seen. In some women, as in this woman, the pores may be prominent throughout the skin surface (**A** and **B**).

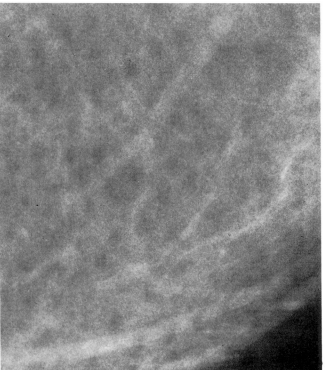

B

Figure 1.23.
Mammogram: Left craniocaudal view. The smooth ovoid density located posteriorly in the breast *(arrow)* represents the pectoralis major muscle. The muscle is usually not seen on the craniocaudal view, but the medial insertion may be seen and, when focally prominent, may simulate a mass.

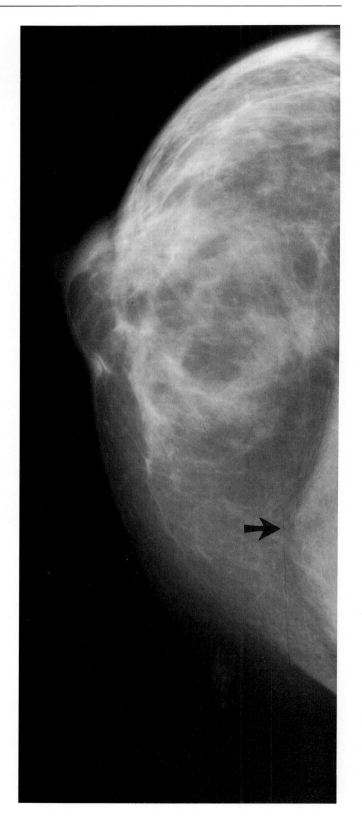

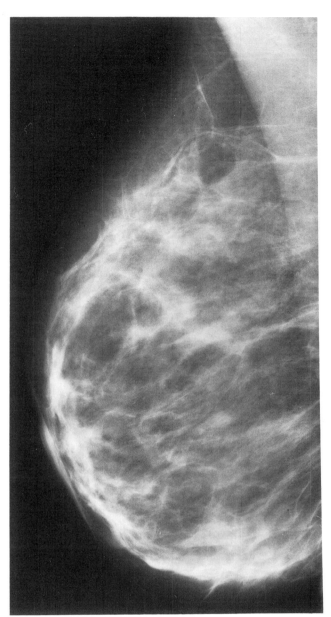

A

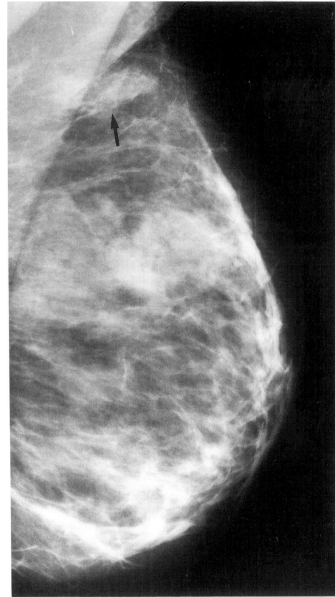

B

Figure 1.24.

Clinical: 49-year-old woman with a family history of breast cancer, for routine screening.

Mammogram: Left oblique (**A**) and right oblique (**B**) views. There is mild to moderate glandularity bilaterally. Focal slightly irregular amorphous tissue is noted in the right upper outer quadrant in the low axillary area *(arrow)* (**B**). This area was nonpalpable and was unchanged from prior examinations. The finding is consistent with ectopic or accessory tissue in the axillary tail.

Impression: Focal asymmetric tissue in the right axillary tail.

References

1. Osborne M. Breast development and anatomy. In: Harris JR, et al., eds. Breast diseases. Philadelphia: JB Lippincott, 1987.

2. Adler DD, Rebner M, Pennes DR. Accessory breast tissue in the axilla: mammographic appearance. Radiology 1987; 163:709–711.

3. Hughes ESR. The development of the mammary gland. Ann R Coll Surg Engl 1950;6:99–105.

4. Parks AG. The micro-anatomy of the breast. Ann R Coll Surg Engl 1959;25:235–251.

5. Wellings SR, Jensen HM, and Marcum RG. An atlas of subgross pathology of the human breast with special reference to precancerous lesions. JNCI 1975;55:231–273.

6. Jensen HM. On the origin and progression of human breast cancer. Am J Obstet Gynecol 1986;154:1280–1284.

7. Wellings SR, Wolfe JN. Correlative studies of the histological and radiographic appearance of the breast parenchyma. Radiology 1978;129:299–306.

8. Netter F. The reproductive system. In: Oppenheimer E, ed. The CIBA collection of medical illustrations. Summit, New Jersey: CIBA, 1965;2.

9. Fewins HE, Whitehouse GH, Leinster SJ. Changes in breast parenchymal patterns with increasing age. Breast Dis 1990;3:145–151.

10. Vogel PM, Georgiade NG, Fetter BF, Vogel FS, McCarty KS. The correlation of histologic changes in the human breast with the menstrual cycle. Am J Pathol 1981;104:23–34.

11. Fanger H, Ree HJ. Cyclic changes of human mammary gland epithelium in relation to the menstrual cycle—an ultrastructural study. Cancer 1974;34:574–585.

12. Pock DR, Lowman Rm. Estrogen and the postmenopausal breast. JAMA 1978;240:1733–1735.

13. Stomper PC, VanVoorhis BJ, Ravnikar VA, Meyer JE. Mammographic changes associated with postmenopausal hormone replacement therapy: a longitudinal study. Radiology 1990; 174:487–490.

14. Trapido EJ, Brinton LA, Schairer C, Hoover R. Estrogen replacement therapy and benign breast disease. JNCI 1984; 73:1101–1105.

15. Ouimet-Oliva D, Van Campenheut J, Hebert G, Ladouccur J. Effect of danazol on the radiographic density of breast parenchyma. J Can Assoc Radiol 1981;32:159–161.

TECHNIQUES AND POSITIONING IN FILM-SCREEN MAMMOGRAPHY

During the past two decades there has been significant improvement in the equipment and image recording systems for mammography. In addition to providing better images, these developments have resulted in a significant reduction in radiation dose. With the importance of and emphasis on mammography in the role of early detection of breast cancer, it is of utmost importance that meticulous techniques be used. Factors that affect the image quality include equipment, image recording system, processing, compression of the breast, and the technologist's skill in positioning the patient. Adherence to strict quality assurance guidelines is critical in mammography to maintain optimum image quality (1, 2). The interpretation skills of the radiologist are limited by a suboptimal image. A poor-quality mammogram or poor positioning can account for many of the cancers missed by mammography (3, 4), and technical errors should not be overlooked or accepted. For the radiologist to detect subtle signs of malignancy, high-quality images are a must. The emphasis of this book is on interpretation and pattern recognition, but it is important to review briefly the technical factors that affect the mammographic image.

Equipment

Only dedicated units should be used for film-screen mammography. Dedicated units are those with special focal spots, target and filter materials, low kilovoltage, and compression devices designed to optimize the mammographic image at low radiation doses. Under no circumstances can nondedicated equipment produce images of similar quality to those performed with dedicated units (Fig. 2.1).

There are two types of target materials being used currently: molybdenum and tungsten. With molybdenum targets, 0.03-mm molybdenum filtration is used; the molybdenum targets are particularly well suited for mammography because of the low kiloelectron volt x-rays produced. The characteristic peaks for molybdenum are 17.9 and 19.5 keV, which provide high-contrast images for breasts of average thickness.

When the 0.03-mm molybdenum filter is used, the photons at energies greater than 20 keV are suppressed, and a larger number of low-energy photons are used in recording the image (5). The kilovolt peak (kVp) setting for molybdenum targets is generally at 25–28 kVp (6).

With tungsten targets, a beryllium window and minimal aluminum filtration are recommended. In comparison with a molybdenum target, even at low kVp settings, the tungsten target produces more high-energy photons, and the subject contrast is, therefore, lower. Generally, settings of 22–26 kVp should be used for tungsten targets (5–7). A newer type of tube for mammography utilizes a tungsten target with a beryllium window and a molybdenum or a rhodium k edge filter to produce high-contrast images. For most patients a 0.06-mm molybdenum filter is automatically in place at low kVp settings; to penetrate thick dense breasts, the 0.05-mm rhodium filter is used at higher kVp settings (2).

The size of the focal spot of the tube is of particular importance in mammography because of the high resolution required for this work. To reduce geometric blurring, the focal spot size and the distance between the breast and image receptor should be kept as small as possible, and the object-to-focal-spot distance should be maximized (8). The size of the focal spot becomes even more important in magnification work (5), where it is generally recommended that the measured focal spot size be no greater than 0.3 mm (9) and preferably in the range of 0.1–0.2 mm (10, 11).

The use of grids in mammography improves image quality by reducing scatter, thus increasing contrast; there is a concomitant increase in radiation dose to the patient (12). Grids are of particular advantage in imaging the more dense, thick breast in which more scatter radiation is present, but because of the improvement in image quality with a grid, most radiologists routinely utilize the grid for all routine mammography. Many of the newer dedicated units have incorporated a reciprocating grid with a ratio of 5:1 (5). If an older dedicated unit is being used, a focused stationary grid with ultrahigh strip density and a ratio of 3.5:1 (5) can be purchased separately and will improve the images to some degree. The grids used in mammography are thinner than conventional grids and contain carbon fiber interspace material for lower absorption. Typical reciprocating grids are composed of 16-μm lead strips separated by 300-μm carbon-fiber resin interspaces (6). The increase in the radiation dose with a grid is about two times that of a nongrid film, but this may be compensated for by using faster screen-film combinations.

Dedicated mammography units should be equipped with a firm radiolucent compression device that forms a 90° angle with the chest wall. No rounded or curved edge compression devices should be used because the posterior aspect of the breast will not be adequately visualized (13). Vigorous compression of the breasts during mammography is extremely important in terms of producing an image of satisfactory diagnostic quality. Compression of the breasts is a very important factor in reducing scatter radiation, which degrades the image. With compression, there is spreading of the tissues apart, and small lesions are more easily identified within the parenchyma. The immobilization of the breasts decreases motion blurring, and the location of structures in the breast closer to the film receptor decreases geometric blurring. There is less variation in the density of the areas of the breast with compression to a uniform thickness from nipple to chest wall. Importantly, the radiation dose to the breast is decreased with compression (6).

Image Recording System

It is important that a screen-film system specifically designed for mammography be utilized in order to obtain the proper diagnostic quality of the images. With the newer dedicated units and the common use of grids and magnification techniques, it is also important that the film-screen combination chosen have the lowest radiation dose while the quality of the images is maintained. Single-emulsion film is recommended for contact mammography because of the image degradation secondary to crossover in double-emulsion systems. In 1972, DuPont introduced the LoDose screen-film systems, which was followed by the DuPont LoDose 2 system. Kodak introduced the MinR system in 1976 and OM film in 1980. Several new films and screens are available for mammography. Among these films are: Kodak OM-SO177, Konica CM, DuPont Microvision, and Fuji MiMa films (14). Some of these films have been specifically developed to be used in either standard 90-second or the extended 3-minute processors. The screens used for most routine mammography are single-back screens. The film and screen are in intimate contact, with the emulsion in contact with the top of the screen (15). Mammographic film-screen combinations have a much higher resolution than that of conventional radiography systems (2). Kimme-Smith et al. (14) found that the screens are of primary importance for good resolution, whereas contrast is affected more by type of film and processing (2, 14).

Cassettes specifically designed for mammography are most commonly used, but polyethylene envelopes that are vacuum sealed are also available. The cassette and its screen should be cleaned daily to maintain proper quality control and to reduce dust artifacts.

Quality control of film processing is of great importance in mammography. It is important to follow the manufacturer's recommendations for film processing in terms of the chemicals used, replenishment rate, development time, temperature, and processor maintenance (2). Developer temperature that is lower than that recommended by the manufacturer for mammography causes a loss in film speed and contrast (2), thereby necessitating a higher dose to produce films of satisfactory optical density (16). There is increasing utilization now of extended-cycle processing for single-emulsion films (2, 17). With extended-cycle processing, the film spends more time in the developer, thereby increasing the total processing time to 3 minutes. It is important that the processor be dedicated to mammography if extended-cycle processing is used. A reduction in radiation dose by 30% (2, 17) and an increase (17) in contrast of 11% were found when Kodak Om1-SO177 film was tested in 3-minute rather than 90-second processing.

Radiation Dose

The parenchyma of the breast, not the skin, is the area that is of greater concern regarding exposure. Therefore, the absorbed glandular dose, not the skin entrance dose, is the more important measurement (5). For a 5-cm-thick average breast the mean absorbed dose using OM film at 28 kVp with a molybdenum target is approximately 0.05 rad (5). Factors that affect radiation dose include: breast-tissue composition and thickness, x-ray tube target materials, filtration, kVp, grid use, film-screen combination, and processing (2). With the development of dedicated mammography equipment and the improvement in film-screen systems, there has been a tremendous decrease in the radiation dose from mammography.

Positioning

Most authors agree that two views should be performed for routine mammography (18, 19). The craniocaudal view and the lateral oblique view (20) are recommended as standard projections. Additional views may be necessary to evaluate specific areas within the breast (21–23), and the techniques for positioning the patient for these various views are described in this chapter. For all views, it is of utmost importance that the breast be compressed tightly with the compression device.

Craniocaudal View

The craniocaudal view is a standard transverse view of the breast (Fig. 2.2). The patient stands or is seated facing the mammographic unit with the head turned away from the breast being examined. The patient should lean slightly forward in order to include the upper posterior aspect of the breast on the film. The breast is pulled forward over the cassette, and the cassette holder is raised until the inframammary crease is smooth. Skin folds and wrinkles should be smoothed out; rotating the shoulder slightly back helps to smooth out the skin folds and the anterior axillary line. The nipple should be in profile if at all possible (Fig. 2.3). The film is marked in the axillary region, and vigorous compression is applied to the breast.

Occasionally, a lesion is seen only on the craniocaudal view and not on the sagittal view. A rolled craniocaudal view can be obtained by sliding the superior aspect of the breast medially or laterally and the inferior aspect of the breast in the opposite direction (22). If the ''lesion'' persists, the direction of its movement relative to its position on the standard craniocaudal view indicates its relative vertical position in the breast.

Lateral Oblique View

When the patient is positioned properly, the oblique view will demonstrate the pectoralis major muscle and the entire breast, including the inferior portion and the axillary tail, on one film. The pectoralis major muscle has a triangular shape with the apex at the level of the nipple (Fig. 2.4). The oblique view is performed by angling the film, compression cone, and cassette 45–60° caudal from the vertical position; the patient leans 45–60° laterally toward the ipsilateral side (Fig. 2.5). The degree of obliquity depends on the patient's body habitus; a thin patient needs a steeper oblique, and a heavy patient may be examined with a lesser degree of obliquity. The patient sits or stands, facing the mammographic unit, with the ipsilateral arm elevated to no more than 90°. The cassette is placed behind the breast, high into the axilla, and the patient may grasp the cassette holder or handle.

In this position, the pectoralis major muscle can be most easily pulled forward from the chest wall, enabling greater visualization of the posterior aspects of the breast (Figs. 2.6–2.8). The patient should not be allowed to tense the arm, since this will also tighten the pectoral muscle and prevent the breast from being pulled forward easily. All aspects of the lateral side of the breast and the axilla should be in contact with the cassette; if the opposite breast is in the radiographic field, the patient should press it up and against the chest wall. If this is not done, the opposite nipple can project into the radiographic field, simulating a nodule (24). Vigorous compression must be applied without allowing the breast to sag on the cassette. Any of the described positions can be performed with the patient sitting or standing. It often is more comfortable for the patient to sit during mammography, but for patients with a prominent abdomen, the standing position may yield a better image, with less overlap of tissue inferiorly.

Mediolateral View

The mediolateral view may not demonstrate the posterior and axillary portion of the breast in entirety; therefore, the oblique view is recommended instead for the routine examination (20). The mediolateral view, however, is essential in localizing a lesion and may also be of help in differentiating a true lesion from superimposition of glandular tissue. With the cassette placed against the lateral aspect of the breast and compression applied from the medial direction (Fig. 2.9), the mediolateral view is a true sagittal view. The mediolateral view may also be extremely useful in demonstrating a lesion located high in the upper inner quadrant, an area sometimes not included on the oblique view (Fig. 2.10) or a lesion deep near the chest wall in the inferomedial or inferolateral aspect of the breast (Fig. 2.11). The mediolateral view can be used to locate a lesion demonstrated on an oblique view but not on a craniocaudal view. A lesion that is lower in position on the mediolateral view than on the oblique view is located laterally; a lesion that is higher in position on the mediolateral view than on the oblique view is located medially.

Medial Oblique View

The advantage of performing the medial oblique view is to image lesions located far medioposteriorly that are seen on the craniocaudal view only or to image palpable lesions in the inner quadrants that are not seen on mammography. To position the patient for this view (Fig. 2.12), the tube and cassette holder are titled 45° toward the contralateral breast. The medial aspect of the breast to be examined is placed against the cassette holder, and the ipsilateral arm rests over the cassette tunnel. The breast is elevated so that it does not droop, and compression is applied from the lateral direction (Fig. 2.13).

Exaggerated Craniocaudal Views

The tissue in the extreme lateroposterior (Fig. 2.14) or medioposterior (Fig. 2.15) aspects of the breast may not be visualized in entirety on the routine craniocaudal view. When a lesion is found on the routine lateral oblique view deep in the breast and is not seen on the craniocaudal view, an exaggerated lateral or medial craniocaudal view will be of help in defining the location of the abnormalities. For the exaggerated lateral craniocaudal view, the lateral aspect of the breast is placed forward on the cassette in the craniocaudal position (Fig. 2.16). For the axillary tail of the breast to be in good contact with the film, the patient must lean backward slightly, keeping the ipsilateral arm extended over the top of the cassette. For the exaggerated medial craniocaudal view (Fig. 2.17), the patient is rotated anteriorly, extending her chest forward, with the far medioposterior aspect of the breast being imaged. If the lesion is located high in the upper inner quadrant, it may be necessary to elevate the cassette holder and compress the uppermost aspect of the breast (Figs. 2.18–2.21).

Spot Compression

Most mammographic units have a smaller compression paddle that can be used for spot compression. The area of concern, identified on the standard view, is spot compressed, with the surrounding normal tissue pushed away by the compression device. The technologist must estimate the location of the lesion in the breast from the initial images, and care must be taken to be certain that the area of concern is included in the spot field. Spot compression is particularly useful for the evaluation of the borders of nodules and for focal densities that may represent either true lesions or overlapping tissue. Another use of spot compression is in the evaluation of a palpable nodule not clearly seen on mammography. The technologist rotates the palpable lesion into tangent with the beam and spot compresses the area (21). Magnification may be combined with spot compression, particularly in the evaluation of small nodule or calcifications (Fig. 2.22).

Axillary View

Although the axillary tail of the breast and the inferior aspect of the axilla are seen on the oblique view, it may be necessary to obtain an additional view to evaluate the upper axilla. The tube and cassette are angled 45–60°, from the superomedial to the inferolateral direction. The patient is turned 15° away from the mammographic unit, and the ipsilateral arm is placed at a 90° angle to the breast. The cassette is placed behind the ribs with the edge just above the patient's humeral head, and the patient leans slightly backward to optimize contact with the cassette (Fig. 2.23). The axilla is the only area to be included on the film (Fig. 2.24). Vigorous compression will not be obtained because of the many structures interposed.

Imaging the Patient with Implants

The presence of breast implants for augmentation poses particular difficulty in obtaining adequate mammographic images of the surrounding parenchyma. Standard oblique and craniocaudal views using manual techniques are necessary

in order to image the posterior aspects of the breast and the implant.

Eklund et al. (25) described a modified positioning technique that allows for better compression and imaging of the anterior parenchymal structures. In positioning the patient for the modified technique, the technologist first palpates the anterior margin of the implant (Fig. 2.25). The breast tissue anterior to the implant is pulled forward and placed over the cassette. For the craniocaudal view, the cassette tray is raised more than for standard positioning, and the inferior edge of the implant is displaced behind the cassette tray. As the compression plate is brought down, the technologist gently pulls the parenchyma forward and displaces the implant posteriorly, guiding the superior margin of the implant behind the descending compression device. For the oblique view (Fig. 2.26) the same procedure is used; the lateral edge is placed behind the cassette holder, and the compression is guided over the medial aspect of the implant (Fig. 2.27).

Magnification Mammography

Direct radiographic magnification results in improved sharpness and detail (26), compared with conventional mammography (Fig. 2.28). There is an improvement in the effective resolution of the recording system, reduction of the effective noise, and reduction of scatter radiation (8). Small focal spots are used for magnification; because of this there is a decrease in tube output and an increase in exposure time (8). This produces an increase in blur from patient motion and an increase in radiation dose (8). Magnification is of help in defining the borders of mass lesions, in defining the morphology and number of microcalcifications (Figs. 2.29 and 2.30), and in determining the existence of multicentric tumor (27). There is an increase in radiation dose to the breast of 1.5–4 times that of conventional mammography (26).

Even with good techniques, 5–10% of breast cancers are not detected by mammography. It is of utmost importance that the radiologist maintain high standards of quality assurance, be certain that good positioning is performed, and correlate the clinical examination with the mammogram (Fig. 2.31) in determining that the region of interest is included on the film. By maintaining these standards, the number of cancers not detected by mammography will be kept to a minimum.

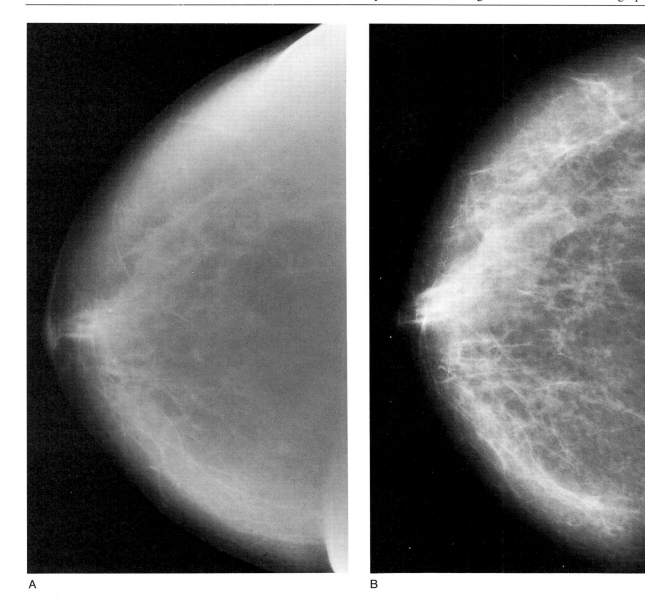

A

B

Figure 2.1. Left craniocaudal projections performed on a nondedicated unit (**A**) and a dedicated unit (**B**) show the marked improvement in image quality on the dedicated equipment. There is loss of contrast and detail as well as inadequate compression on the nondedicated equipment.

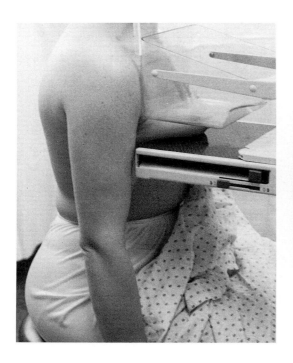

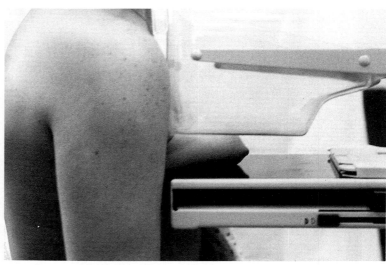

Figure 2.2. Proper positioning for the craniocaudal view.

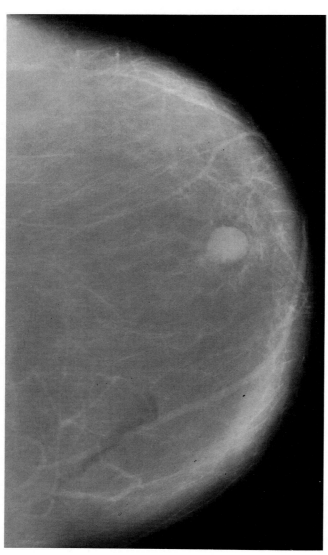

A

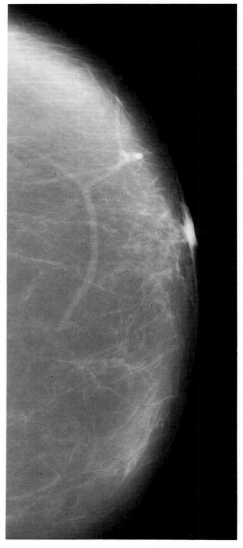

B

Figure 2.3. On the initial right craniocaudal view (**A**), a well-defined mass, which represents the nipple not in profile, is seen. When the patient is repositioned with the nipple in profile (**B**), the "mass" disappears.

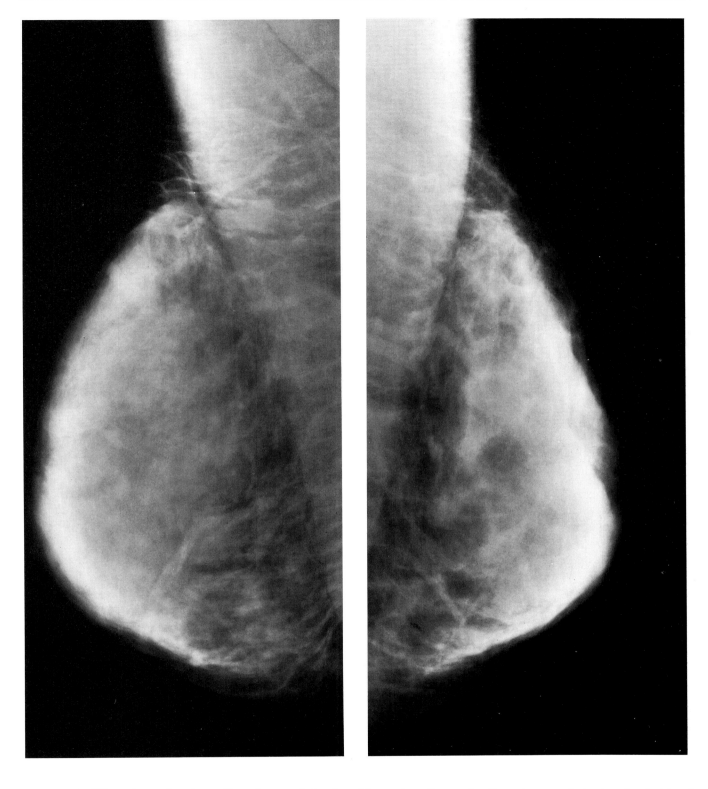

Figure 2.4.   When the patient is positioned properly for the oblique view, the pectoralis major muscle is visualized at least down to the level of the nipple.

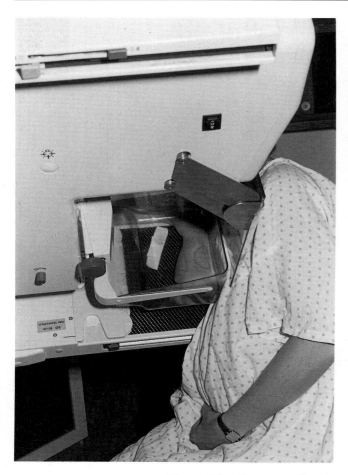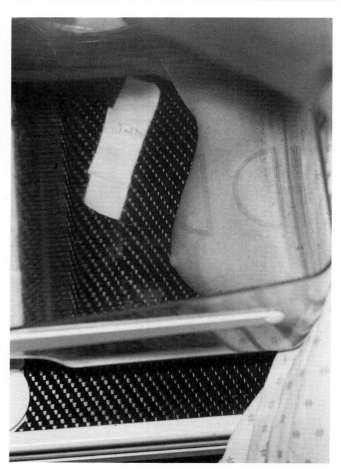

Figure 2.5.   Proper positioning of the patient for the oblique view.

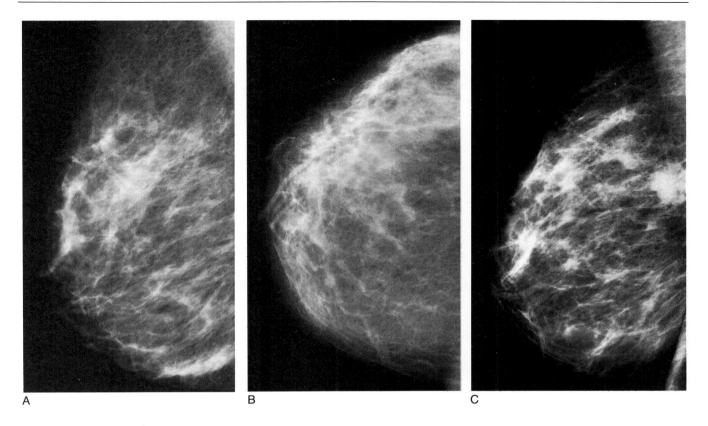

A   B   C

Figure 2.6.

Clinical: 50-year-old woman with a lump deep in the left breast.

Mammogram: Left mediolateral (**A**), craniocaudal (**B**), and oblique (**C**) views. No abnormalities are seen on the craniocaudal or mediolateral views. However, on the oblique view, there is a high-density nodular mass deep in the breast near the chest wall. This emphasizes the importance of performing the oblique view routinely in order to visualize the posterior aspects of the breast adequately.

Impression: Carcinoma.

Histopathology: Infiltrating ductal carcinoma.

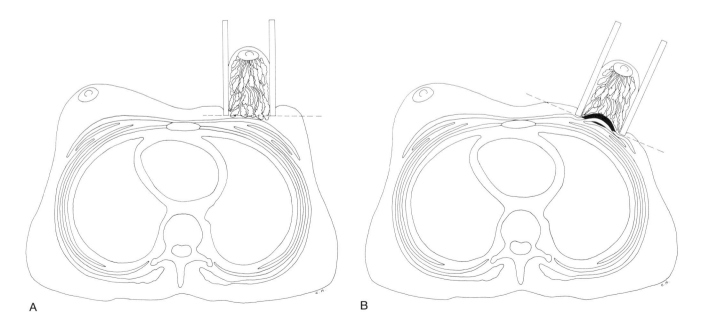

A   B

Figure 2.7.   Cross sections through the thorax show that the axillary tail of the breast may not be included on a mediolateral projection (**A**), but on the oblique projection (**B**) the axillary tail and pectoralis major muscle are imaged.

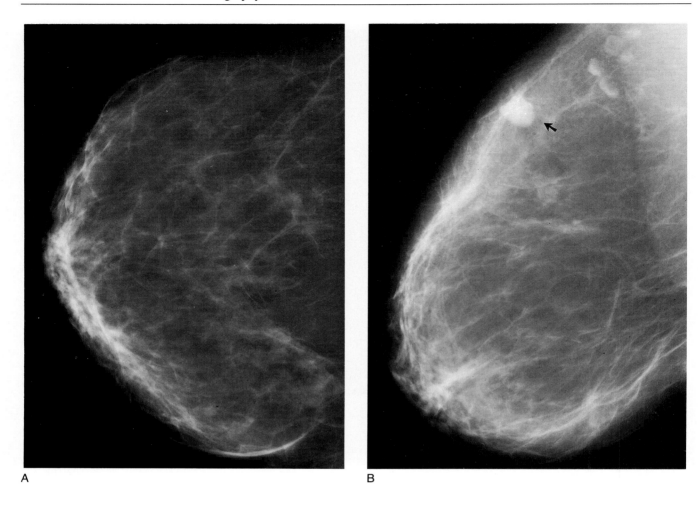

A

B

Figure 2.8. The craniocaudal view (**A**) shows no focal abnormalities. The oblique view (**B**), however, shows a calcifying fibroadenoma *(arrow)* in the upper quadrant. The oblique view should be performed routinely because the tissue located posteriorly, particularly in the axillary tail, is visualized best with this view.

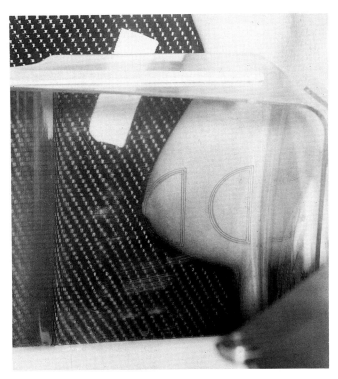

Figure 2.9. Proper positioning for the mediolateral view.

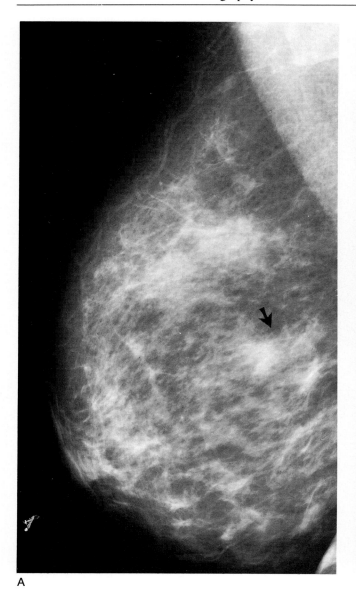

A

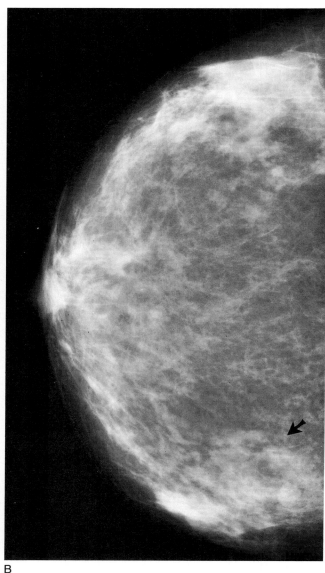

B

Figure 2.10.

Clinical: 50-year-old woman with a family history of breast cancer, for routine screening.

Mammogram: Left oblique view (**A**), craniocaudal view (**B**), mediolateral view (**C**), and ultrasound (**D**). On the initial views (**A** and **B**), a focal area of increased density *(arrows)* in the inner midportion of the left breast was seen. A mediolateral view (**C**) was performed for further evaluation of this density. The asymmetric density appears less prominent, but a second area, a nodular mass, is noted deep in the upper aspect of the left breast. This lesion could not be identified on ad-

ditional exaggerated craniocaudal views. Three-dimensional imaging is necessary occasionally to identify the location of a deep lesion. Ultrasound (**D**) was performed and identified the mass *(arrow)* in the upper inner quadrant. In retrospect, with the guidance of ultrasound, it could be palpated.

Impression: Carcinoma, left upper inner quadrant.

Note: The mediolateral view may visualize a mass that is located high in the upper inner quadrant better than does the oblique or craniocaudal view.

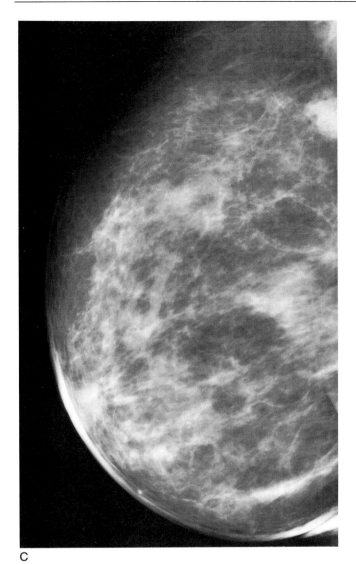

C

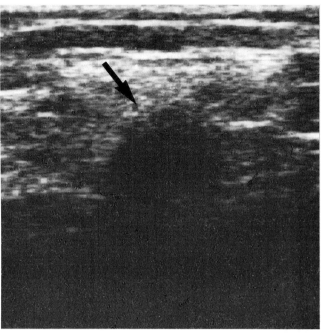

D

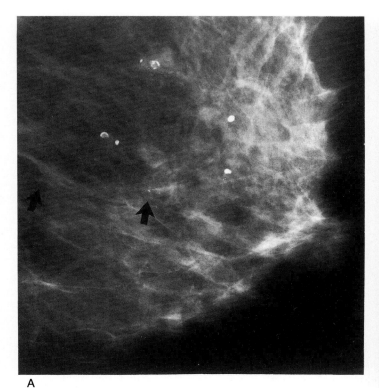

A

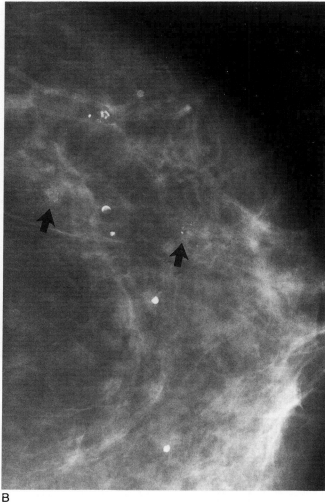

B

Figure 2.11.

Clinical: 56-year-old woman with a history of multiple benign breast biopsies, presenting now with nystagmus and neurologic findings suggesting a paraneoplastic syndrome. An outside mammogram had been interpreted as nonsuspicious for a primary breast cancer.

Mammogram: Enlarged right oblique (**A**) and magnification (2×) (**B**) views and right lateral oblique craniocaudal (**C**) and mediolateral (**D**) views from a needle localization. The breast is moderately dense. There are two clusters *(arrows)* of microcalcifications, irregular in contour and separated by approximately by 2 cm in the right lower outer quadrant (**A** and **B**). These calcifications were considered highly suspicious

for malignancy, and needle localizations were performed prior to excisional biopsy. The two views from the needle localization (**C** and **D**) show a spiculated 8 mm-mass *(arrow)* deep in the lower outer quadrant near the chest wall.

Histopathology: Infiltrating ductal with multicentric intraductal carcinoma.

Note: The mediolateral view may demonstrate a lesion near the chest wall in the inferior aspect of the breast better than the routine oblique view may. In this case, the demonstration of the mass was serendipitous, since the final films for the localization included a standard mediolateral view on which the lesion was seen.

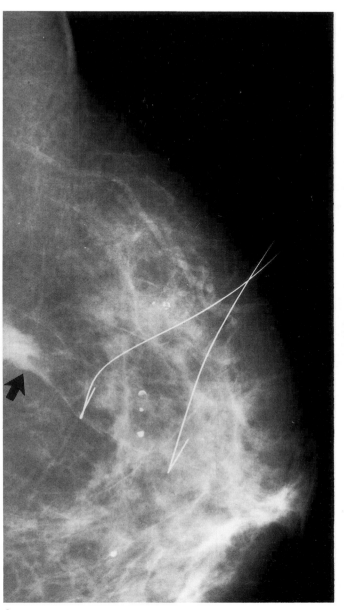

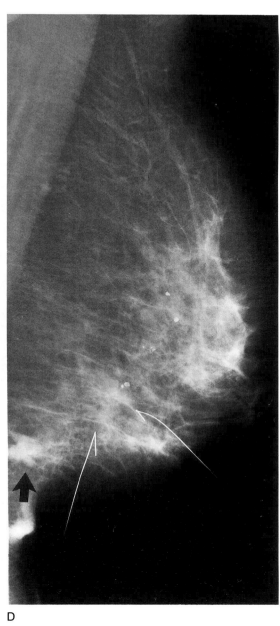

C

D

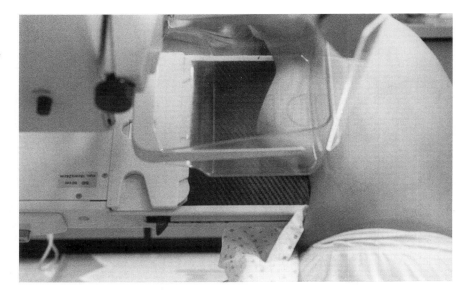

Figure 2.12. Proper positioning for the medial oblique view.

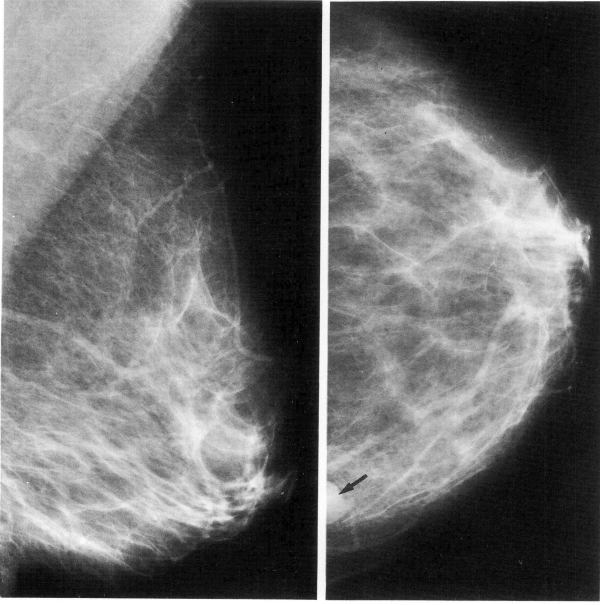

A

B

Figure 2.13.

Clinical: 44-year-old G3, P2, Ab1 woman with no palpable findings, for screening.

Mammogram: Right oblique (**A**), craniocaudal (**B**), medial oblique craniocaudal (**C**) and medial oblique (**D**) views. Although on the routine oblique view (**A**) no abnormality is seen, the edge of a well-circumscribed mass *(arrow)* is present far medioposteriorly on the craniocaudal view (**B**). An exaggerated medial oblique craniocaudal view (**C**) demonstrates the lesion more clearly. To identify the exact position of the mass, the medial oblique view (**D**) was performed and showed the mass to be in the upper inner quadrant.

Note: The medial oblique is particularly useful for demonstrating lesions located medially, near the chest wall.

Histopathology: Fibroadenoma.

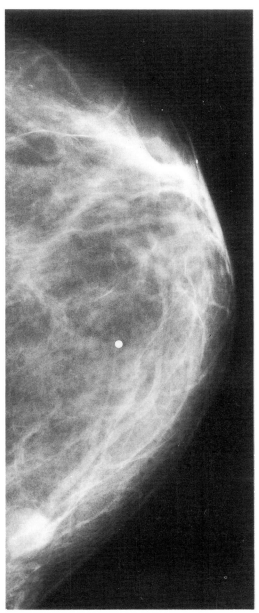

C

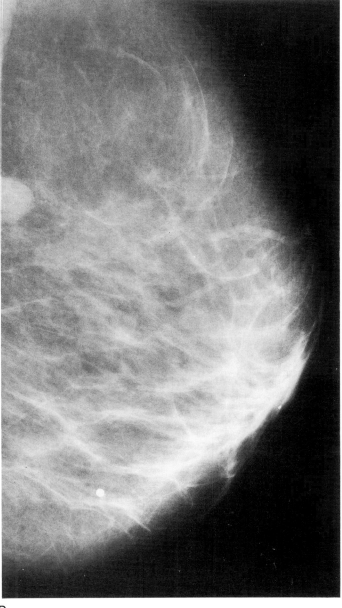

D

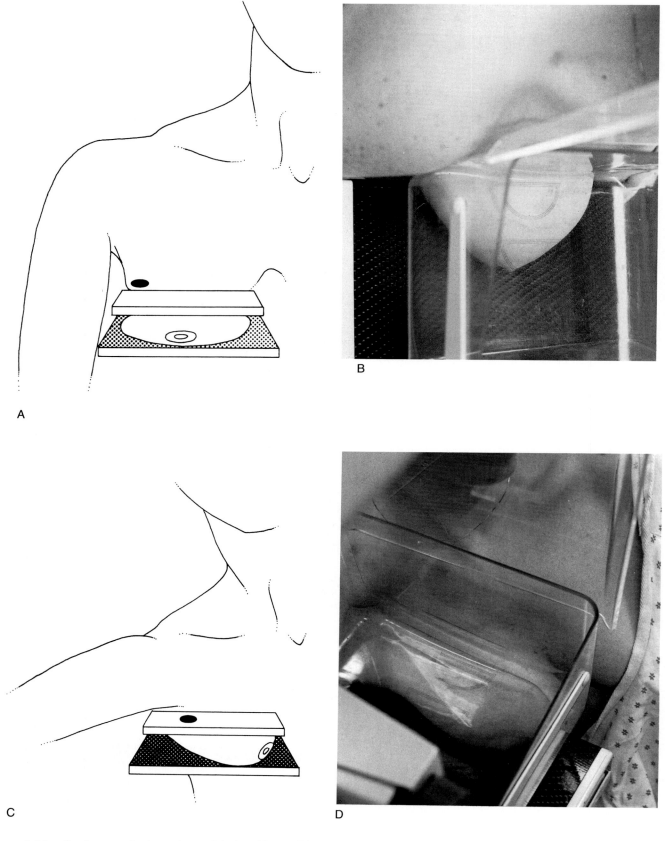

Figure 2.14.   On the standard craniocaudal view (**A** and **B**), a lesion located posterolaterally may not be included on the image, but by rotating the patient for the exaggerated lateral craniocaudal view (**C** and **D**), the lesion projects into the radiographic field.

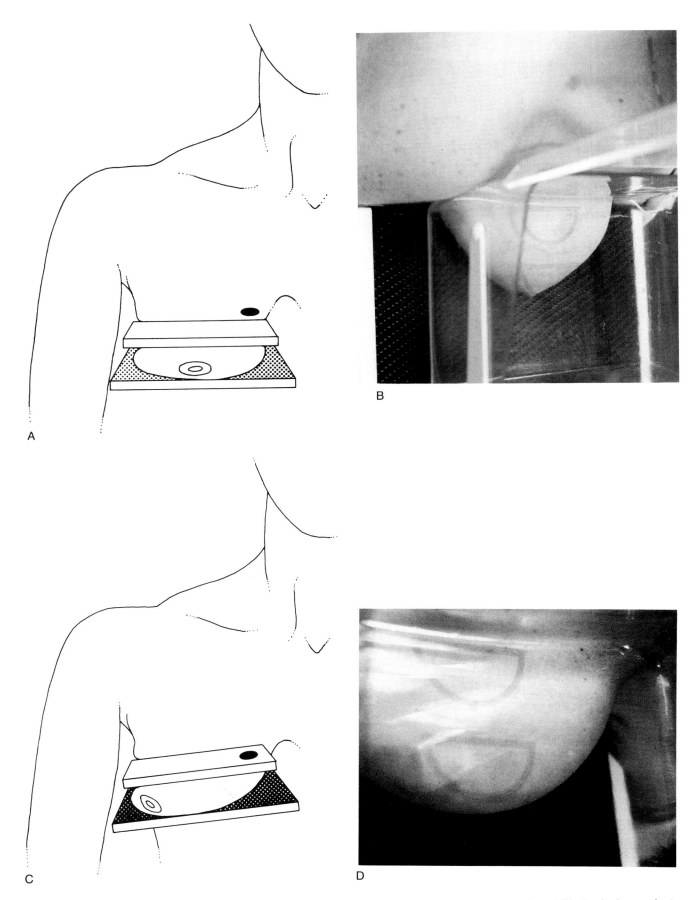

Figure 2.15. On the standard craniocaudal view (**A** and **B**), a lesion located posteromedially may not be included on the image, but by rotating the patient forward for the exagger- ated medial craniocaudal view (**C** and **D**), the lesion projects into the radiographic field.

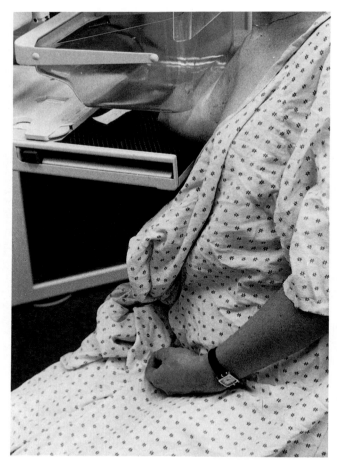

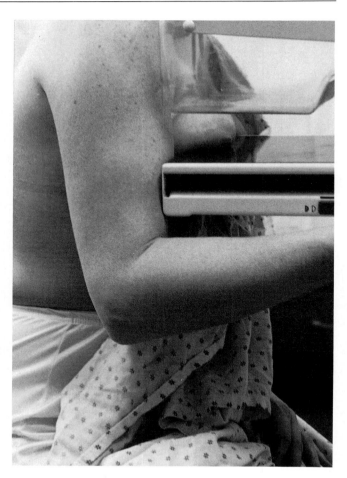

Figure 2.16.   Positioning for the exaggerated lateral cranio-caudal view.

Figure 2.17.   Positioning for the exaggerated medial cra-niocaudal view.

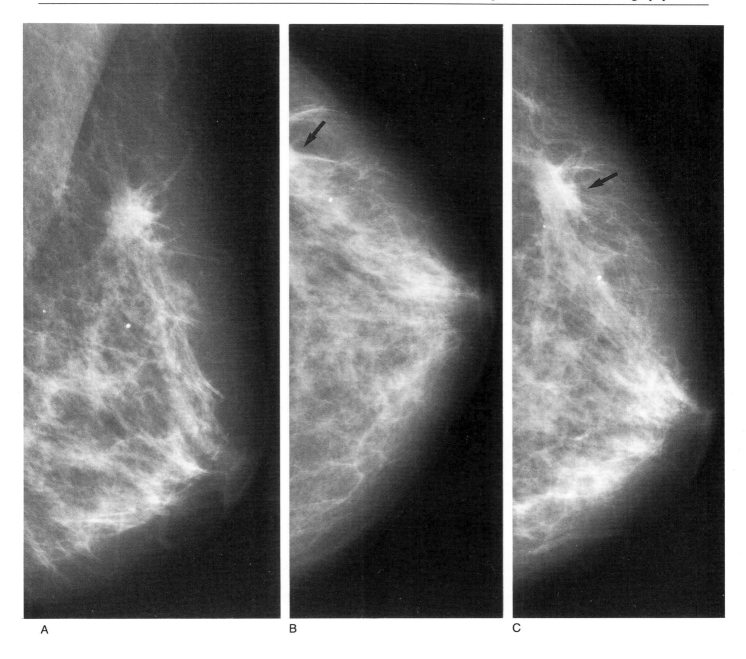

A   B   C

Figure 2.18.

Clinical: 65-year-old G4, P3, AB1 woman for screening.

Mammogram: Right oblique (**A**), craniocaudal (**B**), and lateral oblique craniocaudal (**C**) views. The breast is moderately dense. There is a focal spiculated lesion in the upper aspect of the breast on the oblique view (**A**), but this lesion is faintly seen *(arrow)* on the craniocaudal view (**B**). The lateral oblique craniocaudal view (**C**) is performed to demonstrate the location and the appearance of the lesion *(arrow)*.

The lateral oblique craniocaudal view is performed first if a lesion is seen only on the oblique, since more carcinomas occur laterally than medially. If a lesion is not found in the exaggerated lateral position, then the medial oblique craniocaudal view is performed.

Impression: Spiculated lesion located posteriorly in the upper outer quadrant, highly suspicious for malignancy.

Histopathology: Infiltrating lobular carcinoma.

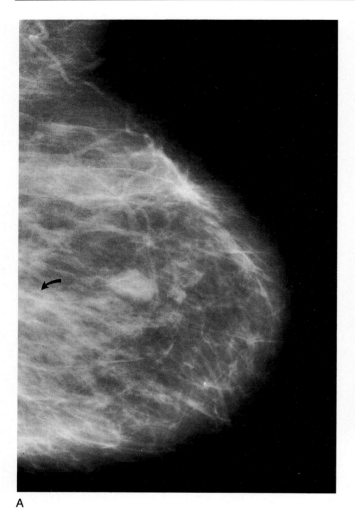

A

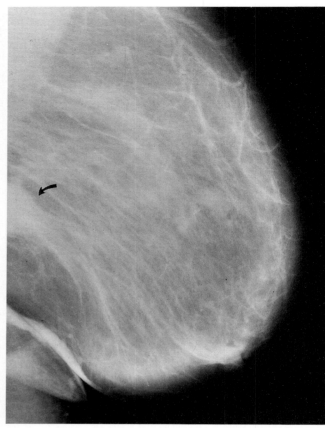

B

Figure 2.19.

Clinical: 48-year-old woman with a palpable 4.5-cm mass in the right upper inner quadrant.

Mammogram: Right oblique (**A**), mediolateral (**B**), and exaggerated medial craniocaudal (**C**) views. The oblique view is not of optimum quality because the posterior aspect of the breast and the pectoralis muscle are not visualized completely. There is a relatively well defined mass in the midportion of the breast. Posterior to this mass there is an ill-defined area of increased density extending to the edge of the film

(arrow). It is important that if one identifies an area of increased density such as this, the breast posterior to it be evaluated with additional views. On repositioning the breast (**B**), the 3.5-cm high-density mass is identified near the chest wall *(arrow)*. An exaggerated medial craniocaudal view (**C**) demonstrates the spiculated lesion in the far posteromedial aspect of the breast.

Impression: Carcinoma of the breast.

Histopathology: Infiltrating ductal carcinoma.

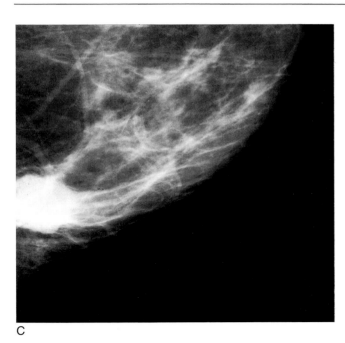

C

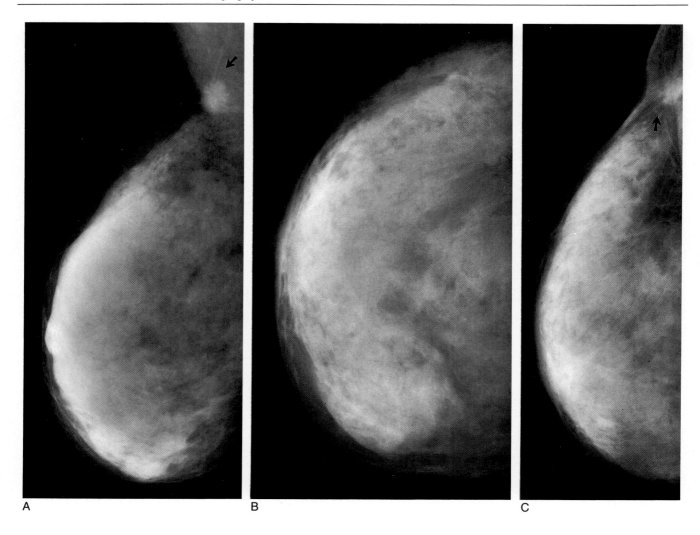

A   B   C

Figure 2.20.

Clinical: 56-year-old woman with thickening in the left axillary tail.

Mammogram: Left oblique (**A**), craniocaudal (**B**), and exaggerated lateral craniocaudal (**C**), views. On the oblique view there is a 1.5-cm spiculated mass in the upper aspect *(arrow)* of the left breast. The mass was not seen on a routine craniocaudal view (**B**). An exaggerated lateral oblique craniocaudal view demonstrates that the mass is situated laterally and is producing skin thickening and retraction *(arrow)* (**C**).

Histopathology: Infiltrating ductal carcinoma.

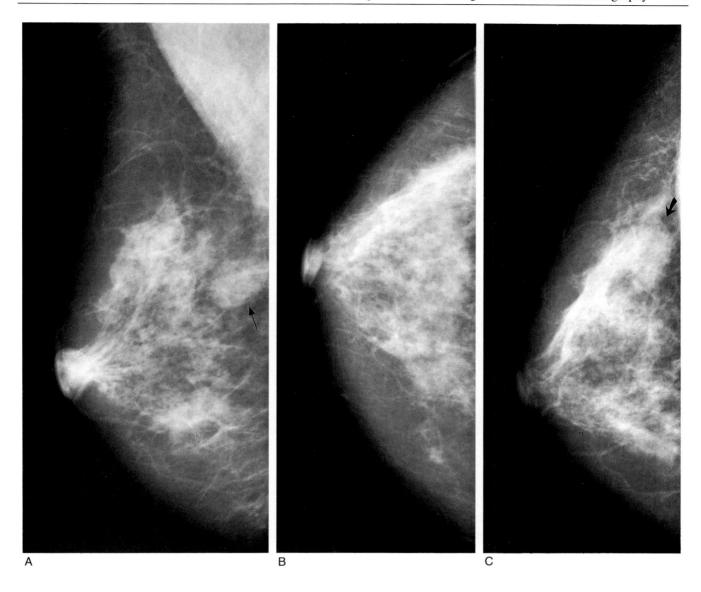

A   B   C

Figure 2.21.
Mammogram: Left oblique (**A**), craniocaudal (**B**), and exaggerated lateral craniocaudal (**C**) views. There is a relatively well defined 2-cm mass *(arrow)* deep in the left breast that is not seen on the routine craniocaudal view (**B**). An exaggerated lateral oblique craniocaudal view demonstrates the mass *(arrow)* in the outer aspect of the breast (**C**).

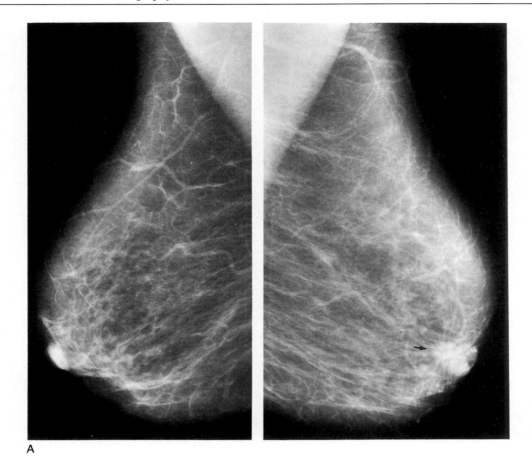

A

Figure 2.22.

Clinical: 56-year-old G10, P10 woman for screening.

Mammogram: Bilateral oblique (**A**), right craniocaudal (**B**), and spot compression (**C**) views. There is asymmetry between the breasts (**A**), with irregular increased density *(arrow)* being noted in the right subareolar area. The area *(ar-row)* appears somewhat spiculated on the craniocaudal view (**B**). However, a spot compression of the area (**C**) demonstrates clearly the spiculated mass beneath the nipple. The appearance is highly suspicious for carcinoma.

Histopathology: Infiltrating ductal carcinoma.

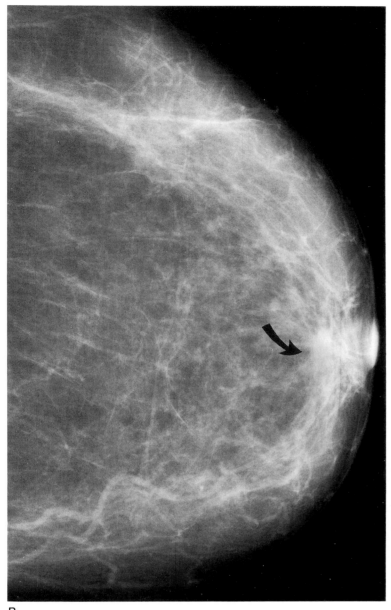

B

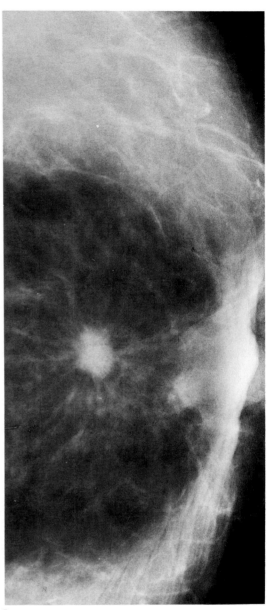

C

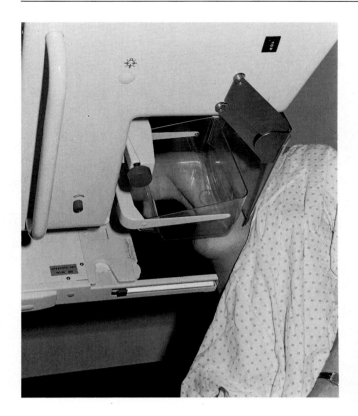

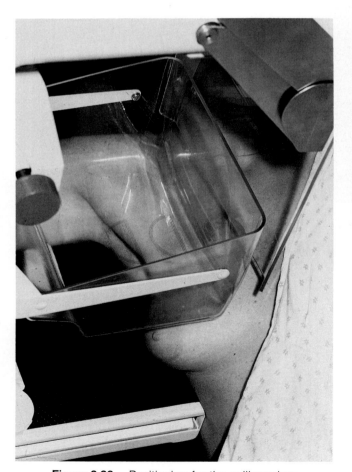

Figure 2.23. Positioning for the axillary view.

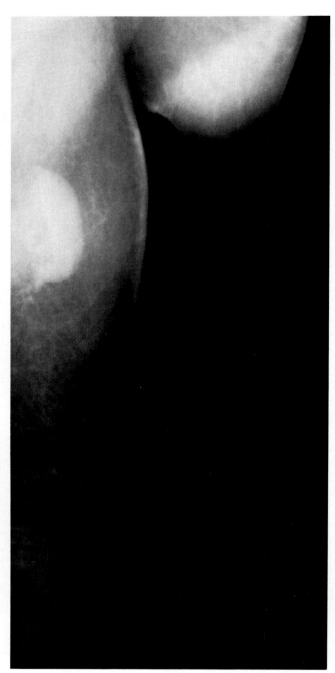

Figure 2.24. Proper positioning and contrast on the axillary view demonstrate an enlarged axillary node.

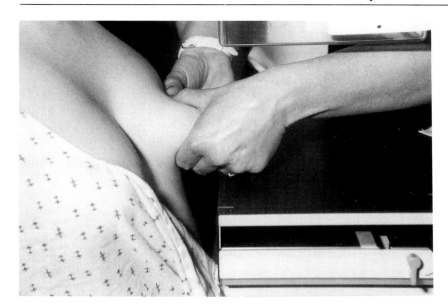

Figure 2.25. Proper positioning of the patient with implants for the craniocaudal view involves identification of the anterior surface of the implant (**A**), placing the anterior parenchyma over the cassette holder (**B**), and compression of the breast parenchyma with the prosthesis displaced posteriorly (**C**).

A

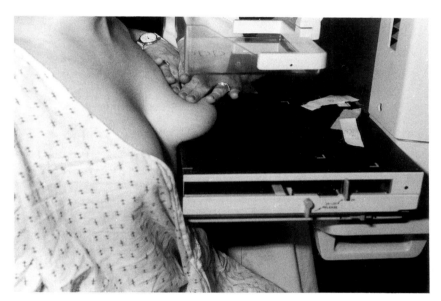

B

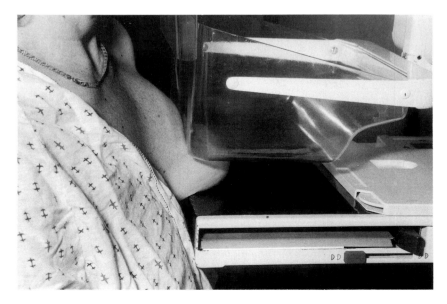

C

Figure 2.26. To position the patient with implants for the oblique view, the medial surface of the prosthesis is identified (**A**), and compression is applied to the parenchyma (**B**), displacing the implant toward the chest wall.

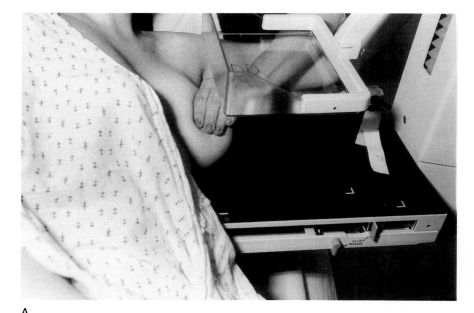

A

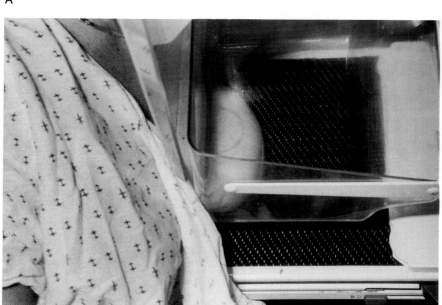

B

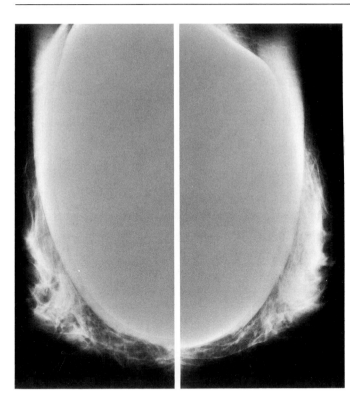

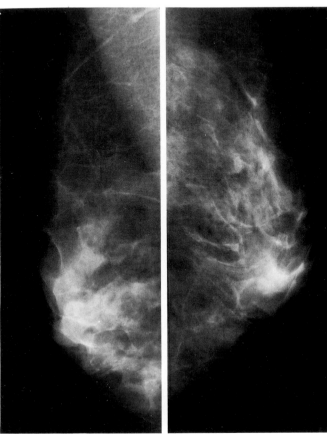

B

Figure 2.27.

Clinical: 42-year-old woman for routine mammography after augmentation mammoplasty.

Mammogram: Bilateral oblique views (**A**) and bilateral oblique views via the Eklund technique (**B**). On the standard views (**A**), bilateral subpectoral implants are present. The implants obscure much of the overlying breast parenchyma that is moderately dense. With the Eklund technique (**B**), the implants are greatly pushed back out of the field of compression, and the overlying parenchyma is seen to a much better advantage.

Impression: Normal breast postaugmentation, demonstrating the advantage of the Eklund technique. (Case courtesy of Dr. Cherie Scheer, Richmond, VA.)

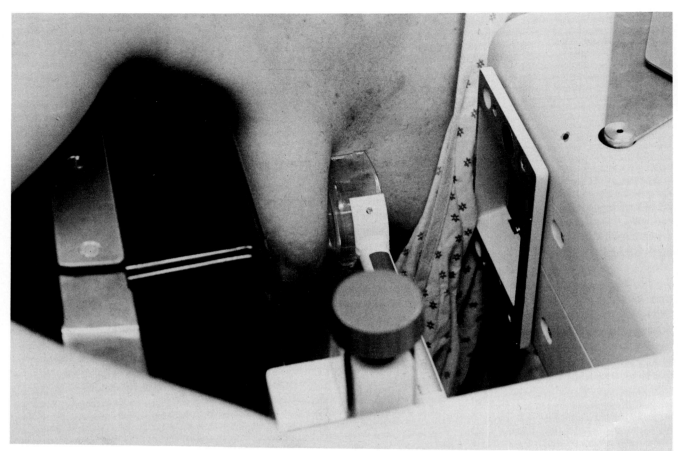

Figure 2.28. Positioning for spot magnification.

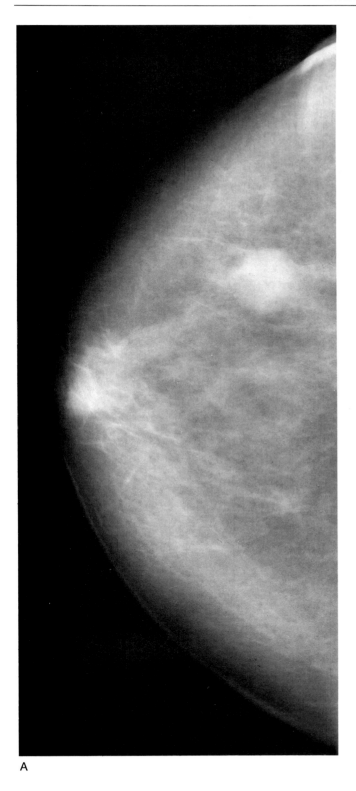

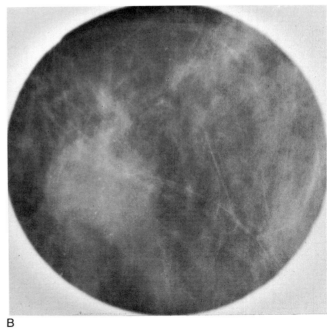

Figure 2.29.   On the craniocaudal view (**A**) of the left breast, there is a high-density mass situated laterally, appearing to have somewhat well-defined margins in some areas. On a spot magnification view (**B**), the irregularity of the margins is shown, as well as the numerous microcalcifications in this malignant mass.

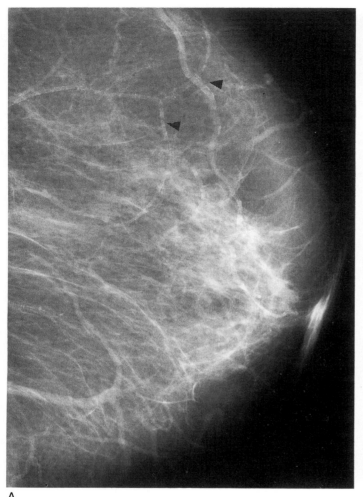

A

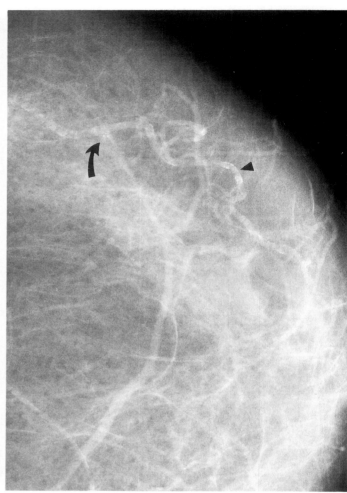

B

Figure 2.30.

Clinical: 72-year-old G6, P4, Ab2 woman for routine screening.

Mammogram: Right mediolateral (**A**), enlarged (1.5×) craniocaudal (**B**), spot magnification (2×) (**C**), and specimen (**D**) views. There is mild glandularity present. Extensive vascular calcifications are seen *(arrowheads)* (**A**, and **B**). On the initial craniocaudal view (**B**), there are microcalcifications *(arrow)* that appear to project beyond the lumen of the calcified vessel. These microcalcifications *(arrow)* are better evaluated with the spot compression magnification view (**C**),

on which they are clearly displaced away from the calcified vessel *(arrowhead)*. Their contour is slightly irregular, and they are, therefore, of moderate suspicion for malignancy. These were biopsied after needle localization (**D**), and the specimen film demonstrates their clustered nature and slightly irregular morphology.

Impression: Moderately suspicious calcifications demonstrated on a spot compression magnification view.

Histopathology: Intraductal carcinoma.

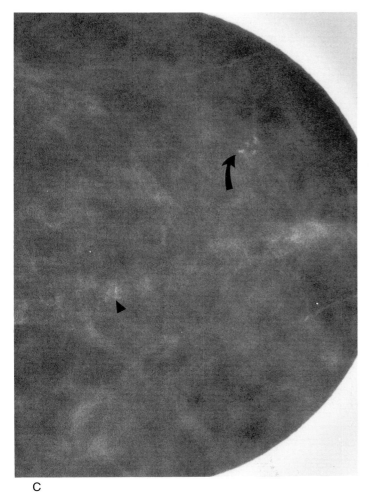

C

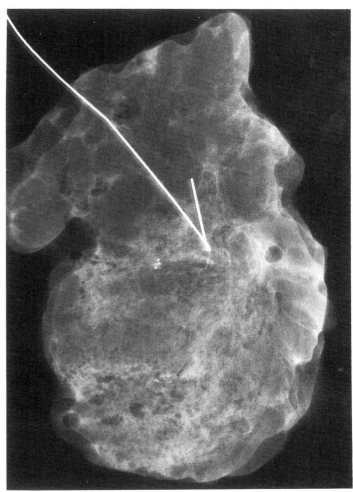

D

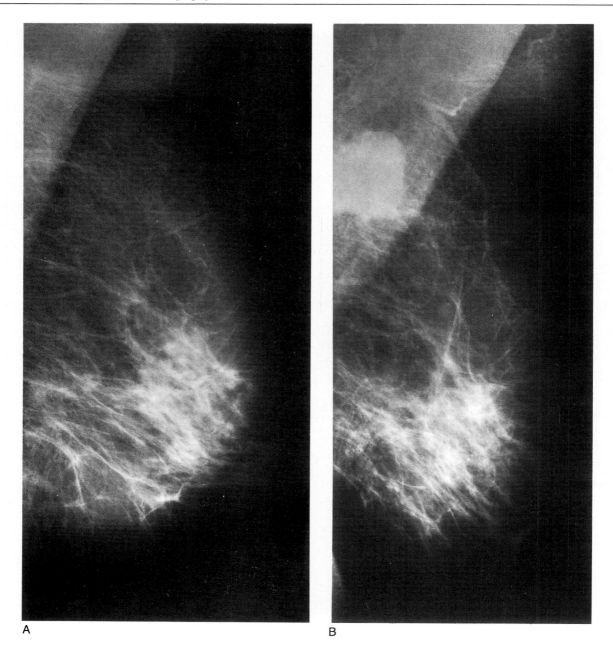

A   B

Figure 2.31.

Clinical: 55-year-old G2, P2 woman with a large tender mass in the right axillary tail.

Mammogram: Right oblique (**A**) and repositioned right oblique (**B**) views. On the initial view (**A**), the breast is moderately dense, and no suspicious abnormalities are seen. The patient did have a palpable lump in the axillary tail, and for this reason the technologist repositioned her to bring the mass forward into the field of view (**B**). More of the axillary area is seen on this view (**B**), but the breast proper is not compressed as well on the standard oblique (**A**). A large partially

circumscribed mass with nodular borders is present in the right axillary tail and is most consistent with breast carcinoma, although a metastatic node is another consideration.

Impression: Carcinoma, right axillary tail, demonstrated on repositioning of the breast.

Histopathology: Poorly differentiated adenocarcinoma.

Note: It is critical that the technologist palpate any masses noted by the clinician or patient and be certain that the area of palpable concern is included in the field of view.

References

1. Shaw de Paredes E, Frazier AB, Hartwell GD, et al. Development and implementation of a quality assurance program for mammography. Radiology 1987;163:83–85.
2. Haus AG. Technologic improvements in screen-film mammography. Radiology 1990;174:628–637.
3. Martin JE, Moskowitz M, Milbrath JR. Breast cancer missed by mammography. AJR 1979;132:737–739.
4. Kalisher L. Factors influencing false negative rates in xeromammography. Radiology 1979;133:297–301.
5. Haus AG. Screen-film mammography update: x-ray units, breast compression, grids, screen-film characteristics, and radiation dose. In: Mulvaney JA, ed. Medical imaging and instrumentation '84. (Proceedings of the SPIE). Bellingham, WA: International Society for Optical Engineering, 1984;486.
6. Feig SA. Mammography equipment: principles, features, selection. Radiol Clin North Am 1987;25:897–911.
7. National Council on Radiation Protection and Measurements: Mammography—a user's guide (NCRP Report No. 85). Bethesda, MD: National Council on Radiation Protection and Measurements, 1986.
8. Haus AG. Recent advances in screen-film mammography. Radiol Clin North Am 1987;25:913–928.
9. Muntz EP, Logan WW. Focal spot size and scatter suppression in magnification mammography. AJR 1979;133:453–459.
10. Tabar L, Dean PB. Screen/film mammography: quality control. In: Feig S, McClelland R, eds. Breast carcinoma: current diagnosis and treatment. New York: Masson Publishing USA, 1983:161–168.
11. Fajardo LL, Westerman BR. Mammography equipment: practical considerations for the radiologist. Appl Radiol 1990;19:12–15.
12. Egan RL, McSweeney MB, Sprawls P. Grids in mammography. Radiology 1983;146:359–362.
13. Logan WW. Screen/film mammography: technique. In: Feig S, McClelland R, eds. Breast carcinoma: current diagnosis and treatment. New York: Masson Publishing USA, 1983:141–160.
14. Kimme-Smith C, Bassett LW, Gold RH, et al. New mammography screen/film combinations: imaging characteristics and radiation dose. AJR 1990;154:713–719.
15. Yaffe MJ. Physics of mammography: image recording process. RadioGraphics 1990;10:341–363.
16. Haus AG. Recent trends in screen-film mammography: technical factors and radiation dose. Presented at the Third International Copenhagen Symposium on Detection of Breast Cancer, Copenhagen, Denmark, August 1985.
17. Skubic SE, Yagan R, Oravec D, Shah Z. Value of increasing film processing time to reduce radiation dose during mammography. AJR 1990;155:1189–1193.
18. Bassett LW, Bunnell DH, et al. Breast cancer detection: one versus two views. Radiology 1987;165:95–97.
19. Schmitt EL, Threatt B. Tumor location and detectability in mammographic screening. AJR 1982;139:761–765.
20. Bassett LW, Gold RH. Breast radiography using the oblique projection. Radiology 1983;149:585–587.
21. Logan WW, Janus J. Use of special mammographic views to maximize radiographic information. Radiol Clin North Am 1987;25:953–959.
22. Sickles EA. Practical solutions to common mammographic problems: tailoring the examination. AJR 1988;151:31–39.
23. Feig SA. The importance of supplementary mammographic views to diagnostic accuracy. AJR 1988;151:40–41.
24. Gilula LA, Destouet JM, Monsees B. Nipple simulating a breast mass on a mammogram. Radiology 1989;170:272.
25. Eklund GW, Busby RC, Miller SH, Job JS. Improved imaging of the augmented breast. AJR 1988;151:469–473.
26. Sickles EA. Magnification mammography. In: Feig S, McClelland R, eds. Breast carcinoma: current diagnosis and treatment. New York: Masson Publishing USA, 1983:177–182.
27. Sickles EA. Microfocal spot magnification mammography using xeroradiographic and screen-film recording systems. Radiology 1979;131:599–607.

AN APPROACH TO
MAMMOGRAPHIC ANALYSIS

Because the mammographic appearance of the breasts is quite variable from patient to patient, it is important that films be placed as mirror images during interpretation. In this way, one will be able to identify most easily a subtle nodule or asymmetry that may be the only sign of carcinoma. With the films placed as mirror images (Fig. 3.1), a systematic comparison of the various areas of each breast should be carried out.

Selection of Appropriate Views

It is important first to correlate any clinical findings with the mammographic findings. The location of skin lesions, scars, or palpable masses should be indicated by the technologist, and the radiologist must correlate the position of such findings with the images (Fig. 3.2).

The mammographic examination should be tailored to the individual patient (1). Particular attention should be paid to the deep aspects of the breasts, and if breast parenchyma extends posteriorly to the edge of the film on both views, exaggerated craniocaudal views should be obtained also to evaluate the deep areas completely. In thin patients with small dense breasts, the posterior lower aspects of the breasts may not be adequately visualized on the lateral oblique view; an additional mediolateral view often demonstrates this posterior tissue.

In the evaluation of each breast, attention should be paid to the skin thickness, the symmetry of the subcutaneous fat, and the presence of asymmetric tissue, nodules, or calcifications (2). The architecture of the breasts should be symmetrical with the fibroglandular tissue oriented to the nipple and with the Cooper's ligaments appearing as thin arcs traversing the fat. Correlation with clinical examination and the location of any scars is important in assessing the presence of an area of asymmetry or architectural distortion. Focal distortion, including linear densities oriented in a different direction from the other structures, or focal puckering in or out of the glandular tissue may indicate an underlying carcinoma.Carcinomas may infiltrate into the fat and parenchyma, producing thickening of Cooper's ligaments. Such involvement can produce skin thickening or retraction that

may first be evident on mammography. Central carcinomas also may fix the nipple-areolar complex, which is evident to the technologist on compression of the breast as nipple retraction but which is not evident in the noncompressed state.

If a nodule or focal area of distortion is found, spot compression views will displace the surrounding tissue and aid in identifying the presence of an underlying lesion (Figs. 3.3 and 3.4). Berkowitz et al. (3) found spot compression was of more help in the analysis of 75 lesions in rendering them more or less suspicious than was the routine view. The spot compression view is useful to determine (a) if a focal density is superimposed tissue or a true lesion, (b) if the borders of a nodule appear to be relatively circumscribed on the routine view, and (c) if a focal area of architectural distortion is being produced by a stellate lesion.

Additional positioning, including mediolateral, lateromedial oblique, or rolled craniocaudal views, may be necessary to determine the presence of and location of a lesion. A mediolateral view may rotate a lesion in tangent, demonstrating distortion or nodularity obscured by glandular tissue on the oblique view (Fig. 3.5). The mediolateral view is also advantageous to demonstrate (a) the relative medial or lateral location of a lesion based on how it moves in relationship to the oblique position, (b) the posteroinferior aspect of the breast, and (c) the medioposterior aspect of the breast. The lateromedial oblique view is performed for palpable lesions deep in the inner quadrant and is not seen on mammography or for lesions identified on mammography deep in the medial aspect of the breast on the craniocaudal view. The rolled craniocaudal view is performed to determine the relative inferior or superior position of a lesion seen on the craniocaudal view but not demonstrated on the oblique. If the superior aspect of the breast is rolled laterally and the lesion moves laterally from its position on the craniocaudal view, it is located in the superior aspect of the breast.

Evaluation of Breast Nodules

In the evaluation of a mass lesion, an assessment of its margins (4, 5), density, location, orientation, the presence of a fatty halo, contour, and size is made. Lesions may be divided into four groups based on their density—radiolucent, mixed density, medium density, or high density. Fatty and mixed-density circumscribed lesions are benign, whereas medium- to high-density masses may be of benign or malignant origin. Benign lesions tend to be of medium to low density, with very well defined margins, and surrounded by a fatty halo (Fig. 3.6), but this is certainly not diagnostic of benignancy (6). The halo sign is a fine radiolucent line that surrounds circumscribed masses. Gordenne and Malchair (7) described a Mach band effect creating a hyperlucent zone around malignant lesions, but this hyperlucency had an average diameter of 5–10 mm.

A spot compression view is important to define the borders of a small circumscribed nodule as either completely or partially well defined (Fig. 3.7). Lack of a complete halo should warrant further investigation. The likelihood of a well-defined mass being benign is great, but various series (8–10) report significant numbers of occult carcinomas presenting as at least partially defined nodules. Sickles (9) found that in a series of 300 nonpalpable cancers, only one half of the noncalcified lesions were spiculated and the remainder were well defined or poorly defined nodules or areas of architectural distortion. Swann et al. (6) found at least a partial halo sign to be associated with 25 of 1000 breast cancers, and in 60% of lesions the halo was complete.

Nodules that are completely well defined and less than 1 cm in diameter are often followed at 6-month intervals for years because of their relatively low risk of being malignant. Ultrasound may demonstrate cysts in some of these lesions but may not be confirmatory because of their small size. If ultrasound does not confirm a cyst, mammographic follow-up is necessary. It is important that in the follow-up of such lesions, the subsequent examinations should be tailored to allow accurate comparisons with the initial study (11). Fine-needle aspiration biopsy of such lesions is an alternative to open biopsy or follow-up, particularly if fine-needle aspiration biopsy can prove that the nodule is a cyst or a fibroadenoma (11). When a round or ovoid well-defined nodule of 1 cm or greater is found, determination of the internal characteristics should follow with ultrasound or aspiration. If the lesion is not a cyst or an intramammary node and is solid, biopsy is often indicated. Occasionally, the mammographic appearance of a carcinoma is that of a non-calcified nodular mass. The borders are not smooth or lobulated but are multinodular (Fig. 3.8).

A lesion that is ill defined or spiculated and in which there is no clear history of trauma to suggest hematoma or fat necrosis suggests a malignant process. The presence of a central high density with surrounding fine spiculation creates a highly suspicious appearance. Spot compression may be of help in elucidating such an appearance with dense parenchyma. Stomper et al. (10) in the evaluation of specimen films and histology of noncalcified nonpalpable carcinomas found that gross spiculation of >2 mm was microscopically found to represent islands of neoplastic cells surrounded by dense collagenous stroma. Biopsy is usually necessary in the evaluation of a poorly defined or spiculated lesion identified on two views (Figs. 3.9–3.12).

Evaluation of Asymmetric Densities

In analyzing an ill-defined area of asymmetric tissue without other associated findings, one should first determine if, in fact, the asymmetry is present on two views or if it merely represents overlapping glandular tissue on one view (Fig. 3.13). If the patient has a scar or has had trauma to the area, the density may be fat necrosis. If a palpable thickening or mass corresponds to an asymmetric density, the density, particularly if large, is regarded with a greater degree of suspicion for malignancy. Kopans et al. (12) found that asymmetric glandularity occurred in 3% of patients for mammography and carcinoma was found in only 3 patients with breast asymmetry without other signs of malignancy but in which there were concurrent palpable findings. If the patient is premenopausal, particularly if she has other fibrocystic changes on mammography, a nonpalpable ill-defined asymmetry may often be followed in 2–3 months, immediately after a menstrual cycle, and may diminish in size or disappear completely. In a postmenopausal patient, if there are no old films for comparison, a focal nonpalpable asymmetric density may be followed or biopsied, depending on the degree of asymmetry and other glandularity in the breast, the risk factors, and the clinical examination. Occasionally, a large area of asymmetry on histopathologic examination is found to contain an in situ or small invasive cancer surrounded by a larger area of fibrocystic changes accounting for the density on mammography (Figs. 3.14–3.16).

Evaluation of Calcifications

Calcifications of some type are present on a majority of mammograms, and it is necessary to exclude those that are characteristically benign to avoid unnecessary biopsies. Microcalcifications rather than macrocalcifications are the form most often presenting as, or associated with, a carcinoma and represent a greater diagnostic dilemma. An analysis of the calcifications as to their distribution, size, morphology, variability, and the presence of associated findings, such as ductal dilatation or a nodule, will assist one in deciding which are benign, which should be followed carefully, and which should be biopsied. In conjunction with the analysis of the pattern of calcification, the radiologist must keep in mind the patient's history and risk factors. A woman with a synchronous contralateral breast cancer or who is otherwise at high risk may be biopsied more readily for clustered microcalcifications of indeterminate nature.

Calcifications that are malignant tend to lie in the abnormal ducts and assume shapes that are casts of the irregular epithelial lining of the duct (13). Malignant calcifications can be identified as such when they are linear or branching, with irregular, jagged, sharp margins. When this morphology is identified on the mammogram, whether in a tight cluster or distributed in several groups or even throughout an entire quadrant or an entire breast, biopsy is indicated (Figs. 3.17–3.20). Many malignant calcifications, however, may not have these classic features and may be more rounded in contour, although they do tend to have variability of size and shape.

Homogeneous round, smooth microcalcifications, which may be clustered, diffuse, or in tiny florets, usually represent lobular calcifications (13) (Fig. 3.21). Often, such calcifications occur in multiple quadrants and are bilateral. Most often, these represent benign fibrocystic disease—adenosis, sclerosing adenosis, lobular hyperplasia—but they may also occur in lobular neoplasia or lobular carcinoma in situ. For these reasons, such calcifications when focal or clustered should be at least followed up carefully with mammography, if not biopsied. There are a variety of opinions concerning the recommendation for follow-up about this finding. If a decision is made to follow a patient with mammography rather than to biopsy calcifications, mammograms should be obtained at 6-month intervals for at least 2 years and annually thereafter to assess for any increase in number.

Magnification views are particularly useful in the evaluation of the morphology of microcalcifications as well as in the more accurate determination of their distribution. The analysis of calcifications should include careful attention to all areas in each breast. There may be a variety of benign calcifications as well as malignant calcifications occurring synchronously in the same breast, and one must inspect carefully all areas to avoid overlooking an occult calcified malignancy (Fig. 3.22).

The Changing Mammogram

Comparison with a baseline mammogram is of great help in the decision about a focal mammographic abnormality. The development of a new nodule, an area of asymmeteric soft tissue density, an area of distortion, or calcifications should alert the radiologist that there is activity in the area identified and that further evaluation is necessary. Similarly, the change in size, density, or margination of a nodule or density or an increase in the number of microcalcifications focally are of concern. Comparison with multiple previous studies, not just the most recent, is important in the determination of any change in a region that is being followed. The doubling times of breast carcinomas vary greatly, from 44 to 1869 days (14), and therefore, the changes that occur at 6 months or a year may be quite variable. Although not common, it is not unusual to see the development of a 1-cm lesion in a 1-year interval, nor is it unusual to identify lack of perceptible change in a lesion over a year. For these reasons, follow-up at 6-month intervals initially, followed by annual mammography after 2 years of stability, is a reasonable approach (Figs. 3.23–3.26).

When a lesion suspicious for malignancy is identified, great care in the evaluation of the remainder of the breast containing the abnormality and of the opposite breast is necessary (Figs. 3.27 and 3.28). A patient with multicentric carcinoma in one breast is generally not considered a good candidate for tylectomy and radiation therapy because of the greater risk of recurrence. Contralateral synchronous carcinoma occurs in 0.1–2.0% of patients (15) and therefore, careful attention must be paid to both breasts when an obvious carcinoma is found.

Mammography has a significant role to play preoperatively in the presence of a palpable breast mass. The presence of a neoplasm can be confirmed; a clearly benign lesion, such as a lipoma or an oil cyst, which does not require biopsy, can be identified; an ipsilateral multicentric cancer is demonstrated; an occult contralateral cancer can be detected; and an occult malignancy in a breast in which a palpable mass is to be excised can be demonstrated (16).

Breast ultrasound provides considerable additional information to film mammography in several circumstances. Ultrasound should not be considered a screening tool for breast cancer but serves as an adjunct to mammography (17–21). Sonography can be performed with high-resolution—7.5 or 10 MHz—real-time transducers or with dedicated automated scanners.

The normal breast on ultrasound is composed of low-echogenicity fat lobules interposed with highly echogenic Cooper's ligaments. The pectoralis major muscle is a band of low-level echoes, and it is an important landmark in determining if a lesion is within the breast or posterior to it (22). The breast parenchyma is composed of medium-level echoes interposed with the more echogenic Cooper's ligaments.

Ultrasound is most helpful in differentiating a cyst from a solid mass when a well-defined mammographic lesion is identified. If a palpable mass is present and mammography demonstrates a dense breast only, ultrasound of the palpable area demonstrates the internal characteristics of the lesion and can determine if it is cystic or solid. In a patient with multinodular breasts that are dense and are nodular on mammography, ultrasound also demonstrates the characteristics of the palpable findings. For lesions that are located far posteriorly and cannot be demonstrated on two views, ultrasound may be used to locate the lesion in the second plane. Sonography may also be used for guidance in interventional procedures including cyst aspiration, fine-needle aspiration biopsy, and needle localization (Figs. 3.29–3.36).

Cysts on sonography are well-circumscribed anechoic lesions with a well-defined posterior wall and increased through-transmission of sound (19, 23). If a lesion appears relatively cystic but contains internal echoes, aspiration is indicated. Otherwise, aspiration is not necessary for simple cysts confirmed on ultrasound (21, 23).

Solid benign and malignant masses cannot be reliably differentiated by sonography, but there are features suggestive of malignancy rather than of fibroadenomas. Malignant masses tend to have an irregular wall, nonhomogeneous internal echoes, and distal acoustic shadowing (24). Fibroadenomas are most often hypoechoic with a homogeneous echotexture, and they produce no change in the distal echoes (25). Well-circumscribed carcinomas may have a sono-graphic appearance similar to that of fibroadenomas, and therefore, confirmation of histology cannot be made by ultrasound.

Careful attention to subtle areas of asymmetry, nodules, and the presence of architectural distortion or microcalcifications is necessary in order to detect breast cancers at an early stage. Correlation with the history and physical findings is of help in determining recommendations about equivocal mammographic findings. The use of ultrasound and interventional techniques such as aspiration, pneumocystography, and galactography as an adjunct to mammography allows the radiologist to make a more accurate diagnosis or recommendation.

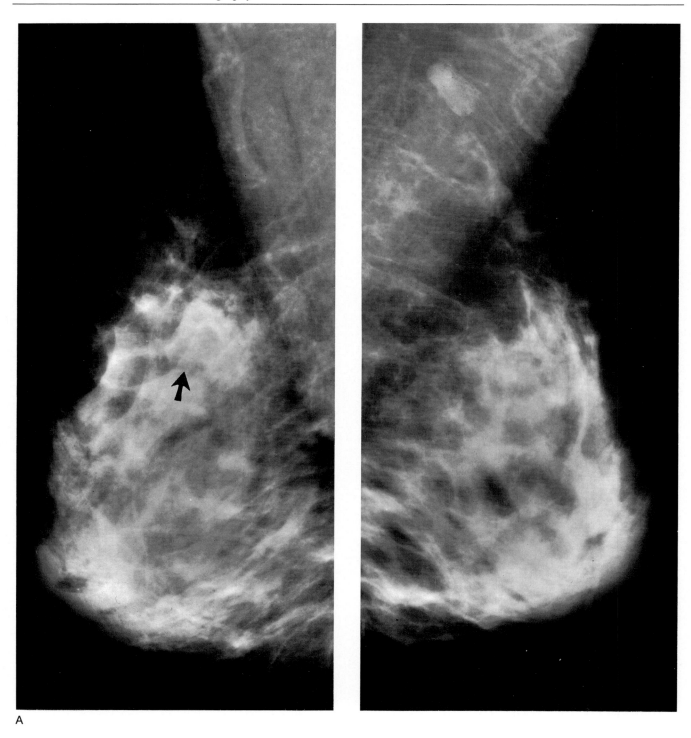

A

Figure 3.1. The initial step in evaluation of the mammogram, after determining that the quality is adequate, should be to assess the symmetry of the breasts. This can be accomplished best by placing the films together, as mirror images of each other. The viewer should make a systematic comparison of the breasts from side to side, determining if there are any asymmetries. In (**A**), both oblique views are shown, and there is a masslike area of asymmetry in the left upper quadrant *(arrow)*. On the craniocaudal views (**B**), the mass is more clearly seen as being asymmetric *(arrow)* in comparison with the opposite breast. This lesion was an infiltrating carcinoma.

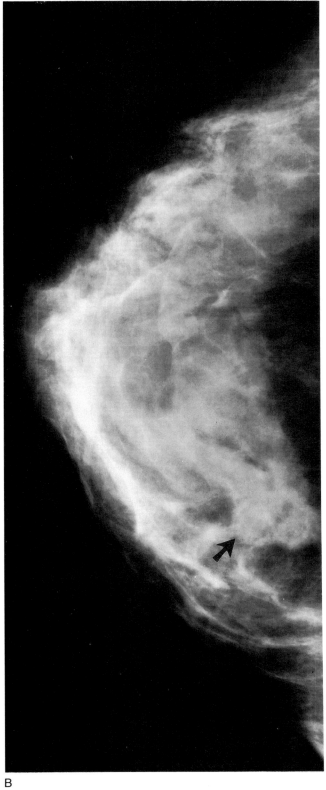
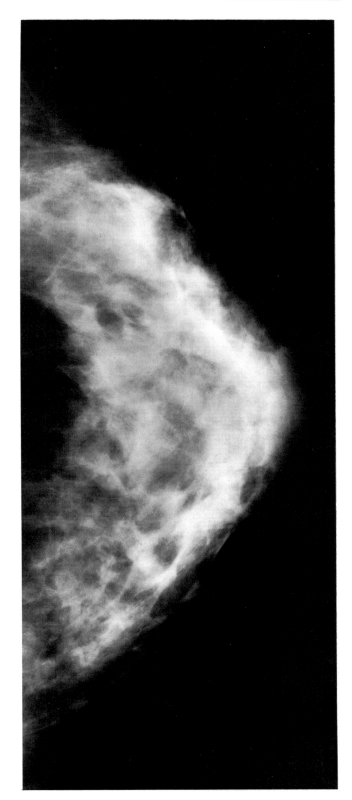

B

Figure 3.2.

Clinical: 73-year-old G2, P1, Ab1 woman for screening. Physical examination showed an accessory nipple inferiorly on the left breast.

Mammogram: Left craniocaudal (**A**) and spot oblique (**B**) views. There is a well-defined lobulated nodule superimposed over the lower central aspect of the left breast *(arrows)* (**A** and **B**), corresponding in location to the accessory nipple.

Impression: Accessory nipple.

Note: It is important for the technologist to document the location of any scars or skin lesions; these may superimpose over the breast on two views and simulate an intraparenchymal lesion.

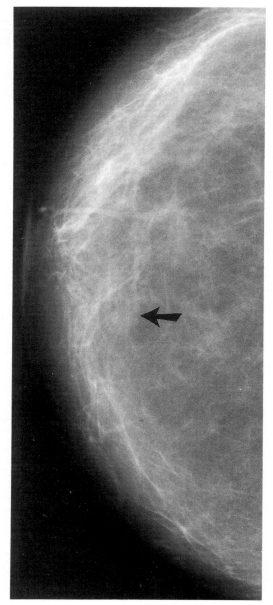

A

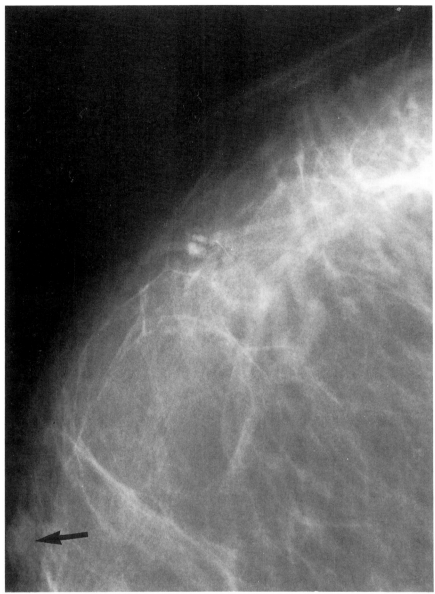

B

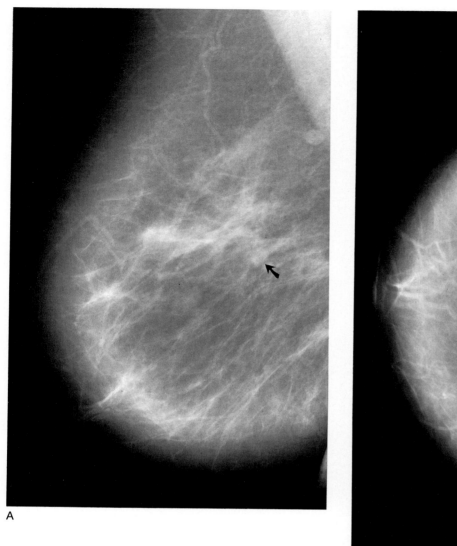

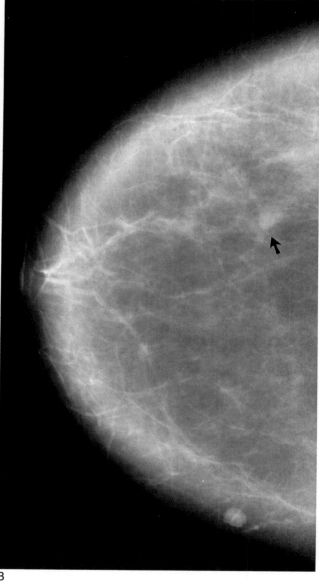

Figure 3.3.

Clinical: Left oblique (**A**), craniocaudal (**B**), and spot magnification (**C**) views. There is a 5-mm nodular density *(arrow)* in the left upper outer quadrant. With the spot compression of the area, the surrounding parenchyma is displaced away from the nodule, and the poor definition and spiculation of the borders of the nodule are better seen. Incidental note is made of a very well circumscribed nodule medially (**B**), which represented a nevus on the skin.

Impression: 5-mm nodule suspicious for carcinoma.

Histopathology: Infiltrating ductal carcinoma.

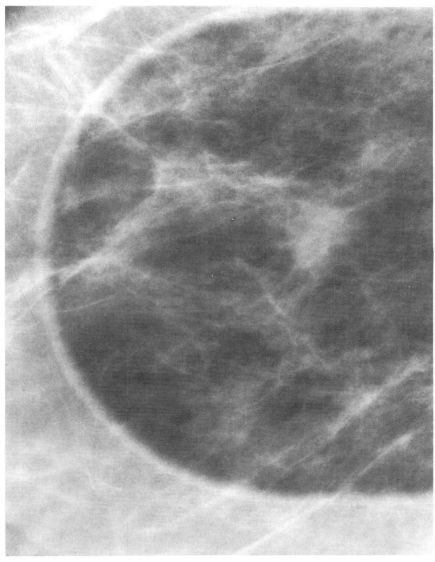

C

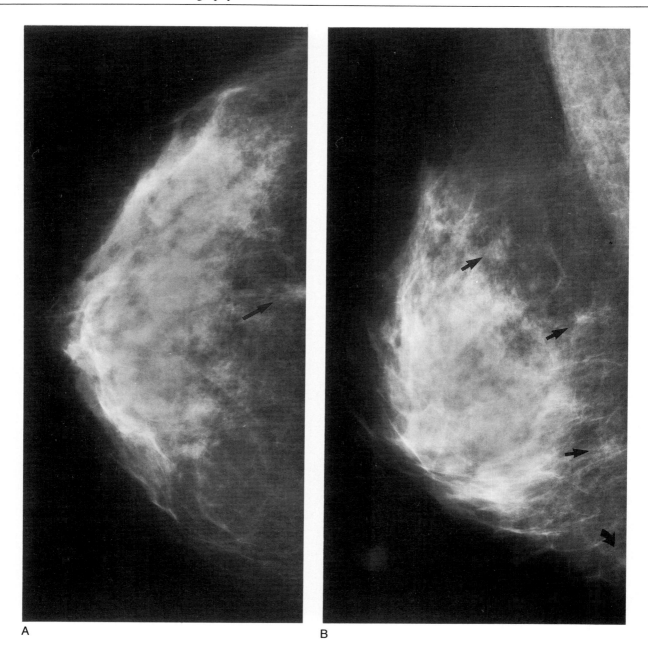

A

B

Figure 3.4.

Clinical: 53-year-old G3, P0, Ab3 woman with a positive family history of breast cancer, for screening mammography.

Mammogram: Left craniocaudal, oblique (**B**), mediolateral (**C**), and enlarged (3×) spot compression (**D**) views. The breast is dense for the age of the patient. Deep in the central aspect of the breast on the craniocaudal view (**A**) is a small, high-density irregular nodule *(arrow)*. On the oblique view (**B**), several nodular densities are seen *(arrows)*, any of which could correspond to the lesion. A mediolateral view (**C**) was ob-

tained but again does not clearly identify the lesion. Spot compression views were obtained in the mediolateral position, along the plane of the nodules. The spot view (**D**) of the lowermost density of the oblique view (**B**) *(curved arrow)* revealed the lesion.

Impression: Irregular nodule at the 6 o'clock position of the left breast, highly suspicious for carcinoma.

Histopathology: Well-differentiated infiltrating ductal carcinoma.

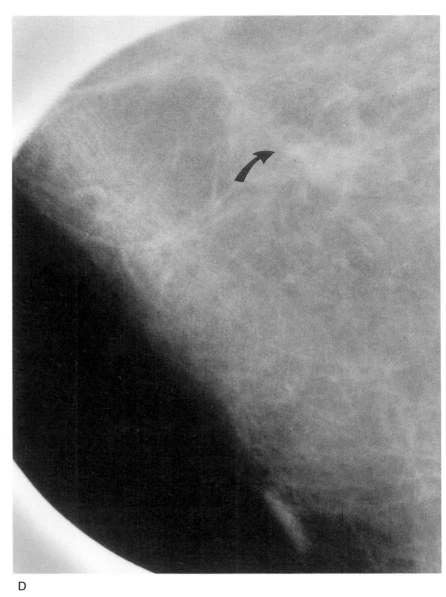

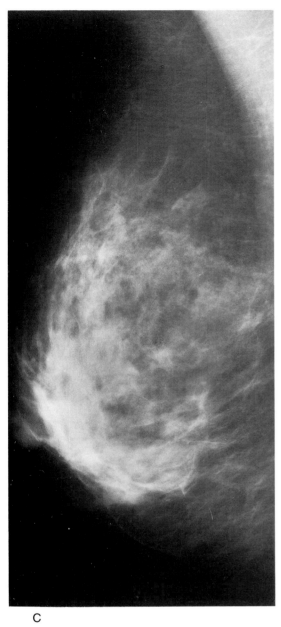

C

D

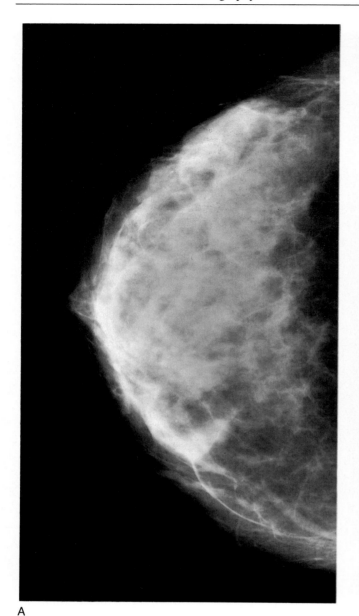
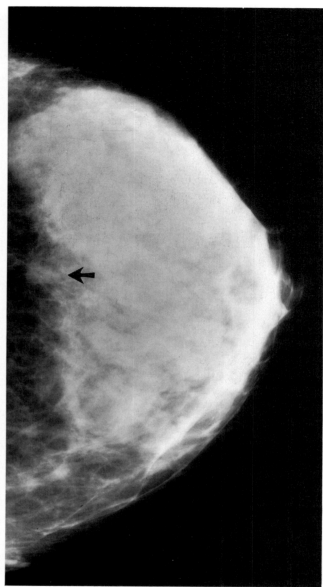

A

Figure 3.5.

Clinical: 56-year-old woman with a history of fibrocystic disease on three biopsies within the previous 2 years, referred for evaluation of microcalcifications found on an outside mammogram.

Mammogram: Bilateral craniocaudal (**A**), right oblique (**B**), and mediolateral (**C**) views. The breasts are very dense and nodular, compatible with fibrocystic changes. There were diffuse areas of microcalcifications bilaterally, which also are most likely of fibrocystic origin. On the right craniocaudal view (**A**), an irregular nodule is noted deep in the midportion of

the breast *(arrow)*. On the routine oblique view (**B**), the area is superimposed over the dense glandular tissue, and there is a suggestion of architectural distortion around it *(arrow)*. A 90° mediolateral view (**C**) is of help, in that the density is positioned differently and can be readily identified in the upper quadrant *(arrow)*. A third view is often useful in elucidating the exact location of an area visualized clearly on one view only.

Impression: Carcinoma of the breast.

Histopathology: Infiltrating ductal carcinoma, negative nodes.

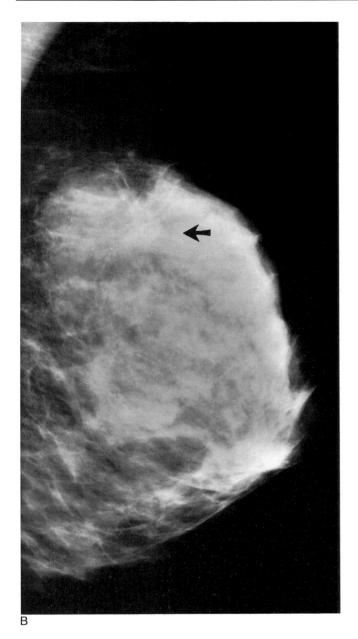

B

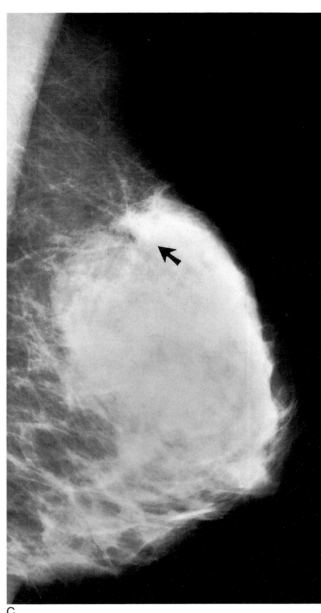

C

Figure 3.6.

Clinical: 41-year-old woman with normal physical examination.

Mammogram: Left oblique (**A**) and exaggerated lateral craniocaudal (**B**) views. There is a 4×6 cm, moderately dense lobulated mass oriented toward the nipple. A fine fatty halo *(arrows)* surrounds the mass in entirety. Normal stromal markings can be seen through the mass. Sonography demonstrated the anechoic lesion to be a simple cyst.

Impression: Cyst.

Aspiration: Clear cyst fluid.

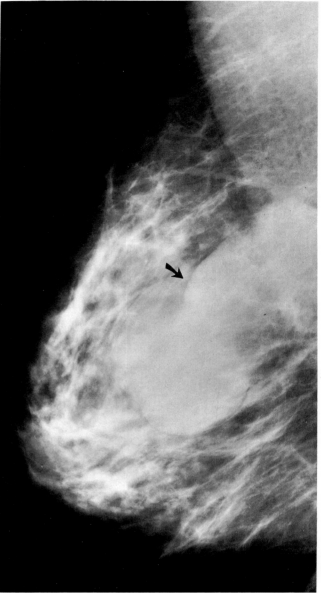

A

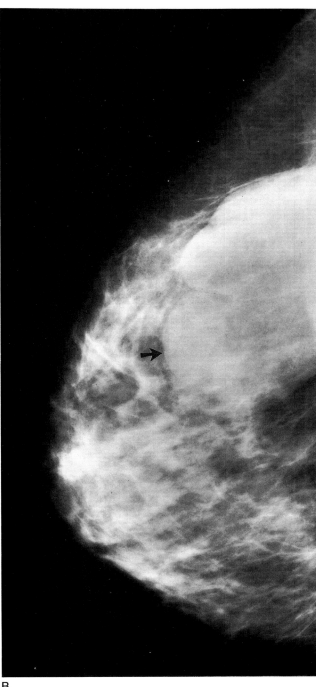

B

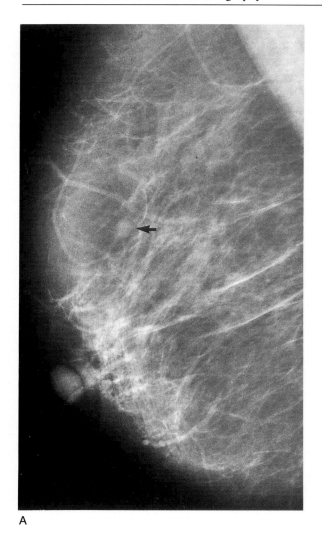

A

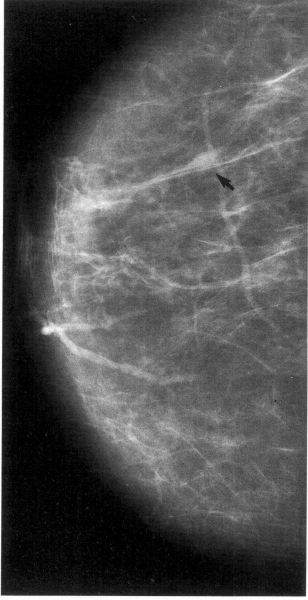

B

Figure 3.7.

Clinical: 68-year-old G2, P2 woman for screening.

Mammogram: Left oblique (**A**), craniocaudal (**B**), and spot compression magnification (1.5×) (**C**) views. The breast shows fatty replacement. In the upper outer quadrant there is a 5-mm, relatively well circumscribed, medium-density nodule *(arrows)* (**A** and **B**). The spot compression view (**C**) shows the nodule to be smooth and ovoid posteriorly but to have a

linear extension anteriorly *(arrow)*. Because of this finding it is of mild to moderate suspicion for malignancy.

Histopathology: Infiltrating ductal carcinoma.

Note: In the evaluation of a small circumscribed nodule, it is important to perform spot compression to evaluate the margins. If the margins are not completely smooth and round, the lesion should be biopsied.

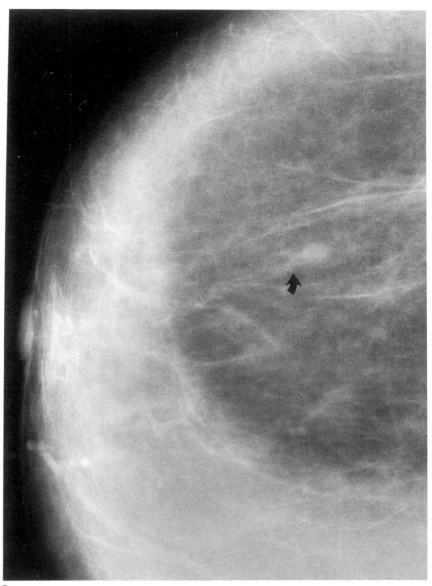

C

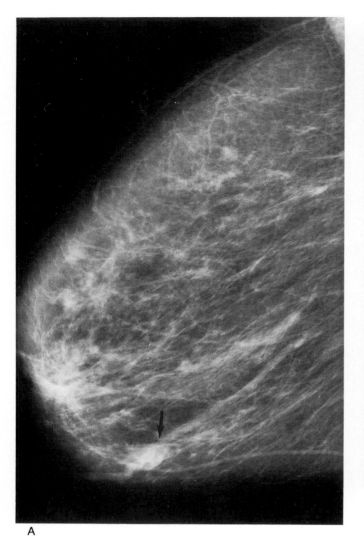

A

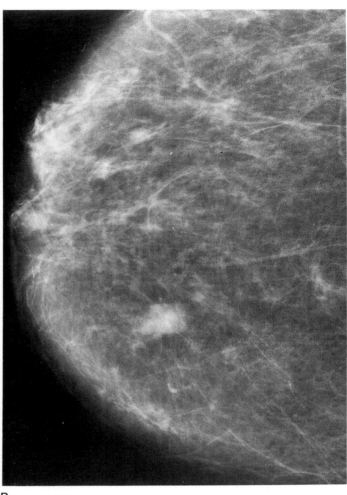

B

Figure 3.8.

Clinical: 72-year-old G1, P1 woman for screening.

Mammogram: Left oblique (**A**) and craniocaudal (**B**) views. The breast is mildly glandular. In the lower inner quadrant there is a multinodular medium- to high-density mass *(arrow)* (**A**). The nodularity on the borders of the lesion are a finding suspicious for carcinoma. A needle localization was performed prior to biopsy.

Impression: Multinodular mass suspicious for carcinoma.

Histopathology: Infiltrating ductal carcinoma with multiple foci of intraductal carcinoma.

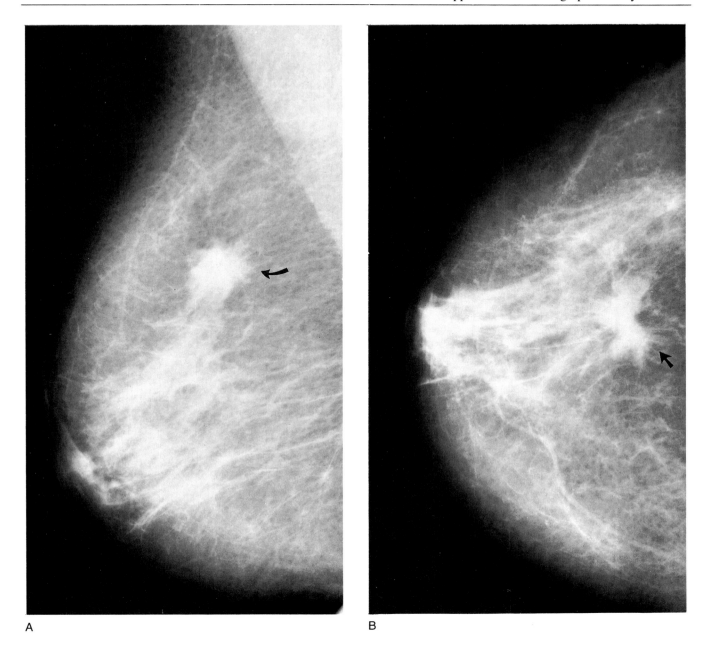

A   B

Figure 3.9.
Clinical: 73-year-old woman with an indurated left breast.
Mammogram: Left oblique (**A**) and craniocaudal (**B**) views. There is a high-density irregular mass in the 12 o'clock po-

sition. Fine spicules surround the nodular mass *(arrows)*, characteristic of malignancy.
Impression: Carcinoma.
Histopathology: Intraductal and infiltrating ductal carcinoma.

Figure 3.10.

Clinical: 67-year-old G0 woman with a left breast lump. No nipple retraction was noted.

Mammogram: Left oblique (**A**) and craniocaudal (**B**) views. There is a 2.5-cm spiculated high-density mass in the left subareolar area. Retraction of the left nipple and skin retraction of the areola *(arrows)* are noted with compression of the breast during mammography. It is not unusual for a central carcinoma to produce nipple retraction during compression of the breast, even when it is not evident during clinical examination.

Histopathology: Infiltrating ductal carcinoma, with macrometastases in 1 of 16 nodes.

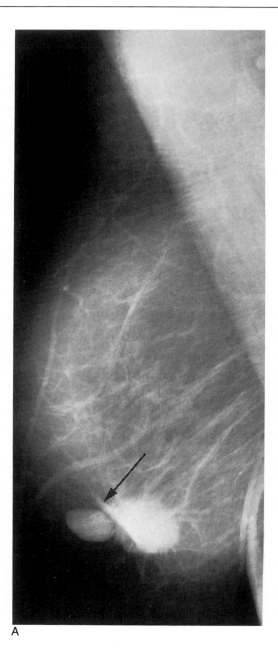

A

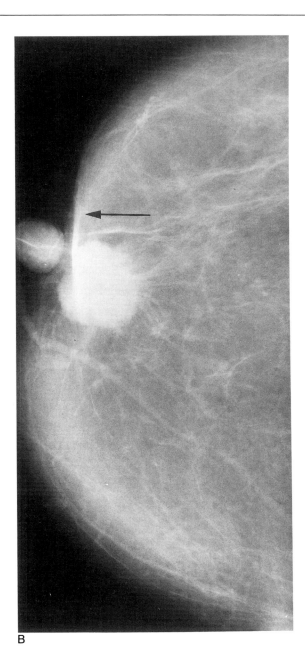

B

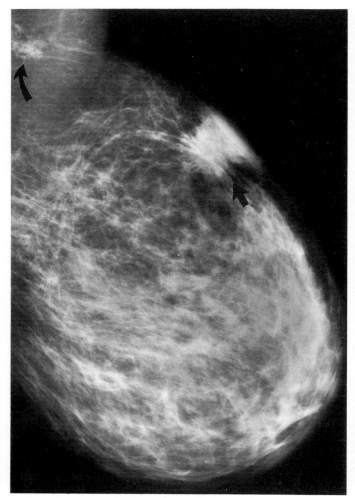

A

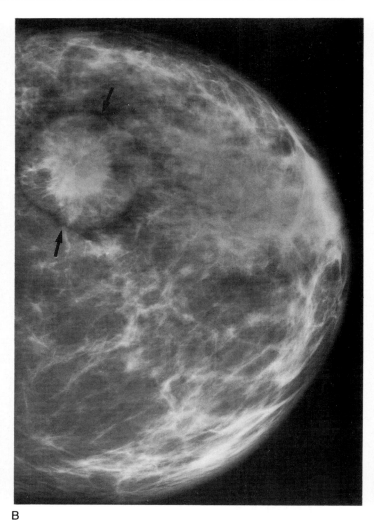

B

Figure 3.11.

Clinical: 52-year-old G3, P3 woman with a large ulcerating mass in the right upper outer quadrant.

Mammogram: Right oblique (**A**), craniocaudal (**B**), and enlarged (**C**) views of the mass. In an otherwise moderately glandular breast, there is a high-density spiculated mass *(arrow)* (**A**) that is attached to the skin and is associated with overlying skin thickening *(arrow)* (**C**). The mass does not compress as does the normal surrounding tissue, so on the craniocaudal view (**B**) an air halo *(arrow)* surrounds the bor-

der of the ulcer. Incidental note (**A**) is made of a second, smaller irregular density in the right axillary area *(curved arrow),* which probably represents metastatic involvement in a node.

Impression: Ulcerating carcinoma of the breast with probable involvement of the axillary nodes.

Histopathology: Infiltrating ductal carcinoma; 3 of 3 axillary nodes contained metastatic tumor that was invading the axillary fat.

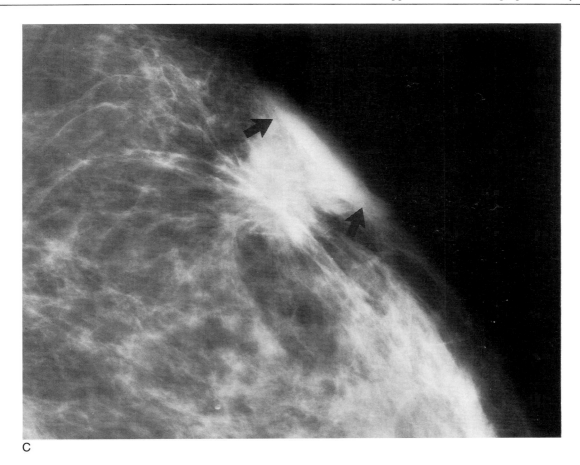

C

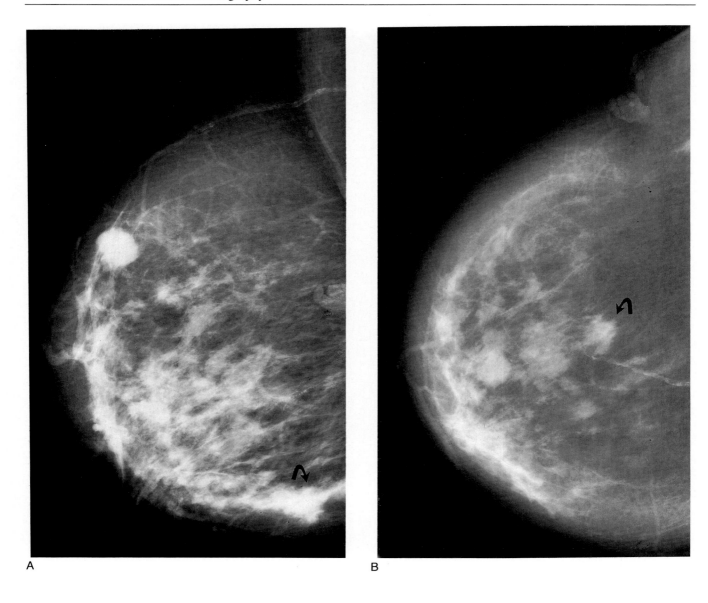

A

B

Figure 3.12.

Clinical: 82-year-old woman with a palpable mass at the 12 o'clock position in the left breast.

Mammogram: Left oblique (**A**) and craniocaudal (**B**) views. There is a high-density circumscribed mass above the left nipple corresponding to the palpable mass. An analysis of the margins of the mass shows that although the lesion is relatively well defined, the borders are nodular and lumpy, highly suspicious for malignancy. A second lesion is present

at the 6 o'clock position *(curved arrow)*. Analysis of this mass shows that the density is moderately high and the borders are ill defined. This lesion is characteristic for malignancy. When a palpable carcinoma is being evaluated, it is very important that a second lesion in the same breast not be overlooked.

Histopathology: Infiltrating ductal carcinoma, infiltrating lobular carcinoma.

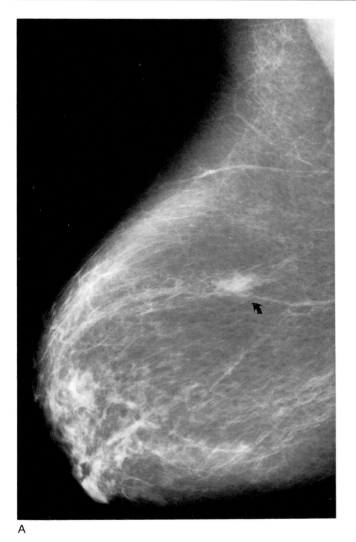

A

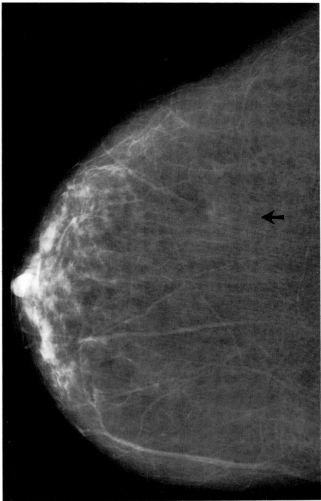

B

Figure 3.13.

Clinical: 62-year-old woman for screening.

Mammogram: Left oblique (**A**) and craniocaudal (**B**) views. There is an ill-defined area of moderately high density on the oblique view (**A**). On the craniocaudal view (**B**), however, the "lesion" disappears, having represented telescop-ing of low-density glandular tissue *(arrow)*. Before an asymmetric density or ill-defined lesion is considered abnormal, requiring biopsy, it must be identified as having a similar appearance on two different projections.

Impression: Overlying glandular tissue simulating a breast mass on one view.

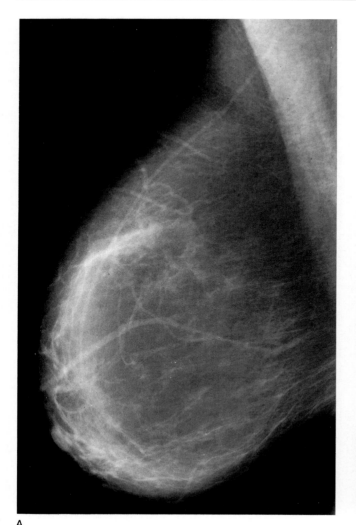

A

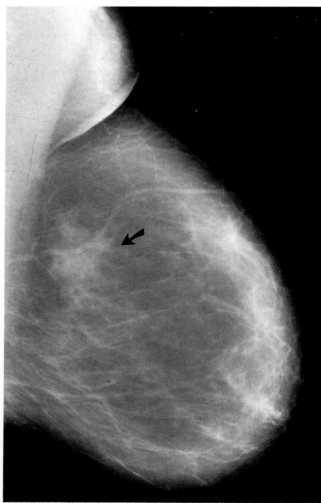

Figure 3.14.

Clinical: 65-year-old woman with a family history of breast cancer, for initial mammogram.

Mammogram: Bilateral oblique (**A**) and craniocaudal (**B**) views. The breasts show fatty replacement. Deep in the right upper outer quadrant is an amorphous area of increased density *(arrows),* which'has a similar configuration on both projections. No microcalcifications or secondary signs of malignancy are present, and although the area is irregular,

there are no radiating spicules. The findings suggest either a focal area of residual glandular tissue or an area of activity in the parenchyma. In situ carcinomas may be present in such an area of asymmetry. Because of the patient's age, risk factors, and the persistent appearance of the area on two views, biopsy was performed.

Histopathology: Intraductal small cell carcinoma, lobular neoplasia.

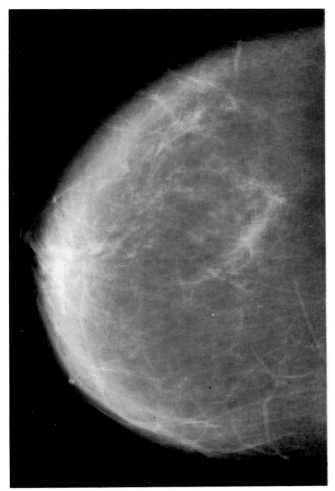
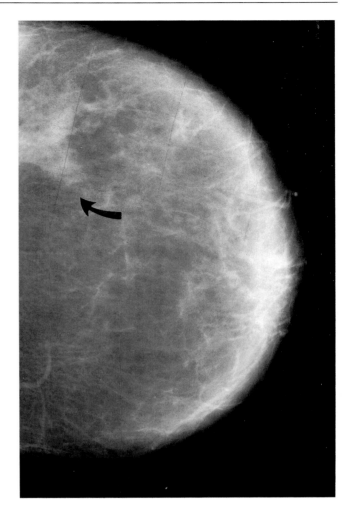

B

Figure 3.15.

Clinical: 67-year-old G3, P3 woman with a palpable mass in the left upper inner quadrant.

Mammogram: Bilateral oblique (**A**) and craniocaudal (**B**) views. The breasts are dense for the age and parity of the patient. In the left upper inner quadrant there is an ill-defined mass *(arrows)* that corresponded to the palpable finding. On the oblique view (**A**) the mass is perceptible only as a focal area of increased asymmetric density *(arrow),* but on the craniocaudal view (**B**) it is clearly evident *(arrow).*

Impression: Irregular mass, highly suspicious for carcinoma.

Histopathology: Infiltrating ductal carcinoma.

Note: Especially when the breasts are dense and glandular, a mass may be obscured by parenchyma on one view. If the area is not palpable, spot compression, mediolateral views, or ultrasound may be of help in locating the lesion.

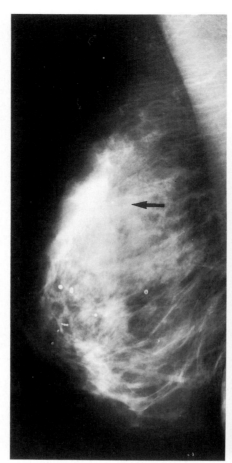
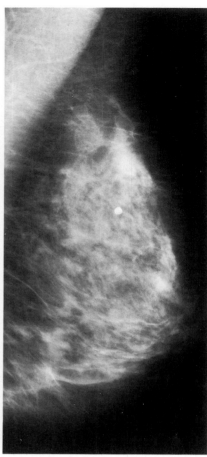

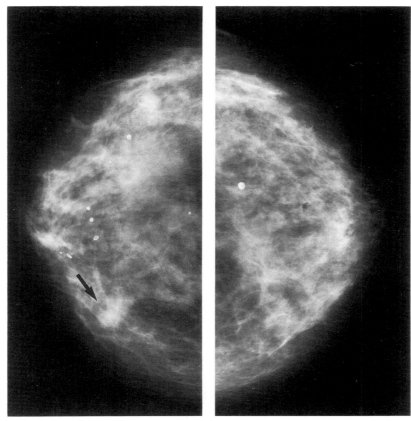

B

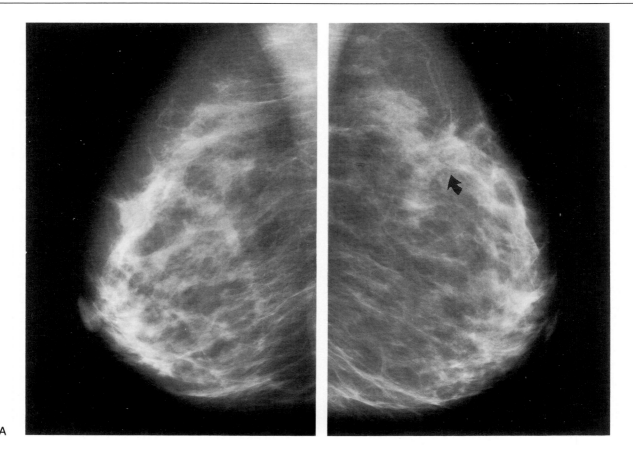

A

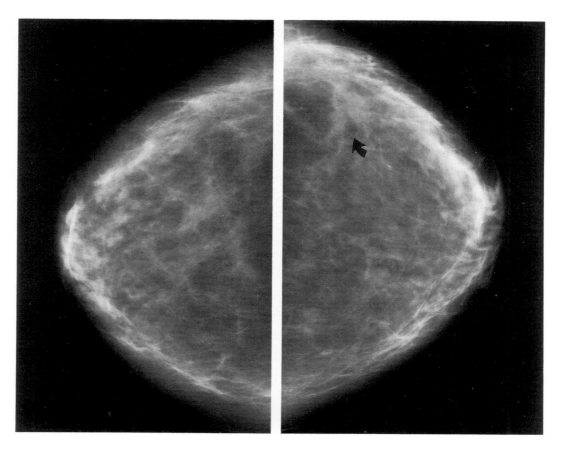

B

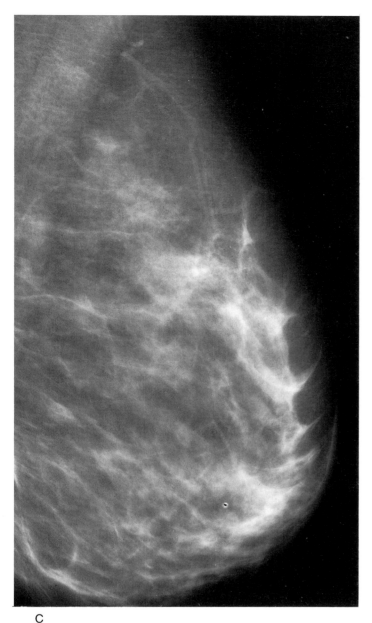

C

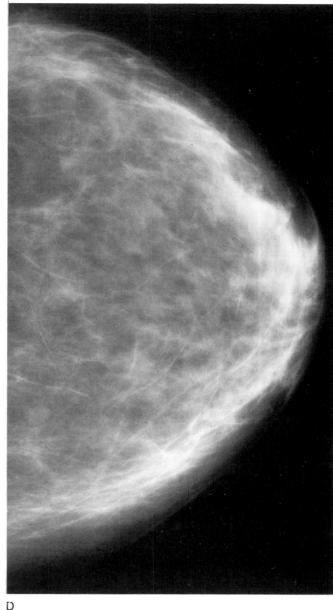

D

Figure 3.16.

Clinical: 67-year-old G3, P3 woman who has been on estrogen replacement therapy for 3 years and who presents with a questionable new palpable thickening in the right upper outer quadrant.

Mammogram: Bilateral oblique (**A**) and craniocaudal (**B**) views from 1989 and right oblique (**C**) and craniocaudal (**D**) views from 1988. The breasts are moderately dense with small areas of nodularity bilaterally. In the right upper outer quadrant *(arrows)* there is a focal irregular area of increased density with slight architectural distortion (**A** and **B**). This density had appeared from the previous examination (**C** and **D**) and was located in the region of the thickening. For these reasons the region was considered suspicious and biopsy was performed.

Histopathology: Infiltrating ductal carcinoma.

Note: The normal changes that may be seen when a patient is placed on estrogen replacement therapy are a diffuse increase in density and nodularity. When the changes are focal, or asymmetric, as in this case, and particularly if there is any change in clinical examination, one should not assume that the area represents an estrogen effect, and biopsy may be warranted.

Figure 3.17. A specimen radiograph shows a cluster of typically malignant ductal calcifications. There are irregular jagged punctate and linear forms in bizarre distribution and tightly clustered.

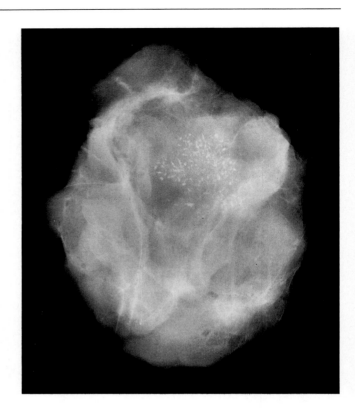

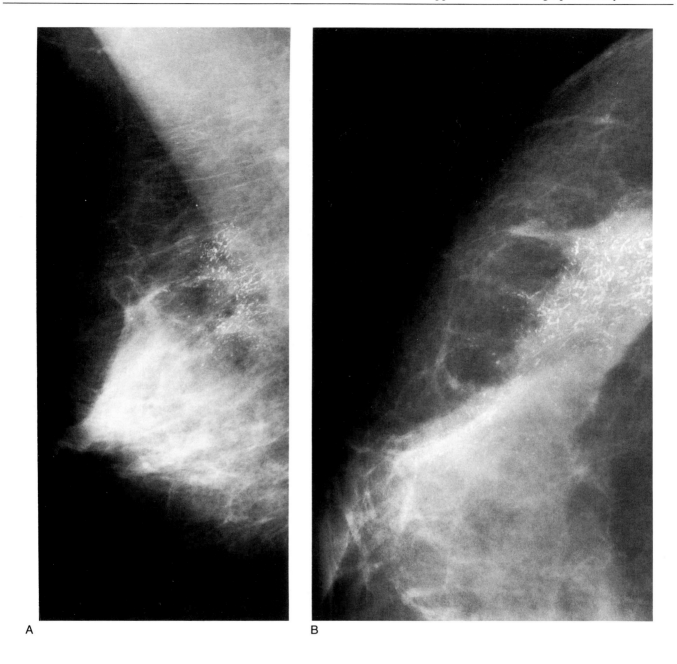

A   B

Figure 3.18.

Clinical: 56-year-old woman with a family history of premenopausal breast cancer; there was tenderness in the left breast without palpable findings.

Mammogram: Left oblique (**A**) and coned-down craniocaudal (**B**) views. There is an extensive area of innumerable, irregular, mixed morphology ductal microcalcifications extending throughout the left upper outer quadrant. The calcifications extend from the subareolar area to the axillary tail.

The appearance is typical of comedocarcinoma.

Histopathology: Extensive comedocarcinoma with foci of invasion (negative axillary nodes).

Note: It is important to describe in the mammographic report the extent of calcifications, as this affects the type of therapy that may be planned. Calcifications that extend over a large area, such as in this case, would not generally be treated with breast conservation therapy.

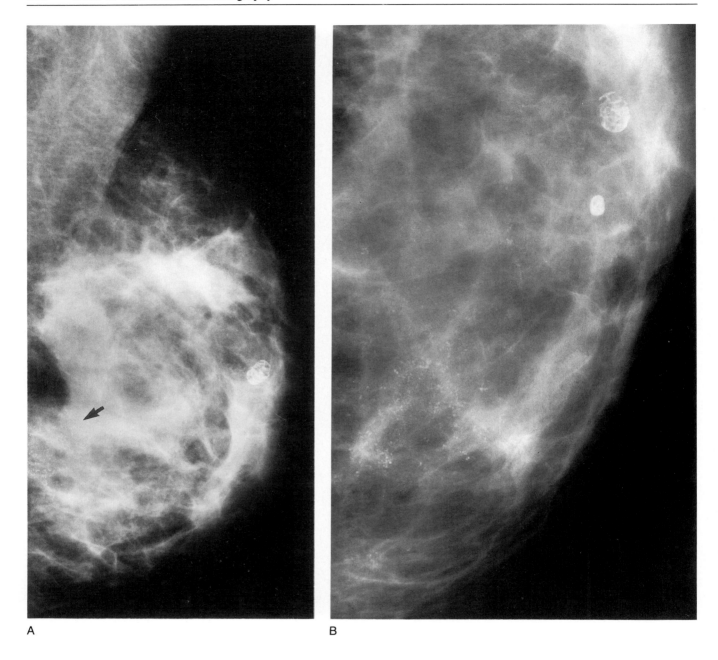

A   B

Figure 3.19.

Clinical: 26-year-old woman with a palpable thickening in the right lower inner quadrant.

Mammogram: Right oblique (**A**) and magnified (2×) (**B**) views. There are extensive irregular microcalcifications throughout the right lower inner quadrant *(arrow)* (**A**). Although the distribution is extensive, the morphology of these

is highly malignant. Even if the area were nonpalpable, it should be considered highly suspicious for carcinoma.

Impression: Extensive calcifications highly suspicious for carcinoma.

Histopathology: Comedocarcinoma and infiltrating ductal carcinoma.

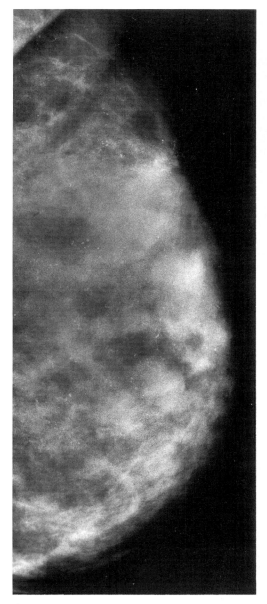

A

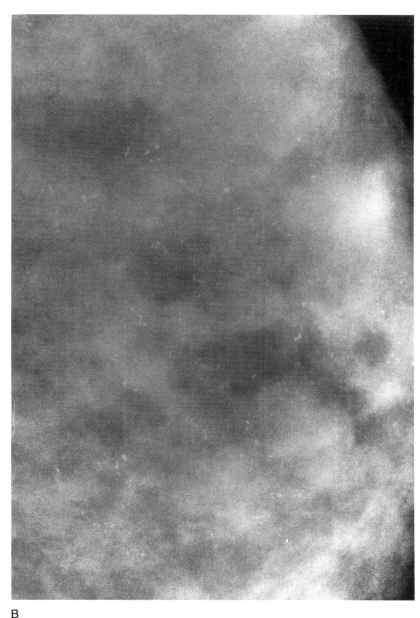

B

Figure 3.20.

Clinical: 33-year-old woman with a diffusely thickened right breast.

Mammogram: Right oblique (**A**) and enlarged (2×) cranio-caudal (**B**) views. The breast parenchyma is dense but consistent with the age of the patient. There are extensive micro-calcifications (**A**) involving all quadrants of the right breast (none were present on the left). The morphology of these calcifications is mixed and highly irregular with variability in sizes (**B**). Even though the distribution is diffuse, which is more compatible with a benign nature, the morphology is highly malignant.

Impression: Highly malignant-appearing calcifications throughout the right breast, consistent with a diffuse carcinoma.

Histopathology: Infiltrating ductal carcinoma, comedocarcinoma, lobular carcinoma in situ, negative axillary nodes.

Figure 3.21.

Clinical: 52-year-old-woman for screening mammography.

Mammogram: Left oblique (**A**) and right oblique (**B**) views. The breasts are dense for the age of the patient. There are bilateral coarse microcalcifications and macrocalcifications involving all quadrants. The relatively rounded morphology, the coarse size, and the bilateral distribution suggest a benign etiology as most likely.

Impression: Bilateral rounded microcalcifications, probably of fibrocystic origin.

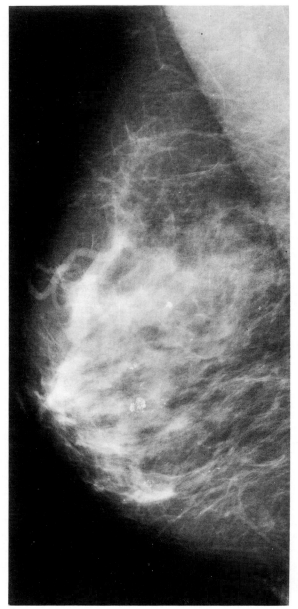

A

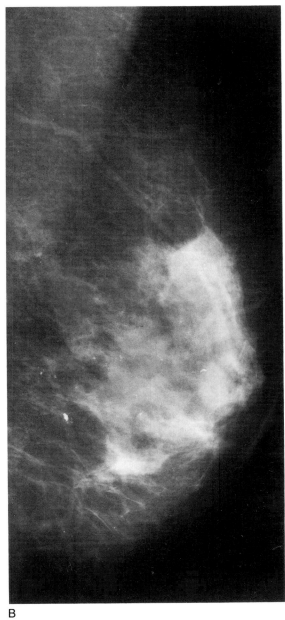

B

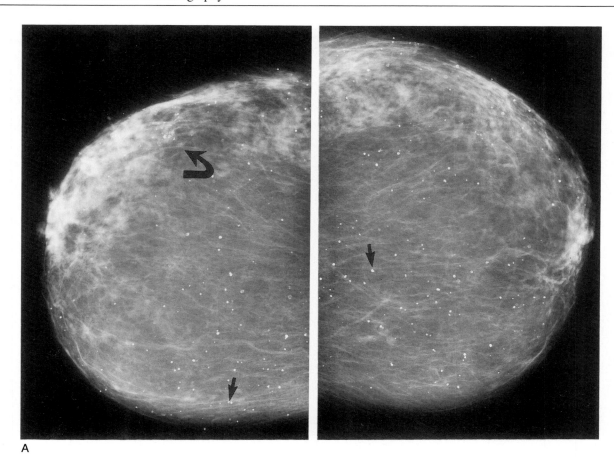

A

Figure 3.22.

Clinical: 75-year-old G0 woman for routine screening mammography.

Mammogram: Bilateral craniocaudal view (**A**), left mediolateral view (**B**), and specimen film (**C**). There are extensive calcifications of fat necrosis bilaterally *(arrows)* (**A** and **B**). In addition, in the left lower outer quadrant *(curved arrows)* (**A** and **B**) there are irregular linear ductal-type microcalcifications extending from the nipple posteriorly. Because of this linear irregular morphology and orientation, these calcifica-

tions have an appearance typical of comedocarcinoma. The area was removed following a needle localization procedure, and the specimen film demonstrates some of the calcifications.

Histopathology: Extensive intraductal carcinoma of comedo type, with residual carcinoma in the mastectomy specimen.

Note: It is important for the radiologist to evaluate all areas of calcifications independently, since there can be two or more etiologies present.

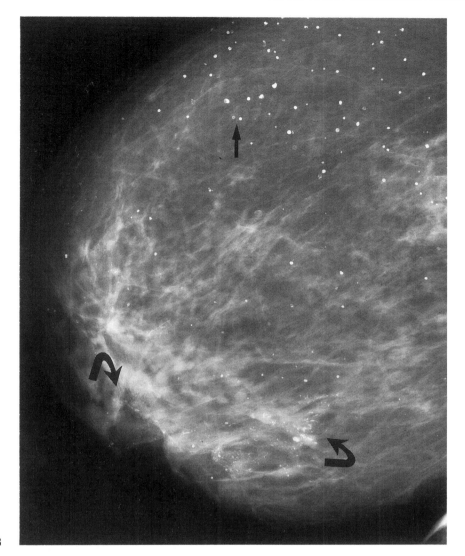

B

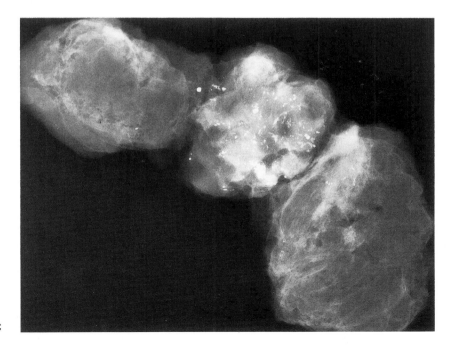

C

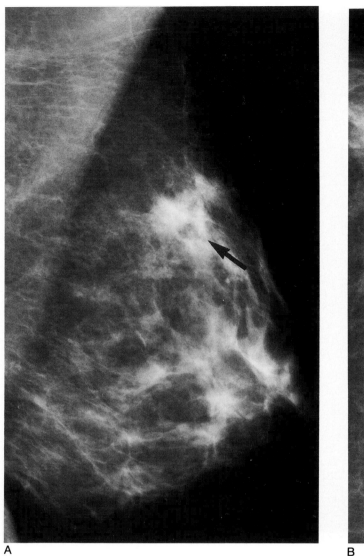

A

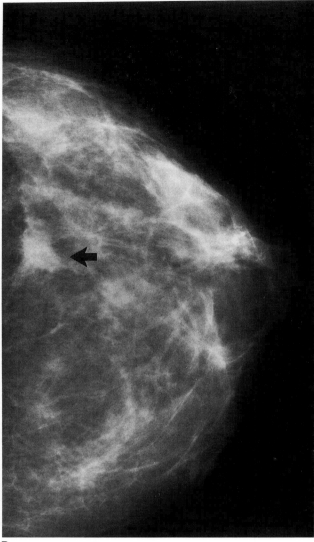

B

Figure 3.23.

Clinical: 53-year-old G0 woman presenting with a new 1-cm mass in the right breast at the 12 o'clock position.

Mammogram: Right oblique (**A**) and craniocaudal (**B**) views from April 1990 and a right craniocaudal (**C**) view from March 1989. On the current study (**A** and **B**), there is a high-density irregular mass *(arrows)* in the upper aspect of the right breast, corresponding in location to the palpable nodule. The mass has a highly suspicious mammographic appearance. Comparison with the previous study (**C**) shows development of the mass over a 1-year interval. There is considerable vari-

ability in the doubling times of breast carcinomas, some of which may be followed for several years without definite change, while others develop over a period of months. For these reasons it is important not only to perform mammography regularly to detect interval changes but also to compare with studies prior to the last one in order to detect subtle changes of slowly growing cancers.

Histopathology: Intraductal and infiltrating ductal carcinoma, grade II or III, with peritumoral lymphatic invasion.

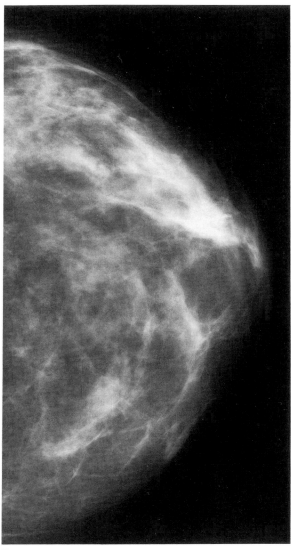

C

Figure 3.24.

Clinical: 61-year-old woman for routine screening.

Mammogram: Left craniocaudal view (**A**) from 1989 and left craniocaudal view (**B**) from 1986. The breast is mildly glandular. In the subareolar area there is a relatively well circumscribed 5-mm medium- to high-density nodule *(arrow)* (**A**). The nodule was not present on the mammogram (**B**) 3 years earlier. Ultrasound was performed but did not demonstrate the nodule. A nodule of this size and in a superficial location would probably be seen on ultrasound if it were cystic; it, therefore, is presumed to be solid. Because of the interval change from the prior study, the nodule should be considered moderately suspicious for malignancy. It can be approached by fine-needle aspiration or needle localization prior to excisional biopsy. In this case, the nodule was excised following a needle localization procedure.

Impression: New nodule, left breast, moderately suspicious for malignancy.

Histopathology: Infiltrating ductal carcinoma, comedocarcinoma.

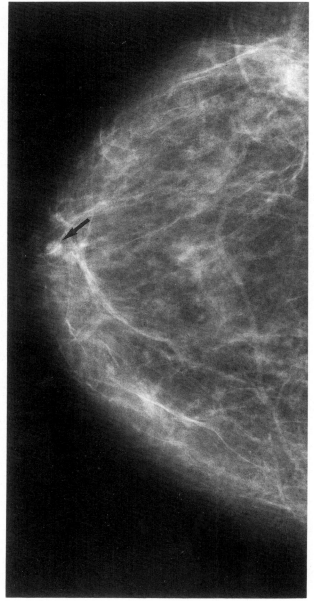

A

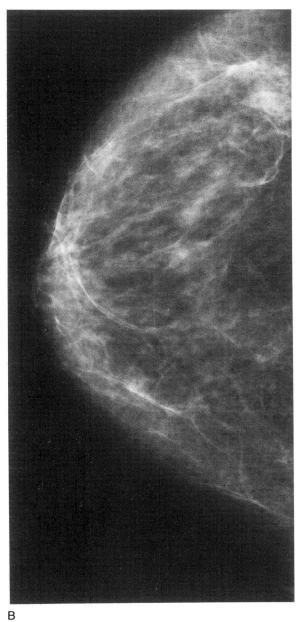

B

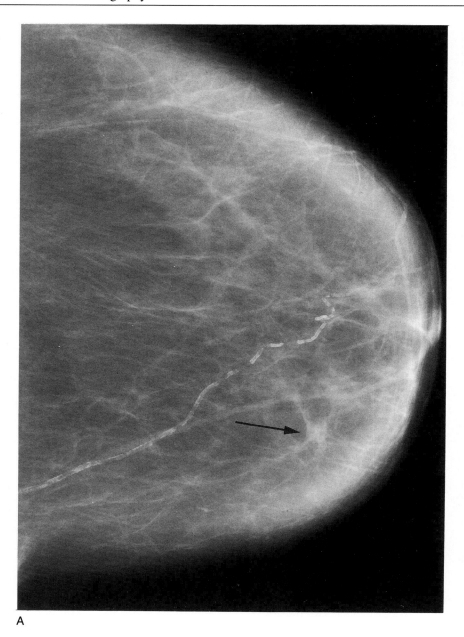

A

Figure 3.25.

Clinical: 84-year-old woman after treatment of left breast cancer, for screening of the right breast.

Mammogram: Right craniocaudal view (**A**) from February 1987, right craniocaudal view (**B**) from December 1988, and right craniocaudal view (**C**) from November 1989. The breast shows fatty replacement. There is a small irregular density located medially *(arrow),* which was not identified on the original mammogram (**A**). Eighteen months later (**B**) it was noted but was unchanged in size and density, and biopsy was not recommended. It was followed at 24 months and remained unchanged, but at 30 months (**C**) it increased in

size. The lesion was considered suspicious, and biopsy was recommended.

Impression: Irregular lesion, suspicious for carcinoma.

Histopathology: Infiltrating ductal carcinoma, intraductal carcinoma.

Note: The lack of change in a nodule over 1 or even 2 years does not confirm a benign nature but suggests it. Carcinomas may grow slowly, and the changes mammographically may be subtle from 6-month interval to 6-month interval. It is important that comparison be made from the most current mammogram and the earliest study to be able to perceive the slight changes that occur in some malignant lesions.

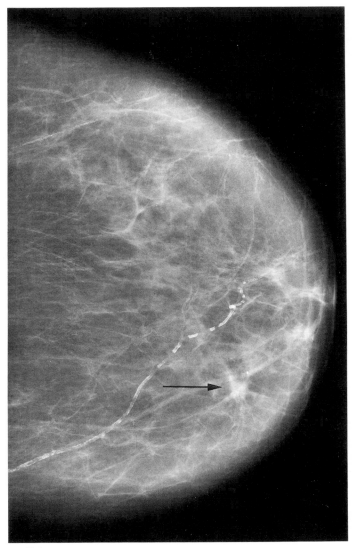

B

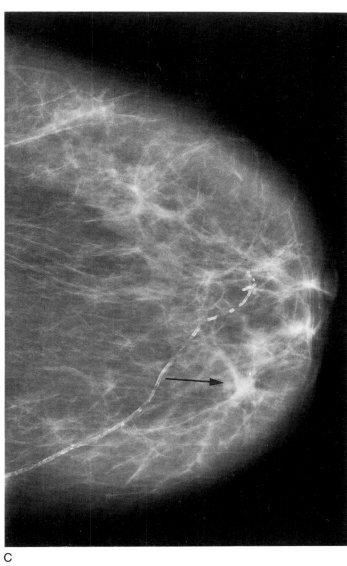

C

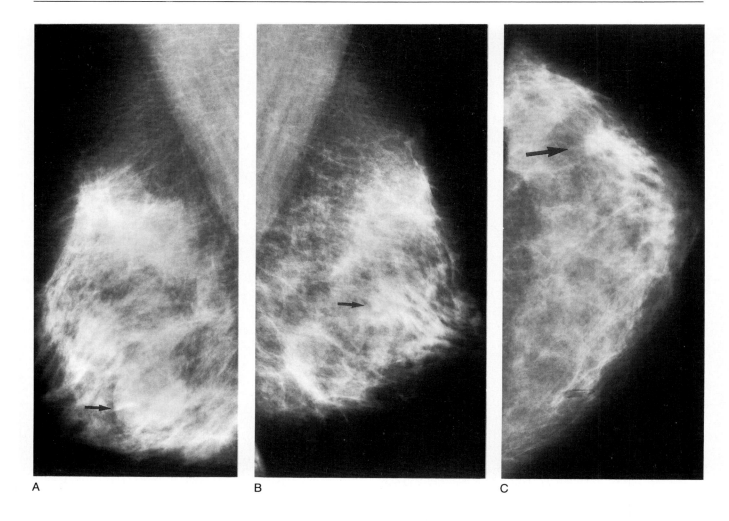

A   B   C

Figure 3.26.

Clinical: 48-year-old G3, P3 woman with a history of multiple cysts, for routine screening.

Mammogram: Left oblique view (**A**), right oblique view (**B**), right craniocaudal view (**C**), and ultrasound (**D**) from 1990 and right craniocaudal views from 1989 (**E**) and 1987 (**F**). The breasts are dense for the age and parity of the patient. In the left lower inner quadrant (**A**), a well-circumscribed medium-density mass *(arrow)* was noted that was confirmed to be a simple cyst on ultrasound. In the right upper outer quadrant (**B** and **C**) there is an irregular area of increased density *(arrows)* surrounded by a broad band of lucency. An ultrasound image (**D**) in this area demonstrated an irregular

mass *(arrow)* with dense shadowing, suspicious for carcinoma. Although the previous studies 1 (**E**) and 3 (**F**) years earlier demonstrated a similar irregular lesion *(arrows)*, the current study shows it to be slightly larger and more spiculated. The minimal change in size of a lesion over several years should not dissuade one from suggesting biopsy, particularly if there are other features (i.e., palpable, sonographic findings, increasing spiculation) that make it suspicious.

Impression: Irregular lesion highly suspicious for carcinoma.

Histopathology: Infiltrating ductal carcinoma (8 mm in diameter).

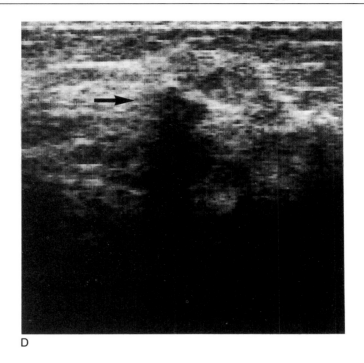

D

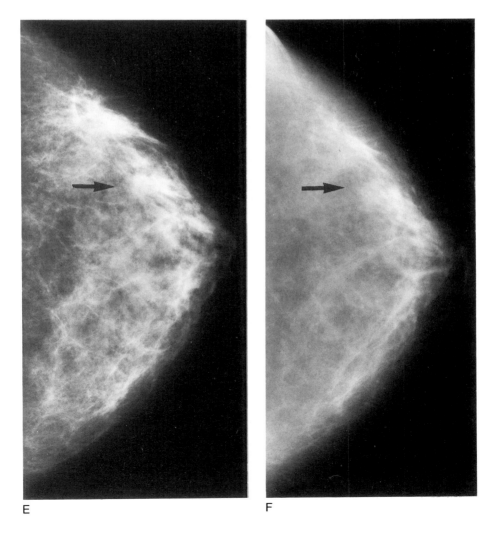

E   F

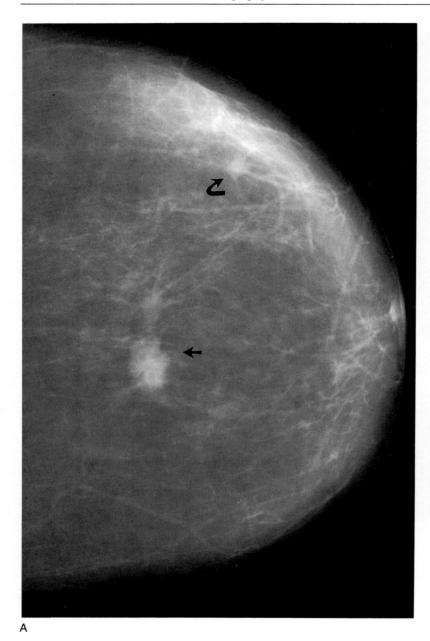

A

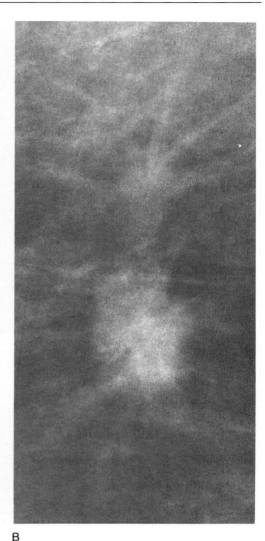

B

Figure 3.27.

Clinical: 45-year-old woman with generalized breast tenderness and no palpable abnormality.

Mammogram: Right craniocaudal (**A**) view and magnified images (**B** and **C**). In a breast that otherwise shows fatty replacement there are two spiculated ill-defined masses. In the central portion of the breast the larger mass is of high density, is irregular, and has an extension laterally with spiculation *(arrow)* (**B**). Lateral to this lesion, a second smaller lesion

(curved arrow) has a similar appearance (**C**). The density and irregularity of the lesions are highly suspicious for carcinoma. It is critical that the radiologist identify not only the obvious carcinoma but also the smaller lesion in the same breast, particularly if the patient may consider lumpectomy and radiation therapy for treatment.

Impression: Multicentric carcinoma.

Histopathology: Multicentric infiltrating ductal carcinoma.

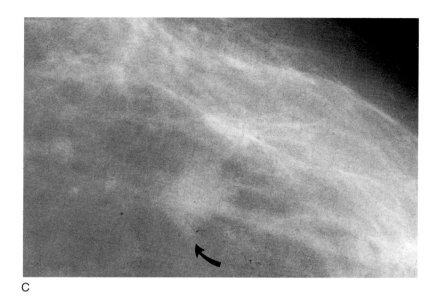

C

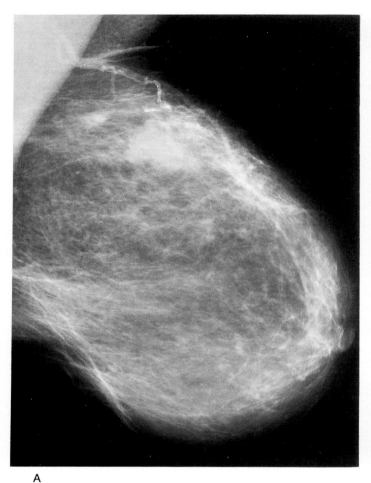

A

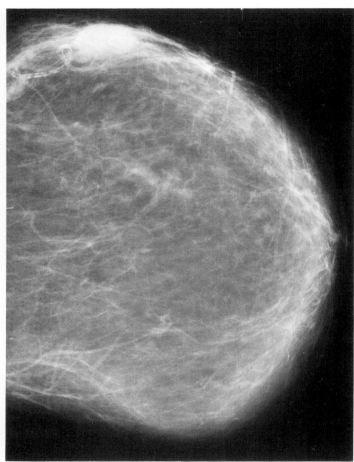

B

Figure 3.28.

Clinical: 58-year-old G5, P5 woman with a firm, tender mass in the right breast.

Mammogram: Right oblique (**A**) and craniocaudal (**B**) views and left oblique (**C**) and craniocaudal (**D**) views. There is a high-density spiculated mass with associated microcalcification in the right upper outer quadrant (**A** and **B**). This lesion has an appearance highly suggestive of carcinoma. In the left upper outer quadrant there is an 8-mm ill-defined nodule *(arrows)* of medium density (**C** and **D**). Although the

nodule appears less distinct and dense on the craniocaudal view (**D**), it nonetheless persists and is therefore of moderate suspicion for a contralateral carcinoma.

Impression: Carcinoma of the right breast, moderately suspicious nodule of left breast.

Histopathology: Right breast: infiltrating lobular carcinoma. Left breast: Widespread intraductal carcinoma, lobular carcinoma in situ.

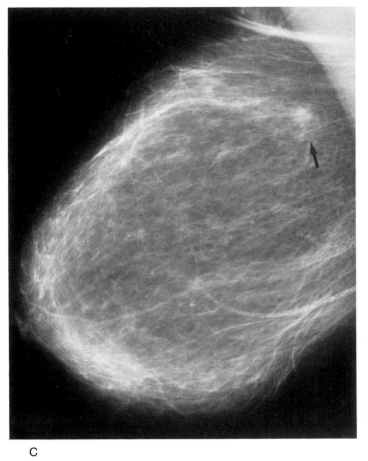

C

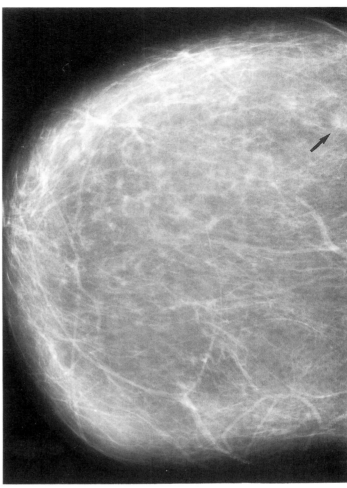

D

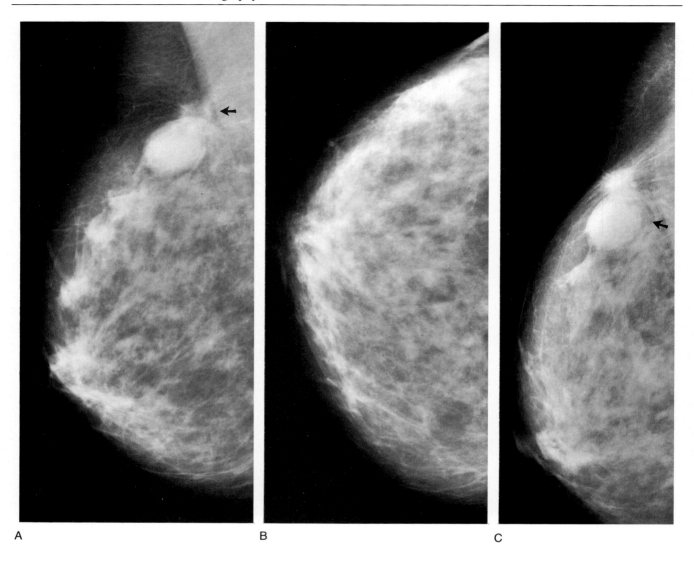

A   B   C

Figure 3.29.

Clinical: 60-year-old G1, P1 woman with a positive family history for breast cancer, for a screening mammogram. (Note: After the mammogram was performed, a mass was palpable in retrospect in the left upper outer quadrant.)

Mammogram: Left oblique view (**A**), craniocaudal view (**B**), exaggerated lateral craniocaudal view (**C**), and ultrasound (**D** and **E**). There is a relatively well defined 2.5-cm mass with an irregular density on its posterior margin *(arrow)* on the oblique view (**A**); this is not demonstrated on a routine cra-

niocaudal view (**B**). An exaggerated lateral craniocaudal view shows the lateral position of the two masses (**C**). Real-time sonography demonstrates the well-defined anterior mass to be a simple cyst (**D**). The smaller posterior spiculated density (**E**) is hypoechoic and irregular on ultrasound, and there is some distal shadowing, which are features of carcinoma.

Impression: Cyst and adjacent carcinoma in the left upper outer quadrant.

Histopathology: 1-cm carcinoma, fibrocystic changes, cyst.

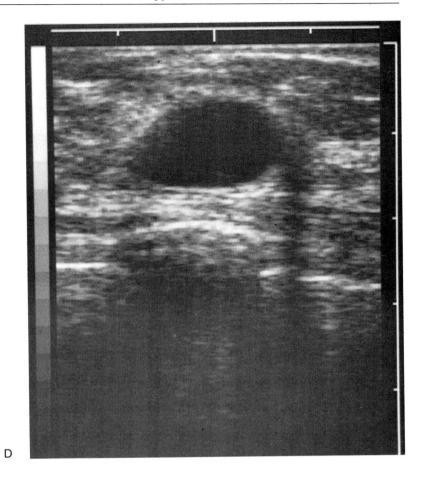

D

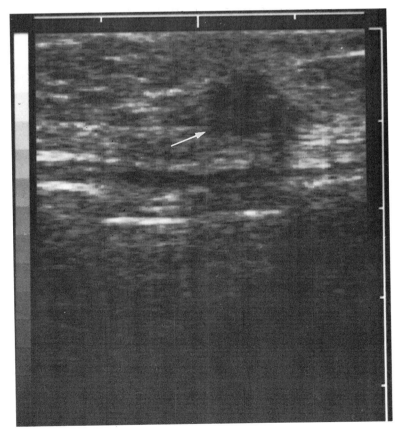

E

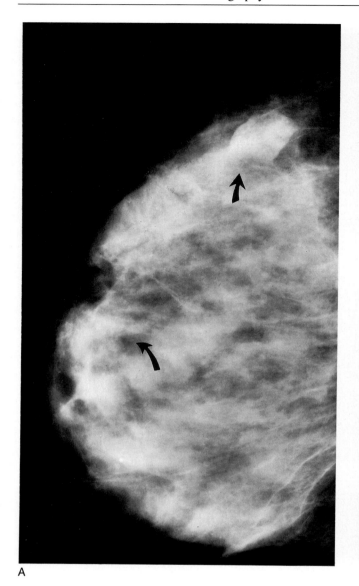

A

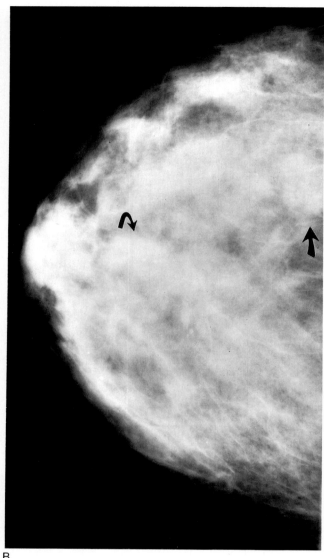

B

Figure 3.30.

Clinical: 49-year-old G3, P3 woman sent for screening mammography. The mammography technologist found an area of dimpling above the patient's left nipple.

Mammogram: Left oblique view (**A**), craniocaudal view (**B**), and ultrasound (**C** and **D**). The left breast is quite dense and glandular with diffuse round calcifications consistent with fibrocystic changes and probably cystic hyperplasia. There is a well-defined lobulated mass *(arrow)* in the left upper outer quadrant, which was shown to be a cyst on sonography (**C**). Anterior to this mass is a focal area of very slightly increased density *(curved arrow)* (**B**) without other signs of malignancy.

This density was directly above the area of skin dimpling. Sonography of this area (**D**) revealed an irregular hypoechoic mass *(arrows)* with shadowing, highly suspicious for malignancy. This case demonstrates the value of sonography as an adjunct to mammography in the patient with a dense and nodular breast.

Impression: Fibrocystic changes, mass in the left upper quadrant highly suspicious for carcinoma.

Histopathology: Infiltrating ductal carcinoma, 2 of 27 nodes positive for malignancy.

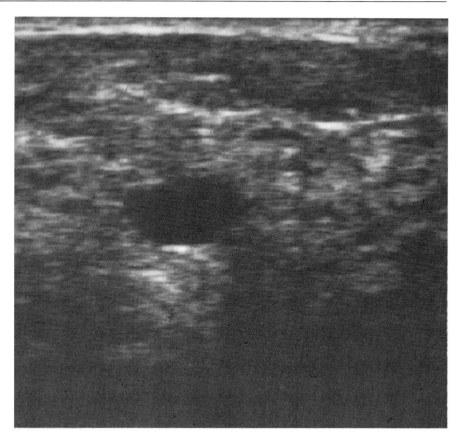

C

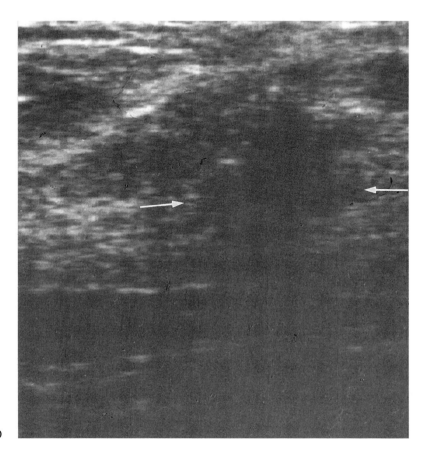

D

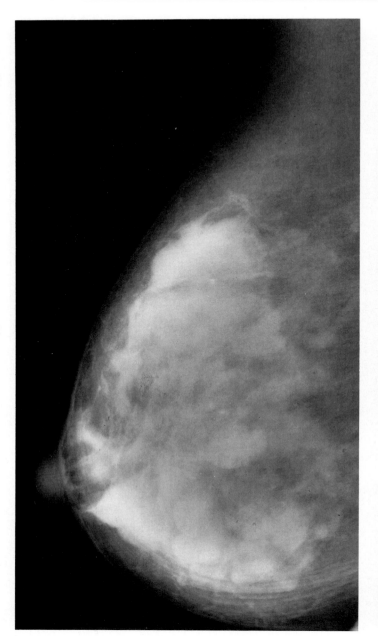
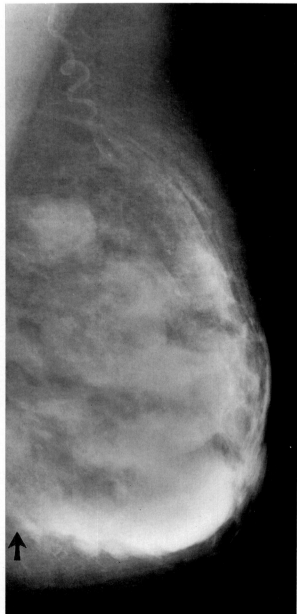

A

Figure 3.31.

Clinical: 71-year-old debilitated woman with a history of cysts and multiple lumps on clinical examination, none of which was identified as suspicious.

Mammogram: Bilateral oblique views (**A**) and ultrasound of the right breast (**B** and **C**). The examination was limited by the patient's inability to cooperate well for positioning. The breasts are very dense for the age of the patient, and there are multiple well-defined nodules bilaterally. Note that in the right breast inferiorly, dense tissue extends posteriorly to the edge of the film *(arrow)*. Whole-breast ultrasound (**B**) shows multiple cysts in both breasts. In the right lower outer quadrant deep near the chest wall there is an irregular hypoechoic area with posterior shadowing (**C**) *(arrow),* highly suspicious for carcinoma.

Histopathology: Infiltrating ductal carcinoma.

Note: It is important to image the entire breast, and parenchyma should not extend beyond the border of the film. A cancer near the chest wall can easily be missed if improper positioning is done. Additionally, sonography is of help in the evaluation of a dense multinodular breast.

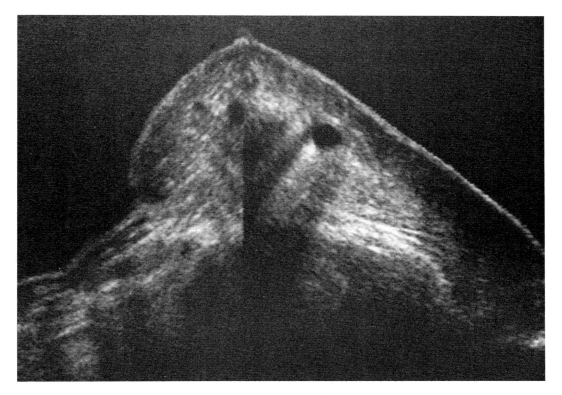

B

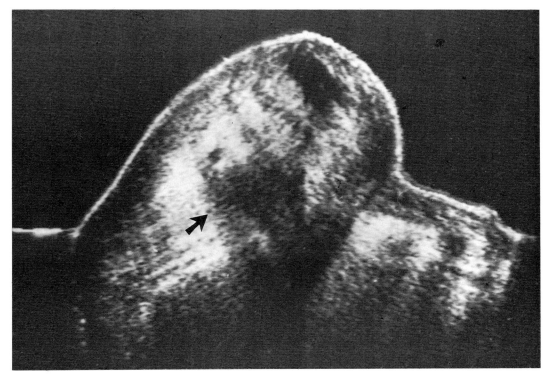

C

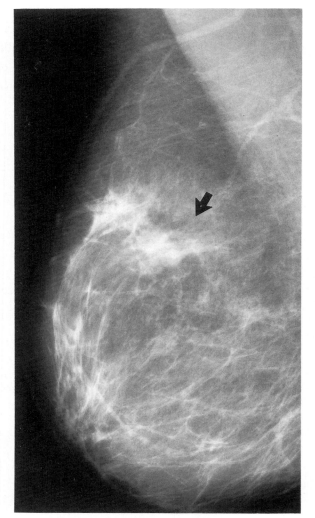

A

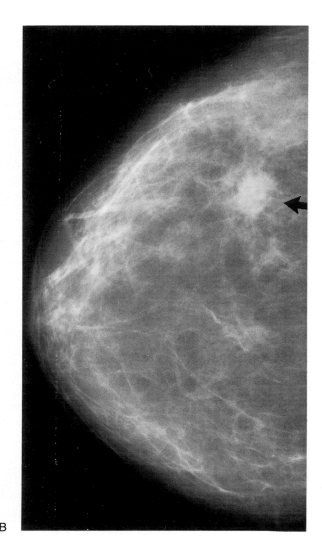

B

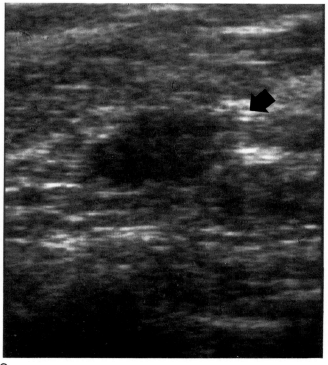

C

Figure 3.32.

Clinical: 45-year-old woman after mastectomy for breast cancer on the right and treatment for colon cancer, for routine screening.

Mammogram: Left oblique (**A**) and craniocaudal (**B**) views and ultrasound (**C**). There is a high-density mass with indistinct margins in the upper outer quadrant of the left breast *(arrows)* (**A** and **B**). The mass has a slightly different shape on the two views but nonetheless persists as a high-density lesion. On ultrasound (**C**), characteristically malignant features are present *(arrow):* mixed hypoechogenicity, ill-defined borders, and faint shadowing.

Impression: Carcinoma, left breast.

Histopathology: Infiltrating ductal carcinoma, with 13 negative axillary nodes.

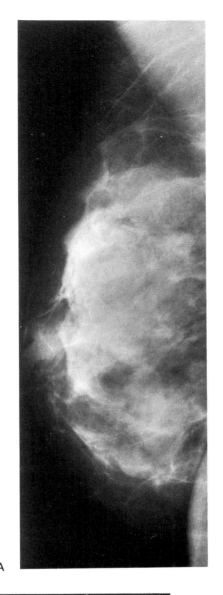

A

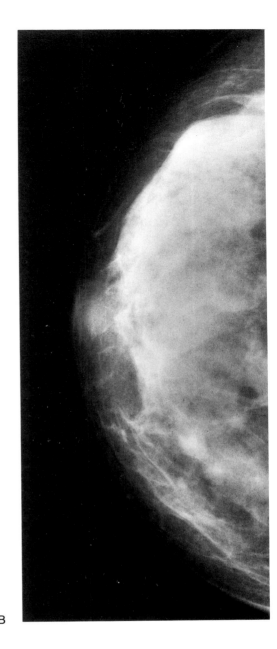

B

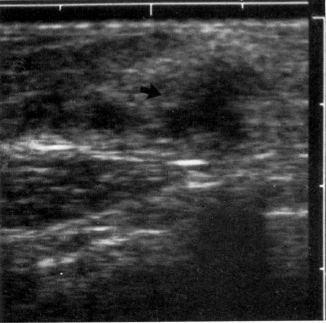

C

Figure 3.33.

Clinical: 53-year-old woman after treatment of right breast cancer, with a history of cysts on the left, for routine follow-up. The left breast was nodular, but no focal palpable masses of suspicion were noted.

Mammogram: Left oblique (**A**) and craniocaudal (**B**) views and ultrasound (**C**). The left breast is dense and nodular for the age of the patient. Because of the palpable nodularity and the nodular pattern, ultrasound was performed. Sonography demonstrated multiple cysts as well as an irregular solid mass *(arrow)* (**C**) in the upper outer quadrant, highly suspicious for carcinoma. The lesion was marked under sonographic guidance for excision.

Impression: Irregular solid mass highly suspicious for carcinoma.

Histopathology: Infiltrating ductal carcinoma.

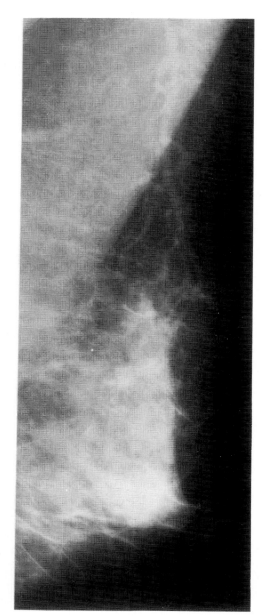

A

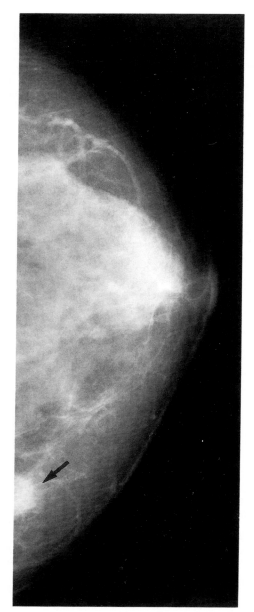

B

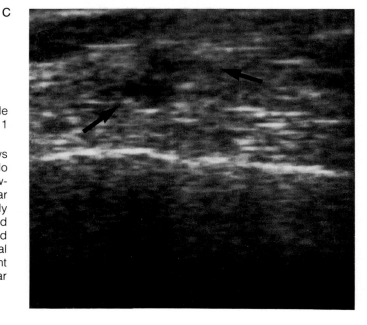

C

Figure 3.34.

Clinical: 44-year-old G1, P1 woman with a questionable thickening medially in the right breast. The mammogram 1 year earlier was normal.

Mammogram: Right oblique (**A**) and craniocaudal (**B**) views and ultrasound (**C**). The breast is moderately glandular. No focal abnormality is present on the oblique view (**A**). However, on the craniocaudal view (**B**) a high-density irregular mass *(arrow)* is present near the chest wall. This has a highly malignant appearance mammographically. The mass could not be demonstrated on additional sagittal views. Ultrasound was performed to locate the mass and mark it for surgical excision. The mass *(arrows)* also appears typically malignant on ultrasound (**C**), having mixed echogenicity and irregular margins.

Histopathology: Infiltrating ductal carcinoma.

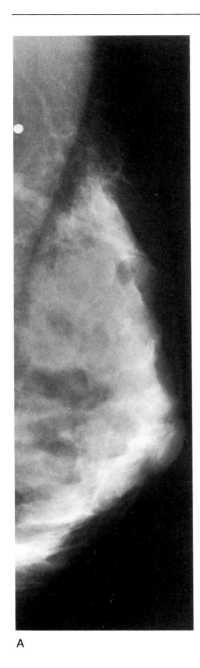

A

Figure 3.35.

Clinical: 36-year-old woman with a questionable small palpable nodule high in the right upper inner quadrant.

Mammogram: Right oblique view (**A**) and ultrasound (**B**). There is a metallic marker overlying the palpable lump (**A**). No abnormality is seen on the mammogram. The palpable lesion is probably lying posterior to the edge of the film. Lesions high in the upper inner quadrant are difficult to image with the routine oblique and craniocaudal views. Ultrasound is of help in documenting the location and characteristics of a palpable lesion not seen on mammography. On the sonogram (**B**) the nodule, which lies just anterior to the pectoralis major muscle, is hypoechoic, somewhat irregular, and therefore suspicious in nature *(arrow)*. The area was marked under ultrasound guidance for confirmation prior to excision.

Impression: Solid mass suspicious for carcinoma.

Histopathology: Infiltrating ductal carcinoma.

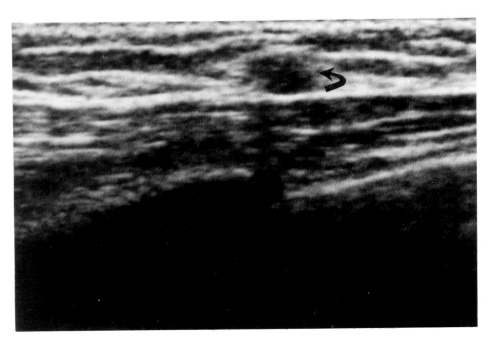

B

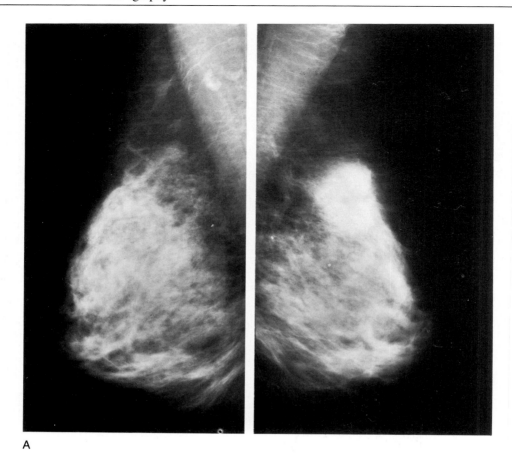

A

Figure 3.36.

Clinical: 52-year-old G2, P2 woman with a large palpable mass in the right breast.

Mammogram: Bilateral oblique (**A**) and craniocaudal (**B**) views and ultrasound (**C**). The breasts are dense for the age and parity of the patient. There is a large high-density round mass in the upper outer quadrant of the right breast (**A** and **B**). Although areas of the lesion are well circumscribed, other margins are indistinct. On ultrasound (**C**) the mass is hypoechoic, with fine irregularity of the margins, which is suspicious for carcinoma.

Impression: Carcinoma.

Histopathology: Poorly differentiated infiltrating ductal carcinoma, with invasion of parenchymal lymphatics and metastatic carcinoma in 3 of 20 axillary nodes.

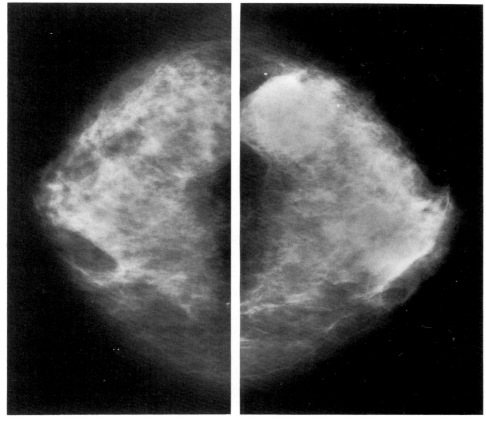

B

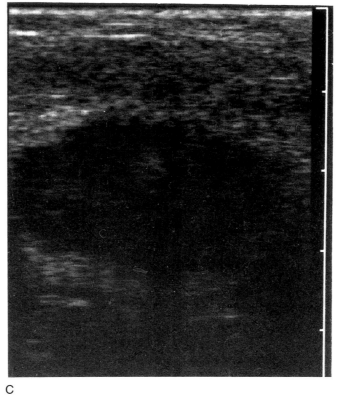

C

References

1. Sickles EA. Practical solutions to common mammographic problems: tailoring the examination. AJR 1988;151:31–39.
2. Egan RL. Fundamentals of mammographic diagnoses of benign and malignant diseases. Oncology 1969;23:126–148.
3. Berkowitz JE, Gatewood OMB, Gayler BW. Equivocal mammographic findings: evaluation with spot compression. Radiology 1989;171:369–371.
4. Gold RH, Montgomery CK, Rambo ON. Significance of margination of benign and malignant infiltrative mammary lesions: roentgenographic pathological correlation. AJR 1973;118:881–895.
5. Sickles EA, et al. Evaluation of breast masses. Radiology 1989;173:297–303.
6. Swann CA, Kopans DB, et al. The halo sign of malignant breast lesions. AJR 1987;149:1145–1147.
7. Gordenne WH, Malchair FL. Mach bands in mammography. Radiology 1988;169:55–58.
8. Marsteller LP, Shaw de Paredes E. Well defined masses in the breast. RadioGraphics 1989;9(1):13–37.
9. Sickles E. Mammographic features of 300 consecutive nonpalpable breast cancers. AJR 1986;146:661–663.
10. Stomper PC, Davis SP, Weidner N, Meyer JE. Clinically occult, noncalcified breast cancer: serial radiologic-pathologic correlation in 27 cases. Radiology 1988;160:621–626.
11. Adler DD, Helvie MA, Ikeda DM. Nonpalpable, probably benign breast lesions: follow-up strategies after initial detection on mammography. AJR 1990;155:1195–1201.
12. Kopans DB, Swann CA, White G, et al. Asymmetric breast tissue. Radiology 1989;171:639–643.
13. Tabar L, Dean PB. Teaching atlas of mammography. Stuttgart: Georg Thieme Verlag, 1983.
14. Fournier DV, Weber E, Hoeffken W, et al. Growth rate of 147 mammary carcinomas. Cancer 1980;45:2198–2207.
15. Kinne DW. Management of the contralateral breast. In: Harris JR, et al, eds. Breast diseases. Philadelphia: JB Lippincott, 1987:620–621.
16. Kopans DB, Meyer JE, Cohen AM, Wood WC. Palpable breast masses: the importance of preoperative mammography. JAMA 1981;246:2819–2822.
17. Kopans DB, Meyer JE, Steinbock RT. Breast cancer: the appearance as delineated by whole breast water-path ultrasound scanning. J Clin Ultrasound 1982;10:313–322.
18. Kopans DB. Nonmammographic breast imaging techniques: current status and future developments. Radiol Clin North Am 1987;25(5):961–971.
19. Rubin E, Miller VE, Berland LL, et al. Hand-held real-time breast sonography. AJR 1985;144:623–627.
20. Ikeda DM, Adler DD, Helvie MA. Breast ultrasound. App Radiol 1991;20(2):19–24.
21. Jackson VP. The role of US in breast imaging. Radiology 1990;177:305–311.
22. Hilton SvW, Leopold GR, Olson LK, Willson SA. Real-time breast sonography: application in 300 consecutive patients. AJR 1986;145:479–486.
23. Sickles EA, Filly RA, Callen PW. Benign breast lesions: ultrasound detection and diagnosis. Radiology 1984;151:467–470.
24. Harper AP, Kelly-Fry E, Noe JS, et al. Ultrasound in the evaluation of solid breast masses. Radiology 1983;146:731–736.
25. Fornage BD, Lorigan JG, Andry E. Fibroadenoma of the breast: sonographic appearance. Radiology 1989;172:671–675.

CHAPTER

4

WELL-DEFINED MASSES

Masses or nodules with well-circumscribed margins are a common finding on mammography. Well-defined lesions are more commonly benign, but it is imperative that the radiologist evaluating a mass differentiate those that are characteristically benign from the indeterminate or suspicious lesions. Sonography (1) plays a key role in the differentiation of solid from cystic masses and greatly facilitates the recommendations for follow-up or further evaluation of the patient.

An approach to the evaluation of a well-defined mass on mammography includes an assessment of the density, margins, size, orientation, contour, presence of a fatty halo, and presence of other findings (i.e., calcifications). Benign lesions tend to be of medium to low density and to have very well defined margins, whereas malignant masses are more often of greater density and have fine irregularity or nodularity on their borders (Table 4.1).

A basic division of well-circumscribed masses based on their density is of help in determining possible etiologies of and approach to such lesions. Masses that are fatty—lipomas, oil cysts, and galactoceles—and circumscribed masses that are of mixed density are benign. Medium-density circumscribed masses include benign and malignant lesions, and an evaluation of the borders is made to help differentiate these etiologies.

Any notching, waviness, or irregularity of the margins of a lesion should be regarded with suspicion (2). The presence of a halo sign, i.e., a fine radiolucent ring surrounding a well-defined mass, has long been considered to be a mammographic sign of benignancy (3). The halo may be due to compression of fat by the mass (4) or to the Mach effect (5). Swann et al. (6) have, however, described 25 malignant lesions, from approximately 1000 breast cancers, in which a halo sign was present. The presence of a halo suggests but does not guarantee a benign process (6).

The growth rates of breast cancers are quite variable; in two series, the mean doubling time for mammary carcinoma has been found to be 212 (7) and 325 (8) days. The lack of interval change suggests that a well-defined lesion is more likely benign, but this is not confirmatory. Meyer and Kopans (9) reported five cases of occult cancers that did not change in size on follow-up mammography over a minimum of 2 years and a maximum of 4.5 years from the original study. Therefore, if a nodule is followed and there is no

Table 4.1. Differential Diagnosis of Well-Defined Masses

Type of Lesion	Mammographic Characteristics
Cyst	Medium density, round, any size, oriented toward the nipple
Fibroadenoma	Medium density, lobulated, any size, coarse calcification
Carcinoma	Medium to high density, slightly irregular, microcalcification
Papilloma	Medium density, small, may calcify
Hematoma	Medium to high density, slightly irregular, skin thickening
Hamartoma	Mixed density, encapsulated
Lipoma	Low density, encapsulated
Metastases	Medium density, round, superficial location
Inclusion cyst	Medium density, round, superficial location
Intramammary node	Mixed density, small, lateral location
Cystosarcoma phylloides	Medium to high density, large, lobulated
Abscess	Medium to high density, skin thickening
Fat necrosis (oil cyst)	Radiolucent with calcific rim
Galactocele	Fat density or mixed density
Skin lesion (neurofibroma, nevus, keratosis)	Medium density or mixed density, crenulated surface, extremely well defined (air halo)
Nipple out of profile	Medium to high density, different appearance on orthogonal view

interval change in size at 6 months or 1 year, continued follow-up is necessary.

Well-Defined Masses of Fat Density

Lipomas are benign, well-circumscribed radiolucent masses (Figs. 4.1–4.3). Clinically, lipomas either are nonpalpable or, if palpable, are soft and freely mobile. Lipomas are visualized more easily in an otherwise dense, glandular breast because of the difference in density. In a fatty breast, this radiolucent mass is perceived because it is surrounded by a thin capsule and, if large, displaces the normal breast around it (10). Lipomas may develop coarse calcification, probably secondary to infarction.

Posttraumatic oil cysts, a form of fat necrosis, may occur as early as 6 months after breast trauma or surgery. Clinically, an area of fat necrosis may be asymptomatic, or it may be an indurated mass with thickening or retraction of the overlying skin. Histologically, the fat necrosis is characterized by anuclear fat cells, histiocytic giant cells, and foamy phagocytic histiocytes. The necrotic focus may cavitate, forming an oil cyst (11). The ringlike calcification (Figs. 4.4 and 4.5) in the wall of an oil cyst as originally described by Leborgne (12) is characteristic of this form of fat necrosis.

Galactoceles also are radiolucent masses. Galactoceles are benign breast masses that contain inspissated milk; they are commonly found during or after lactation (10) (Fig. 4.6). Mammographically, they are small, round, often multiple, radiolucent or mixed-density lesions, and they often occur in the retroareolar area (10). The retention or lactiferous material accounts for the low density of these lesions (13) (Fig. 4.6). A fat-water level within a well-defined mass is characteristic of a galactocele (14).

Mixed-Density Well-Defined Masses

Fibroadenolipoma

A hamartoma or fibroadenolipoma is a benign tumor composed of normal or dysplastic mammary tissue—including adipose and fibrous tissues—and ducts and lobules of varying amounts. The lesion is relatively uncommon, with a frequency of 16 in 10,000 mammograms in a series by Hessler et al. (15). Clinically, the patients ranged in age from 27 to 88 years and presented with a breast mass of a consistency similar to that of the adjacent tissue (15).

On mammography (Figs. 4.7–4.12), the appearance of a fibroadenolipoma may be pathognomonic (15–18). Helvie et al. (19), however, found the mammographic findings of hamartomas to range from the mixed-density circumscribed mass to the medium-density irregular lesions that were biopsied because of the concern of possible malignancy. Depending on the amount of fat versus parenchymal tissue, the lesion may vary from a relatively radiolucent mass to a relatively radiodense mass. The borders are very well defined, and a thin pseudocapsule may be evident. There is a loss of normal architecture of the mammary tissue with lack of orientation of glandular elements toward the nipple. The hamartoma displaces away the normal parenchyma of the breast, which appears to be draped over the lesion. On sonography, the lesion is well defined and composed of lobulated sonolucent areas mixed with irregular echogenic planes (20). If large and cosmetically a problem or if not clearly of mixed density mammographically, the lesion is treated with complete excision and enucleation. No association with malignancy has been described.

Intramammary Nodes

Intramammary lymph nodes have an appearance similar to that of axillary nodes, namely, they are well-defined, mixed-density or medium- to low-density, round or ovoid nodules

with a fatty notch or center (Figs. 4.13–4.16). Intramammary nodes can be found throughout the breast (21) but most commonly are located in the middle to upper outer aspect of the breasts and are often multiple and bilateral. Most intramammary nodes are less than 1 cm in diameter. Nodes may increase in diameter and be benign, although if the nodule does not have a fatty hilum, biopsy may be necessary to confirm its etiology. In a study of 158 whole-breast specimens with primary operable carcinoma, Egan and McSweeney (22) found intramammary lymph nodes in 28% and metastatic deposits in intramammary nodes in 10%. Although nodes involved with metastatic disease may enlarge and become more rounded and dense (21), this is not necessarily the case, and nodes of less than 1 cm in diameter can be malignant (22).

Other benign conditions also may be associated with the presence of intramammary nodes as well as axillary adenopathy. These include rheumatoid arthritis (23), sarcoidosis (24), psoriatic arthritis, and systemic lupus erythematosus (21).

Skin Lesions

It is critical that the technologist indicate any skin lesions on the patient's breasts. Moles, keratoses, retracted nipples, and neurofibromas may appear as very well defined masses of mixed or medium density on at least one of the projections (Figs. 4.17–4.19). As the lesion is compressed against the breast, air is trapped around it, creating an especially lucent halo. If the surface is irregular, a crenulated appearance is noted, creating a mixed density on mammography. By turning the breast with the lesion in tangent, the well-defined mass disappears or projects at the skin surface. Artifacts on the patient's skin, including electrocardiogram pads and various patches for transdermal medications, may trap air underneath, producing a ''mixed-density'' appearance on mammography (Fig. 4.20).

Medium- to High-Density Masses

There is considerable overlap between the lesions that are of medium density or isodense with the background parenchyma and the lesions that are of high density. Cysts and fibroadenomas tend to be of medium density, and background stromal markings may be visualized through the masses. Carcinomas tend to be of high density, but these divisions are not absolute, and several benign lesions, including fibroadenomas, hematomas, and abscesses, may be of high density. Margination of the mass is important in suggesting a malignant etiology. Also, a multimodality approach to these masses, including physical examination, mammography, and ultrasound, is important in determining the approach for further evaluation (25).

Cysts

One of the manifestations of fibrocystic disease is simple cysts that vary from 3 mm to several centimeters in diameter. Cysts are more commonly seen in women 30–50 years old. Pain and tenderness may accompany the development of a cyst, and the symptoms may occur just prior to and with the menstrual cycle. Cysts are derived from the lobules and may be lined by ordinary mammary epithelium or by an apocrine-type epithelium (26). A tension cyst is an apocrine cyst that contains fluid under pressure, secondary to obstruction of the outflow tract (26). Clinically, cysts are tender circumscribed masses that are mobile, ranging from soft to firm, depending on the degree of distension.

On mammography, cysts (Figs. 4.21–4.30) are very well defined, round or ovoid masses that may vary from several millimeters to 5 cm or more in diameter (27). The density is usually equal to or slightly greater than that of the parenchyma. A halo sign is often present, and the orientation of the cyst is along the path of the ducts. Cysts may be multilocular or multiple and may be associated with other findings of fibrocystic disease. It is important, when multiple masses are present, that each lesion be evaluated individually so that a well-defined carcinoma not be missed.

On sonography, cysts are well defined and anechoic, with well-defined walls and good through-transmission of sound. If a few echoes are present within a lesion thought to be a cyst, aspiration and pneumocystography should be performed for complete evaluation. Papillomas and intracystic papillary carcinomas may develop within a cyst and usually cannot be differentiated radiographically (28). Invasive papillary carcinomas tend to present as multiple, relatively well defined masses. If a cyst contains an intracystic lesion, lobulation or slight irregularity of the wall may be seen on mammography. On pneumocystography, papillary lesions are seen as a polypoid filling defect within the cyst cavity.

Fibroadenoma

A fibroadenoma is a benign tumor of the breast, usually presenting as a well-defined mass. Being estrogen-sensitive tumors, fibroadenomas usually appear in adolescents and young women before the age of 30 years. Their growth may be enhanced by pregnancy or lactation (29). After menopause, these tumors undergo mucoid degeneration, hyalinize, and eventually develop characteristic coarse calcifications.

On histology, fibroadenomas are composed of dense connective tissue stroma surrounding canaliculi or tubules lined with ductal epithelium (30). On clinical examination, these tumors are smooth and of a firm or rubbery consistency and freely movable. In young patients, fibroadenomas may reach a very large size.

The mammographic findings (Figs. 4.31–4.43) of a fibroadenoma are a medium-density, very well defined, round, ovoid, or smoothly lobulated mass (31). A fatty halo surrounds the lesion and may be the key to identifying a fibroadenoma in a young dense breast. Calcifications may vary from punctate peripheral deposits to the typical coarse pop-

corn-like densities that are characteristic. On ultrasound, fibroadenomas are usually smooth, hypoechoic masses of homogeneous echo-texture, with well-defined margins and no attenuation or enhancement of sound posteriorly (32). Rarely, a fibroadenoma may contain or be associated with malignancy (33, 34), usually in situ carcinomas. Fibroadenomas containing malignancy may be indistinguishable from benign fibroadenomas, but features that Baker et al. (35) found of concern were the large size of the mass, indistinct margins, and clustered microcalcifications. Particularly in a patient over 30 years, a solid mass having an appearance consistent with a fibroadenoma is often removed because a well-circumscribed malignancy can have a similar appearance.

Cystosarcoma Phylloides

Cystosarcoma phylloides is a fibroepithelial breast tumor that has malignant potential. The term refers to the leaflike pattern of growth of the epithelial elements, and not to prognosis. Most cystosarcomas are benign or have limited invasion into the surrounding parenchyma. If the tumors are not completely excised, they may recur (36); when the lesions are malignant, metastases most often occur to lung, pleura, and bone (37).

Cystosarcoma phylloides is a rare tumor presenting at a mean age of 40.5 years (38). On palpation, a firm, mobile, smooth mass is found; the lesion may be rapidly enlarging. Mammographically, the tumor is well circumscribed, large, and dense, having an appearance similar to that of a large fibroadenoma (39) (Figs. 4.44 and 4.45). Coarse calcification within a large circumscribed tumor should suggest, more likely, a fibroadenoma. If calcification occurs in a cystosarcoma, it has been described as plaquelike (10). Histologically, a cystosarcoma phylloides has a more cellular, pleomorphic connective tissue component than a fibroadenoma. Epithelially lined clefts are present within the lesion. The microscopic features of the connective tissue component determine if the lesion is considered benign or malignant (40).

Other Benign Masses

Other benign lesions that may present mammographically as well-defined medium-density masses include focal fibrocystic lesions, papillomas, hematomas, abscesses, and epidermal inclusion cysts. Occasionally, focal fibrosis, sclerosing adenosis (Fig. 4.46), or areas of ductal hyperplasia can present as well-circumscribed masses; the mammographic appearance is nonspecific, and many of these lesions are associated with microcalcifications. Biopsy is usually necessary to exclude a malignant process.

Solitary intraductal papillomas are often not evident on the mammogram and are instead detected on galactography. When small, these lesions present typically with a nipple discharge, usually sanguineous or serosanguineous (41). If papillomas are identified on mammography (Figs. 4.47 and 4.48), they generally are small, well-defined lesions oriented along the path of the ducts and located often in the subareolar area. A tubular shape should suggest the possibility of a papilloma. Because papillomas have a delicate blood supply via their stalk, they have a tendency to infarct (41). Calcification that is nonspecific may occur in infarcted papillomas.

A hematoma may be loculated and appear as a well-defined mass or be interstitial and dissect through the tissues, creating a diffuse density (Figs. 4.49–4.52). The density of a hematoma is the same or slightly greater than that of the parenchyma. The margins of the lesion are often slightly irregular. Overlying skin edema is usually present in the acute stage with the bruising noted on clinical examination. Follow-up examinations will show gradual resolution of the lesion.

Epidermal inclusion cysts or sebaceous cysts are of skin origin and therefore superficially located. Sebaceous cysts are palpated as smooth, firm cutaneous nodules. These very well defined lesions are often located in the areolar area or in the lower aspect of the breast and are contiguous with the skin on mammography (3) (Figs. 4.53–4.55). Calcification may occur within the lesion. On ultrasound, a complex mass is visualized with varying amounts of debris. Moles and skin lesions, if smoothly marginated, appear as medium-density superficial masses on mammography. A normal structure that may stimulate a well-defined mass is the nipple out of profile. With care taken to keep the nipple in profile on both views or at least on one view, there should not be any doubt as to whether a well-defined lesion represents the nipple (Figs. 4.56–4.61).

An acute breast abscess is usually suspected in clinical examination because of the associated findings of inflammation—a painful tender breast, redness of the skin, fever. With the inflammation associated with an acute abscess, skin thickening and an edema pattern are present and may obscure the abscess itself. Mammography with good compression is difficult to perform because of the severe breast tenderness present. When the abscess is visualized, it is usually a relatively well defined mass (10) (Fig. 4.62).

Well-Circumscribed Carcinoma

Primary breast carcinoma characteristically presents mammographically as a spiculated mass. However, some carcinomas are relatively well defined or even very sharply marginated, and these lesions may be confused with benign masses, such as fibroadenomas, radiographically.

It has been said (10) that approximately 2% of carcinomas are very well defined masses (Figs. 4.63–4.76). Moskowitz (42) found 2% of carcinomas to be very well defined and 5–10% to be partially well defined. Marsteller and Shaw de Paredes (43) found that 5.1% of relatively circumscribed lesions were carcinomas and an additional 4% were atypical hyperplastic lesions. If one considers nonpalpable breast cancers only, however, a greater percentage (4%) appear very sharply marginated (44). Most relatively circumscribed carcinomas are ductal carcinomas, which are the most frequently occurring primary carcinomas of the breast. Intraductal or infiltrating ductal carcinomas can be well defined on mammography, although there is usually some indistinctness of the margins of the infiltrating lesions. In a series of 350 cases of intraductal carcinomas, Mitnick et al. (45) found that 13 lesions were sharply circumscribed lesions simulating benign masses. Calcifications within these nodules tend to be asymmetric and located within the nodules.

The types of carcinomas that more characteristically appear as well-defined masses are medullary or mucinous cancers. Medullary carcinoma accounts for 3% of all breast cancers (46). Clinically, the lesions are soft and movable, and unlike the irregular scirrhous carcinomas, medullary carcinomas do not necessarily palpate as larger than they appear mammographically. The lesions tend to be located either deep in the breast or in the subareolar or subcutaneous areas (47). Histologically, medullary carcinoma is a variety of ductal carcinoma characterized by a growth pattern of syncytial, solid sheetlike areas of malignant cells. Necrosis is frequent; calcification does not usually occur (48). The mammographic appearance is of a well-circumscribed, medium- to high-density noncalcified mass. Faint irregularity of the borders may be detected, indicating a suspicious nature. On ultrasound, medullary carcinomas are well-defined inhomogeneous hypoechoic masses that show enhanced through-transmission (49).

Mucinous carcinomas also may present as well-circumscribed masses (47). The density of these lesions tends to be medium to low because of the presence of mucin (47). Mucinous carcinomas, like medullary cancers, tend to be peripherally located.

Metastases

Metastases from extramammary primary carcinomas are unusual, accounting for about 1–2% (50) of all breast malignancies. The mammographic presentation of a metastasis may be as a very well defined mass having an appearance similar to that of fibroadenoma. Although it is more common for a patient presenting with a metastatic lesion in the breast to have a known carcinoma, that is not necessarily the case (50). The most common sites of origin of metastases to the breast are lymphoma, melanoma, sarcoma, lung, stomach, prostate, and ovary (51). In most series (51–53), a solitary well-defined mass is the most common presentation, with multiple masses and diffuse involvement of the breast being less likely; others have described diffuse involvement more frequently (53). The lesions tend to be superficially located (51) and may have an appearance similar to that of a sebaceous cyst (Figs. 4.77 and 4.78). Lymphomas may produce axillary or intramammary adenopathy or may present with circumscribed or poorly marginated breast nodules (Figs. 4.79 and 4.80).

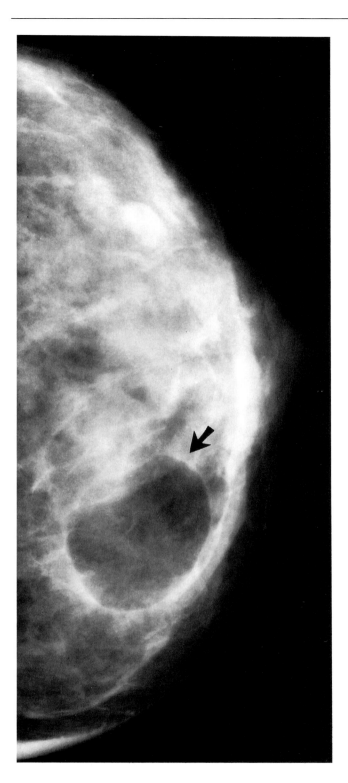

Figure 4.1.

Clinical: 34-year-old G1, P1 woman with a family history of breast cancer and a history of bilateral nipple discharge.

Mammogram: Right craniocaudal view. The breast is dense, consistent with the age and parity of the patient. There is a well-circumscribed radiolucent mass in the inner quadrant of the breast most consistent with a lipoma *(arrow)*. The density of the breast allows the more radiolucent lipoma to be easily visualized.

Impression: Lipoma.

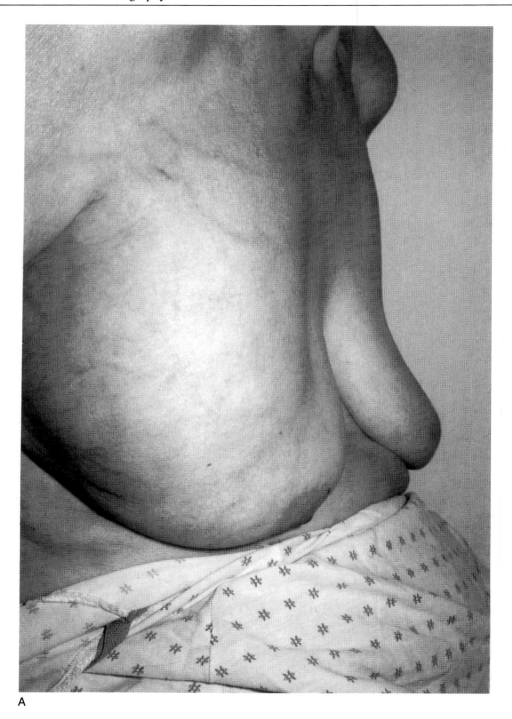

A

Figure 4.2.

Clinical: 79-year-old G3, P3 woman with a history of the right breast being larger than the left for years (**A**).

Mammogram: Bilateral mediolateral views (**B**). There is marked asymmetry in the size of the breasts. There is a large radiolucent mass surrounded by a thin capsule *(straight arrow)* in the right upper outer quadrant. The mass compresses and drapes the normal parenchyma around it. These findings are characteristic of a lipoma. The ovoid nodules present in the superior aspect of the breast *(curved arrow)* are lymph nodes superimposed over the large lipoma.

Impression: Lipoma.

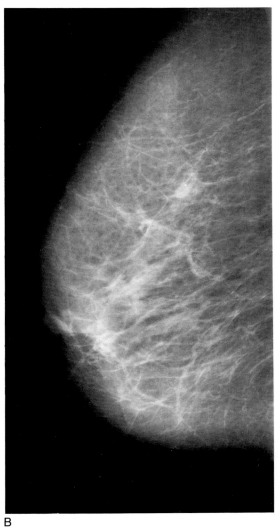

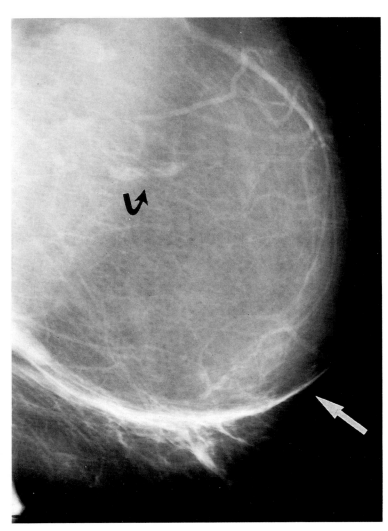

B

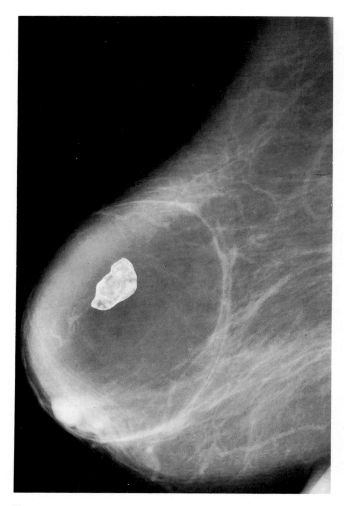

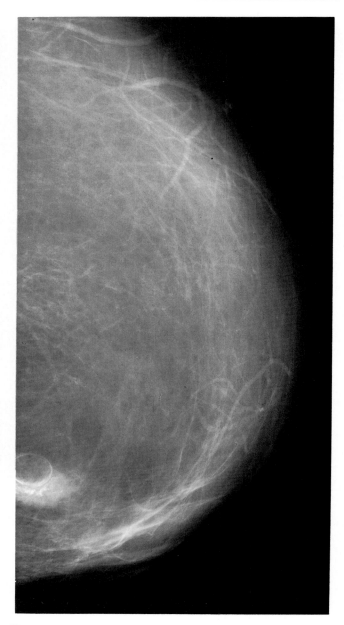

Figure 4.3.

Clinical: 67-year-old woman with a history of a left breast mass for years.

Mammogram: Left mediolateral view. In the left subareolar area, there is a large lucent mass that is surrounded by a thin capsule. The normal breast tissue is draped around the lesion. A large coarse central calcification is present, suggesting old infarction or fat necrosis in a large lipoma.

Impression: Lipoma.

Figure 4.4.

Clinical: 32-year-old woman after reduction mammoplasties who presents with a hard lump beneath the scar on the right breast.

Mammogram: Right mediolateral view. There is a well-defined radiolucent mass with circumlinear calcification in its wall, characteristic of a posttraumatic oil cyst. Surrounding increased density with coarse calcifications are other manifestations of fat necrosis.

Impressions: Oil cyst, fat necrosis.

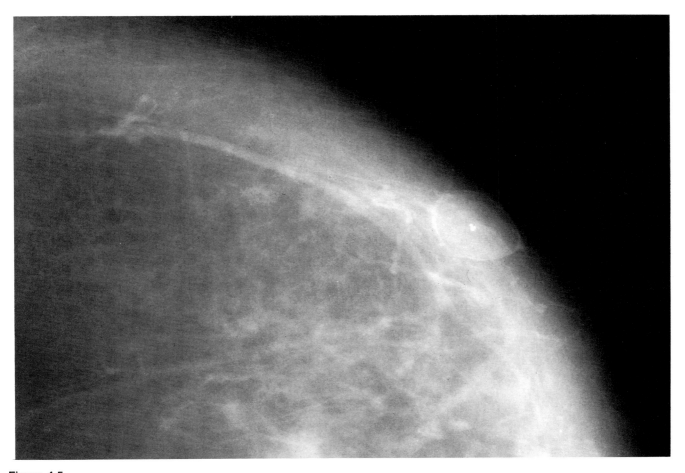

Figure 4.5.

Clinical: 73-year-old woman who has had a palpable nodule in the right outer quadrant for years.

Mammogram: Right craniocaudal view. There is a very well defined radiolucent mass in the subcutaneous area of the breast. Rimlike calcification is present around part of the border of this lesion. The findings are typical of a posttraumatic oil cyst.

Impression: Posttraumatic oil cyst.

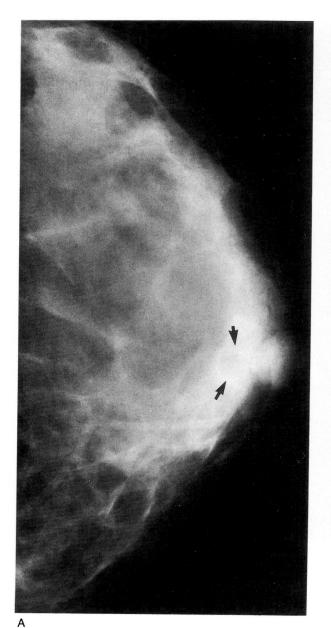

A

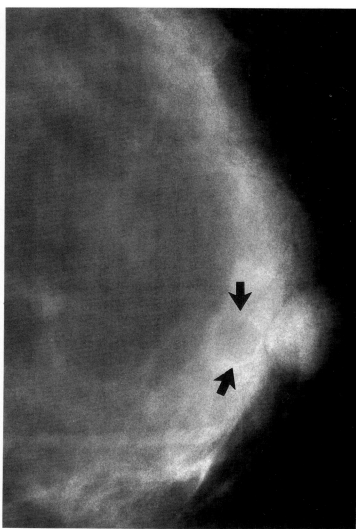

B

Figure 4.6.

Clinical: 32-year-old G1, P1 patient who stopped nursing 4 months earlier, presenting with a small right subareolar nodule.

Mammogram: Right craniocaudal (**A**) and enlarged (2×) craniocaudal (**B**) views. The breast is quite dense, consistent with the patient's age and her recent lactating state. In the subareolar area, corresponding to the palpable nodule, there is a small circumscribed radiolucent nodule *(arrows)*. The differential for this nodule includes a lipoma, an oil cyst, or a galactocele, and given the clinical history, a galactocele is most likely. The lesion appears radiolucent because of the fat content of the milk it contains.

Impression: Galactocele.

Note: The patient was followed clinically, and the nodule resolved.

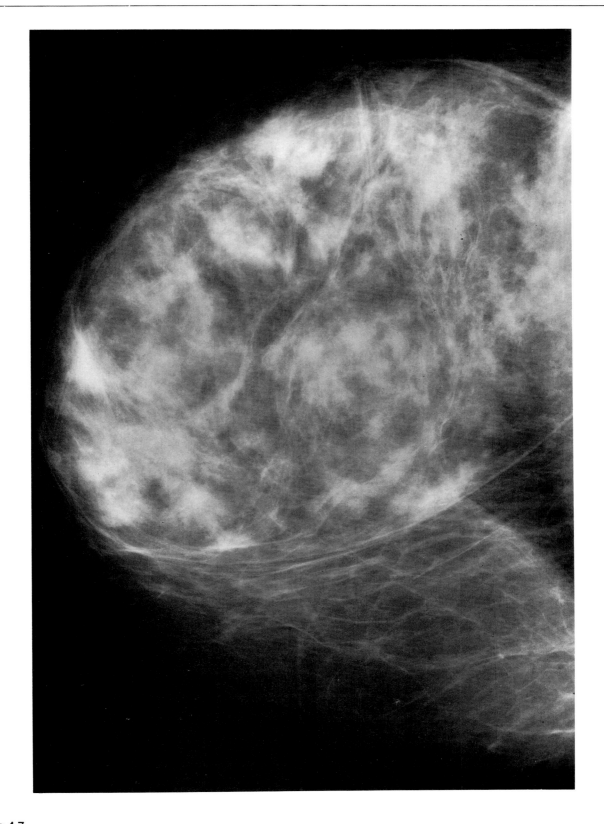

Figure 4.7.

Clinical: 60-year-old woman who has had a left breast mass for years.

Mammogram: Left craniocaudal view. There is a well-defined encapsulated mass of heterogeneous density in the outer quadrant of the left breast. This contains fat and soft tissue elements and is surrounded by a fine pseudocapsule. The features are typical of a fibroadenolipoma or hamartoma of the breast.

Impression: Fibroadenolipoma. (Case courtesy of Dr. A. C. Wagner, Culpeper, VA.)

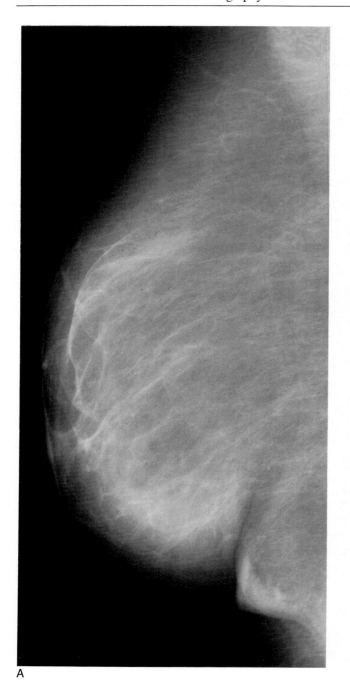

A

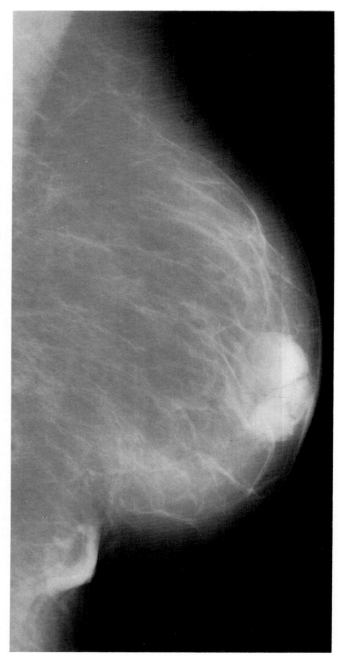

Figure 4.8.

Clinical: 41-year-old woman with a soft mass in the right breast.

Mammogram: Bilateral oblique views (**A**) and magnified image (**B**). There is a well-defined mass of heterogeneous density in the right retroareolar area (**A**). A large portion of the mass is composed of dense lobulated tissue, but fatty strands bisect these solid elements (**B**). The findings are characteristic of fibroadenolipoma or hamartoma of the breast, a benign lesion.

Impression: Hamartoma.

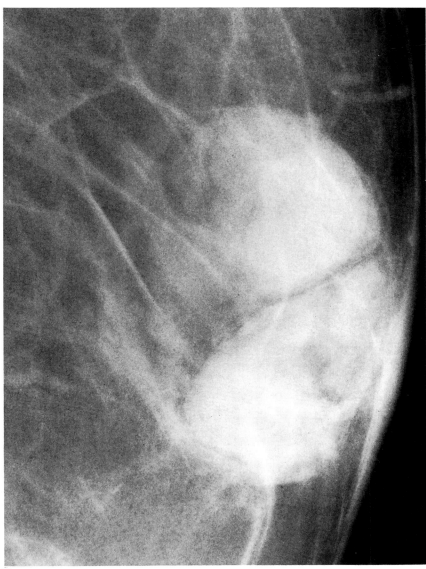

B

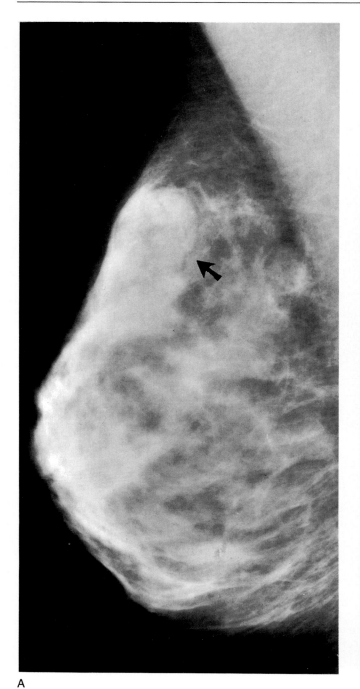

A

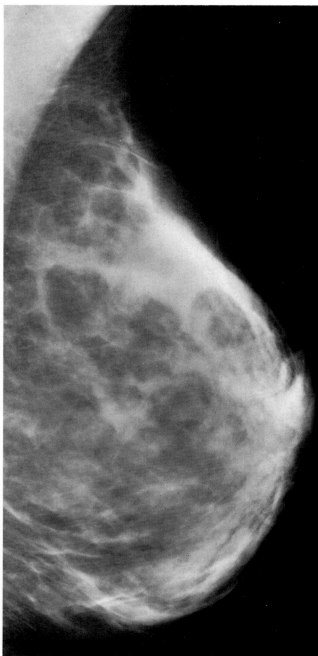

Figure 4.9.

Clinical: 35-year-old woman with a 3-cm firm lump in the left upper outer qudrant.

Mammogram: Bilateral oblique views (**A**) and a left magnification view (**B**). There is a well-defined round mass superficially located in the left upper outer quadrant. A magnifica-tion view of the area (**B**) shows the very well defined margins of the mass and the heterogeneous density. Curvilinear bands of fat *(arrow)* transect the dense elements.

Impression: Fibroadenolipoma.

Histopathology: Fibroadenolipoma.

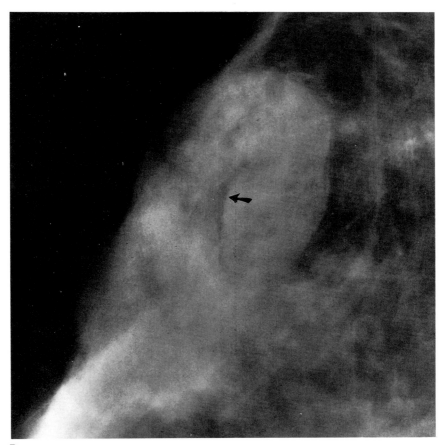

B

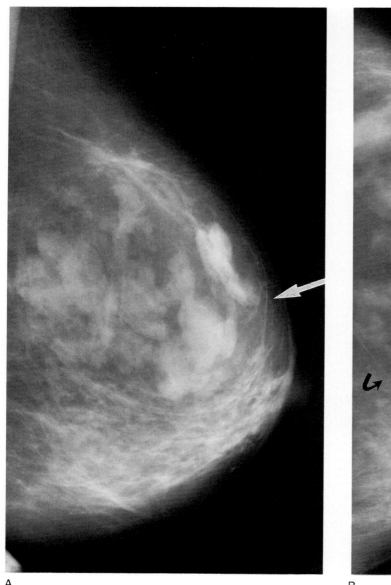

A

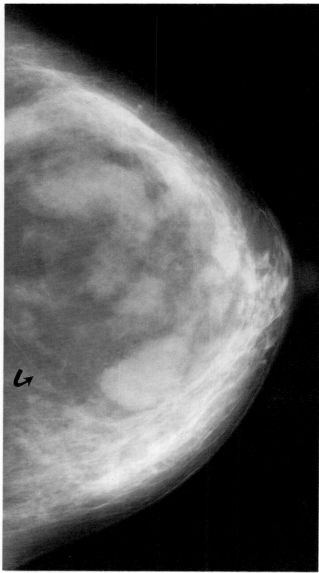

B

Figure 4.10.

Clinical: 50-year-old woman with a normal breast examination.

Mammogram: Right oblique (**A**) and craniocaudal (**B**) views. There is a large well-defined mass of mixed density in the upper central portion of the right breast. This mass contains fat as well as ovoid soft tissue masses, and it is surrounded by a thin pseudocapsule *(arrows)*. The lesion compresses away the normal breast parenchyma. The findings are characteristic of a fibroadenolipoma (hamartoma) of the breast.

Impression: Hamartoma (fibroadenolipoma)

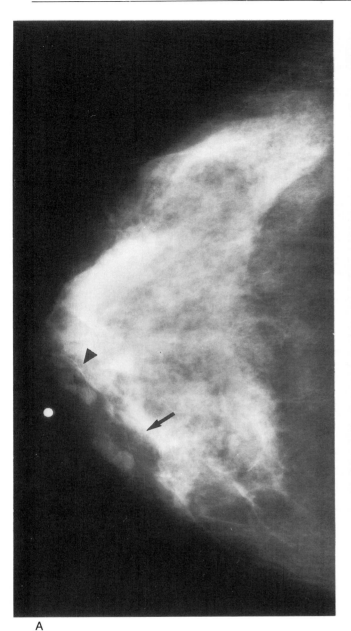

A

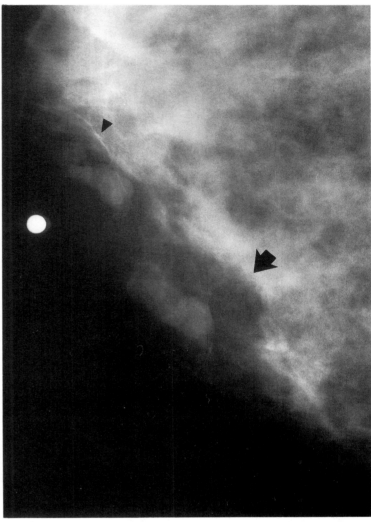

B

Figure 4.11.

Clinical: 53-year-old G8, P4, Ab4 woman with a 4-cm palpable soft mass in the left middle inner quadrant.

Mammogram: Left craniocaudal (**A**) and enlarged (2.5×) craniocaudal (**B**) views. The breast is dense for the age and parity of the patient. A BB was placed over the palpable lesion. Beneath the BB, there is a striking area of asymmetry *(arrow)* that is fatty, in contrast to the background of dense parenchyma; within this fatty mass are two lobulated medium-density nodules. Portions of a capsule are seen *(arrowhead)* surrounding this heterogeneous mass. The appearance is characteristic of a fibroadenolipoma of the breast.

Impression: Fibroadenolipoma (hamartoma).

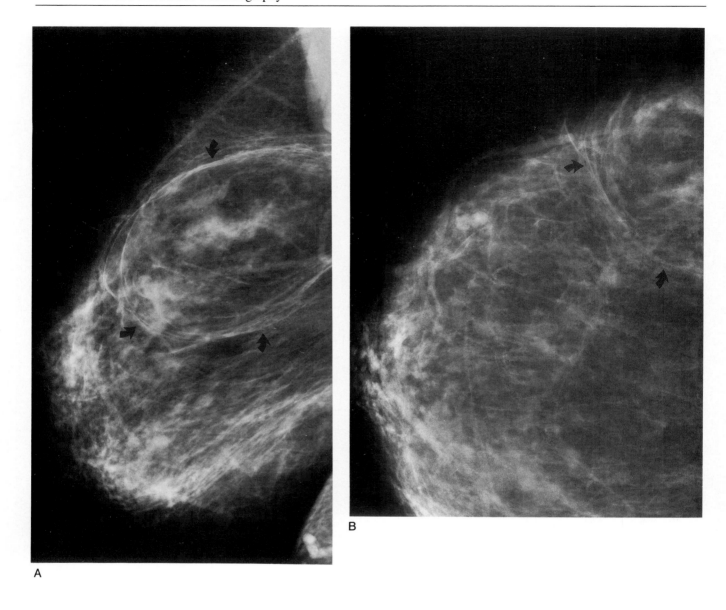

A

B

Figure 4.12.

Clinical: 52-year-old G0 woman for screening.

Mammogram: Left oblique (**A**) and craniocaudal (**B**) views. The breast is mildly glandular. In the upper outer quadrant, there is a large, mixed-density circumscribed mass. A thin pseudocapsule *(arrows)* surrounds the lesion that is primarily fatty but that does contain some glandular elements. The lesion is very smoothly marginated and drapes the background parenchyma over it. The appearance of this lesion is characteristic of a benign hamartoma or fibroadenolipoma.

Impression: Hamartoma.

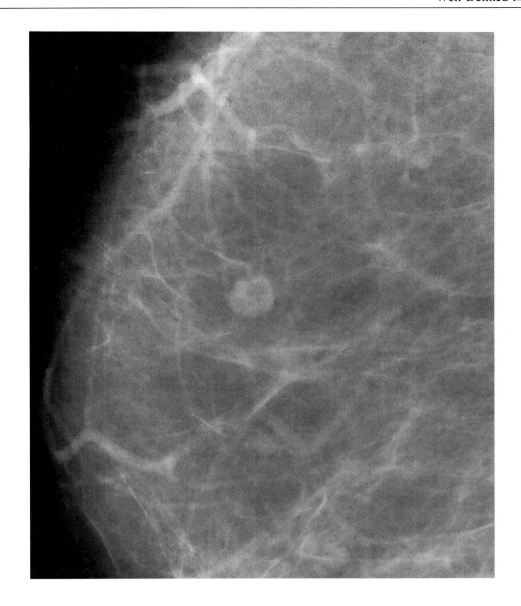

Figure 4.13.

Clinical: 47-year-old woman for screening mammography.

Mammogram: Left craniocaudal view. There is a very well defined round nodule in the upper outer quadrant of the left breast. (Similar nodules were present in the right also.) The nodule has a fatty center representing the hilar area of a normal intramammary lymph node.

Impression: Intramammary node.

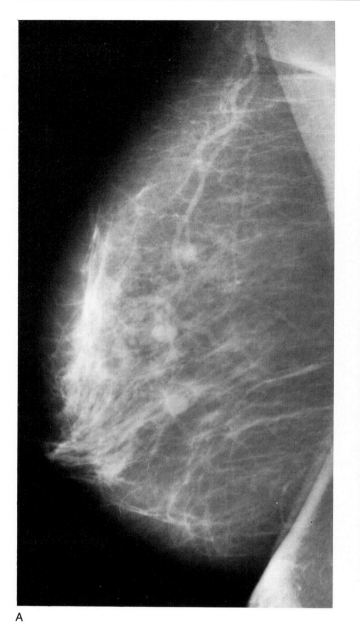

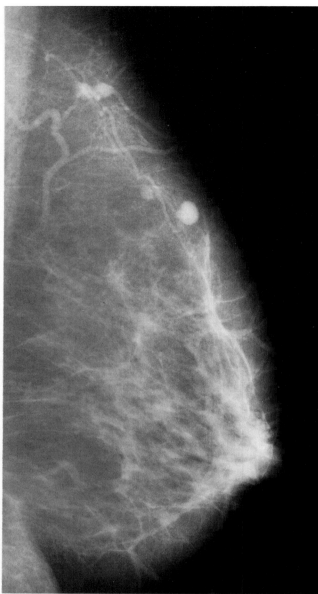

A

Figure 4.14.

Clinical: 53-year-old woman for screening mammography.

Mammograms: Bilateral oblique (**A**) and craniocaudal (**B**) views. The breasts are mildly glandular. There are very well defined nodules in the upper outer quadrants of both breasts

(**A**). The nodules are of moderate density (**B**) but with central lucencies representing the fatty hila of intramammary nodes.

Impression: Intramammary lymph nodes.

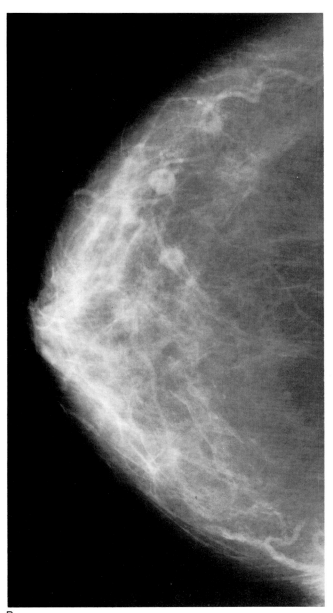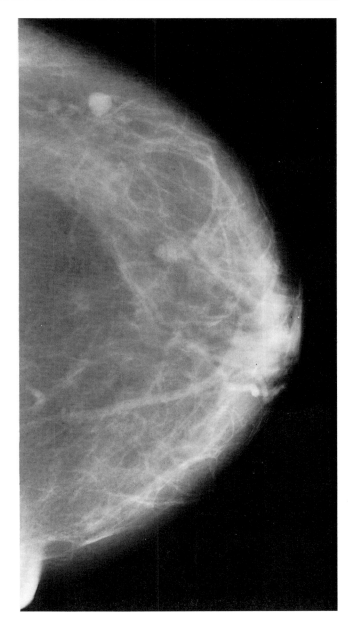

B

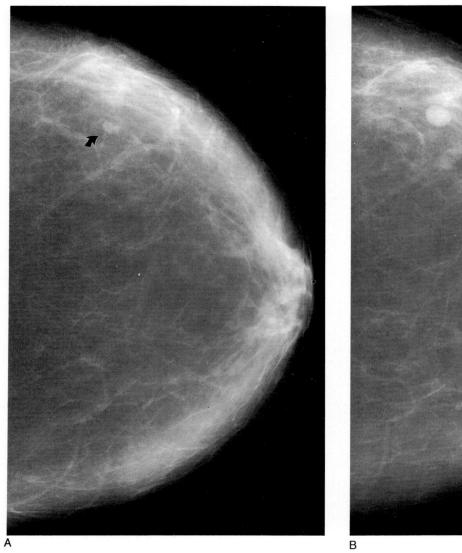

A

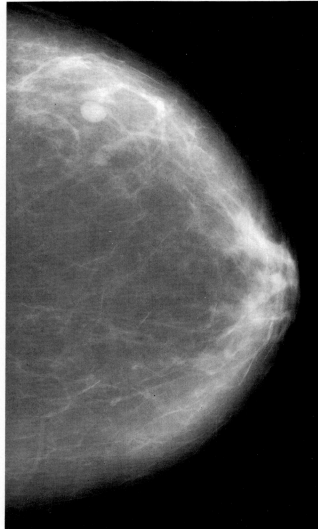

B

Figure 4.15.

Clinical: 39-year-old woman 7 years after left mastectomy for carcinoma.

Mammogram: Right craniocaudal view from 1982 (**A**) and right craniocaudal view 12 months later (**B**). The breast shows fatty replacement. In 1982 (**A**), a small well-defined low-density nodule *(arrow)* was present superficially in the outer aspect of the breast, having the appearance of an intramammary lymph node. In 1983 (**B**), the nodule more than doubled

in size but remained very well defined. For this patient with a history of carcinoma, there was concern that the increase in size could represent metastatic involvement of the node.

Impression: Enlarging nodule, favoring intramammary node, with possible metastatic involvement.

Histopathology: Intraparenchymal lymph node without pathologic change.

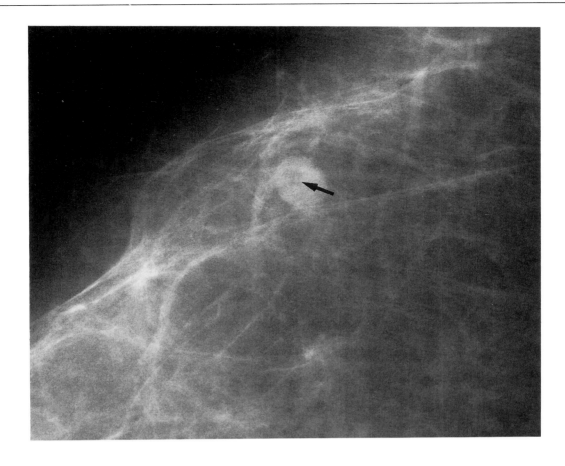

Figure 4.16.
Clinical: 54-year-old woman for screening.
Mammogram: Right craniocaudal magnification (1.5×) view. There is a well-defined nodule located superficially in the outer aspect of the breast. The fatty hilum *(arrow)* is characteristic of an intramammary lymph node.
Impression: Intramammary lymph node.

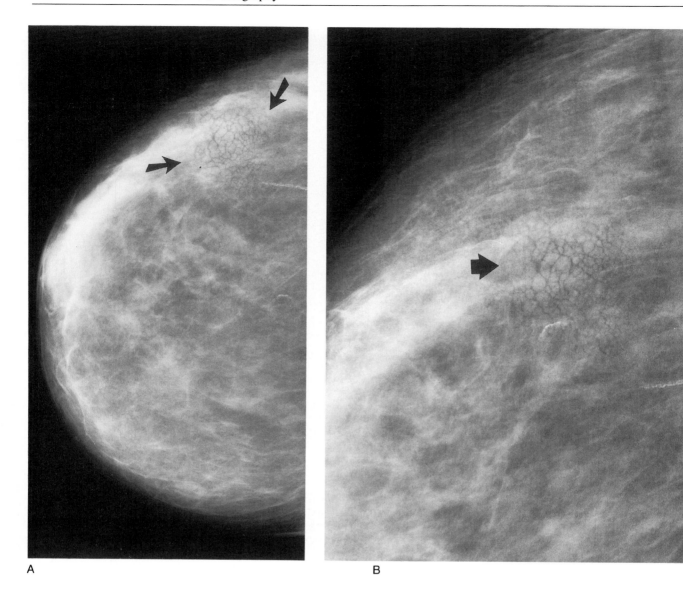

A

B

Figure 4.17.

Clinical: 77-year-old G3, P3 woman for screening mammography.

Mammogram: Left craniocaudal (**A**) and enlarged (2×) (**B**) views. The breast is moderately glandular. There is a mixed-density lesion (*arrows*) in the outer aspect of the breast. The crackled appearance is typical of air in the surface of a skin lesion.

Impression: Skin lesion (seborrheic keratosis) simulating a breast nodule.

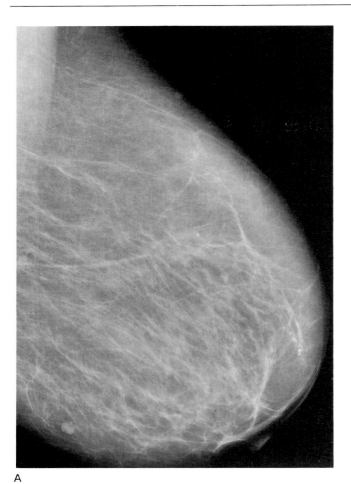

A

Figure 4.18.

Clinical: 81-year-old woman for screening mammography.

Mammogram: Right oblique view (**A**) and magnified image (**B**). There is a very well defined, slightly lobulated nodule in the right lower quadrant (**A**). Magnification (**B**) of this area shows the very discrete borders, more well defined than the fatty halo surrounding a parenchymal lesion. The lesion represented a seborrheic keratosis on the patient's skin.

Note: It is very important for the technologist to document all skin lesions that might be confused with a parenchymal lesion.

Impression: Skin lesion, benign.

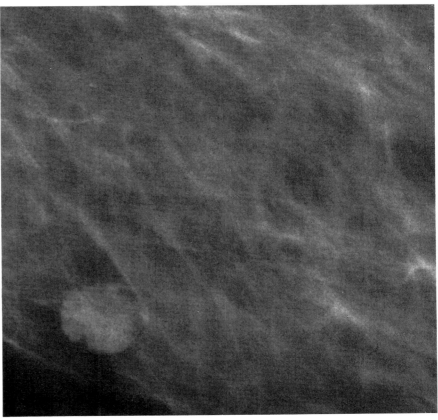

B

Figure 4.19.

Clinical: 52-year-old woman for screening mammography.

Mammogram: Right oblique view (**A**) and magnified image (**B**). There is a very well defined low-density nodule superimposed over the lower aspect of the breast *(arrows)*. A magnified image (**B**) of this area shows the irregular linear lucencies crossing this lesion, corresponding to air within the crenulated surface of a keratosis or nevus.

Impression: Benign lesion consistent with keratosis or nevus.

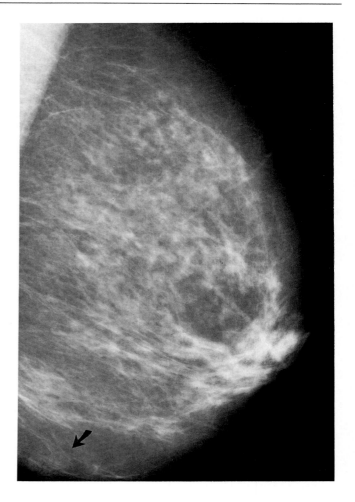

A

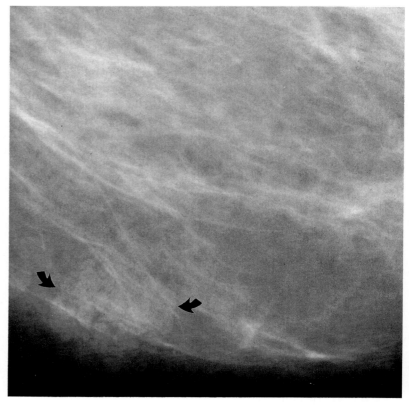

B

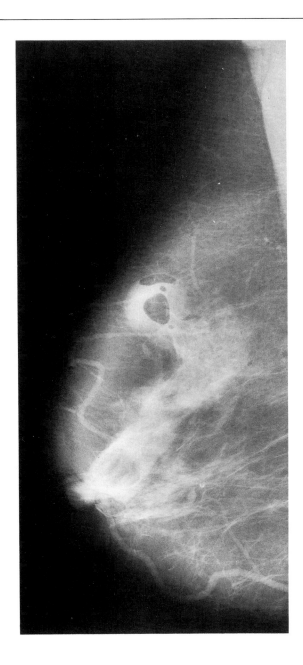

Figure 4.20.

Clinical: 65-year-old woman with angina, for screening mammography. She had had no recent breast interventional procedures.

Mammogram: Left oblique view. There is a very well circumscribed mixed-density mass superimposed over the upper aspect of the left breast. The lucencies within the mass are more radiolucent than fat, suggesting air beneath a device on the skin. An unusual appearance of a pneumocystogram or air within a mass or hematoma from recent biopsy would also be a consideration with an appropriate clinical history.

Impression: Air trapped beneath a Nitro-Bid patch on the skin, simulating a breast lesion.

Note: The patient had placed the new patch on her breast just before the mammogram and refused to have the technologist remove it for the study.

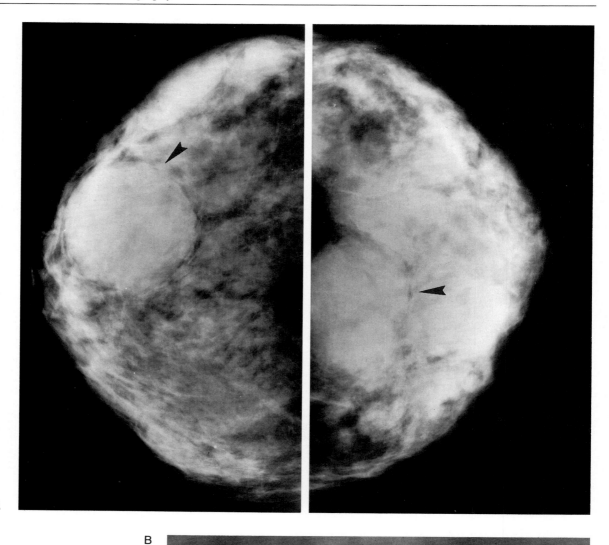

A

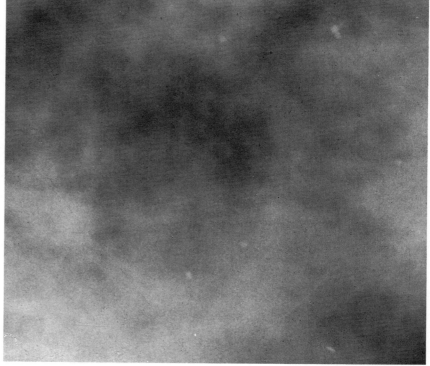

B

Figure 4.21.

Clinical: 51-year-old G1, P2 woman with a history of fibrocystic disease and lumpy breasts on physical examination.

Mammograms: Bilateral craniocaudal views (**A**) and magnification (**B**). The breasts are dense and glandular for the age and parity of the patient. There are bilateral, well-defined round masses surrounded by fatty haloes *(arrow)* and oriented in the direction of the ducts. There are also scattered round microcalcifications in both breasts, suggesting a lobular origin (**B**). The multiplicity of findings and the similarity in appearance of the lesions suggest fibrocystic changes. Ultrasound confirmed the cystic nature of the masses.

Impression: Bilateral cysts, diffuse fibrocystic changes.

Histopathology (of area of microcalcifications): Fibrocystic changes with lobular hyperplasia.

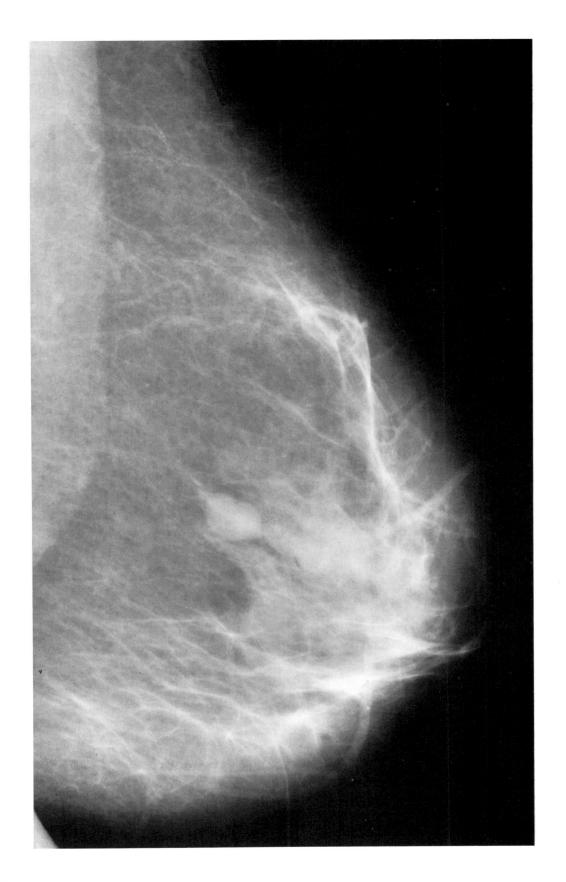

Figure 4.22.

Clinical: 59-year-old woman for screening mammography.

Mammogram: Right oblique view. There is a well-defined lobulated nodule in the upper outer quadrant of the right breast. A fatty halo surrounds the mass, and the nodule is oriented along the direction of the ducts. Sonography showed the mass to be a cyst.

Impression: Cyst.

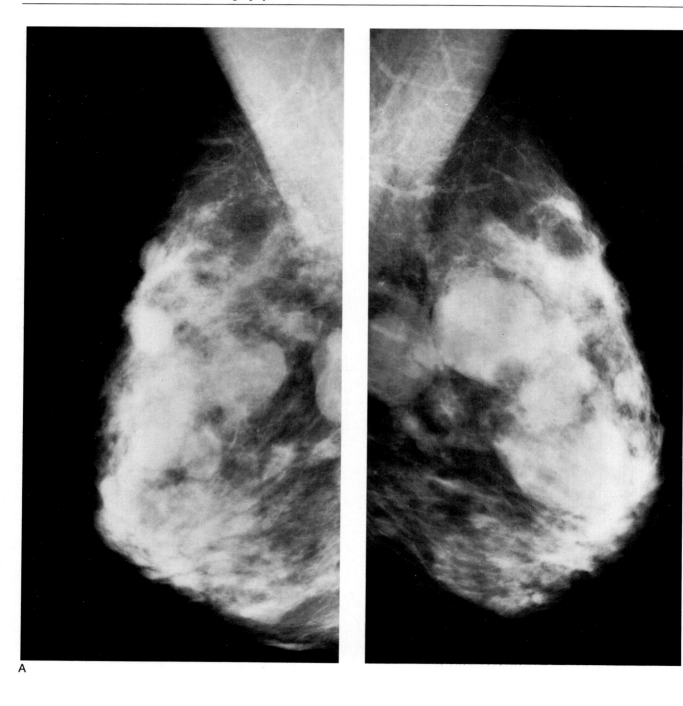

A

Figure 4.23.

Clinical: 49-year-old G2, P3 woman with nodular breasts.

Mammogram: Bilateral oblique (**A**) and craniocaudal (**B**) views. There are multiple, very well defined, round, moderately dense masses of varying size, oriented in the direction of the nipples in both breasts. Fatty haloes surround each of these lesions. The appearance, orientation, and multiplicity of findings are most consistent with numerous cysts.

Impression: Many cysts (confirmed by ultrasound).

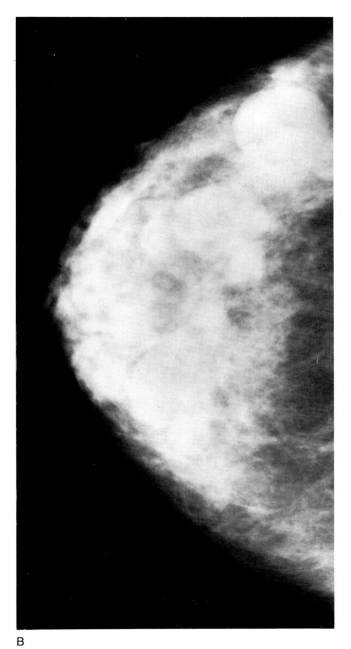
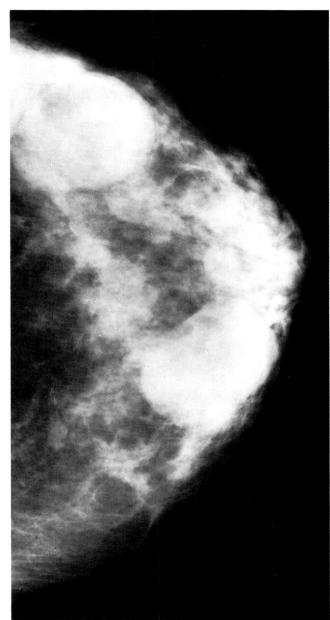

B

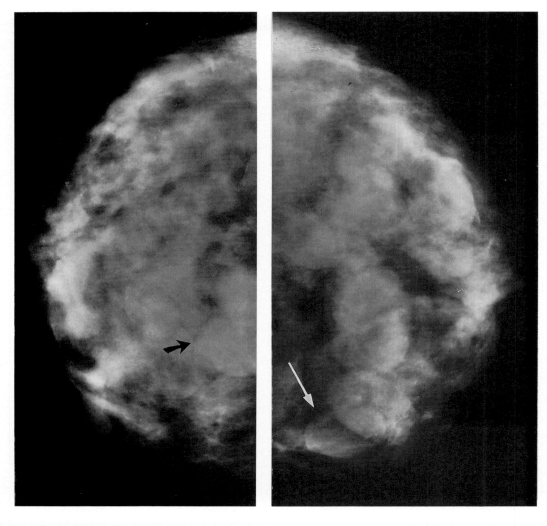

A

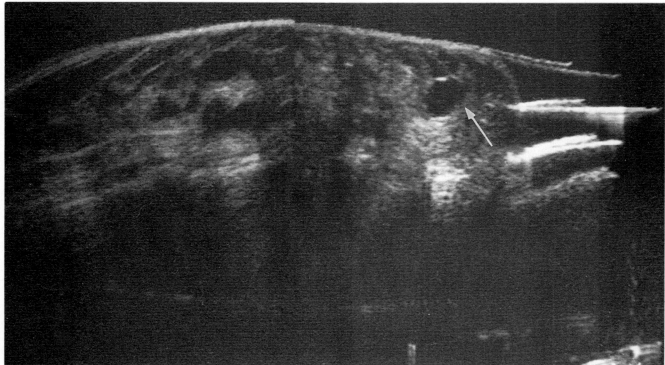

C

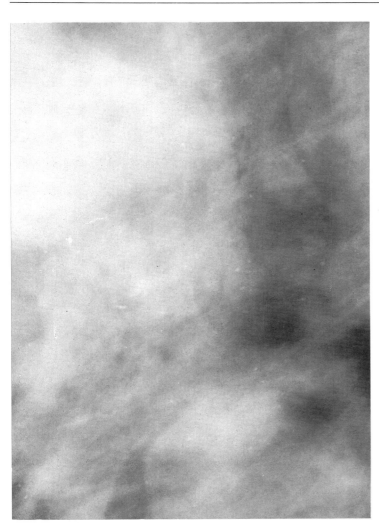

B

Figure 4.24.

Clinical: 45-year-old G0 woman with a family history of breast cancer, presenting with multiple palpable masses bilaterally.

Mammogram: Bilateral craniocaudal views (**A**), magnified image (**B**), and ultrasound (**C** and **D**). The breasts are quite dense and contain multiple, round well-defined masses. Fatty haloes surround many of these lesions *(arrows)*. Additionally, there are innumerable microcalcifications bilaterally that, on a magnified view (**B**), are noted to be round, punctate, or circumlinear. The diffuse nature and morphology of the calcifications are most compatible with fibrocystic disease. Whole-breast ultrasound (**C** and **D**) shows many cystic masses bilaterally, corresponding to the lesions in mammography.

Impression: Fibrocystic changes, bilateral cysts.

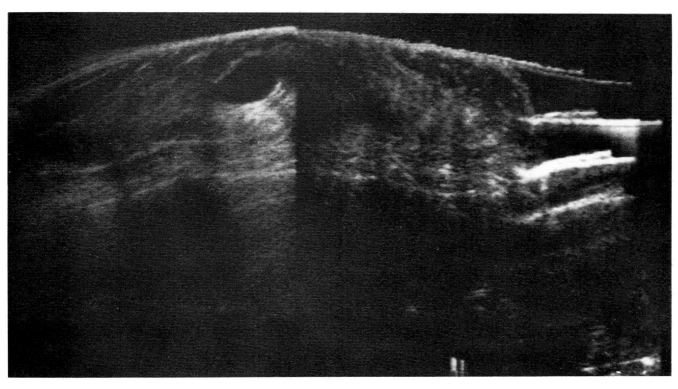

D

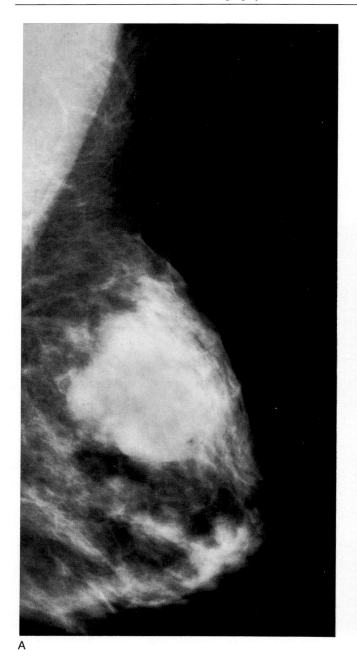

A

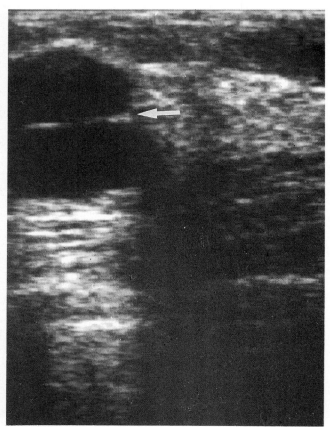

B

Figure 4.25.

Clinical: 45-year-old woman with a tender right breast mass.

Mammogram: Right oblique view (**A**), sonogram (**B**), and pneumocystogram (**C**). There is a large, well-defined lobulated mass in the right breast (**A**). Sonography shows the lesion to be a septated cyst *(arrow)*. Aspiration of the mass

yielded 15 ml of clear yellowish fluid. The pneumocystogram shows multiple connecting lobules and no intracystic mass.

Impression: Multilocular cyst. (Case courtesy of Dr. Patricia Abbitt, Charlottesville, VA.)

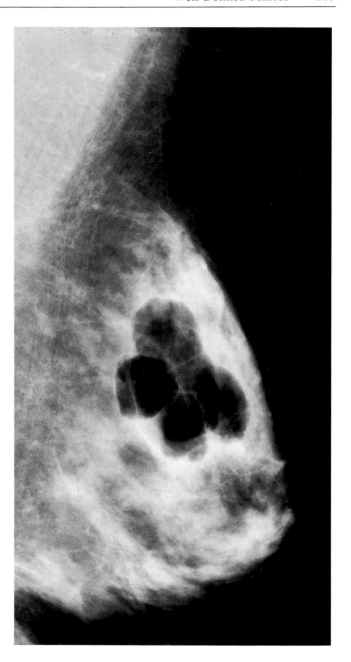

C

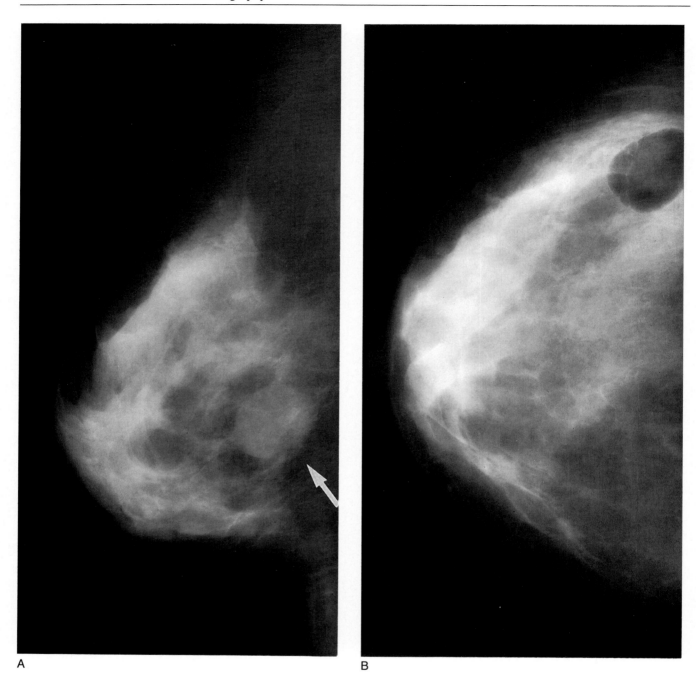

A

B

Figure 4.26.

Clinical: 43-year-old woman with a history of fibrocystic disease, for screening mammography.

Mammograms: Left oblique view (**A**) and left pneumocystogram (**B**). There is a well-defined, medium density, ovoid mass deep in the left breast *(arrow)*. The appearance suggests a benign lesion as more likely. Cyst aspiration produced 8 ml of turbid yellow fluid. Pneumocystography shows no intracystic masses.

Impression: Cyst.

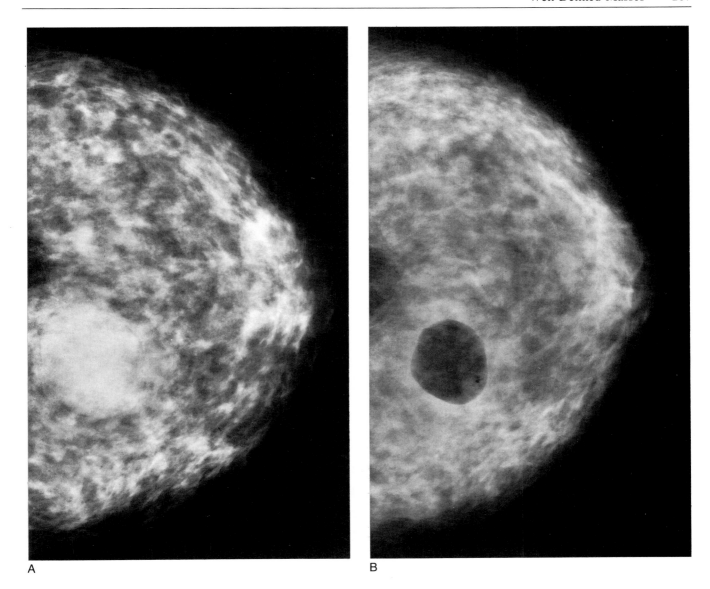

A   B

Figure 4.27.

Clinical: 42-year-old G3, P3 woman with a lump in the right breast.

Mammogram: Right craniocaudal view (**A**) and pneumocystogram (**B**). The breast is dense and diffusely nodular. There is a moderately high density, very well defined round mass surrounded by a fatty halo. Sonography revealed a cyst. The pneumocystogram (**B**) shows a normal, thin-walled cavity.

Impression: Cyst.

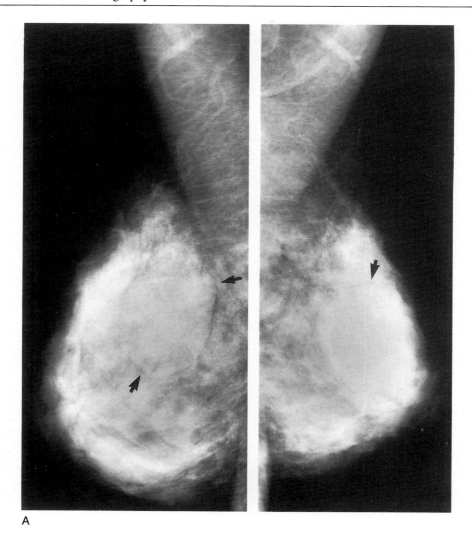

A

Figure 4.28.

Clinical: 43-year-old G2, P2 patient with lumpy breasts.

Mammogram: Bilateral oblique (**A**) and craniocaudal (**B**) views and ultrasound (**C**). The breasts are very dense and glandular for the age and parity of the patient. There are medium-density, round and ovoid, circumscribed masses bilaterally (**A** and **B**). Fatty haloes *(arrows)* surround the margins of these masses, suggesting most likely a benign nature. Ultrasound (**C**), performed to determine the internal nature of these masses, confirms that these are simple cysts. The masses are anechoic with well-defined back walls and good through-transmission.

Impression: Bilateral cysts.

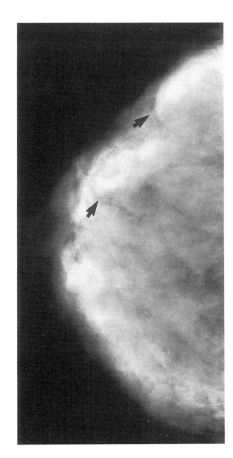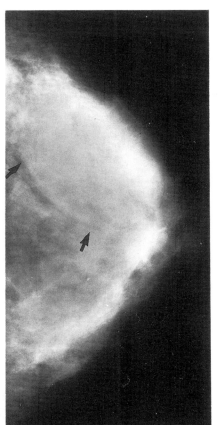

B

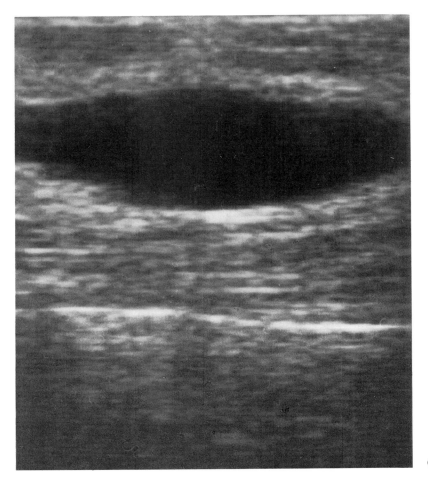

C

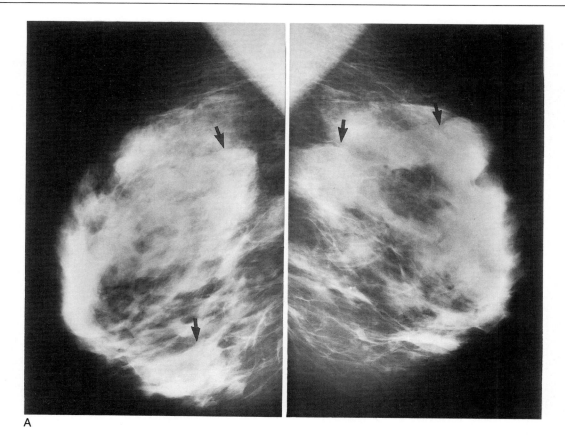

A

Figure 4.29.

Clinical: 45-year-old G1, P1 woman with a history of fibrocystic changes on previous breast biopsies, for routine follow-up. The breasts are nodular on clinical examination.

Mammogram: Bilateral oblique (**A**), left craniocaudal (**B**), right craniocaudal (**C**) views and ultrasound (**D**). The breasts are dense and glandular. Bilateral, well-circumscribed, medium-density masses are present, the largest of which are located in the upper outer quadrants *(arrows)* (**A–C**). The multiplicity of findings and the similarity in appearance suggest that these are most likely cysts; however, ultrasound is necessary for confirmation. Sonography demonstrates cysts—anechoic masses with a well-defined back wall and good through-transmission of sound—to correspond to these masses.

Impression: Bilateral cysts.

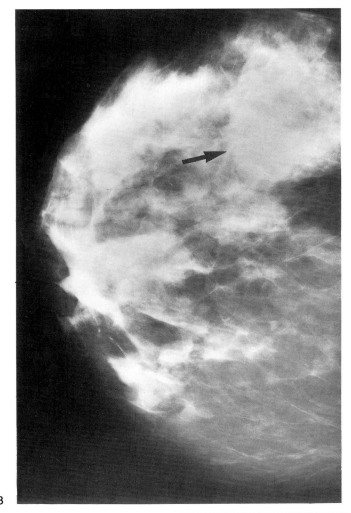

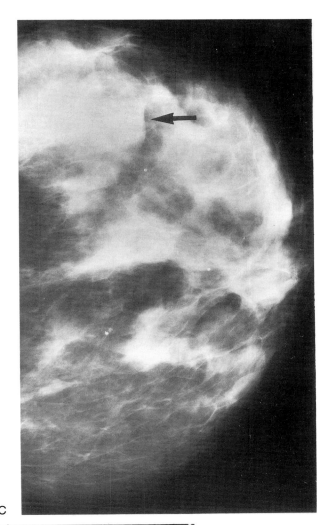

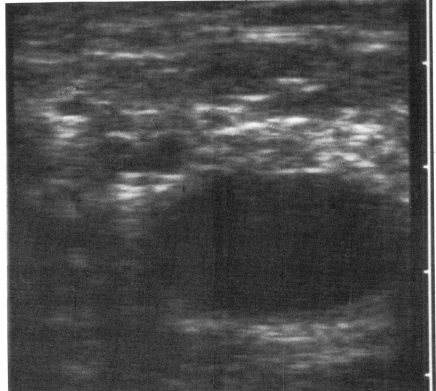

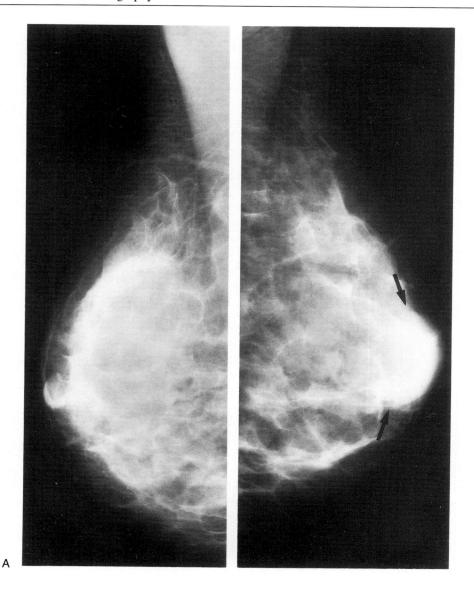

A

Figure 4.30.

Clinical: 41-year-old G3, P4 woman with a right subareolar mass.

Mammogram: Bilateral oblique (**A**) and craniocaudal (**B**) views and ultrasound (**C**). The breasts are dense and glandular for the age and parity of the patient. In the right subareolar area,

there is a medium-density, relatively circumscribed mass *(arrows)* (**A** and **B**). A halo is present around the anterior aspect of the lesion, but its posterior margin is indistinct. Ultrasound (**C**) demonstrates the anechoic nature of the lesion.

Impression: Simple cyst.

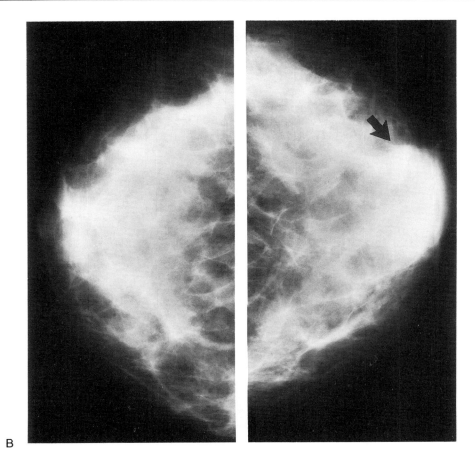

B

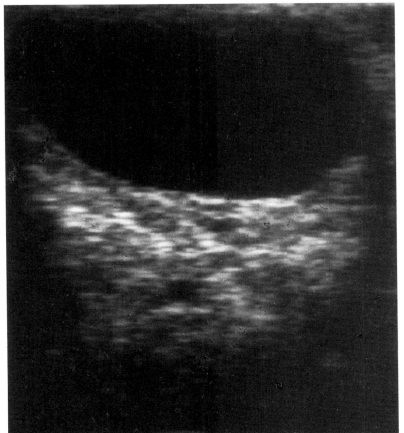

C

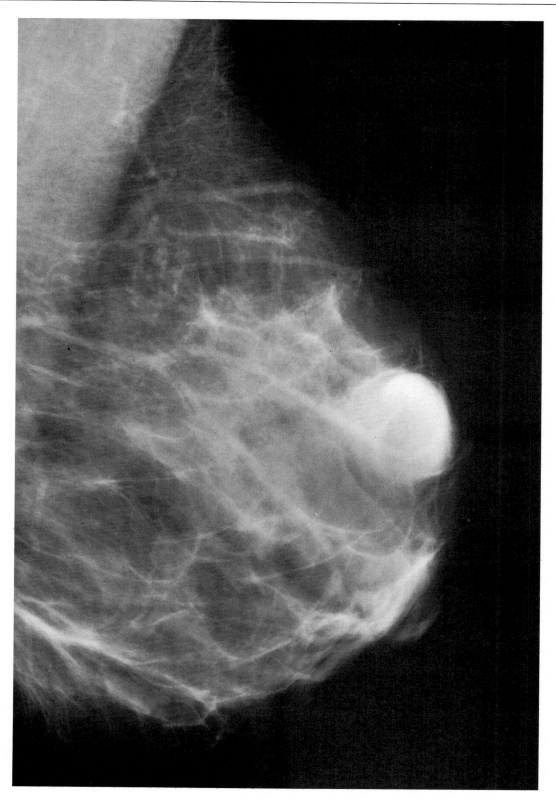

Figure 4.31.

Clinical: 27-year-old woman with 3 × 3 mass at the 12 o'clock position in the right breast.

Mammogram: Right oblique view. In the supra-areolar area, there is an ovoid mass with very well defined margins around greater than one half of its border. Sonography showed it to be solid. The medium-density and well-defined margins sug-

gest a benign nature as most likely. In a patient of this age group, a fibroadenoma is the most common lesion.

Impression: Solid mass in the right breast, probably benign, favoring fibroadenoma.

Histopathology: Fibroadenoma.

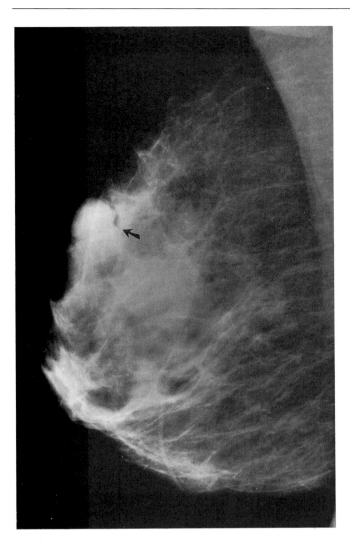

Figure 4.32.

Clinical: 23-year-old woman with a palpable 3-cm mass in the upper aspect of the left breast.

Mammogram: Left oblique view (**A**) and ultrasound (**B**). There is a very well defined lobulated mass of moderate density in the left supra-areolar area. Sonography of the mass (**B**) shows it to be well defined and hypoechoic with no posterior shadowing. The lesion has benign characteristics, and in a patient of this age, a fibroadenoma is most likely.

Impression: Fibroadenoma.

Histopathology: Fibroadenoma.

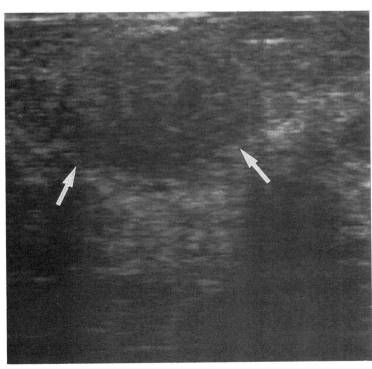

B

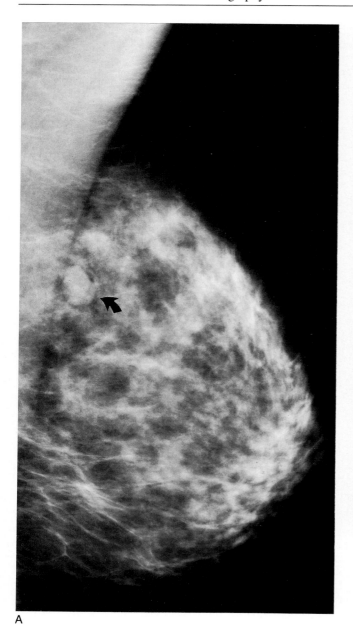

A

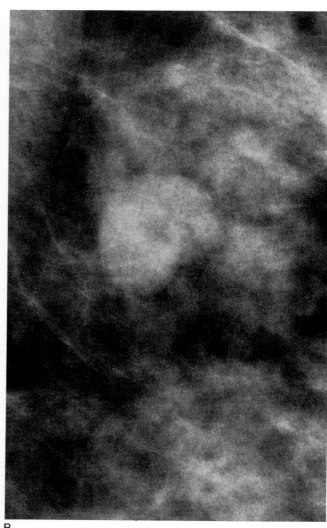

B

Figure 4.33.

Clinical: 54-year-old woman for screening mammography. Her last normal mammogram was 3 years previously.

Mammogram: Right oblique view (**A**) and magnified image (**B**). There is a very well defined lobulated mass in the right upper outer quadrant (**A**). A fatty halo surrounds this mass (**B**), suggesting that it is more likely benign. Sonography did not reveal a cyst. That the mass has developed since a previous mammogram, however, was of some concern.

Impression: Well-defined solid mass, favoring a benign lesion such as a fibroadenoma or lymph node; well-defined carcinoma is less likely but cannot be excluded.

Histopathology: Fibroadenoma.

Note: Although it is thought that fibroadenomas appear in young women, they certainly may also develop in premenopausal or postmenopausal women.

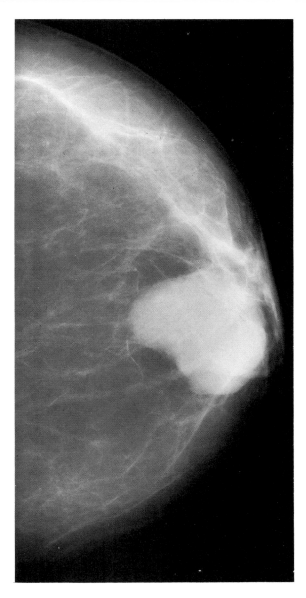

A

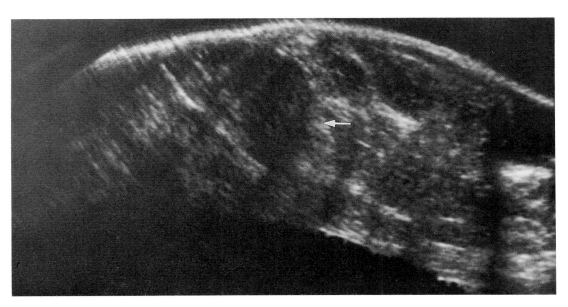

B

Figure 4.34.

Clinical: 28-year-old G4, P3 woman with a 2-year history of a right breast mass, slowly increasing in size.

Mammogram: Right craniocaudal view (**A**) and ultrasound (**B**). There is a large lobulated mass with very well defined margins in the right subareolar area (**A**). The well-defined contour suggests that it is benign, and in a patient of this age, it is most likely a fibroadenoma. Whole-breast sonography (**B**) confirms the solid nature of this mass.

Impression: Probable fibroadenoma.

Histopathology: Fibroadenoma.

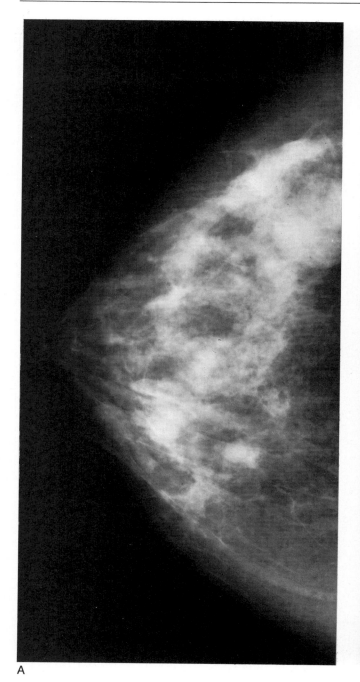
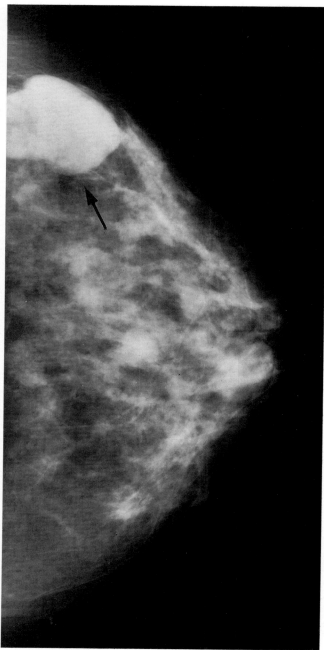

A

Figure 4.35.

Clinical: 46-year-old woman with multiple palpable breast masses bilaterally.

Mammogram: Bilateral craniocaudal views (**A**) and ultrasound images of the right (**B**) and left (**C**) breast. The breasts are moderately dense and glandular. There are multiple well-defined masses in both breasts. The mass in the right outer quadrant *(arrow)* is slightly more dense and more nodular in its margin than the other lesions. Sonography of the large lesion in the right breast (**B**) shows it to be hypoechoic and lobulated. Sonography of all other lesions showed them to be simple cysts (**C**). The solid mass in the right breast had

developed since a previous mammogram 3 years earlier. Although fibroadenomas can develop in perimenopausal women, the high density and large size of the mass were of concern; cystosarcoma phylloides and well-circumscribed carcinoma were considered higher in the differential.

Histopathology: Fibroadenoma.

Note: In the analysis of a mammogram in which multiple masses are present, each lesion needs to be individually evaluated. Ultrasound is very useful in the determination of the internal character of well-defined lesions.

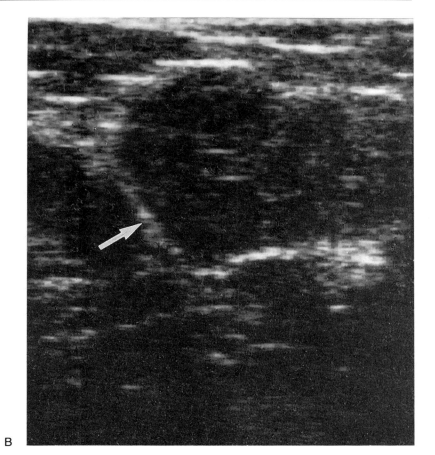

B

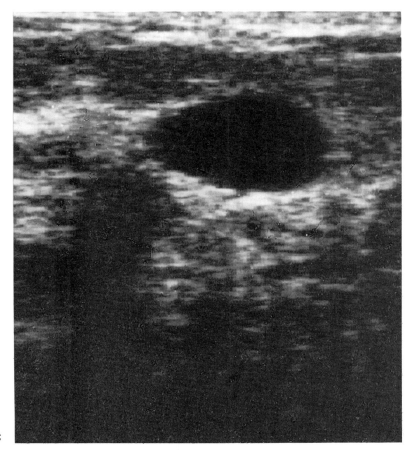

C

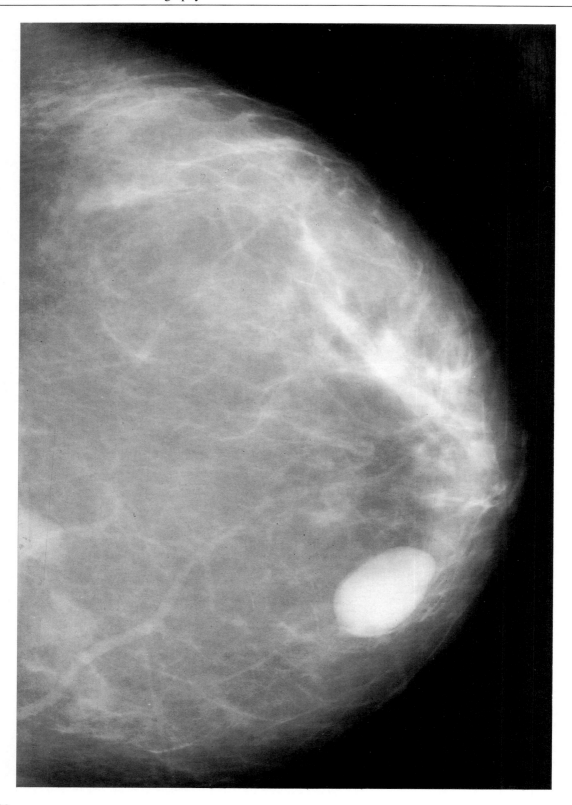

Figure 4.36.

Clinical: 38-year-old G2, P2 woman with a firm mass in the right breast.

Mammogram: Right craniocaudal view. There is a very well defined mass of moderately high density located just medial to the right nipple. The mass has a slightly lobulated contour and is surrounded in entirety by a fatty halo, suggesting that

it is most likely benign. Sonography showed the mass to be solid. Although a well-circumscribed malignancy cannot be excluded, it would be considered far less likely, particularly in this age group.

Impression: Solid mass, probable fibroadenoma.

Histopathology: Fibroadenoma.

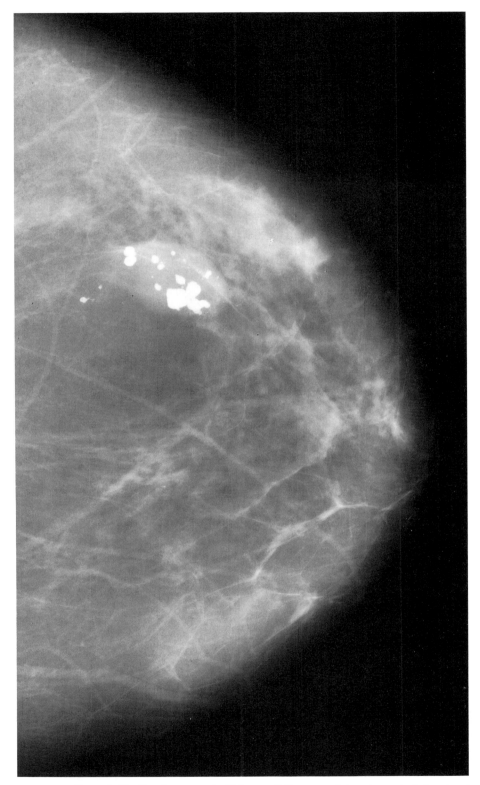

Figure 4.37.   Coarse popcorn-like calcification is present within a soft tissue nodule, characteristic of a degenerated fibroadenoma.

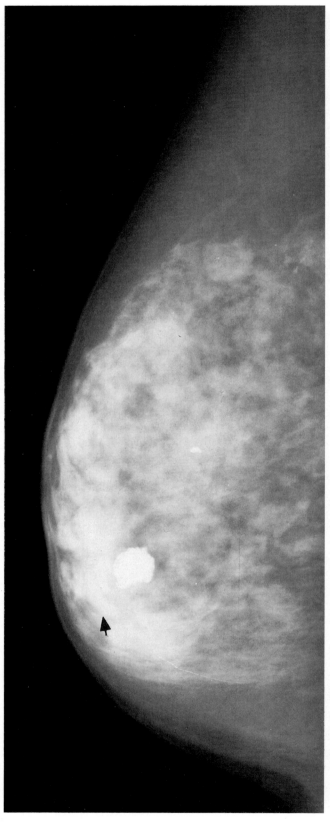

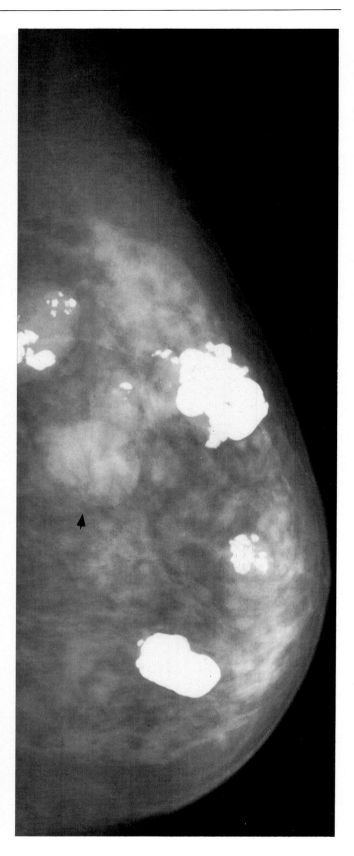

Figure 4.38.

Clinical: 65-year-old woman with multiple palpable masses.

Mammogram: Bilateral oblique views. There are several well-defined noncalcified *(arrow)* as well as calcified masses in both breasts. The popcorn-like calcifications are typical of fibroadenomas.

Impression: Multiple degenerating fibroadenomas.

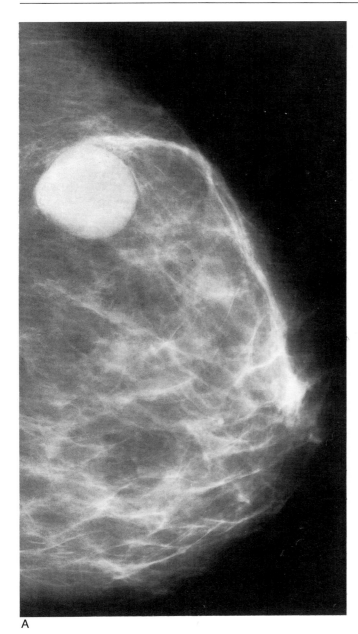

A

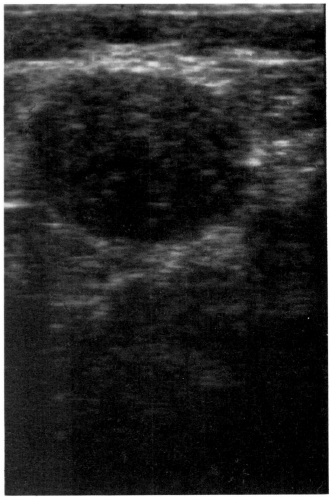

B

Figure 4.39.

Clinical: 30-year-old G2, P2 patient with a right breast mass.

Mammogram: Right craniocaudal view (**A**) and ultrasound (**B**). There is a medium-density, very well circumscribed mass in the right upper outer quadrant. A halo surrounds the lesion. On sonography (**B**), the mass is circumscribed, solid, and of relatively homogeneous hypoechogenicity, suggesting a fibroadenoma.

Impression: Solid mass, favoring fibroadenoma.

Histopathology: Fibroadenoma.

Figure 4.40.

Clinical: 33-year-old G3, P0, Ab3 woman with a palpable mass in the left breast.

Mammogram: Left oblique (**A**) and enlarged craniocaudal (**B**) views. The breast is dense, compatible with the age of the patient. There is a very well circumscribed, lobulated, medium-density mass *(arrow)* in the upper outer quadrant of the left breast. The lobulated contour suggests that this is most likely a fibroadenoma. Ultrasound confirmed the solid nature of the lesion.

Impression: Solid mass, probable fibroadenoma.

Histopathology: Fibroadenoma.

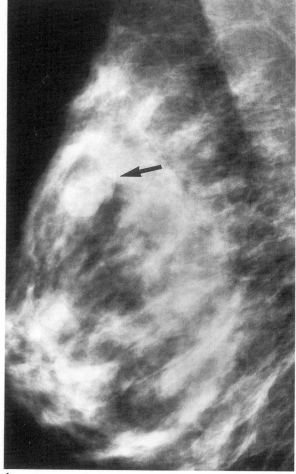

A

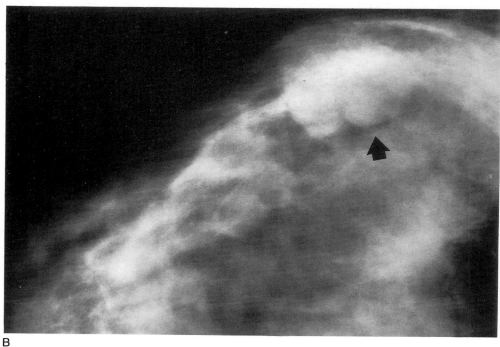

B

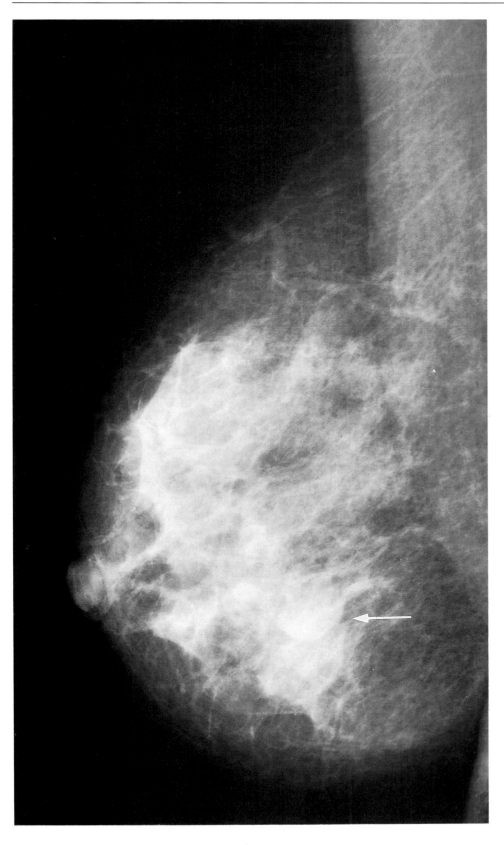

Figure 4.41.

Clinical: 64-year-old G3, P3 woman for screening.

Mammogram: Left oblique view. The left breast is dense for the age and parity of the patient. There is a very well defined round mass in the lower aspect *(arrow)* without associated calcification. Sonography showed no cysts. Since the lesion was not calcified, as one might expect in a fibroadenoma in a postmenopausal woman, biopsy was recommended.

Impression: Well-defined solid mass of indeterminate nature, favoring fibroadenoma.

Histopathology: Fibroadenoma containing a focus of lobular carcinoma in situ.

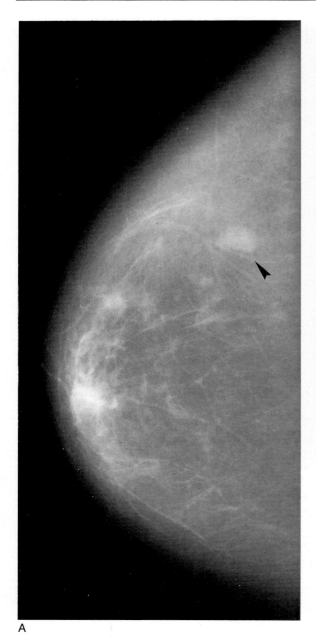

A

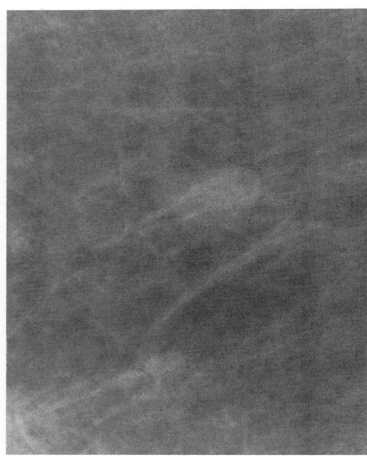

B

Figure 4.42.

Clinical: 56-year-old woman for screening mammography.

Mammogram: Left craniocaudal view (**A**) and magnified image (**B**). In a breast with otherwise fatty replacement, there is a moderate- to low-density, well-defined 1-cm nodule in the outer aspect *(arrow)*. Magnification of the nodule shows a fatty halo surrounding the lobulated lesion. The features of the mass suggest a benign etiology, more likely a fibroadenoma because of the lobulation.

Impression: Probable fibroadenoma.

Histopathology: Fibroadenoma containing intraductal papillary carcinoma.

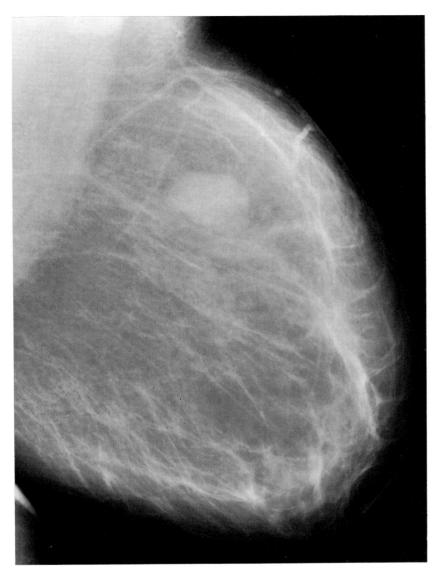

A

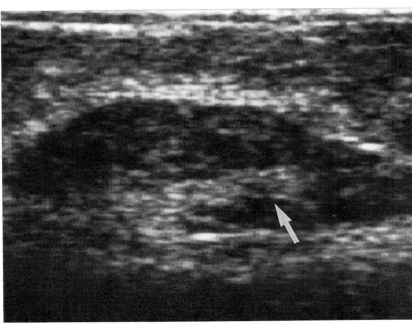

B

Figure 4.43.

Clinical: 23-year-old G2, P1, Ab1 obese woman with a palpable mass in the right breast.

Mammogram: Right oblique view (**A**) and ultrasound (**B**). There is a well-defined, medium-density, lobulated mass in the right upper outer quadrant. This lesion has very smooth margins, suggesting a benign nature. Real-time sonography (**B**) shows the mass to be hypoechoic, with some echogenic bands *(arrow)* traversing it, suggesting that it might be a dense hamartoma.

Impression: Hamartoma versus fibroadenoma.

Histopathology: Sclerosing lobular hyperplasia.

Note: This is a benign lesion typically occurring in young black women. Histologically, there is a proliferation of lobules with surrounding sclerosis (54); the lesion is associated with fibroadenomas.

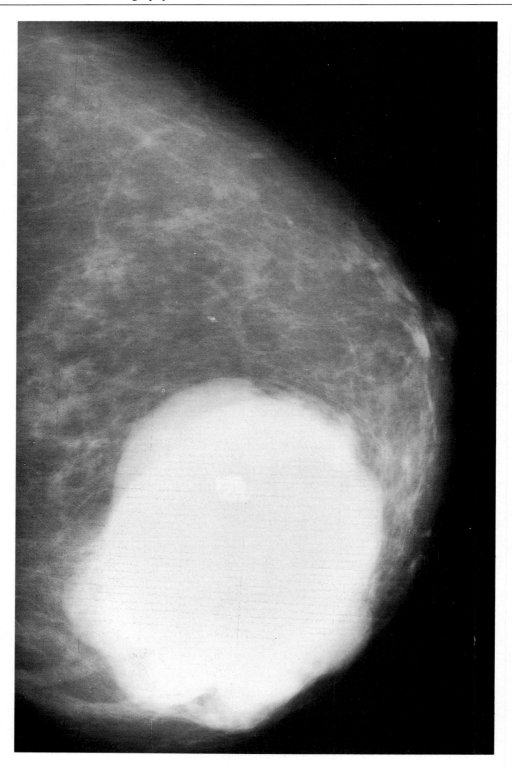

Figure 4.44.

Clinical: 84-year-old woman with a large palpable mass in the right breast.

Mammogram: Right craniocaudal view. There is a large mass in the inner quadrant of the right breast with lobulated but well-defined margins. Some dense coarse calcification is present within the lesion. The well-defined contours and the coarse calcification suggest the possibility of a cysto-sarcoma phylloides, particularly in an elderly patient. Less

likely in the differential diagnosis are a fibroadenoma (which probably would have degenerated to a greater degree and calcified) and a well-circumscribed carcinoma.

Impression: Cystosarcoma phylloides versus fibroade-noma.

Histopathology: Malignant cystosarcoma phylloides.

Note: The calcifications in a cystosarcoma are described as plaquelike and coarse.

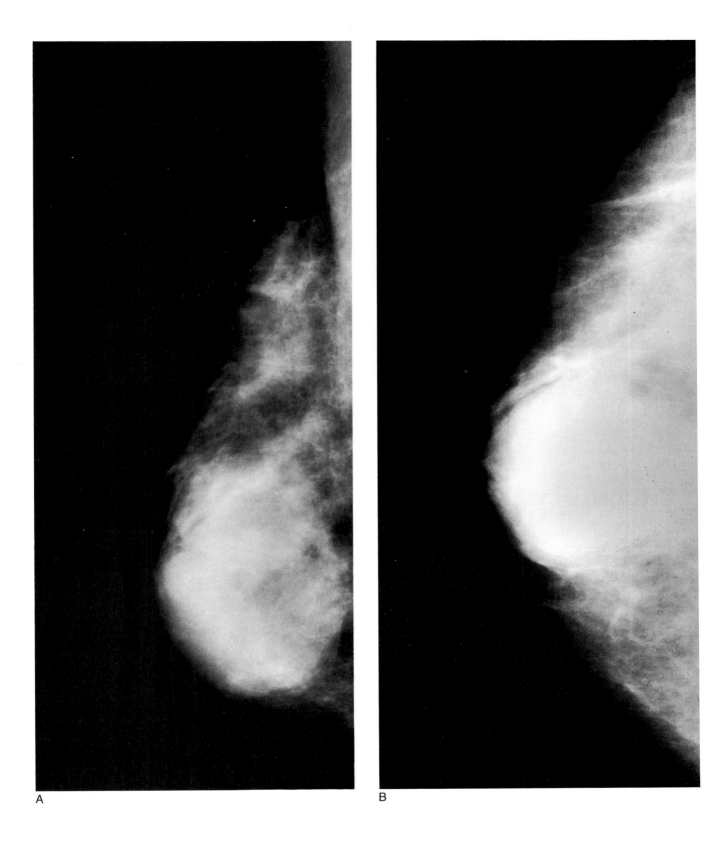

A

B

Figure 4.45.

Clinical: 52-year-old woman with a large smooth mass in the left breast.

Mammogram: Left oblique (**A**) and craniocaudal (**B**) views. There is a large well-defined mass of moderate density, surrounded at least in part by a fatty halo. No calcifications are present. Sonography showed a solid mass. The differential includes primarily a well-defined breast carcinoma, fibroadenoma, and cystosarcoma phylloides. The size of the lesion, lack of calcifications, and very well defined margins suggest more likely a cystosarcoma or a well-defined carcinoma.

Histopathology: Cystosarcoma phylloides. (Case courtesy of Dr. M. C. Wilhelm, Charlottesville, VA.)

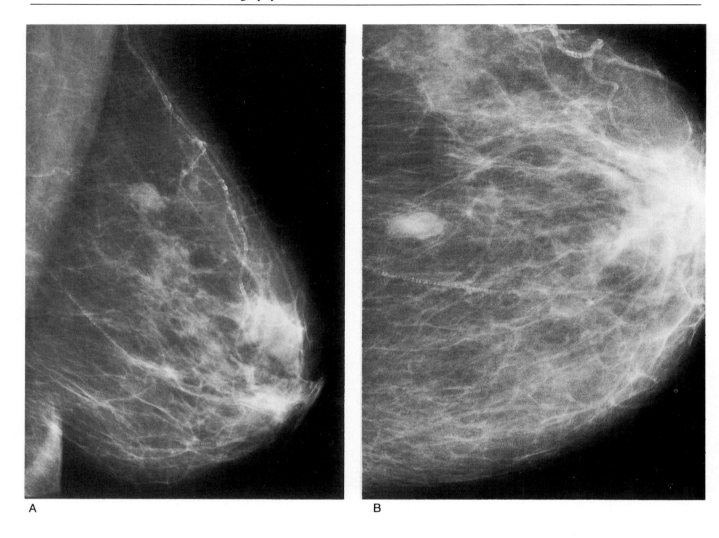

A

B

Figure 4.46.

Clinical: 66-year-old woman for screening mammography.

Mammogram: Right oblique (**A**) and craniocaudal (**B**) views. There is a relatively circumscribed, 1.2-cm-oval, medium-density mass in the 12 o'clock position of the right breast. Sonography did not reveal a solid or cystic lesion. Because of the size of the lesion and the slight indistinctness of some of its margins, it was regarded with a moderate degree of suspicion.

Histopathology: Sclerosing adenosis (adenosis tumor).

Note: It is unusual for sclerosing adenosis to present mammographically as a circumscribed mass. Generally, the appearance is that of an ill-defined lesion with lobular-type microcalcifications.

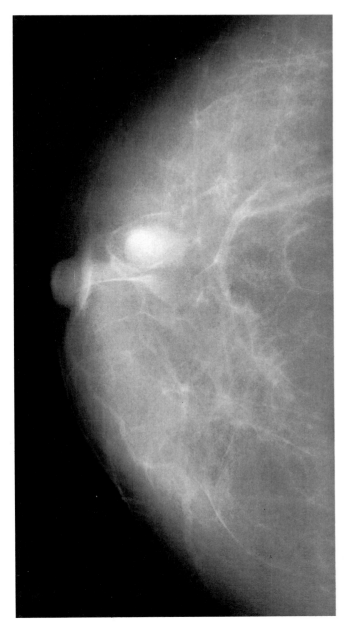

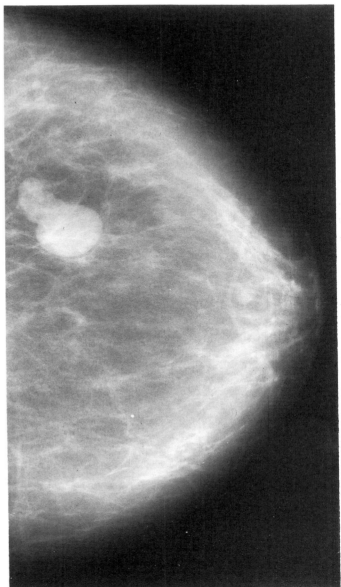

Figure 4.47.

Clinical: 56-year-old woman with bloody discharge from the left nipple and no palpable mass.

Mammogram: Left craniocaudal view. There is a 1.5-cm well-defined ovoid mass oriented in the direction of the ducts in the left subareolar area. The finding suggests a large intraductal papilloma because it is very well defined and because of the history of bloody discharge. An intraductal carcinoma could also present in this way but is less likely because of the well-defined margins of the lesion.

Impression: Intraductal papilloma.

Histopathology: Intraductal papilloma.

Figure 4.48.

Clinical: 52-year-old woman with generalized right breast pain but no palpable masses.

Mammogram: Right craniocaudal view. There is a 2×2.5-cm, bilobed, well-defined medium-density mass in the lower outer aspect of the right breast. A fatty halo surrounds the majority of the lesion. The differential includes a fibroadenoma or a dilated duct secondary to an obstructing lesion, hematoma, or intracystic papillary carcinoma. The tubular shape should suggest the dilated duct as the more likely etiology.

Histopathology: Intraductal papilloma.

Figure 4.49.

Clinical: 49-year-old woman who suffered a seat belt injury to the left breast 2 weeks earlier. She now presents with a firm mass, skin thickening, and some residual bruising of the skin.

Mammogram: Left craniocaudal view (**A**) and sonogram of the left breast (**B**). There is a relatively well-defined mass of moderate to high density in the inner aspect of the breast *(arrow)* (**A**). There is no spiculation, but there is increased density of the stroma and overlying skin thickening. Ultrasound (**B**) shows the mass to be well defined and complex with good through-transmission of sound.

Impression: Loculated and interstitial hematoma.

Note: The mammographic appearance of the lesion might be considered to be suspicious for carcinoma, but the history and physical examination are key in making the diagnosis. This patient was followed and the mass resolved spontaneously.

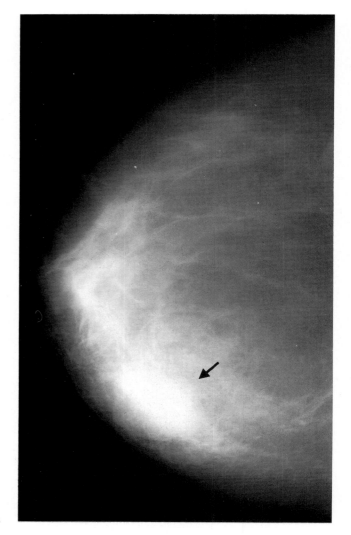

A

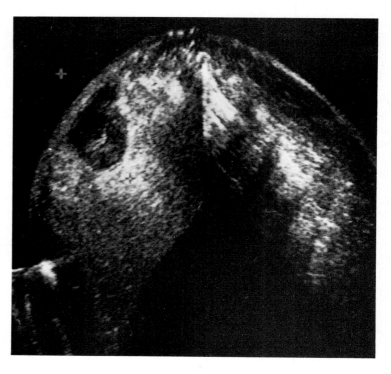

B

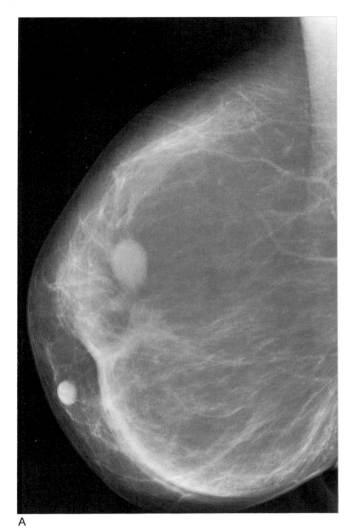

A

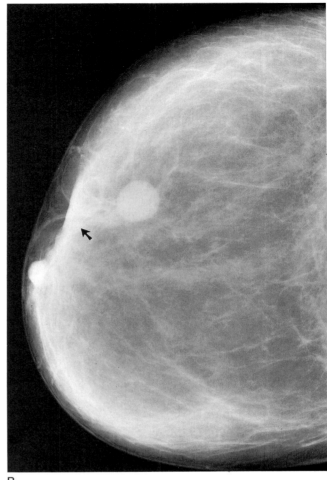

B

Figure 4.50.

Clinical: 76-year-old woman 8 months after a lumpectomy for lobular carcinoma in situ in the left breast, with no palpable masses on physical examination.

Mammogram: Left oblique (**A**) and craniocaudal (**B**) views. There is a well-defined, moderately dense round mass demonstrated on both views. This mass is situated directly be-neath the surgical scar *(arrow)* from lumpectomy. Considering the history of recent biopsy in this region, a well-circumscribed hematoma was considered most likely.

Impression: Hematoma.

Histopathology: Fibrous-walled cyst containing old blood.

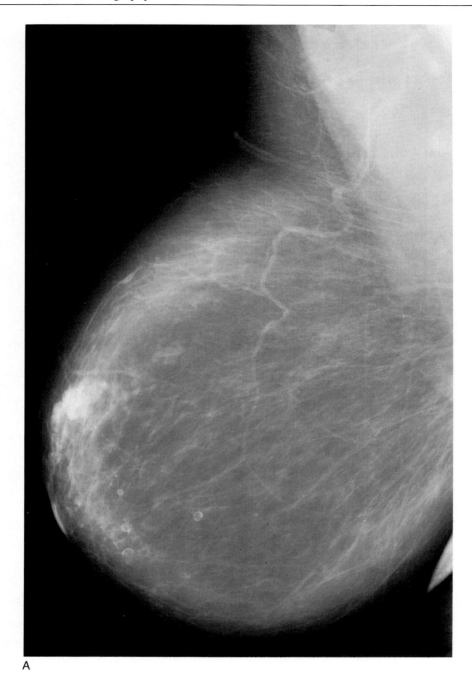

A

Figure 4.51.

Clinical: 68-year-old woman who recently sustained breast trauma to the left breast. Bruising was present in the supra-areolar area.

Mammogram: Left oblique view (**A**), craniocaudal view (**B**), and ultrasound (**C**). There is a lobulated, very well defined medium-density nodule in the supra-areolar area, beneath the area of bruising. Sonography shows the nodule to be slightly irregular and to contain a few internal echoes. The findings are most compatible with a hematoma. Follow-up mammography showed complete resolution of the nodule.

Impression: Hematoma. (Case courtesy of Dr. Jay Levine, Richmond, VA.)

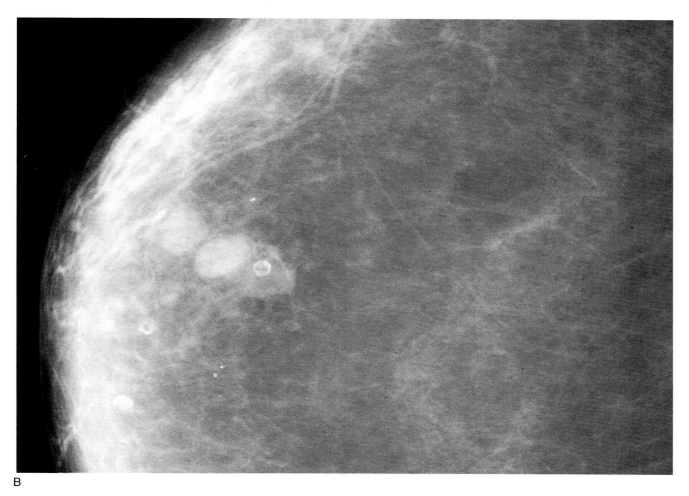

B

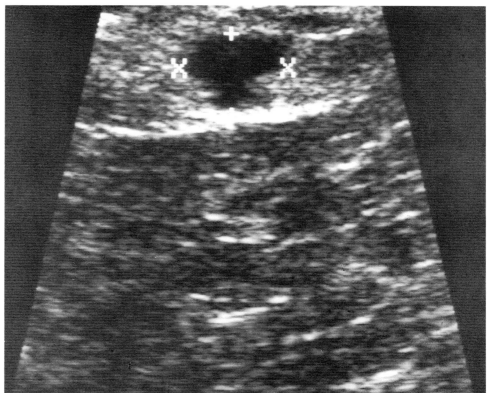

C

Figure 4.52.

Clinical: 81-year-old woman with a history of trauma to the right breast and a palpable mass beneath the right nipple.

Mammogram: Right oblique view (**A**) and magnified image (**B**). There is a relatively well defined, lobulated mass beneath the right nipple *(arrow)* (**A**). Faint indistinctness of some of the margins is seen on magnification. The lesion could represent a loculated hematoma, but in an elderly patient a relatively well defined malignancy cannot be excluded.

Histopathology: Organizing hematoma.

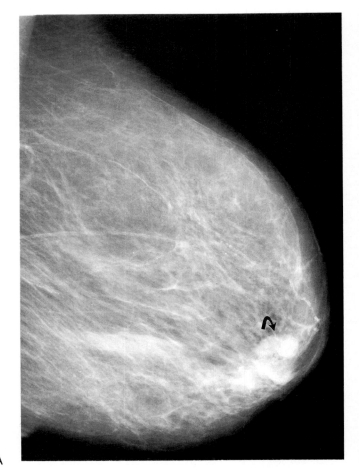

A

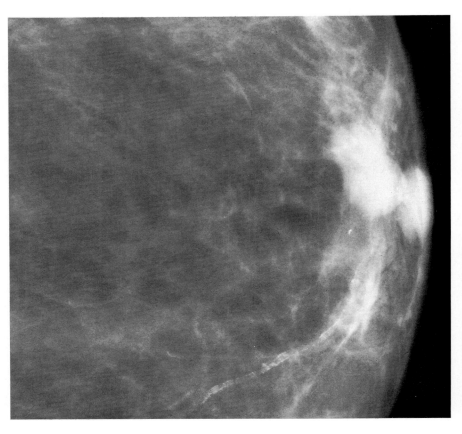

B

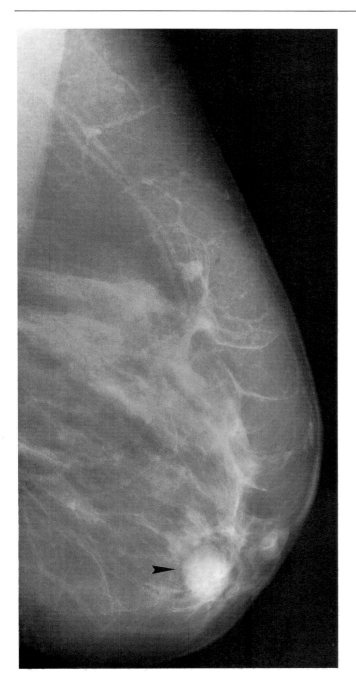

Figure 4.53.

Clinical: 50-year-old woman with a nodule palpable beneath the skin of the right breast.

Mammogram: Right oblique view. There is a well-defined medium-density nodule located superficially in the right breast. The differential is vast, but because of the superficial location, an inclusion cyst, hematoma, or metastasis is most likely.

Histopathology: Epidermal inclusion cyst.

Figure 4.54.

Clinical: 65-year-old G1, P1 woman for routine screening.

Mammogram: Right oblique (**A**) and enlarged (2×) cranio-caudal (**B**) views. There is mild glandularity present. In the right supra-areolar area, there is a well-circumscribed nodule attached to the skin *(arrow)* (**A**). Coarse calcifications are present within this nodule (**A** and **B**). The subcutaneous location of the nodule is key to the diagnosis of a sebaceous cyst. Clinical examination also showed a firm nodule within the skin. The calcifications are dystrophic, related to chronically retained secretions.

Impression: Sebaceous cyst of right breast.

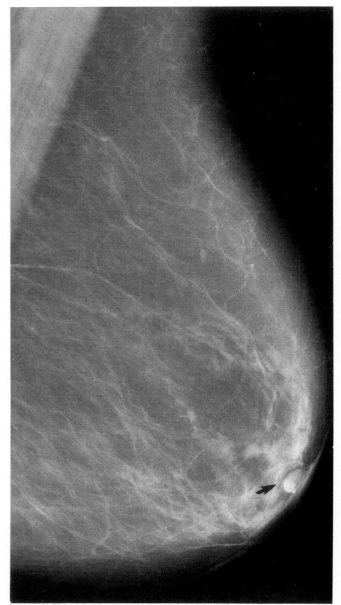

A

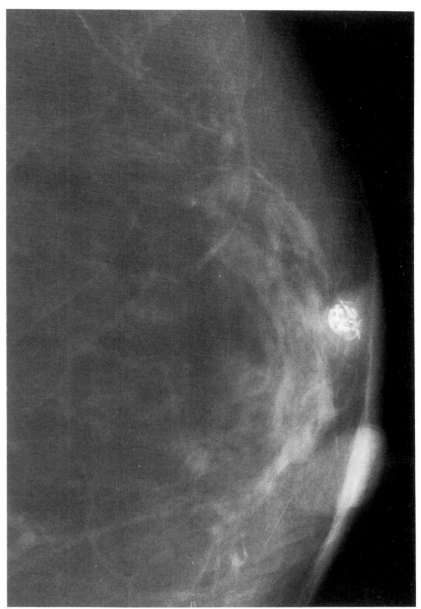

B

Figure 4.55.

Clinical: 57-year-old G7, P7 woman with a palpable nodule in the right lower inner quadrant.

Mammogram: Bilateral craniocaudal view (**A**), right oblique view (**B**), left oblique (**C**) view, and ultrasound of the right (**D** and **E**) and left (**F**) breasts. There are three relatively well circumscribed masses present. In the right inner quadrant (**A** and **B**), there is a very well marginated high-density mass *(straight arrow)* located in the subcutaneous area and corresponding to the palpable nodule. On ultrasound (**D**), this mass is complex; there is a fluid component with debris layering in the base. This mass, particularly its location, is most consistent with an inclusion or sebaceous cyst. In the right upper outer quadrant (**A** and **B**), there is a medium-density circumscribed mass *(curved arrow)*, which on ultrasound (**E**) is a simple cyst. In the left upper outer quadrant, a third nodule is noted (**A** and **C**) *(arrowhead)*. This mass is of medium density and has well-circumscribed lobulated margins, suggesting that the lesion may be a fibroadenoma. Sonography (**F**) reveals the lesion to be hypoechoic and well margined, consistent with a fibroadenoma.

Impression: Three circumscribed masses: simple cyst and sebaceous cyst on the right and fibroadenoma on the left.

Histopathology: Right epidermal cyst, left fibroadenoma.

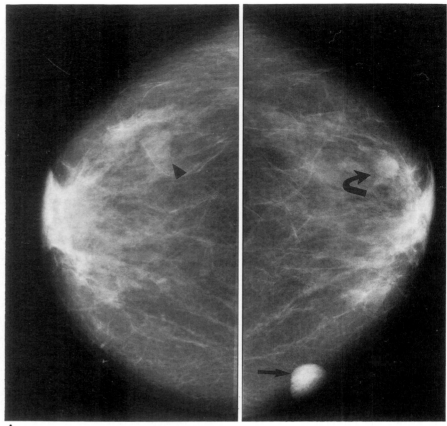

A

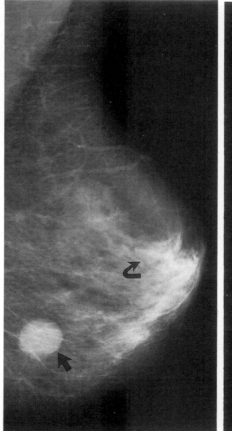

B

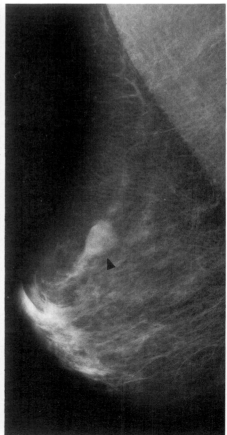

C

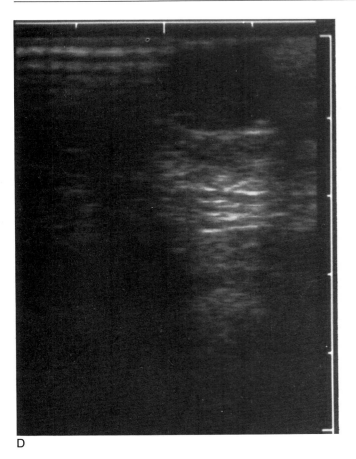

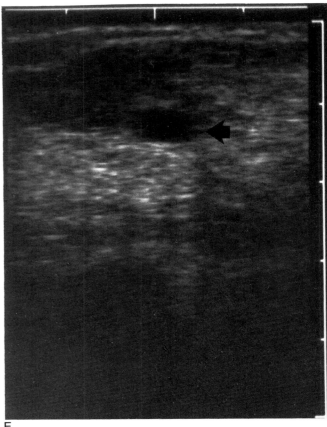

D

E

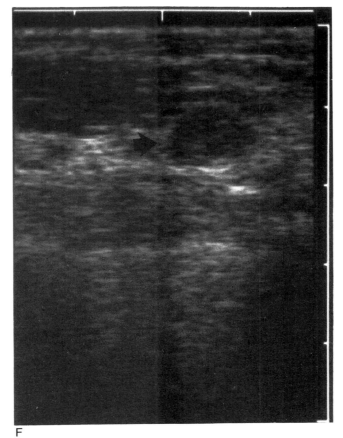

F

Figure 4.56.

Clinical: 56-year-old woman for follow-up of a nonpalpable right breast nodule that had been stable for 5 years.

Mammogram: Right oblique (**A**) and craniocaudal (**B**) views. The breast is mildly glandular. In the central aspect, there is a well-circumscribed ovoid nodule *(straight arrow)* that was stable from prior examinations and presumed to be a fibroadenoma (**A** and **B**). A second nodule *(curved arrow)*, seen superiorly on the oblique view (**A**), disappears on the craniocaudal view (**B**). This represents the nipple out of profile, simulating a breast lesion.

Impression: Nipple out of profile, simulating a breast lesion.

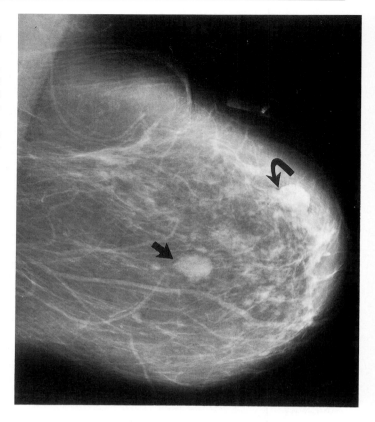

A

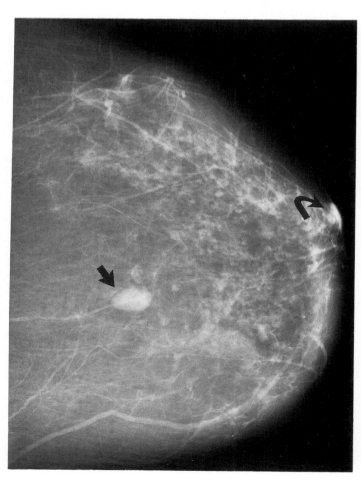

B

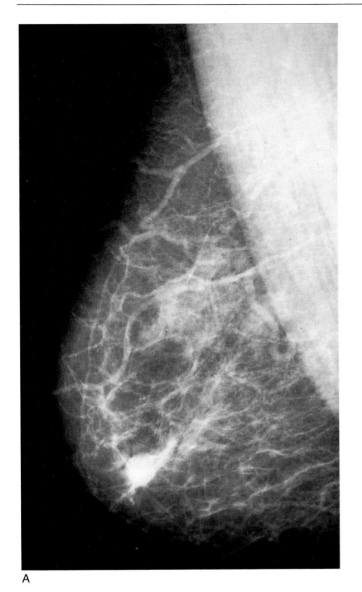

A

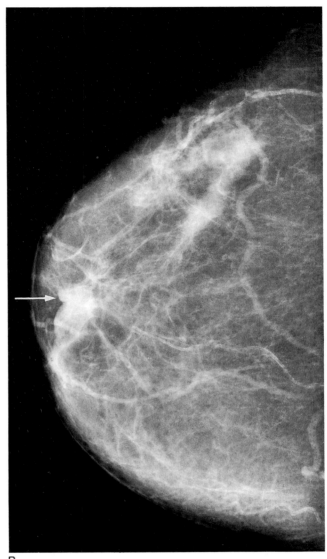

B

Figure 4.57.

Clinical: 73-year-old woman for screening mammography. Left nipple retraction had been present for many years.

Mammogram: Left oblique (**A**) and craniocaudal (**B**) views. There is a well-defined high-density nodule superficially lo-

cated in the left breast. The very lucent halo on the anterior surface of this "lesion" *(arrow)* represents air surrounding the margin of the inverted nipple.

Impression: Inverted nipple simulating a breast mass.

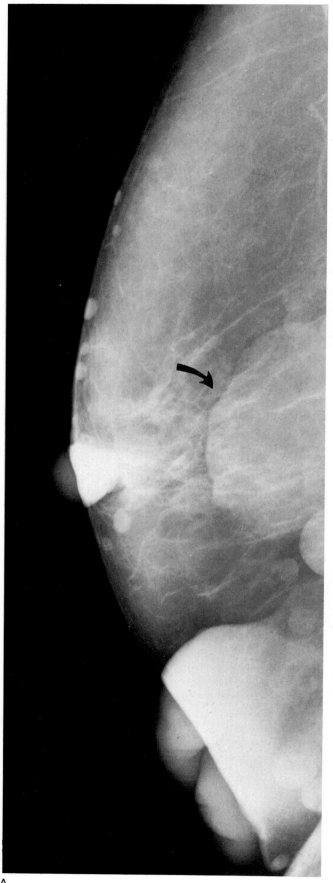
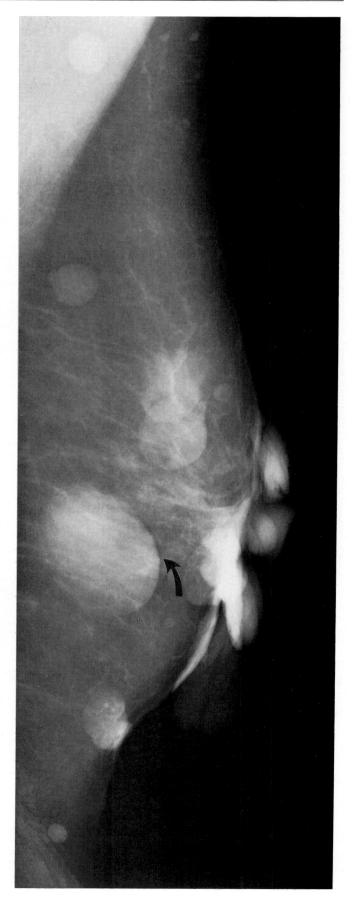

A

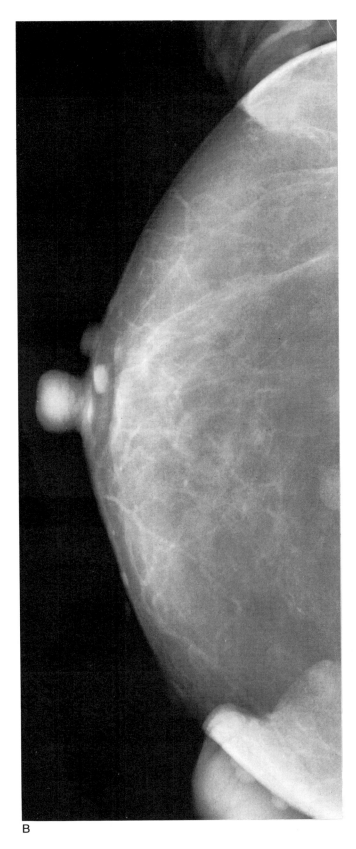

B

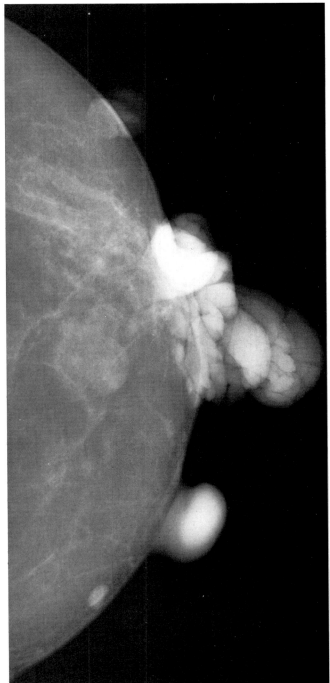

Figure 4.58.

Clinical: 57-year-old woman with neurofibromatosis, for screening mammography.

Mammogram: Bilateral oblique (**A**) and craniocaudal (**B**) views. The breasts show fatty replacement. There are multiple, very well defined masses of varying size projected over the skin surfaces of both breasts, compatible with the obvious cutaneous lesions on physical examination. Note on the oblique view (**A**) that the lesions that superimpose over the breast have strikingly lucent haloes *(curved arrows)*, more lucent than is seen with a fatty halo. This appearance is created by air surrounding the nodule compressed against the surface of the breast.

Impression: Multiple cutaneous lesions of neurofibromatosis.

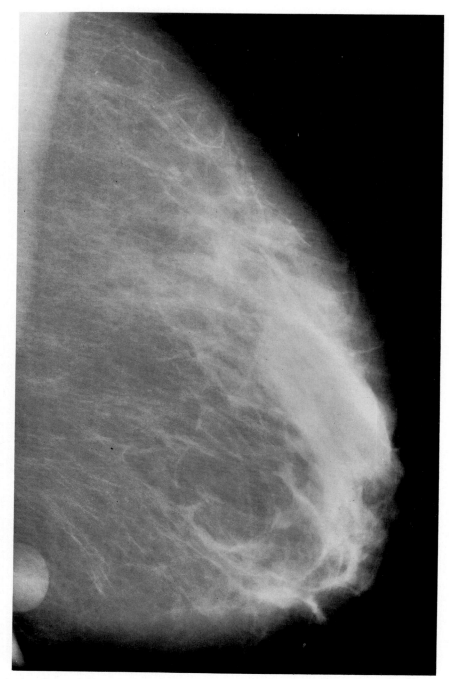

Figure 4.59. A skin lesion (nevus) simulates a breast mass. Note the very lucent air halo surrounding the nodule, characteristic of skin lesions.

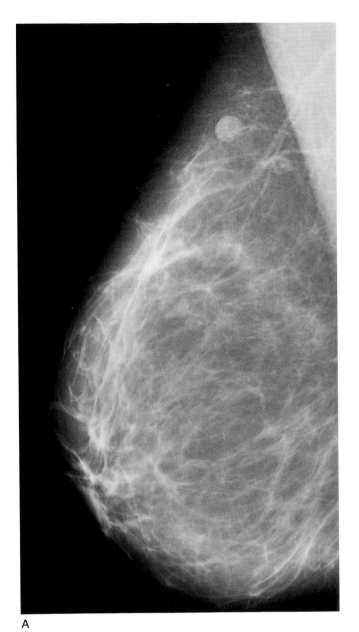

A

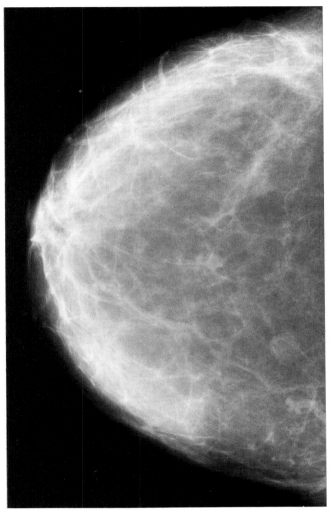

B

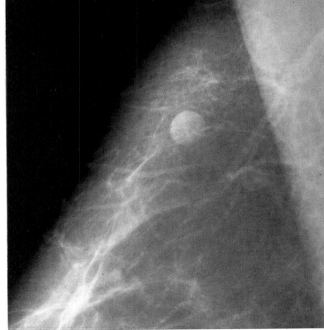

C

Figure 4.60.

Clinical: 51-year-old woman for screening mammography.

Mammogram: Left mediolateral view (**A**), craniocaudal view (**B**), and magnified image (**C**). The breast shows fatty replacement. There is a well-defined nodule of moderate to low density in the area of the upper inner quadrant. The nodule has an extremely well defined margin (**C**) and a strikingly radiolucent halo, typical of the appearance of a skin lesion. This was confirmed on clinical examination.

Impression: Skin lesion, nevus.

Figure 4.61.

Mammogram: Right oblique (**A**) and craniocaudal (**B**) views. On the oblique view, a skin lesion (seborrheic keratosis) simulates a breast mass. On the craniocaudal view, the location on the skin is confirmed *(arrow)*.

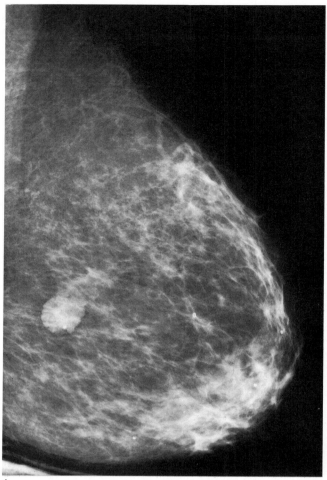

A

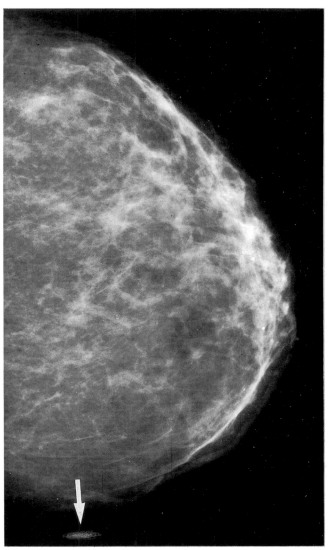

B

Figure 4.62.

Clinical: 46-year-old woman with an acute, very tender, indurated mass in the left subareolar area.

Mammogram: Bilateral oblique (**A**) and craniocaudal (**B**) views and left breast ultrasound (**C**). Asymmetry in the appearance of the breasts is present (**A** and **B**), with the left breast being more dense, particularly in the subareolar area, than the right. Beneath the left nipple is a well-circumscribed medium-density mass *(arrow)*. On ultrasound (**C**) the mass is complex, having an irregular wall and some internal echoes. The combination of findings on imaging and clinical examination is most consistent with a breast abscess.

Impression: Left breast abscess.

Note: The lesion was aspirated of purulent material and resolved after treatment with antibiotics.

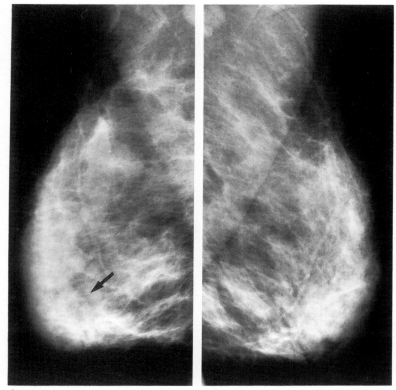

A

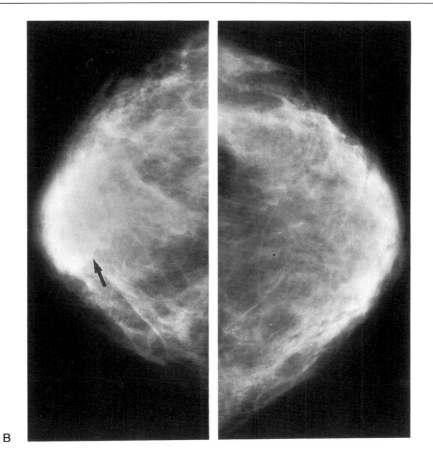

B

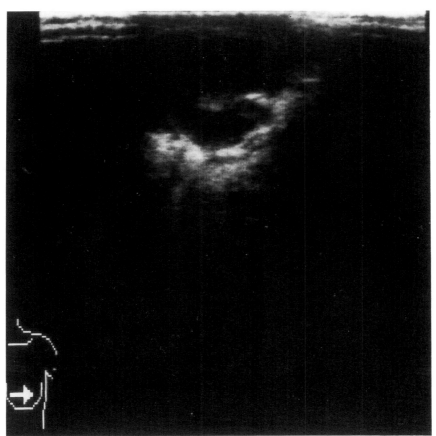

C

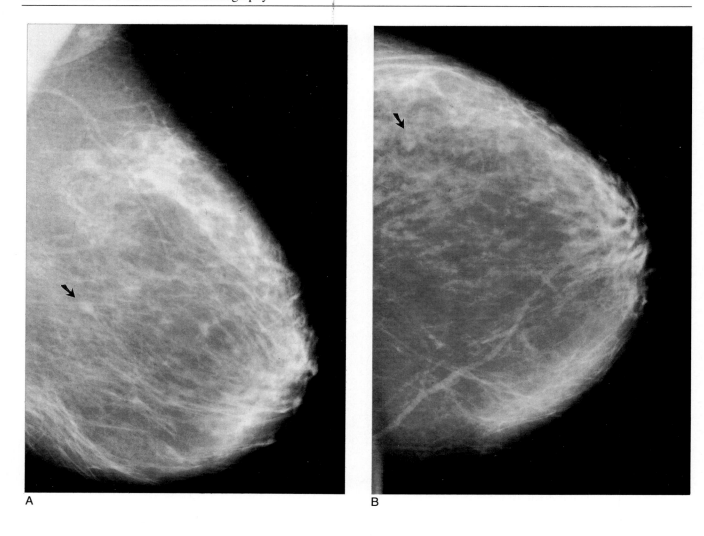

A

B

Figure 4.63.

Clinical: 52-year-old woman for screening mammography.

Mammogram: Right oblique (**A**) and craniocaudal (**B**) views. There is a relatively well-defined nodule deep in the upper outer quadrant *(arrow)*. The density of this nodule is high, particularly for its small size. Slight irregularity on the anterior margin is present. The key to the identification of this lesion is in the perception of its higher density than the parenchyma.

Impression: Relatively well defined nodule moderately suspicious for malignancy.

Histopathology: Infiltrating ductal carcinoma.

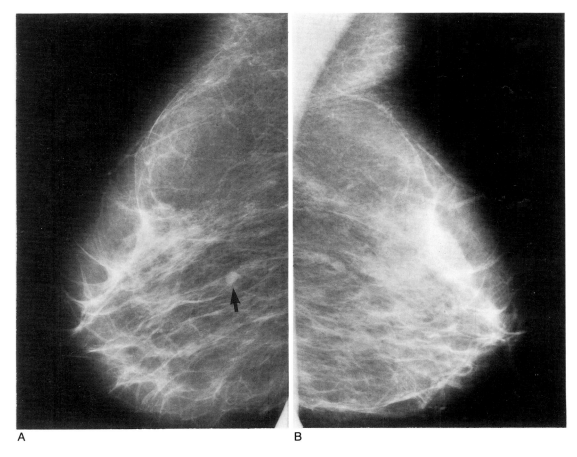

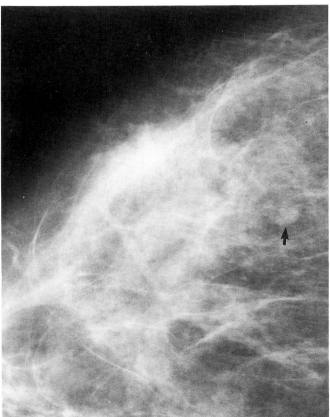

Figure 4.64.

Clinical: 51-year-old G2, P2 patient for screening.

Mammogram: Left oblique view in 1988 (**A**), left oblique view in 1987 (**B**), and left craniocaudal view in 1988 (**(C**). There is a relatively well defined 7-mm nodule in the left upper outer quadrant *(arrow)*. The nodule was identified on the study from 1987 (**B**) and followed. In 1988, it is slightly larger and more dense (**A** and **C**). The nodule is in a deeper location than would be expected for an intramammary node, and portions of the borders are slightly indistinct. For these reasons, biopsy was recommended after needle localization.

Impression: Relatively circumscribed nodule of mild suspicion for malignancy.

Histopathology: Intraductal carcinoma.

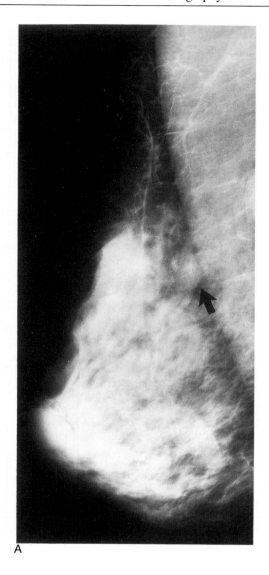

A

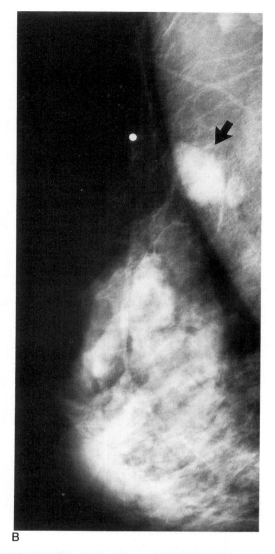

B

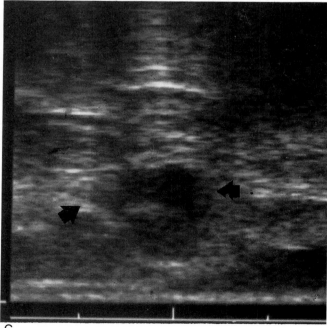

C

Figure 4.65.

Clinical: 37-year-old G1, P1 woman with a positive family history of breast cancer and a palpable 2-cm lump in the left upper outer quadrant.

Mammogram: Left oblique (**A**) and lateral oblique craniocaudal (**B**) views and ultrasound (**C**). There is a relatively well circumscribed mass in the left upper outer quadrant *(arrow)* (**A** and **B**). The mass is of medium to high density; and although it is relatively circumscribed, its borders are nodular, suggesting a malignancy etiology. On ultrasound (**C**) the mass is hypoechoic with mixed echogenicity, and it has irregular borders *(arrow)*. Such findings are more consistent with a malignant lesion than with a benign lesion such as a fibroadenoma.

Impression: Highly suspicious for primary carcinoma.

Histopathology: Adenocarcinoma, with 24 nodes negative.

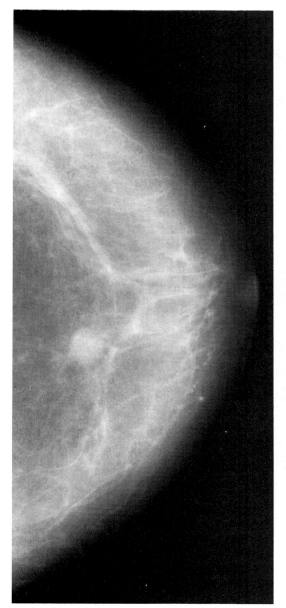

A

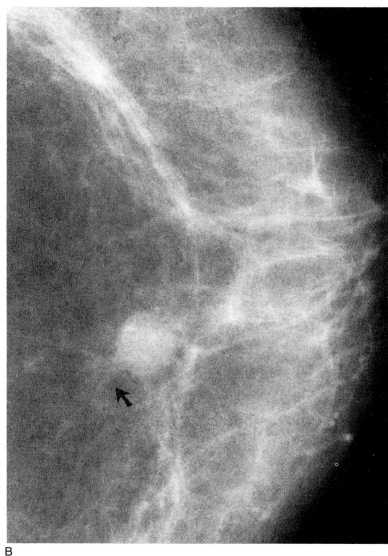

B

Figure 4.66.

Clinical: 54-year-old woman for initial screening mammogram.

Mammogram: Right craniocaudal (**A**) view and magnified image (**B**). There is a relatively well defined round mass of moderate density in the middle portion of the right breast (**A**).

On close inspection (**B**) a fine comet tail is noted *(arrow)* on the posterior aspect of the mass, which is suspicious for carcinoma. Sonography was performed and showed no cystic mass.

Impression: Suspicious for carcinoma.

Histopathology: Infiltrating small cell lobular carcinoma.

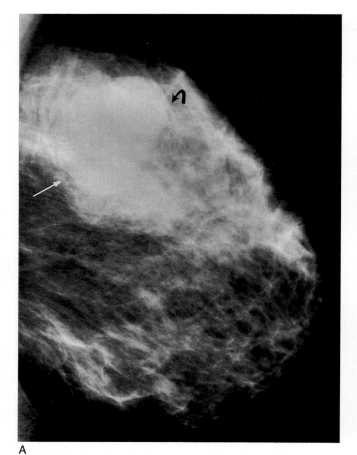

A

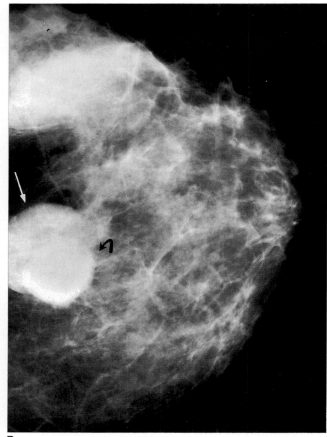

B

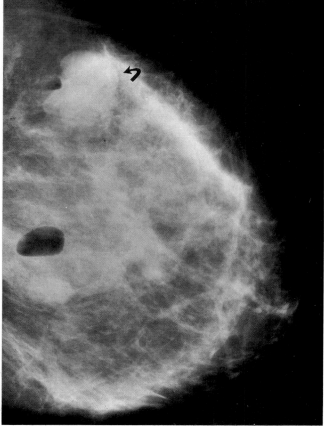

C

Figure 4.67.

Clinical: 39-year-old woman with a history of cystic disease, presenting with multiple palpable lumps in the right breast.

Mammogram: Right mediolateral (**A**) and craniocaudal (**B**) views and mediolateral view after pneumocystography (**C**). There are multiple masses present. In the outer quadrant, a medium- to high-density area of asymmetry is present; sonography showed two cysts within the density. Centrally, there are two lobulated superimposed masses. One lesion is of medium density and is very well defined *(straight arrow)*. The more superior lesion is of higher density and is slightly ill defined anteriorly *(curved arrow)*, producing a suspicious mammographic appearance. Aspiration of the masses was performed. The two lateral lesions were simple cysts, as was the lower-density central lesion. Pneumocystography demonstrated no intracystic masses (**C**). A fine-needle aspirate of the higher density central mass *(curved arrow)* revealed malignant cells.

Impression: Carcinoma, right breast, multiple cysts.

Histopathology: Infiltrating ductal carcinoma.

Note: It is very important, when multiple masses are present, that one not assume that all are cystic, but evaluate each individually.

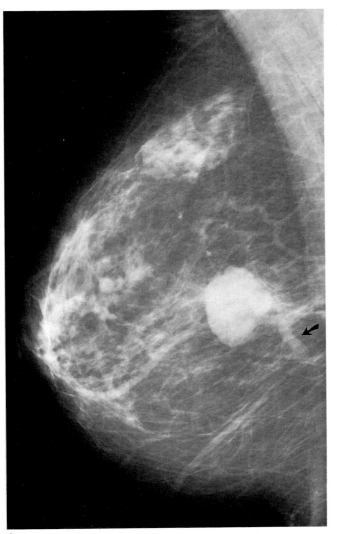

A

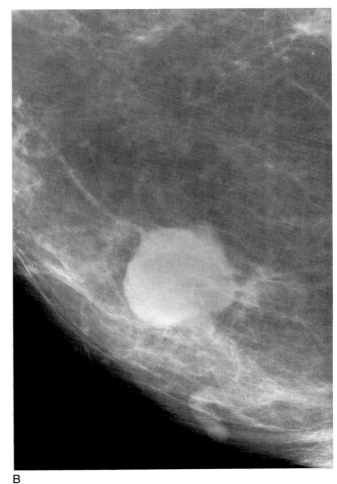

B

Figure 4.68.

Clinical: 46-year-old woman with a left breast mass 4 cm in diameter.

Mammogram: Left oblique (**A**) and magnified craniocaudal (**B**) views. The breast is markedly glandular. There is a 2.5-cm well-defined, medium- to high-density mass in the upper inner quadrant. The lesion has a fatty halo around portions of its borders, but slight irregularity is present elsewhere. A prominent vein *(arrow)* is present in the vicinity of the tumor. The slight irregularity of the margins of this lesion is the finding that makes the mass suspicious for carcinoma. A fibroadenoma is a less likely consideration.

Impression: Left breast mass consistent with carcinoma.

Histopathology: Infiltrating ductal carcinoma.

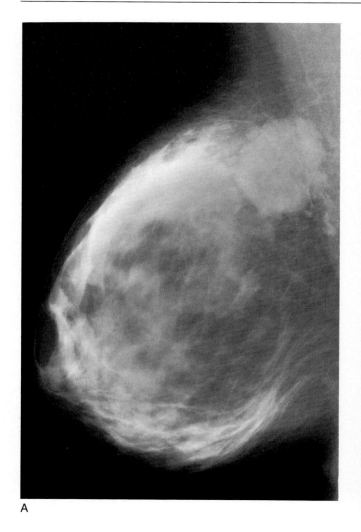

A

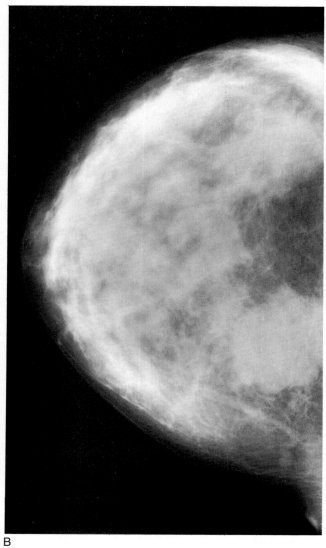

B

Figure 4.69.

Clinical: 34-year-old G3, P2, Ab1 woman with a large left breast mass.

Mammogram: Left oblique (**A**) and craniocaudal (**B**) views. There is a large nodular mass that is relatively well demarcated from the surrounding parenchyma in the upper inner quadrant. The lesion is of the same density as the remainder of the parenchyma. Because of the nodularity along the borders and slight irregularity, this lesion has a mammographic appearance suspicious for malignancy.

Impression: Carcinoma.

Histopathology: Infiltrating ductal carcinoma, negative nodes.

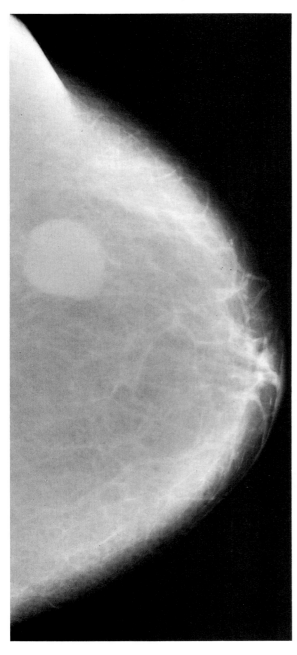

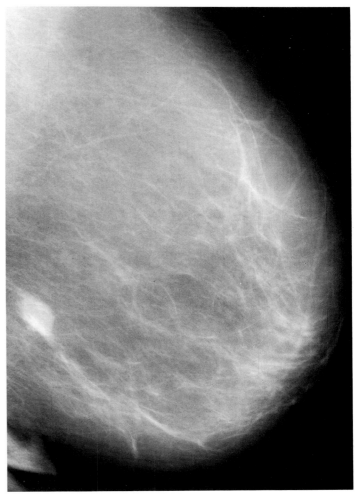

Figure 4.71.

Clinical: 75-year-old woman for screening mammography.

Mammogram: Right oblique view. There is a moderate-density 1.5-cm mass deep in the right breast. Although the lesion is relatively well defined on some of its borders, there is stranding anteriorly and posteriorly, making it suspicious for carcinoma.

Impression: Carcinoma.

Histopathology: Infiltrating ductal carcinoma, negative nodes.

Figure 4.70.

Clinical: 35-year-old G2, P2 woman with a family history of breast cancer in three sisters. On physical examination there was a palpable 2.5-cm lump in the right upper outer quadrant.

Mammogram: Right craniocaudal view. In the upper outer quadrant, there is a relatively well defined, 3×4-cm mass with slight ill definition on some of the borders. Sonography showed the mass to be solid. In a patient of this age, a fibroadenoma would be most likely for a solid well-defined mass. However, because of the strong family history in the patient and the slight ill definition of the anterior margins, the mass was considered to be of moderate suspicion for malignancy.

Histopathology: Atypical medullary carcinoma.

Note: Medullary carcinoma is one of the types of carcinoma that more typically presents as a well-defined mass.

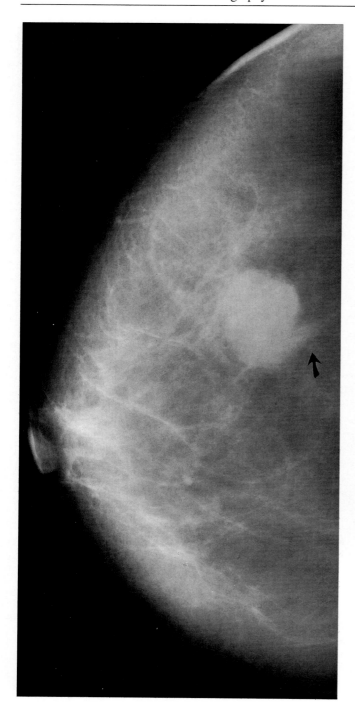

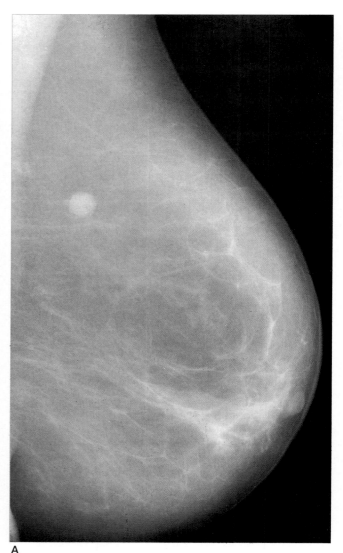

A

Figure 4.72.

Clinical: 66-year-old G1, P1 woman with a family history of breast cancer and a palpable mass in the left upper outer quadrant.

Mammogram: Left craniocaudal view. There is a relatively well defined high-density mass in the outer aspect of the left breast. The axis of the mass is not oriented in the direction of the ducts, and the posterior margin of the lesion is ill defined *(arrow),* making it suspicious mammographically. So-nography showed the mass to be solid.

Impression: Solid mass, favoring carcinoma.

Histopathology: Infiltrating lobular carcinoma, well circum-scribed on gross and microscopic examination.

Figure 4.73.

Clinical: 74-year-old woman with a tender right breast and no palpable findings.

Mammogram: Right oblique (**A**) and craniocaudal (**B**) views and magnified image (**C**). There is a very well defined 1-cm mass in the right upper outer quadrant. A magnified view shows the very well defined margins and fatty halo, suggest-ing a benign nature. Because of the location of the lesion, a primary consideration was an enlarged intramammary lymph node. Other considerations were fibroadenoma, cyst, and well-circumscribed malignancy.

Impression: Well-defined mass of low suspicion for malig-nancy.

Histopathology: Adenoid cystic carcinoma.

Note: The prognosis for a patient with adenoid cystic carci-noma is excellent. Axillary node metastasis is rare, and dis-tant metastases occur in less than 10% of cases.

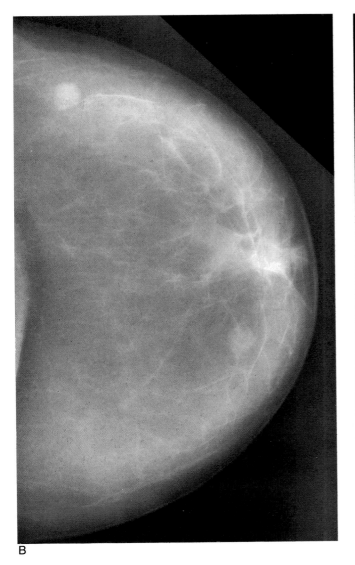

B

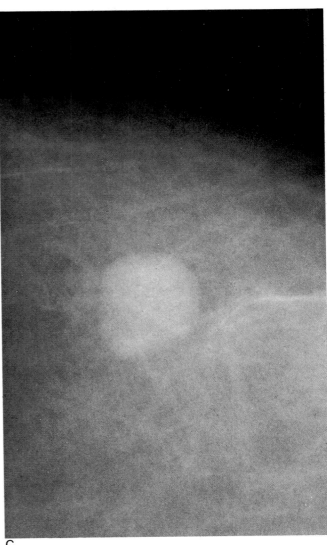

C

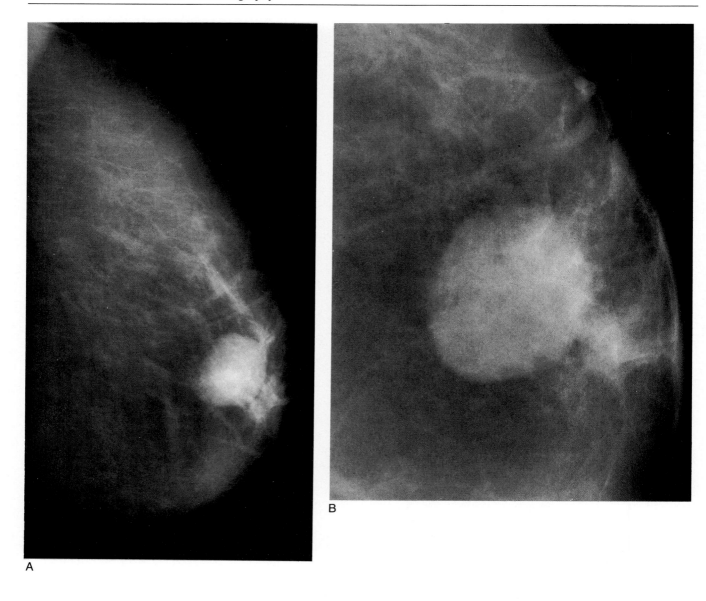

A

B

Figure 4.74.

Clinical: 69-year-old G0 woman with adenocarcinoma in right axillary node.

Mammogram: Right oblique view (**A**) and magnified image (**B**). The breast shows fatty replacement compatible with the age of the patient. There is a relatively well defined, moderately dense 2.5-cm mass in the subareolar area. A magnified image demonstrates fine irregularity of the borders of the le-

sion, rendering it suspicious in nature. Particularly in a patient of this age group, carcinoma is the most likely consideration.

Impression: Well-circumscribed carcinoma, possibly of medullary or mucinous type.

Histopathology: Medullary carcinoma.

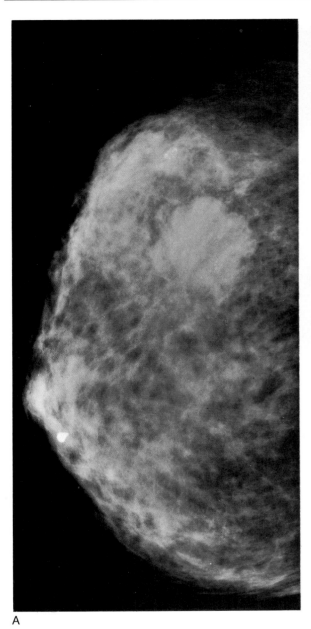

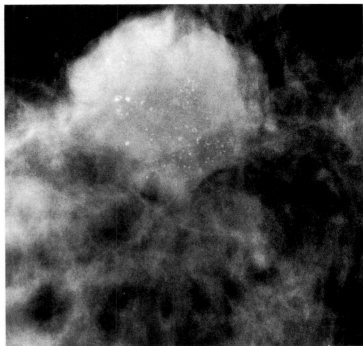

Figure 4.75.

Clinical: Elderly multiparous woman with a hard mass in the left upper outer quadrant.

Mammogram: Left oblique view (**A**) and magnified image (**B**). There is an underlying pattern of prominent ducts and fibroglandular tissue. In the upper outer quadrant of the left breast, there is a relatively well defined but knobby mass containing innumerable microcalcifications (**A**). The borders of the mass are multinodular (**B**), as opposed to the smooth and lobulated contour that might be seen with a fibroadenoma. The features of this lesion are characteristic of malignancy.

Histopathology: Infiltrating ductal carcinoma.

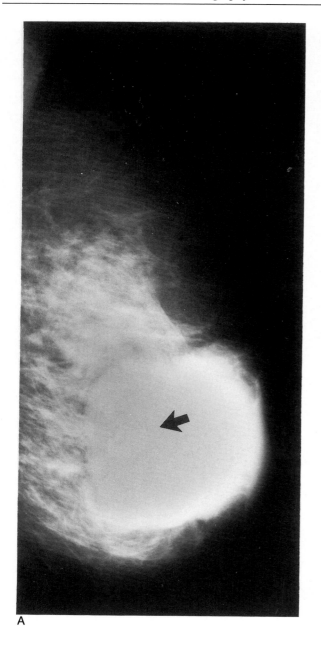

A

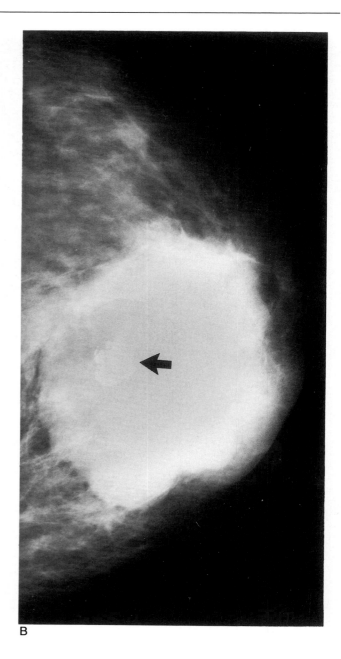

B

Figure 4.76.

Clinical: 73-year-old woman with a large palpable right breast mass.

Mammogram: Right oblique (**A**) and craniocaudal (**B**) views. There is a large, high-density, relatively circumscribed mass in the central aspect of the right breast. The borders of the mass are nodular and poorly defined in areas. A single area of coarse calcification *(arrow)* is present within the lesion.

The differential diagnosis for the mass includes cystosarcoma phylloides, primary breast cancer, and a calcifying fibroadenoma; the favored diagnosis is a cystosarcoma phylloides because of the borders, large size, and the coarse calcification.

Histopathology: Infiltrating ductal carcinoma.

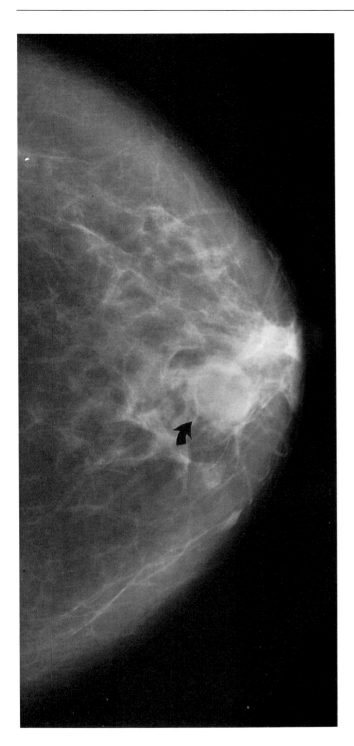

Figure 4.77.

Clinical: 61-year-old woman with a history of ovarian cancer and a firm lump in the right breast.

Mammogram: Right craniocaudal view. There is a 2-cm well-defined radiodense mass *(arrow)* in the right breast at the 12 o'clock position. There is a fatty halo around a portion of the lesion. The primary differential diagnoses include cyst, fibroadenoma, well-defined primary breast cancer, and metastasis to the breast. In a patient of this age, a fibroadenoma would very likely have begun to calcify. Therefore, malignancy, either primary or secondary, is more likely.

Histopathology: Adenocarcinoma metastatic from ovarian primary.

Note: Metastatic disease to the breast may present as a solitary well-defined mass, usually located in the subcutaneous fat layer. More common primary sites for metastases to the breast are melanoma, lymphoma, sarcoma, lung, and gynecologic cancers.

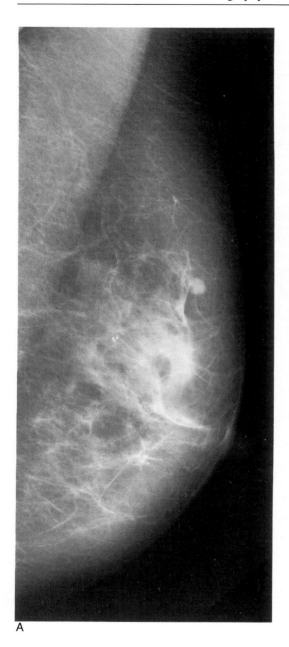

A

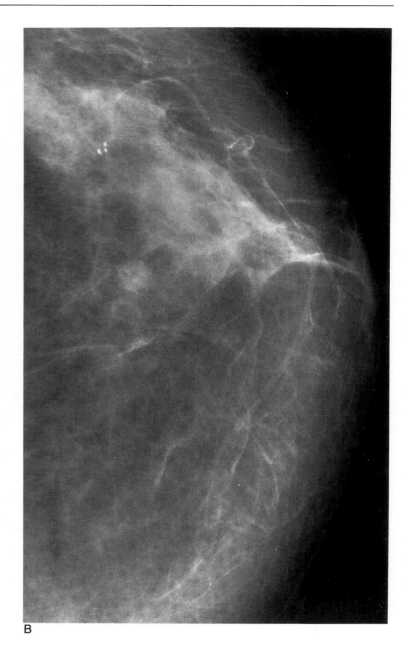

B

Figure 4.78.

Clinical: 69-year-old woman with a history of ovarian cancer and breast cancer, for routine screening.

Mammogram: Right oblique view (**A**), enlarged (2×) cranio-caudal (**B**) view, ultrasound (**C**) from 1988, and right oblique view (**D**) from 1 year earlier. There is a well-circumscribed medium-density 5-mm nodule in the subcutaneous area at the 12 o'clock position (**A** and **B**). The nodule is solid on ultrasound *(arrow)* (**C**) and had developed since the study 1 year earlier ((**D**). Because of the interval change, this nodule

was regarded with a moderate degree of suspicion for malignancy. Although this could represent a primary breast cancer, a metastatic lesion should be considered because of the subcutaneous location.

Impression: New solid nodule, moderately suspicious for malignancy.

Histopathology: Adenocarcinoma metastatic from breast, completely replacing an intramammary node.

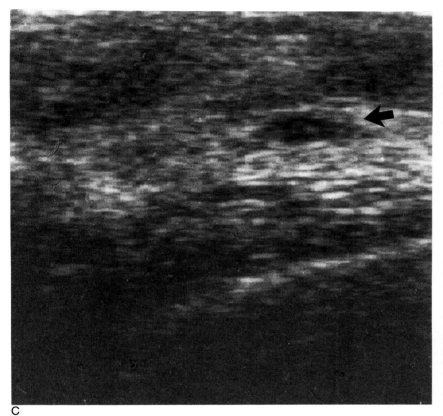

C

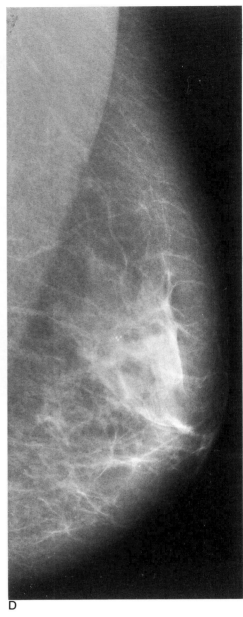

D

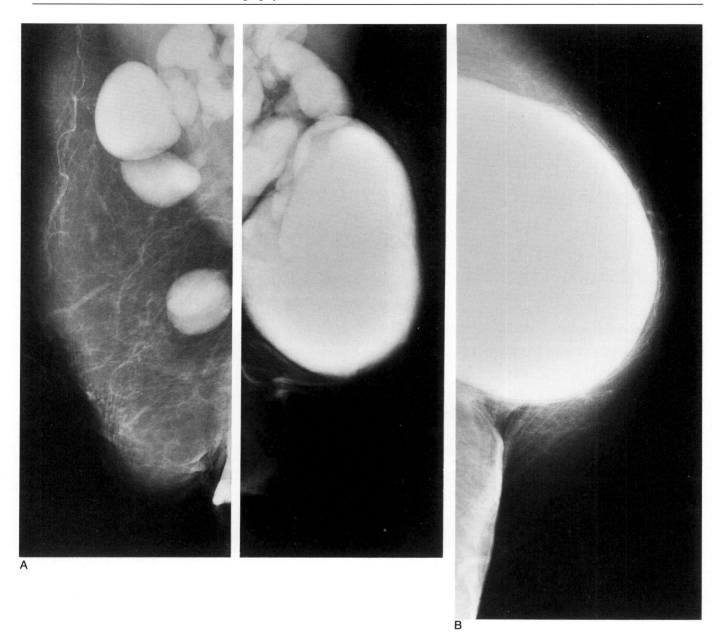

A

B

Figure 4.79.

Clinical: 71-year-old G6, P6 woman with a history of treated lymphoma, presenting with a large indurated mass in the right breast.

Mammogram: Bilateral oblique (**A**) and right oblique cranio-caudal (**B**) views and ultrasound (**C**) of the large right breast mass. The breasts show fatty replacement. Multiple, very well circumscribed, medium- to high-density masses are pre-sented in both axillary tails and axillae. The large mass on the right (**A** and **B**), corresponding to the palpable finding, has a similar appearance, with a halo surrounding all bor-ders. Sonography (**C**) shows the smoothly marginated mass to be hypoechoic, with echogenic strands within it, consis-tent with an enlarged node containing fatty strands. These findings are consistent with recurrence of lymphoma.

Impression: Recurrent lymphoma.

Cytology: Lymphoma.

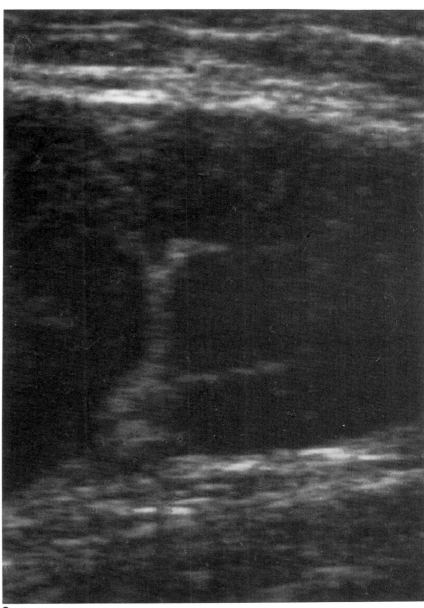

C

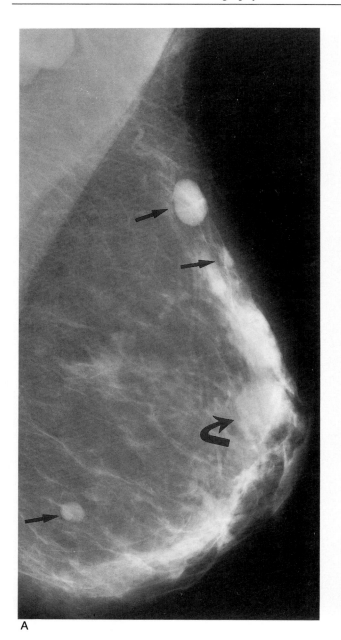

A

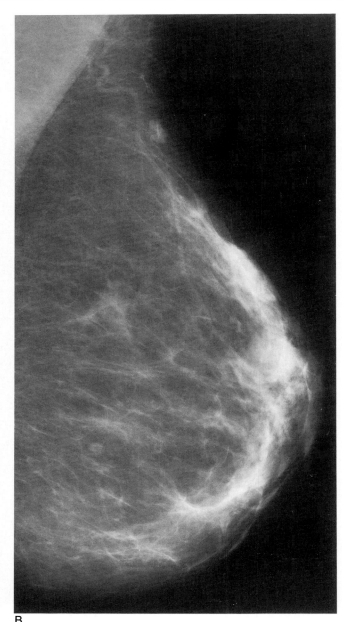

B

Figure 4.80.

Clinical: 45-year-old G3, P3 patient with a history of lymphomas and a palpable nodule in the right retroareolar area.

Mammogram: Right oblique views from April 1989 (**A**) and July 1989 (**B**), after chemotherapy for lymphoma. On the initial study, there are three bean-shaped, very well circumscribed nodules *(straight arrows)* in the right breast, as well as a partially circumscribed, round, medium-density mass *(curved arrow)* in the subareolar area. The subareolar mass was shown to be a simple cyst on ultrasound. The bean-shaped nodules are most consistent with adenopathy related to the patient's known lymphoma. Following chemotherapy (**B**), the nodes decreased in size to a normal range. Mammography may be useful for monitoring the response to chemotherapy in patients in whom there is axillary or intramammary adenopathy.

Impression: Adenopathy secondary to lymphoma.

References

1. Teixidor HS, Kazam E. Combined mammographic-sonographic evaluation of breast masses. AJR 1977;128:409–417.
2. Gershon-Cohen J, Schorr S. The diagnostic problems of isolated circumscribed breast tumors. AJR 1969;106:863–870.
3. Martin JE. Atlas of mammography. Baltimore: Williams & Wilkins, 1982.
4. Wolfe JN. Xeroradiography of the breast. Springfield, IL: Charles C Thomas, 1972.
5. Lane EJ, Proto AV, Phillips TW. Mach bands and density perception. Radiology 1976;121:9–17.
6. Swann CA, Kopans DB, Koerner FC, McCarthy KA, White G, Hall DA. The halo sign and malignant breast lesions. AJR 1978;149:1145–1147.
7. Fournier DV, Weber W, Hoeffken M, Bauer R, Kubli F, Barth V. Growth rate of 147 mammary carcinomas. Cancer 1980;45:2198–2207.
8. Heuser L, Spratt J, Polk H. Growth rates of primary breast cancer. Cancer 1979;43:1888–1894.
9. Meyer JE, Kopans DB. Stability of a mammographic mass: a false sense of security. AJR 1981;137:595–598.
10. Wolfe J. Xeroradiography: uncalcified breast masses. Springfield, IL: Charles C Thomas, 1977.
11. Bassett LW, Gold RH, Cove HC. Mammographic spectrum of traumatic fat necrosis: the fallibility of "pathognomonic" sign of carcinoma. AJR 1978;130:119–122.
12. Leborgne R. Esteato necrosis quistica calcificade de la mama. Torace 1967;16:172–175.
13. Gomez A, Mata JM, Donoso L, Rams A. Galactocele: three distinctive radiographic appearances. Radiology 1986;158:43–44.
14. Salvador R, Salvador M, Jimenez JA, et al. Galactocele of the breast: radiologic and ultrasonographic findings. Br J Radiol 1990;63:140–142.
15. Hessler C, Schnyder P, Ozzello L. Hamartoma of the breast: diagnostic observation of 16 cases. Radiology 1978;126:95–98.
16. Andersson I, Hildell J, Linell F, Ljungqvist U. Mammary hamartomas. Acta Radiol (Diagn) 1979;20:712–720.
17. Ljungqvist U, Andersson I, Hildell J, Linell F. Mammary hamartoma, a benign breast lesion. Acta Chir Scand 1979;145:227–230.
18. Abbitt PL, Shaw de Paredes E, Sloop FB. Breast hamartoma: a mammographic diagnosis. South Med J 1988;8:167–170.
19. Helvie MA, Adler DD, Rebner M, Oberman HA. Breast hamartomas: variable mammographic appearance. Radiology 1989;170:417–421.
20. Kopans DB, Meyer JE, Proppe KH. Ultrasonographic, xeromammographic and histologic correlation of a fibroadenolipoma of the breast. Clin Ultrasound 1982;10:409–411.
21. Andersson I. Mammography in clinical practice. Med Radiogr Photogr 1986;62:2.
22. Egan RL, McSweeney MB. Intramammary lymph nodes. Cancer 1983;51:1838–1842.
23. Andersson I, Marshal L, Nilsson B, Sjoblom KG, Wollheim FA. Abnormal axillary lymph nodes in rheumatoid arthritis. Acta Radiol (Diagn) 1980;21:645–649.
24. Lazarus AA. Sarcoidosis. Otolaryngol Clin North Am 1982;15:621–633.
25. vanDam PA, VanGoethem MLA, Kersschot E, et al. Palpable solid breast masses: retrospective single- and multimodality evaluation of 201 lesions. Radiology 1988;166:435–439.
26. Azzopardi JG. Cystic disease: duct ectasia: fat necrosis: fibrous disease of the breast. In: Problems in breast pathology, vol 11: Major problems in pathology. London: WB Saunders, 1979.
27. Gershon-Cohen J, Ingleby H. Roentgenography of cysts of the breast. Surg Gynecol Obstet 1953;97:483–489.
28. Mitnick JS, Vazquez MF, Harris MN, et al. Invasive papillary carcinoma of the breast: mammographic appearance. Radiology 1990;177:803–806.
29. Hoeffken W, Lanyi M. Fibroadenoma. In: Mammography. Philadelphia: WB Saunders, 1977.
30. McDivitt RW, Stewart FW, Berg JW. Tumors of the breast. Bethesda, MD: Armed Forces Institute of Pathology, 1968.
31. Gershon-Cohen J, Ingleby H. Roentgenography of fibroadenoma of the breast. Radiology 1952;59:77–87.
32. Fornage BD, Lorigan JG, Andry E. Fibroadenoma of the breast: sonographic appearance. Radiology 1989;172:671–675.
33. Buzanowski-Konakry K, Harrison EG, Payne WS. Lobular carcinoma arising in fibroadenoma of the breast. Cancer 1975;35:450–456.
34. McDivitt RW, Stewart FW, Farrow JH. Breast carcinoma arising in solitary fibroadenomas. Surg Gynecol Obstet 1967;125:572–576.
35. Baker KS, Monsees BS, Diaz NM, et al. Carcinoma within fibroadenomas: mammographic features. Radiology 1990;176:371–374.
36. Hajdu SI, Espinosa MH, Robbins GF. Recurrent cystosarcoma phylloides: a clinicopathologic study of 32 cases. Cancer 1976;38:1402–1406.
37. D'Orsi CJ, Feldhaus L, Sonnenfeld M. Unusual lesions of the breast. Radiol Clin North Am 1983;21:67–80.
38. Haagensen CD. Cystosarcoma phylloides. In: Diseases of the breast. Philadelphia: WB Saunders, 1986.
39. Gershon-Cohen J, Moore L. Roentgenography of giant fibroadenoma of the breast (cystosarcoma phylloides). Radiology 1960;74:619–625.
40. Azzopardi JG. Breast sarcomas. In: Breast pathology, vol 11: Major problems in pathology. London: WB Saunders, 1979.
41. Haagenson CD. Solitary intraductal papilloma. In: Diseases of the breast. Philadelphia: WB Saunders, 1986.
42. Moskowitz M. The predictive value of certain mammographic signs in screening for breast cancer. Cancer 1983;51:1007–1011.
43. Marsteller LP, Shaw de Paredes E. Well defined masses in the breast. RadioGraphics 1989;9(1):13–37.
44. Sickles EA. Mammographic features of 300 consecutive nonpalpable breast cancers. AJR 1986;146:661–663.
45. Mitnick JS, Roses DF, Harris MN, Feiner HD. Circumscribed intraductal carcinoma of the breast. Radiology 1989;170:423–425.
46. D'Orsi CJ, Weissman BNW, Berkowitz DM, Stay EJ. Cor-

relation of xeroradiography and histology of breast disease. CRC Crit Rev Diagn Imaging 1978;11:75–119.

47. Martin J. Malignant breast masses. In: Atlas of mammography. Baltimore: Williams & Williams, 1982.

48. Azzopardi JC. Special variants of carcinoma. In: Problems in breast pathology, vol 11: Major problems in pathology. London: WB Saunders, 1979.

49. Meyer JE, Amin E, Lindfors KK, et al. Medullary carcinoma of the breast: mammographic and US appearance. Radiology 1989;170:79–82.

50. Hajdu SI, Urban JA. Cancers metastatic to the breast. Cancer 1972;29:1691–1696.

51. Toombs BD, Kalisher L. Metastatic disease to the breast: clinical, pathologic, and radiographic features. AJR 1977;129:673–676.

52. Bohman LG, Bassett LW, Gold RH, Voet R. Breast metastases from extramammary malignancies. Radiology 1982;144:309–312.

53. McCrea ES, Johnston C, Haney PJ. Metastases to the breast. AJR 1983;141:685–690.

54. Kovi J, Chu HB, Leefall L. Sclerosing lobular hyperplasia manifesting as a palpable mass of the breast in young black women. Hum Pathol 1984;15:336–340.

ILL-DEFINED MASSES

An irregularly marginated mass on mammography is a primary sign of breast carcinoma. The majority of breast carcinomas have an infiltrative, irregular appearance with spiculation (1). A variety of benign lesions, including fibrocystic changes (fibrosis, cysts, hyperplasia), radial scars, fat necrosis, hematomas, abscesses, and plasma cell mastitis, and scar may also present as an ill-defined mass radiographically. Clinical history and physical examination may be of help, in addition to the mammographic findings, in differentiating these lesions. However, in many cases, biopsy is necessary to confirm the etiology of a poorly defined mammographic lesion.

It is important to determine that an ill-defined lesion can be identified on two projections. Overlying glandular tissue can be visualized on one projection as an irregular density but on the orthogonal view is seen to disperse (Figs. 5.1 and 5.2). If a density has a similar configuration on two projections, more complete evaluation is necessary. Spot compression views of the lesion may be of help in evaluating its central density and in displacing the surrounding glandular tissue. The presence of a radiolucent center within a poorly defined density suggests a fibrocystic process as a likely etiology (2), but it is not confirmatory.

Secondary signs of malignancy, such as architectural distortion or microcalcifications associated with an irregular mass, are highly suspicious for carcinoma. Even without secondary signs, if an irregular mass has a high-density center and fine surrounding spicules, it is regarded as suspicious for carcinoma.

Fibrocystic Disease

Sclerosing adenosis is a form of fibrocystic disease characterized by a proliferation of lobules with surrounding fibrous sclerosis (3). When the condition is localized, it may masquerade as cancer mammographically and has been confused with carcinoma on histologic examination. In the early stages, there is a florid proliferation of epithelial cells, which in later stages is followed by a stromal fibrosis in which coalescence of adjacent lobules produces areas of fibroepithelial proliferation and loss of normal lobular architecture (1). If the process is diffuse, the mammographic finding is diffuse; small nodules with increased-density microcalcifi-

cations may be present. If the condition is localized, a mass with ill-defined margins is often seen (1). In a series of 27 cases of sclerosing adenosis, Nielsen and Nielsen (4) reported an irregular density as the most frequent finding, but circumscribed and stellate masses were also seen. Although the density of the center of an area of sclerosing adenosis may not be as great as that of a malignancy and the spicules may not radiate completely around the lesion, it is often impossible on mammography to differentiate such an area with certainty from a carcinoma (Fig. 5.3).

Focal fibrocystic changes of a variety of forms may appear as ill-defined lesions (Figs. 5.4–5.9). Focal fibrosis is a benign condition in which there is dense stromal fibrous tissue without cyst or epithelial changes (5). On mammography, fibrosis appears as dense tissue that is often irregularly marginated (6). Irregular microcalcifications may be associated with fibrosis and may occasionally simulate carcinoma. Although biopsy is often necessary to confirm the nature of the lesion, the lack of fine linear surrounding tendrils around the border of the lesion might suggest malignancy as a less likely diagnosis. An area of epithelial hyperplasia or atypical hyperplasia may similarly present in a variety of ways, including as an ill-defined mass. Even a cyst or collection of cysts associated with surrounding fibrous stroma or inflammation may appear as an ill-defined lesion.

Radial Scar

Radial scar is a rosette-like proliferative breast lesion (7) that has also been described as sclerosing papillary proliferation (8), benign sclerosing ductal proliferation (9), nonencapsulated sclerosing lesion (10), infiltrating epitheliosis, and indurative mastopathy (11). The lesion has been confused with cancer by mammographers (12) and pathologists.

In a study of 32 cases of radial scar, Andersen and Gram (7) found most lesions to be small (mean diameter of 7 mm) and in a stellate configuration. On histology, a fibroelastic center is surrounded by lobules and ducts radiating outward. In 93% of cases, either papillomatosis or a benign epithelial proliferation was present. Small round microcalcifications were seen in 63% of cases (7). Because of the presence of elastosis with sclerosis and ductal distortion, a pseudoinfiltrative pattern occurs, and the lesion may be confused with carcinoma histologically (11).

There is debate as to whether this lesion represents a premalignant lesion (10) or not (7, 8, 11). Fisher et al. (10) raised the concern that the lesion may represent an incipient form of tubular carcinoma. In an average follow-up of 19.5 years of 32 patients treated with local excision of radial scar, Andersen and Gram (7) found no significant increase in the incidence of breast cancer, however.

On mammography, a radial scar is an ill-defined lesion that produces retraction and distortion of surrounding structures (13). Microcalcifications may be associated with radial scar. Mitnick et al. (14) found mammography to be unreliable in differentiating radial scar from infiltrating carcinomas; of 73 nonpalpable stellate cancers, 19% had mammographic features of radial scar, but calcifications were more commonly associated with carcinomas. The presence of small radiolucencies with the lesion are more in favor of a radial scar than of malignancy (2), but histologic examination is necessary to confirm the diagnosis (13, 14) (Figs. 5.10–5.13).

Posttraumatic Changes

Fat necrosis is a nonsuppurative inflammatory response to trauma. Particularly if the area is associated with a desmoplastic reaction, fat necrosis may be confused with carcinoma on clinical examination. One manifestation of fat necrosis mammographically is an irregular mass that simulates carcinoma (1). Thickening and retraction of overlying skin may occur. On histologic examination of an area of fat necrosis, fibrous connective tissue proliferates at the periphery of the necrotic debris. The extent of fibrous response correlates with the mammographic image. A marked response may appear on mammography as a spiculated mass resembling carcinoma, whereas a mild response occurs when a thin-walled radiolucent oil cyst is seen (15). Correlation with clinical history is key in suggesting the presence of fat necrosis. The history of a recent biopsy or severe blunt trauma in the area of abnormality should alert one to the possibility of fat necrosis (Figs. 5.14–5.20).

If there is any doubt about the location of a spiculated mass relative to a surgical scar, lead markers or a wire should be placed over the scar and the film repeated.

Intraparenchymal scars after biopsy appear as poorly defined masses, often with spiculated margins (16). Scars are imaged more frequently in the first 6 months after biopsy and are less prominent after several years (17). A feature of fat necrosis or scars that may help to differentiate them from cancers on mammography is that fat necrosis tends to have a different configuration and density on the orthogonal views of the breast. In patients who have undergone lumpectomy and radiation therapy for treatment of primary breast carci-

noma, fat necrosis at the surgical site may resemble recurrent carcinoma (18, 19). In these patients it is particularly useful to have a mammogram after surgery, before radiation therapy is started (20), to serve as a basis for future comparisons of the irregular density that may be present at the lumpectomy site.

An acute response to trauma, such as a hematoma, may also appear as an ill-defined lesion, although a relatively well-defined mass or a diffuse increase in density is more commonly seen. Another radiographic feature of a hematoma that may simulate a cancer is the overlying skin thickening from the edema and bruising. Hematomas tend to resolve over a period of 3–4 weeks (13) (Figs. 5.21 and 5.22) but may occasionally persist for a longer time, particularly if they are of a large size.

Abscess

A breast abscess is often suspected on clinical examination because of the very tender, red, hot indurated area. Abscesses tend to occur in lactating breasts. If a lesion having the clinical appearance of an abscess is found in a nonlactating patient, it should be regarded with suspicion. Most abscesses occur in the subareolar area (13), and skin and areolar thickening may be present (Fig. 5.23). Because of the extreme tenderness and the level of clinical suspicion in patients with breast abscesses, mammography may not be performed in the acute stages. The clinical appearance of a breast abscess may be difficult to differentiate from an inflammatory carcinoma, and aspiration is usually performed in the acute stages. Mammography is necessary after therapy to evaluate the remainder of the breast. In an older patient, in particular, abscesses are not common and may be associated with a nearby malignancy or a papilloma obstructing a duct.

A chronic abscess, although associated at times with some thickening and induration of the skin, does not present with the redness and tenderness found in the acute stages. A chronic abscess is usually imaged as an ill-defined lesion that may be associated with skin thickening. Sonography may reveal an irregular fluid-filled mass with debris (Fig. 5.24).

Plasma Cell Mastitis

Another cause of an ill-defined mass on mammography is plasma cell mastitis (1). This ductal and periductal inflammatory process occurs in the subareolar areas and tends to be bilateral. Mammographically, a prominent ductal pattern may be seen, or the subareolar area may be involved with an irregular fan-shaped density. In the later stages of plasma cell mastitis, typical benign ductal and periductal calcifications occur.

Granular Cell Myoblastoma

Myoblastoma is a benign tumor that occurs in the tongue or subcutaneous tissues (21), and only 5–6% of myoblastomas occur in the breast (22). The patient often presents with a firm palpable lump that may be suspicious for malignancy on clinical examination. On mammography, a stellate or irregular lesion (21, 22) (Figs. 5.25 and 5.26) having a malignant appearance is seen. These lesions are benign but locally infiltrative and are treated with excision.

Fibromatosis

A rare cause of an ill-defined lesion of the breast is fibromatosis (23). This is a fibroblastic lesion that behaves in a locally invasive but nonmetastasizing manner and may be associated with trauma (24). Also known as desmoid tumors, fibromatosis can occur elsewhere, particularly in the abdominal wall. The involvement of the breast is thought to represent an extension from the pectoralis fascia (23). The ill-defined mass of fibromatosis has an appearance similar to that of carcinoma (Fig. 5.27), namely, a poorly defined or irregular mass.

Carcinoma

A classic appearance of primary breast carcinoma is an ill-defined mass. The density of the lesion is as dense as or more dense than the parenchyma. Fine linear tendrils extend around the border of the lesion (25, 26). These findings are related to the growth patterns of infiltrating carcinomas. Gross examination of these tumors reveals a firm, white, gritty mass with tendrils radiating into the adjacent breast tissue. Histologic examination shows nests and cords of malignant cells associated with fibrous stroma infiltrating into the normal breast tissue (1).

On physical examination, carcinomas usually are palpated as larger than they appear on mammography, because of the surrounding spiculation and reaction. The fine extensions of tumor cells into the surrounding tissue and the fibrotic, desmoplastic reaction account for the larger palpable mass than is evident mammographically (27).

Although an intraductal carcinoma occasionally presents mammographically as a spiculated mass (Figs. 5.28–5.30), this finding is more typical of infiltrating breast cancers. Infiltrating ductal carcinoma accounts for the largest group of malignant mammary tumors and comprises 70–80% of breast malignancies (28). Infiltrating ductal carcinomas can generally be divided into two categories based on their gross appearance: stellate or circumscribed. Tumors that are stellate in configuration have been found to be more likely associated with axillary metastases than are circumscribed tumors (28, 29). Infiltrating ductal carcinomas more typically have the sunburst appearance and the fibrotic response that lends

the name "scirrhous" to these lesions (Figs. 5.31–5.47). Scirrhous carcinomas have a marked amount of fibrous stroma and elastosis, accounting for some of the spiculation seen on mammography.

Other variants of intensive ductal carcinoma include: tubular, medullary, mucinous, metaplastic, adenoid cystic, and colloid carcinomas (28). Tubular (well-differentiated) carcinoma is characterized microscopically by neoplastic elements that resemble normal breast ductules (28). An uncommon form of invasive breast cancer, tubular carcinoma, has a typical appearance of a stellate mass (Fig. 5.48). Tubular carcinomas tend to be detected when small (<1 cm) (30). These lesions are characterized histologically by orderly, elongated tubules arranged in an irregular radiating manner and infiltrating into the surrounding parenchyma (30). There is a marked desmoplastic reaction (30, 31). The lesion must be distinguished microscopically from sclerosing adenosis, which it resembles (28). There has been controversy as to whether (32) or not (33) tubular carcinomas may arise from radial scars. On mammography, a stellate spiculated lesion is seen (30) but may not necessarily have a high-density center, which is more characteristic of malignancy. Medullary carcinoma accounts for about 5% of all breast cancers (28) and tends to be a relatively circumscribed rather than a spiculated lesion (Fig. 5.49). Mucinous or colloid carcinomas represent about 1–2% of breast carcinomas and, like medullary carcinomas, are well circumscribed (28).

Infiltrating lobular carcinomas, representing 3–4% of all breast malignancies, are characterized by a linear arrangement of tumor cells (Indian-file pattern), a tendency to grow circumferentially around ducts and lobules, and an accompanying desmoplastic reaction (28). Bilaterality and multicentricity are twice as common in patients with infiltrating lobular carcinoma than in patients with infiltrating ductal carcinoma (34).

Occasionally, infiltrating lobular carcinomas may produce a scirrhous response (27). A spiculated lesion may extend through the subcutaneous fat to the skin, tethering it and producing the dimpling or puckering noted as secondary signs of malignancy. More often, however, the mammographic appearance is that of a subtle derangement of parenchymal architecture (35). Mendelson et al. (35) found that microcalcifications occurred in 25% of patients with lobular carcinoma, but the pattern of calcification was nonspecific (Figs. 5.50 and 5.51).

In the assessment of nonpalpable breast carcinomas detected by mammography, Sickles (36) found that very small cancers were commonly poorly defined rather than being spiculated, which is characteristic of larger malignancies. Magnification mammography can be of help in better demonstrating the borders of these tiny lesions (37). A small carcinoma may be difficult to detect in a dense breast because of the overlying glandular tissue. Associated distortion of architecture characterized by retraction or puckering of the parenchyma may be the only indication of an underlying carcinoma (36). Placing the breast with the area of retraction in tangent to the beam or performing a spot compression view of the area of distortion may be of help in demonstrating the underlying lesion.

Other Malignancies

An unusual form of infiltrating ductal carcinoma is metaplastic carcinoma. These tumors may have squamous or pseudosarcomatous changes (28). Those tumors with pseudosarcomatous metaplasia may contain areas of cartilage or bone formation and are demonstrated mammographically as unusual patterns of calcification.

Lymphoma of the breast presents as a diffuse increase in density of the breast or as nodules that are either well circumscribed or poorly defined but are not spiculated (38). Other features of lymphoma include enlarged axillary nodes. Calcifications are not associated with masses (Fig. 5.52).

When a nodular density with poorly defined borders or a stellate lesion is found on mammography, the lesion has a high positive predictive value for carcinoma (39). Unless an ill-defined lesion is clearly a scar or area of fat necrosis, biopsy is usually necessary to confirm or exclude malignancy.

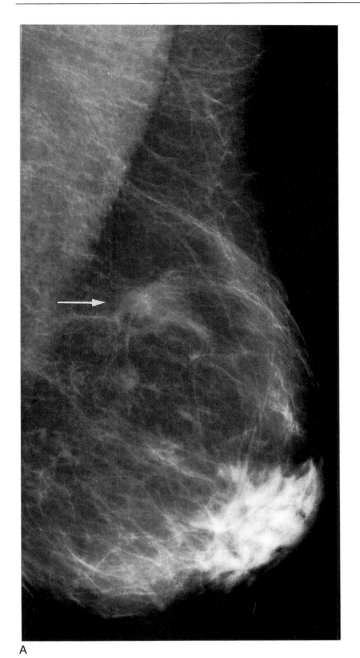

A

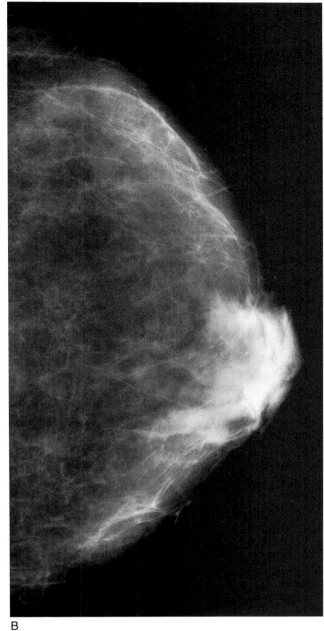

B

Figure 5.1.

Clinical: 55-year-old woman without palpable abnormalities, for screening.

Mammogram: Right oblique (**A**) and craniocaudal (**B**) views. On the oblique view (**A**), there is a prominent focal area of increased density in the upper aspect of the right breast *(arrow)*. On the craniocaudal view (**B**), no similar density is seen. The finding on the oblique view represents overlapping glan-

dular tissue. When an area of asymmetric tissue is seen, it is important that it is identified on two views before it is considered abnormal. Also, clinical examination is important for correlation with a large area of asymmetry on mammography.

Impression: Overlapping glandular tissue simulating a mass on one view.

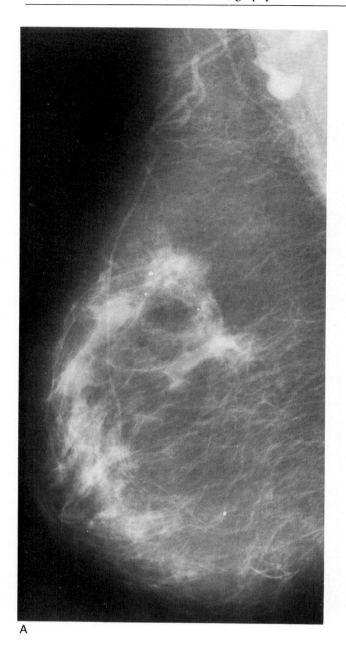

A

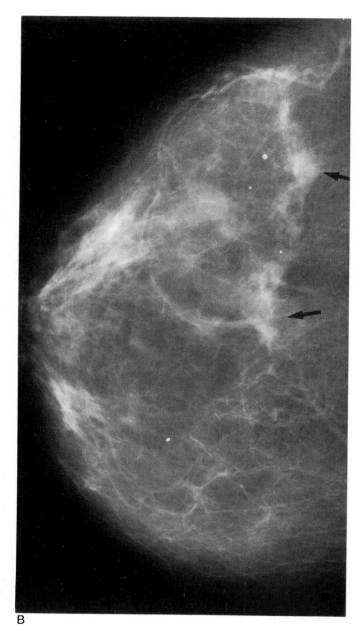

B

Figure 5.2.

Clinical: 63-year-old G3, P3 woman for routine screening.

Mammogram: Left oblique (**A**), craniocaudal (**B**), and mediolateral (**C**) views. On the initial oblique (**A**) and craniocaudal (**B**) views, there is focal dense glandular tissue in the upper outer quadrant. Particularly on the craniocaudal view (**B**), the appearance is that of two spiculated lesions (arrows). Be-

cause of this an additional mediolateral view (**C**) was performed and shows the densities to represent telescoping of tissue and not actual mass lesions. This tissue was unchanged from the earlier outside mammograms.

Impression: Superimposing glandular tissue simulating a breast lesion.

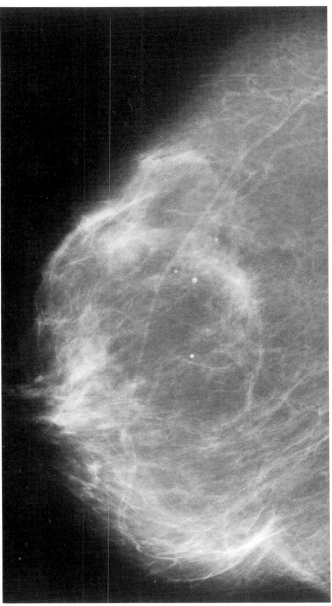

C

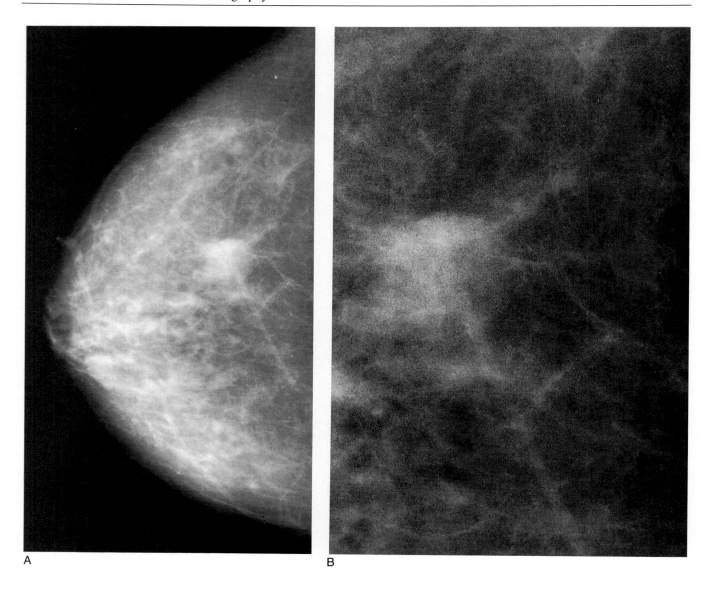

A   B

Figure 5.3.

Clinical: 52-year-old woman with no palpable findings.

Mammogram: Left craniocaudal view (**A**) and magnified image (**B**). The breast is moderately dense. There is an ill-defined 2-cm mass of moderately high density in the outer aspect of the breast. A coned-down image shows the irregularity of the margins but lack of fine surrounding spicula-tions that would be more characteristic of malignancy. This finding suggests more likely a fibrocystic etiology.

Impression: Ill-defined mass, more likely fibrocystic; malignancy cannot be excluded.

Histopathology: Sclerosing adenosis with epithelial hyperplasia.

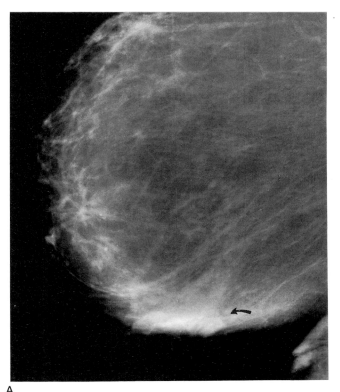

A

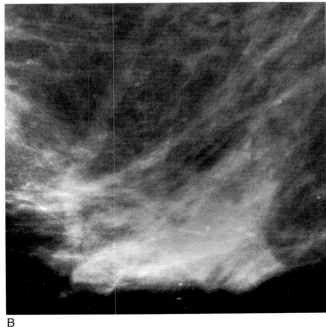

B

Figure 5.4.

Clinical: 61-year-old woman for screening.

Mammogram: Left mediolateral view (**A**) and magnified image (**B**). In the left lower quadrant (**A**), there is a moderately high density, ill-defined, 1.5 × 2.5-cm mass containing microcalcifications *(arrow)*. Although the borders are ill defined, the spiculation is not surrounding the area in radiating strands

(**B**). The microcalcifications are nonspecific. The findings are of mild suspicion for malignancy, and the favored diagnosis was fibrocystic change, possibly sclerosing adenosis.

Histopathology: Fibrocystic disease, intraductal papillomatosis, ductal hyperplasia.

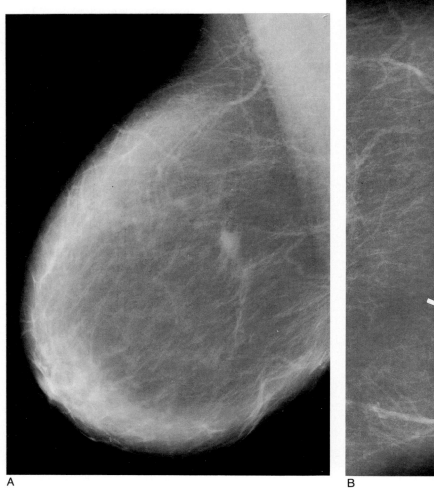

A

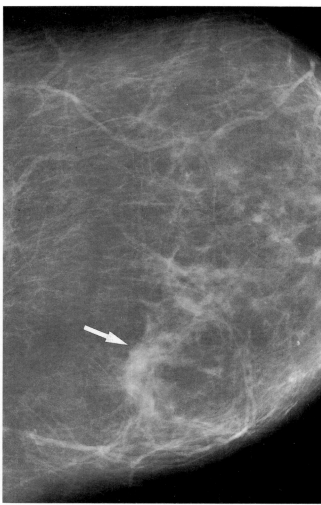

B

Figure 5.5.

Clinical: 61-year-old asymptomatic woman for a screening mammogram.

Mammogram: Left oblique (**A**) and craniocaudal (**B**) views. The breast shows relatively fatty replacement. In the upper outer quadrant, there is an ill-defined mass of moderate to high density with a dense center and fairly coarse spiculation

(arrow). This has a similar appearance on the oblique (**A**) and craniocaudal (**B**) views, suggesting that it is not superimposition of normal glandular structures.

Impression: Moderately suspicious, ill-defined mass: carcinoma versus focal fibrocystic disease.

Histopathology: Fibrocystic changes, fibrosis.

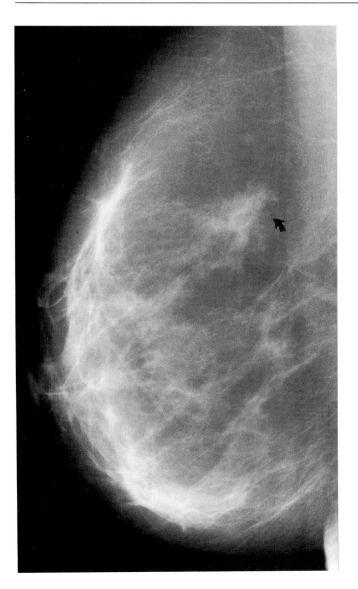

Figure 5.6.

Clinical: 35-year-old G2, P2 woman with a family history of breast cancer in a sister and a normal clinical examination.

Mammogram: Left oblique view. There is an irregular spiculated area of increased density in the upper outer quadrant *(arrow)*. This lesion lies posterior to the remainder of the parenchyma, but its density is no greater than that of the glandular tissue. The margins are irregular, but the spicules do not surround it in its entirety as might be expected in malignancy.

Impression: Ill-defined mass of mild to moderate suspicion for malignancy.

Histopathology: Fibrosis.

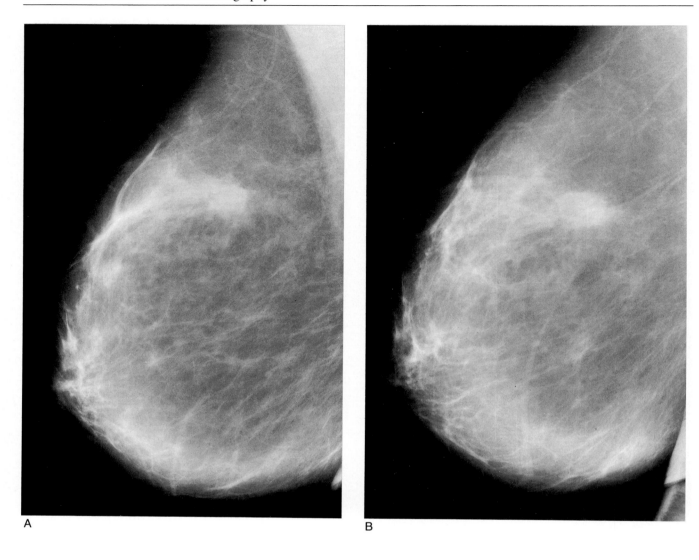

A

B

Figure 5.7.

Clinical: 59-year-old woman with a family history of breast cancer.

Mammogram: Left oblique (**A**) and mediolateral (**B**) views. There is a 2-cm irregular lesion in the left upper outer quadrant of a density greater than that of the parenchyma. There are a few lucencies within the nodule that might suggest that

it is benign; however, because of the overall density and irregular margins, biopsy was performed.

Impression: Irregular lesion, left breast, of mild to moderate suspicion for malignancy.

Histopathology: Microglandular adenosis.

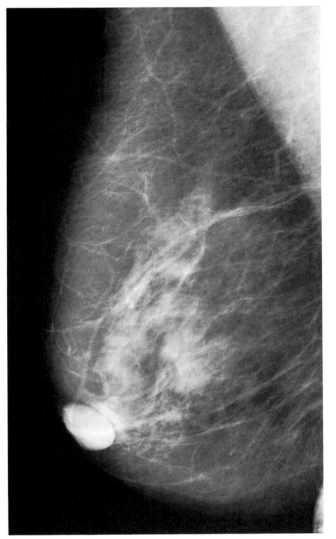
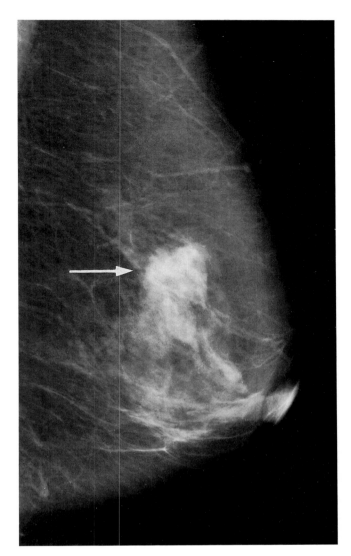

A

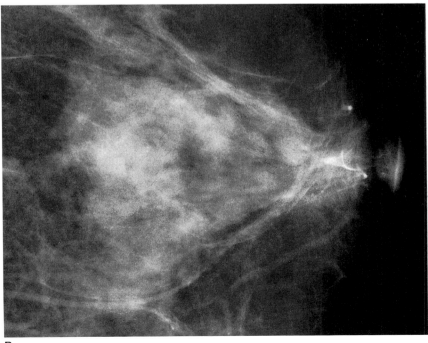

B

Figure 5.8.

Clinical: 74-year-old G2, P2 woman for screening mammography.

Mammogram: Bilateral oblique views (**A**) and magnified image (**B**). There is a prominent ill-defined area of asymmetric tissue in the right supra-areolar area *(arrow)* (**A**). The area is of heterogeneous density (**B**) and, although ill-defined, is not spiculated or distorting the architecture, all features of benignity.

Impression: Ill-defined asymmetry of low suspicion for carcinoma.

Histopathology: Fibrosis.

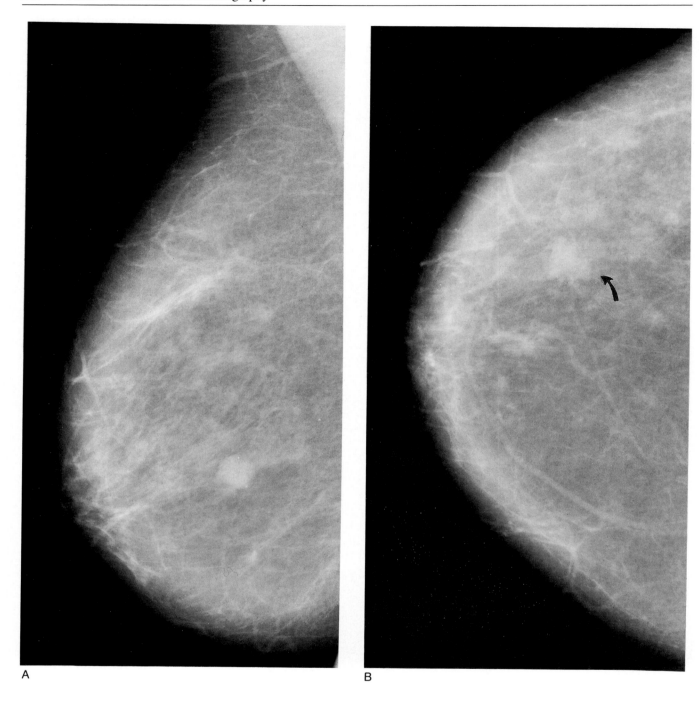

A

B

Figure 5.9.

Clinical: 65-year-old woman for routine screening. Her last mammogram was 4 years previously and was unremarkable.

Mammogram: Left oblique (**A**) and craniocaudal (**B**) views. There is a 1-cm high-density mass in the middle outer aspect of the left breast. On the oblique view the mass appears somewhat well defined, but on the craniocaudal view its margins are much more irregular *(arrow)* (**B**). Sonography showed no cyst in the area of the mass. The mass had appeared

since the previous mammogram, and because of the interval changes as well as the high density and irregular margins of the mass, it was considered of high suspicion for carcinoma.

Histopathology: Fibrocystic changes, ductal hyperplasia.

Note: On histopathologic evaluation the mass represented numerous tiny cystic areas surrounded by dense fibrosis with an area of epithelial hyperplasia.

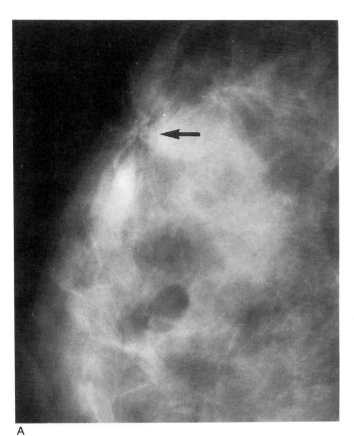

A

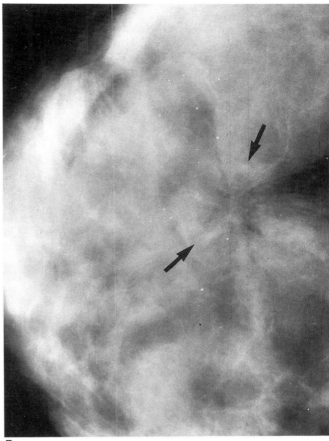

B

Figure 5.10.

Clinical: 30-year-old woman with a positive family history of breast cancer and no palpable findings.

Mammogram: Left enlarged (2×) mediolateral (**A**) and craniocaudal (**B**) views. The background parenchymal pattern is dense and glandular. There is a focal area of architectural distortion *(arrows)* in the 12 o'clock position of the breast, having the appearance of a spiculated lesion. This lesion has a radiolucent center and is associated with some adjacent lobular-type microcalcifications. The differential includes radial scar versus carcinoma; radial scar is favored because of the central lucency.

Histopathology: Radial scar.

Figure 5.11.

Clinical: 39-year-old G1, P1 patient with a clinical history of fibrocystic breasts, for screening.

Mammogram: Right oblique (**A**) and mediolateral magnification (1.5×) (**B**) views. The breast is dense, compatible with the age of the patient. In the upper outer quadrant, there is a 3-cm area of architectural distortion *(arrows)* (**A**) associated with a few microcalcifications *(arrowhead)* (**B**). The lesion is of similar density to the background but has an irregular spiculated margin. The lack of a palpable finding corresponding to a lesion of this size on mammography would decrease the level of suspicion for malignancy from high to moderate. The differential includes radial scar, carcinoma, and sclerosing adenosis.

Impression: Ill-defined density moderately suspicious for malignancy.

Histopathology: Radial scar, fibrocystic change with focal severe atypia.

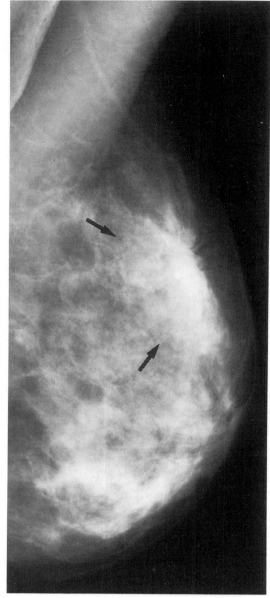

A

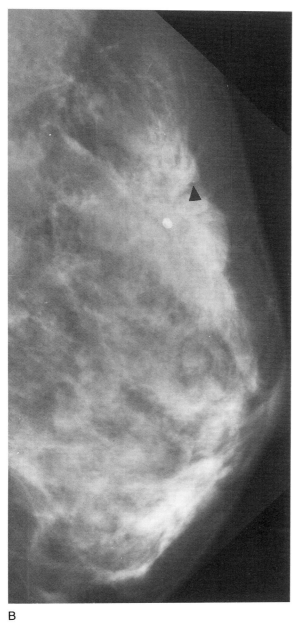

B

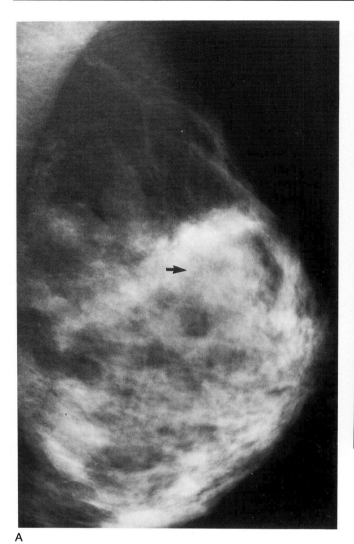

A

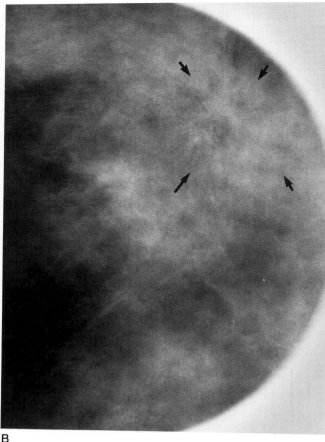

B

Figure 5.12.

Clinical: 45-year-old G2, P2 woman with a history of nodular breasts, for routine mammography. She had no history of breast biopsy.

Mammogram: Right oblique view (**A**), spot compression craniocaudal view (**B**), specimen film (**C**), and histopathology at 10× (**D**) and at 60× (**E**). The breast is very dense for the patient's age and parity. In the upper aspect on the oblique view (**A**), there is a focal spiculated area of architectural distortion *(arrow)*. On spot compression (**B**), the lesion persists and is found to have a central lucency surrounded by dense spicules *(arrows)*. The finding suggests a radial scar as the most likely diagnosis. The central lucency on spot compression is key to suggesting this diagnosis. However, carcino-mas may occasionally have this appearance, and therefore, a biopsy was recommended. The specimen film (**C**) for the needle localization demonstrates well the spiculated lesion *(arrow)*. On the specimen film the lesion appears more dense, and the central lucency is not evident.

Impression: Spiculated lesion, favoring radial scar.

Histopathology: Radial scar, sclerosing adenosis. At 10× magnification the stellate appearance of the lesion is evident. There is a spokewheel pattern of central fibrosis interposed with epithelial proliferation. At high power (60×) there are haphazardly arranged ductules within bands of fibrous tissue. Focal calcification is present in a ductule *(arrow)*.

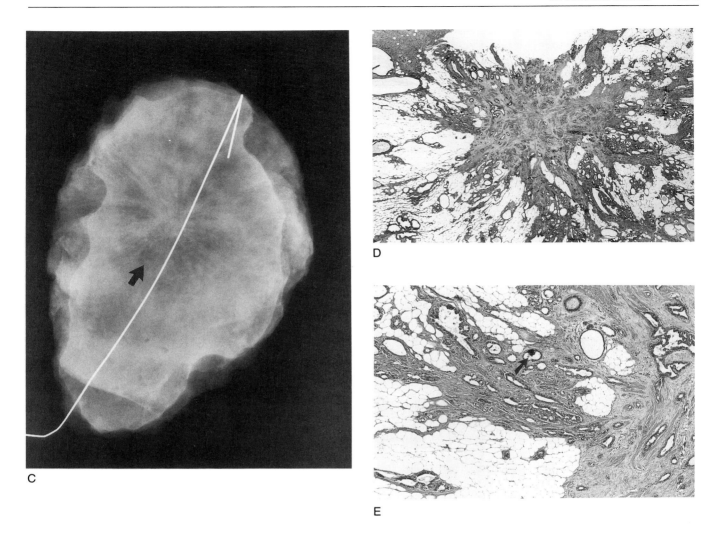

C

D

E

Figure 5.13.

Clinical: 73-year-old woman for screening mammography.

Mammogram: Right oblique view (**A**) and magnified image (**B**). There is a small ill-defined density *(arrow)* deep in the breast near the chest wall. Magnification of this lesion shows irregular margination and the presence of microcalcifications. The differential includes carcinoma, hyperplasia, other fibrocystic changes, and radial scar.

Histopathology: Radial scar.

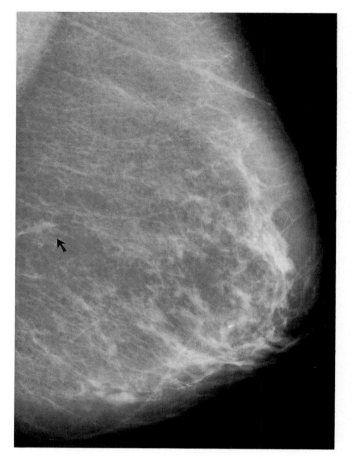

A

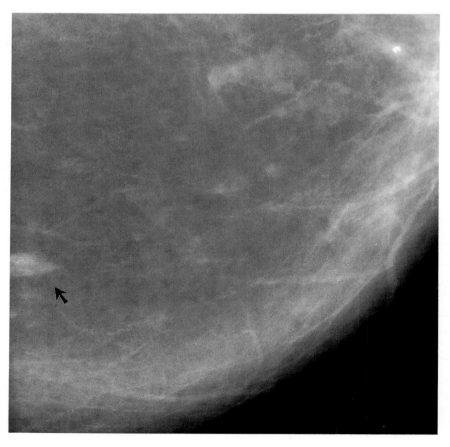

B

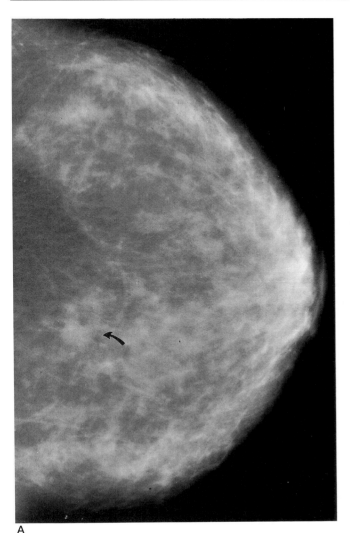

A

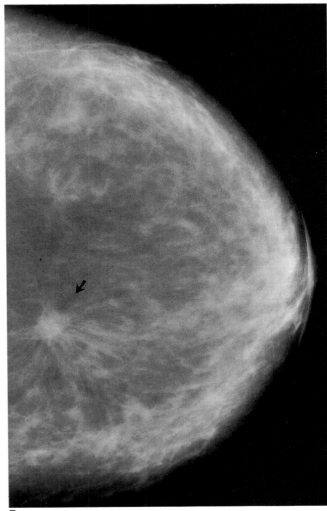

B

Figure 5.14.

Clinical: 50-year-old woman with a family history of breast cancer, 6 months after a right breast biopsy for microcalcifications. Specimen films had confirmed removal of the suspicious area, and the histopathologic diagnosis was fibrocystic disease without atypia.

Mammogram: Right craniocaudal view, October 1986 (**A**); right craniocaudal view, June 1987 (**B**). There is diffuse nodularity present (**A**) with a focal area of increased density with microcalcifications *(arrow)* in the inner quadrant. This area

was removed after needle localization. On the follow-up film 8 months later (**B**) in the area of previous biopsy *(arrow)*, there is a moderately high density spiculated mass. Long tendrils surround the lesion and produce a suspicious appearance. However, because of the clinical history, the area is most consistent with fat necrosis and scar. The area diminished in size on follow-up mammograms.

Impression: Fat necrosis.

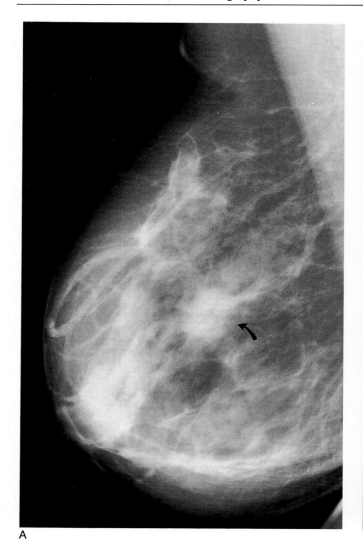

A

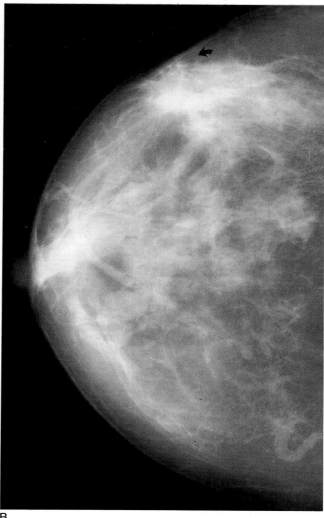

B

Figure 5.15.

Clinical: 58-year-old G12, P12 woman with fibrocystic breasts and a history of biopsy of an area of fibrocystic disease in the left upper outer quadrant 8 months earlier.

Mammogram: Left oblique (**A**) and craniocaudal (**B**) views. There is a high-density spiculated mass in the upper quadrant *(arrow)* on the oblique view (**A**). This area has a different configuration and is less dense on the craniocaudal view (**B**), and it is directly beneath the scar in the subcutaneous fat *(arrow)*. The change in configuration and density on the two views suggests that the area represents a benign process.

Impression: Fat necrosis secondary to previous biopsy.

Note: The patient was followed with mammography, and the area decreased in size and density in 6 months, confirming its benign nature.

→

Figure 5.16.

Clinical: 70-year-old G6, P6 woman for routine screening.

Mammogram: Right mediolateral (**A**) and craniocaudal (**B**) views and left oblique (**C**) and craniocaudal (**D**) views. The breasts show fatty replacement. In the 6 o'clock position of the right breast (**A** and **B**), there is a high-density mass appearing circumscribed on some margins and irregular in other areas. Coarse microcalcifications are present in the periphery of this lesion. On the left (**C** and **D**) in the 6 o'clock position, there is a poorly defined mass having a differing shape and density on the two views. Similar coarse calcifications are associated with this lesion. On both sides, but particularly on the left, some of the calcifications are round or ring-like, suggesting fat necrosis as the etiology of these densities. Because there was no definite history of trauma, biopsy was performed.

Impression: Bilateral masses, favoring fat necrosis.

Histopathology: Bilateral fat necrosis.

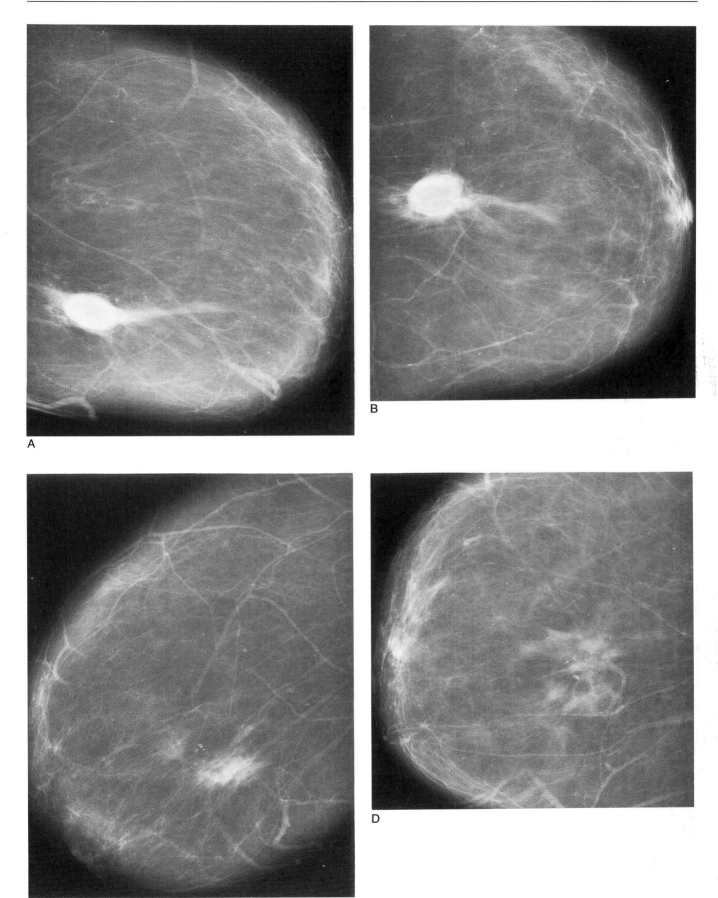

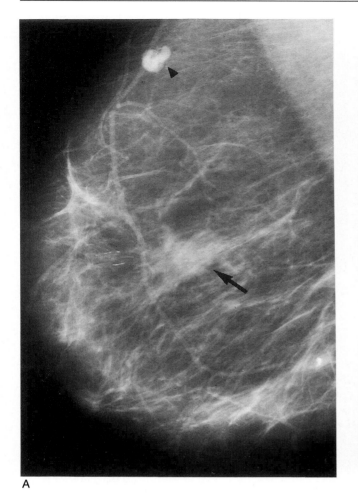

A

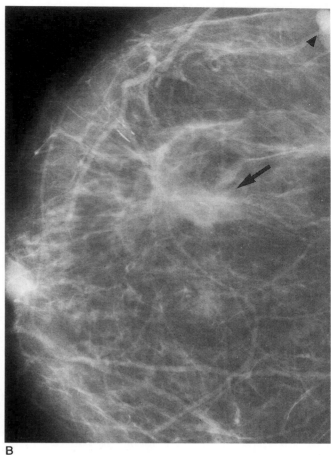

B

Figure 5.17.

Clinical: 52-year-old G7, P7 woman after right breast cancer and left breast biopsy for a benign lesion.

Mammogram: Left oblique (**A**) and enlarged craniocaudal (**B**) views. There is an ill-defined focal 2-cm area of increased density *(arrow)* in the upper outer quadrant of the left breast. This density had increased in size since a prior examination and, because of the interval change, was regarded with a moderate degree of suspicion for malignancy. Benign secretory calcifications are adjacent to the lesion. An enlarged intramammary node *(arrowhead)* is present in the upper outer quadrant.

Impression: New focal area of increased density, of moderate suspicion for malignancy.

Histopathology: Fat necrosis, chronic inflammation.

Note: Areas of fat necrosis are usually most prominent immediately after biopsy and gradually decrease in size and density over time. Occasionally, such an area may increase in size, and biopsy is usually warranted to exclude a neoplastic process.

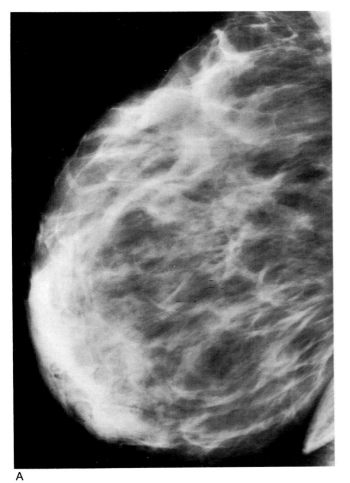

A

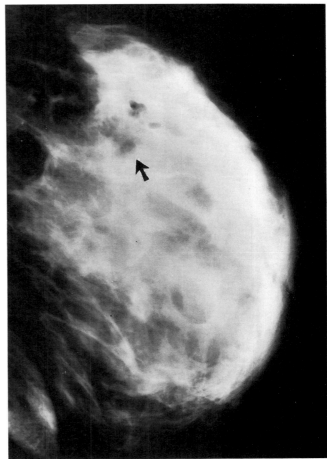

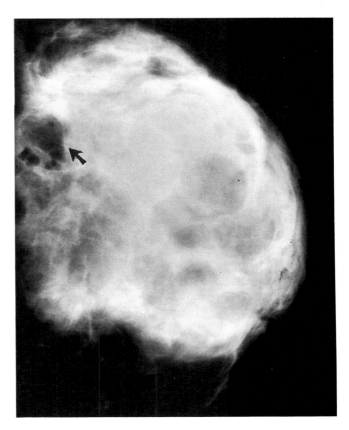

B

Figure 5.18.

Clinical: 33-year-old woman who sustained blunt trauma to the right breast 6 weeks earlier, presenting with a large firm mass with skin ulceration. During mammography the mass ruptured through the skin, draining a large amount of thick fluid.

Mammogram: Bilateral oblique (**A**) and right craniocaudal (**B**) views. There is diffusively increased density throughout the entire right upper outer quadrant. Pockets of air are present within this lesion *(arrow)*. Given the clinical history of this patient, the lesion was thought to represent most likely a large hematoma or area of fat necrosis with formation of a sterile abscess. The air was inspissated into the mass after rupture through the sinus tract.

Impression: Hematoma or fat necrosis.

Histopathology: Chronic inflammation, fat necrosis.

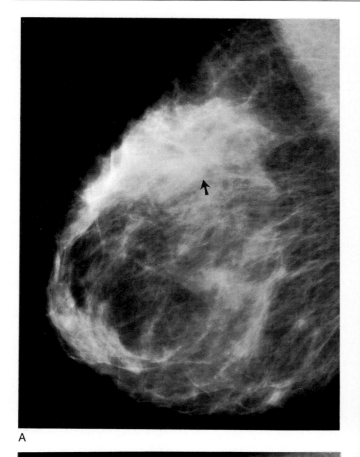

A

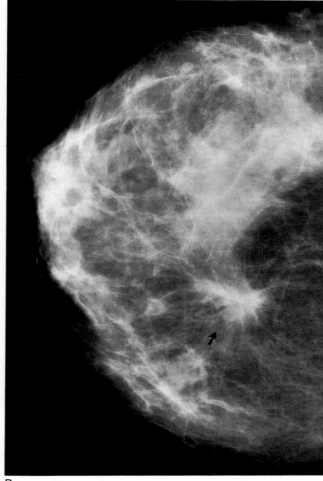

B

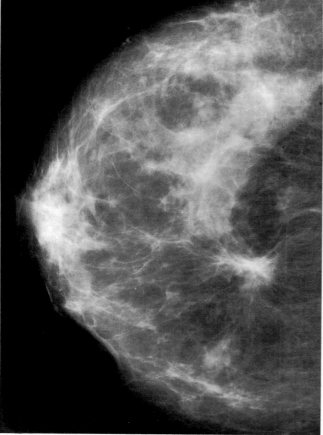

C

Figure 5.19.

Clinical: 54-year-old woman 6 months after left breast biopsy for benign disease.

Mammogram: Left oblique (**A**) and craniocaudal (**B**) views and left craniocaudal view 9 months later (**C**). There is an irregular spiculated 1.5-cm mass of moderately high density in the left upper inner quadrant. The lesion is more apparent on the craniocaudal view (**B**) than on the oblique view (**A**), suggesting that it is less likely malignant *(arrows)*. The lesion was in the area of the recent scar, and because of this and the difference in appearance on the two views, it was thought to be benign, representing hematoma and fat necrosis. A follow-up mammogram 9 months later showed decrease in size of the area, confirming its benign nature.

Impression: Fat necrosis, postsurgical change.

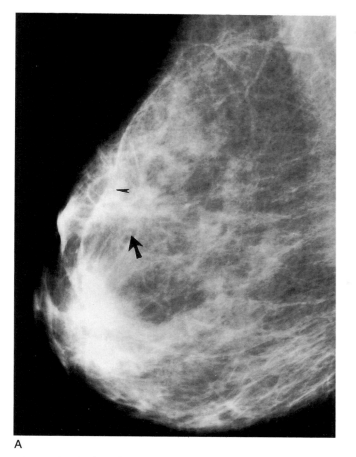

A

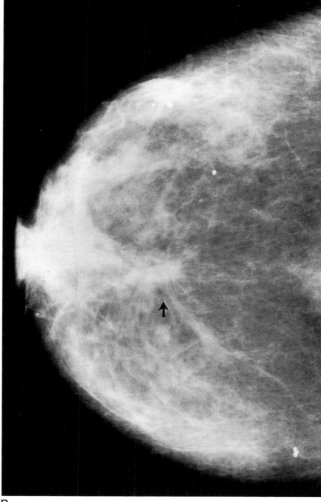

B

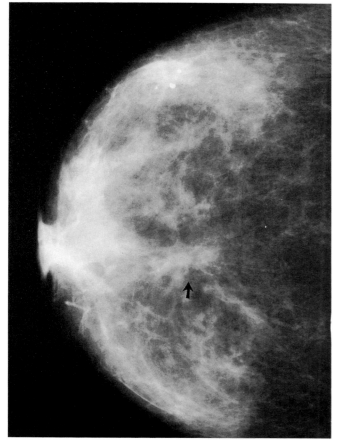

C

Figure 5.20.

Clinical: 63-year-old woman 6 months after removal of a fibroadenoma in the 12 o'clock position of the left breast.

Mammogram: Left oblique (**A**) and craniocaudal (**B**) views and follow-up craniocaudal view 6 months later (**C**). There is a moderately high density spiculated mass *(arrow)* in the 12 o'clock position of the left breast (**A** and **B**). Without a history of recent surgery in this area, this lesion might be considered as suspicious for malignancy. The lesion is situated directly beneath the surgical scar *(arrowhead)* (**A**) and is most consistent with fat necrosis. A follow-up mammogram 6 months later (**C**) shows decrease in size and density of the lesion.

Impression: Fat necrosis.

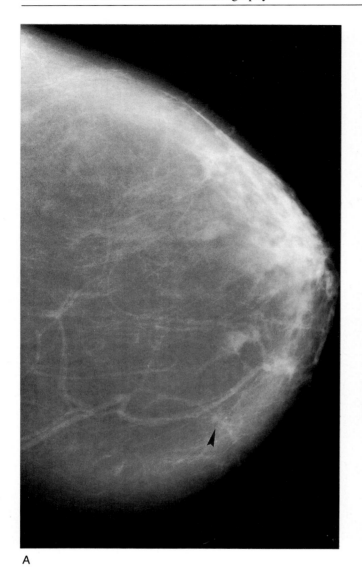

A

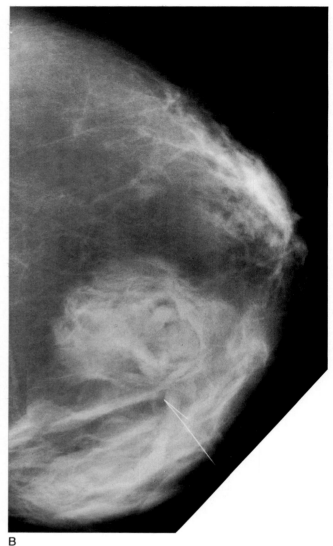

B

Figure 5.21.

Clinical: 53-year-old woman scheduled for needle localization of clustered microcalcifications in the right upper inner quadrant.

Mammogram: Prelocalization craniocaudal view (**A**) and postlocalization right craniocaudal view (**B**). On the preliminary film (**A**), there is a cluster of microcalcifications *(arrow)* near an artery. During localization the vessel was inadvertently punctured, creating a large interstitial hematoma (**B**). The blood dissected through the tissue, creating an ill-defined mass of nonhomogeneous density.

Impression: Interstitial hematoma.

Note: The hematoma was partially evacuated during biopsy.

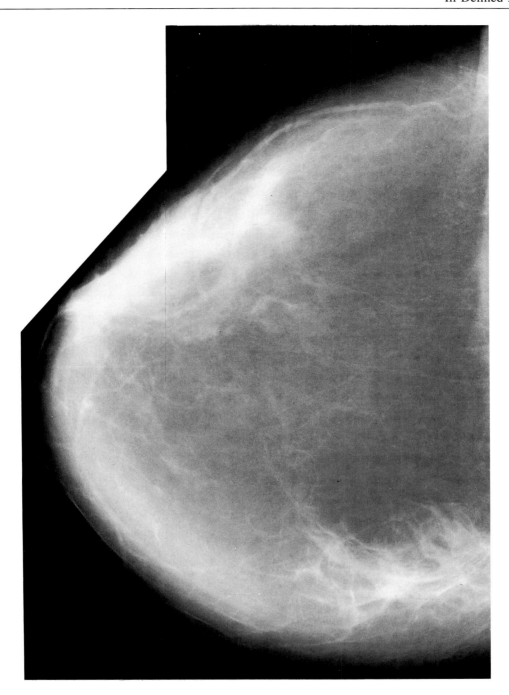

Figure 5.22.

Clinical: 47-year-old woman who sustained recent trauma to the inner aspect of the left breast.

Mammogram: Left craniocaudal view. There is an ill-defined irregular area of focal increased density in the left inner quadrant that corresponded to a bruise noted on clinical examination. The density is stringy, and fat is present within it.

This lesion was not present on a routine screening mammogram 5 months earlier. The finding is not suspicious for malignancy because of the lucencies within it and the lack of fine spiculation.

Impression: Interstitial hematoma.

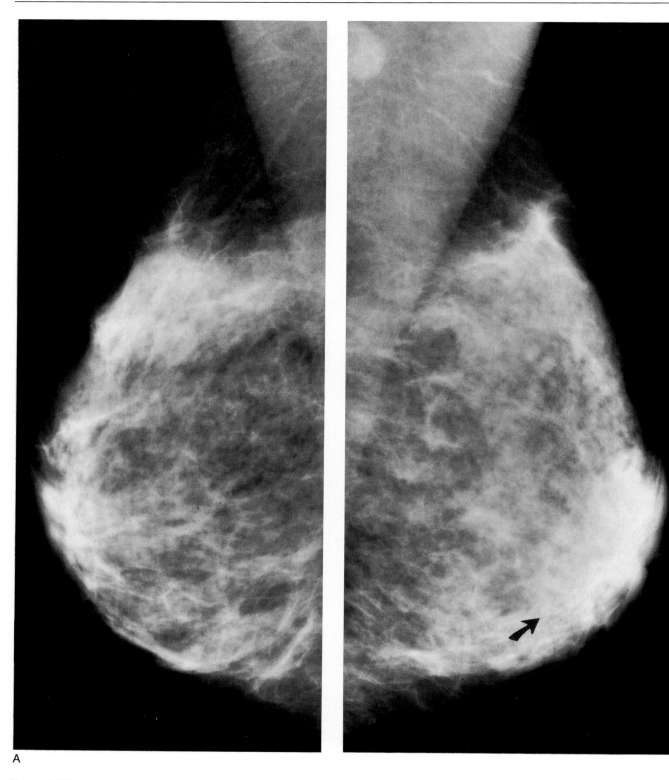

A

Figure 5.23.

Clinical: 32-year-old woman with a strong family history of breast cancer who presented with a firm tender nodular area beneath the right nipple with thickening of the nipple-areolar complex. No nipple discharge was present, but erythema of the skin was noted.

Mammogram: Bilateral oblique (**A**) and craniocaudal (**B**) views. There is asymmetry in the appearance of the breasts with the right subareolar area being more dense, radiating posteriorly from the nipple *(arrows)*. Thickening of the skin over this area is noted. The differential in this patient was mastitis and abscess versus carcinoma. Fine-needle aspiration was performed, showing inflammatory cells; the patient was treated with antibiotics and drainage, and the area resolved.

Impression: Mastitis with breast abscess.

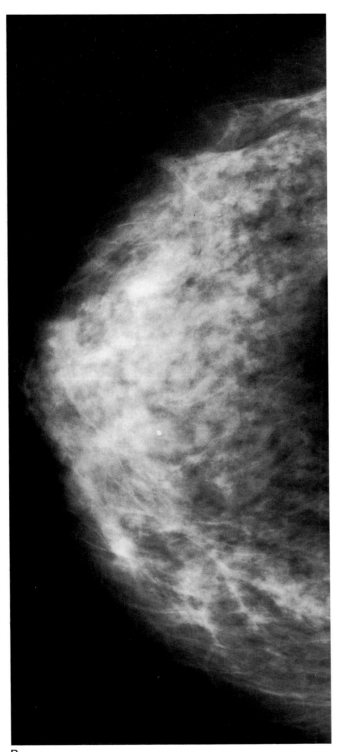
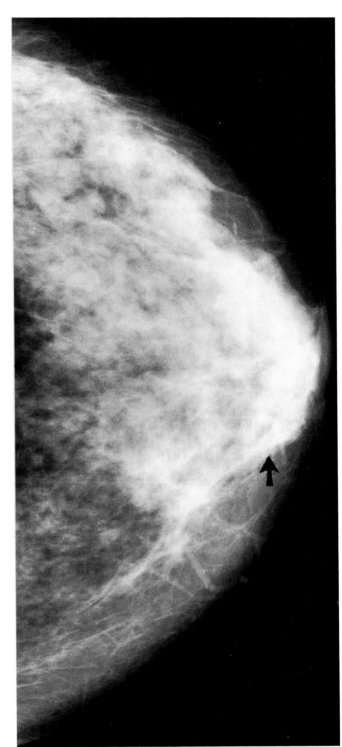

B

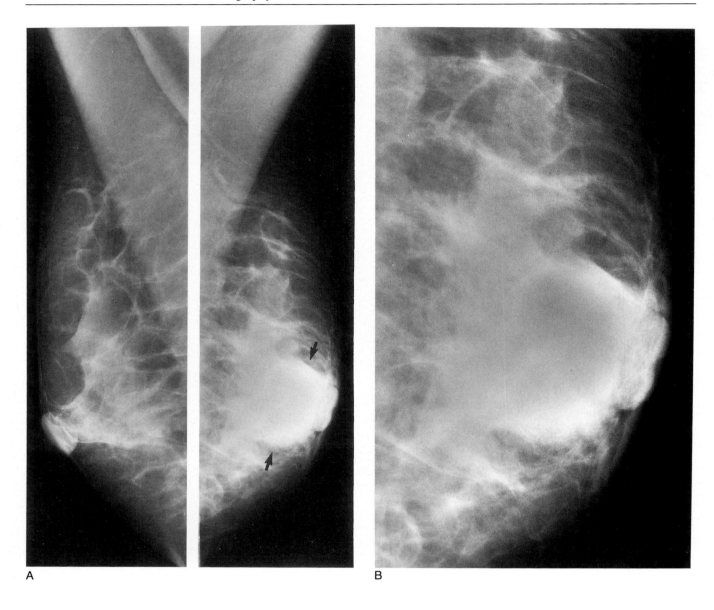

A   B

Figure 5.24.

Clinical: 35-year-old G4, P3, Ab1 woman with a family history of breast cancer who presented with an indurated tender mass in the right subareolar area.

Mammogram: Bilateral oblique views (**A**), right craniocaudal (**B**) view, and ultrasound (**C**). The breasts are moderately dense and glandular, consistent with the age and parity of the patient. Marked asymmetry is present, with an ill-defined mass *(arrows)* in the right subareolar area (**A** and **B**). Nipple retraction and areolar thickening are associated with the mass. Sonography (**C**) shows the mass to be slightly ill defined and to contain some internal echoes suggesting thick fluid. Particularly because of the ultrasound, the favored diagnosis is an abscess; aspiration revealed purulent material.

Impression: Mass in the right breast, favoring abscess.

Histopathology: Acute mastitis, breast abscess.

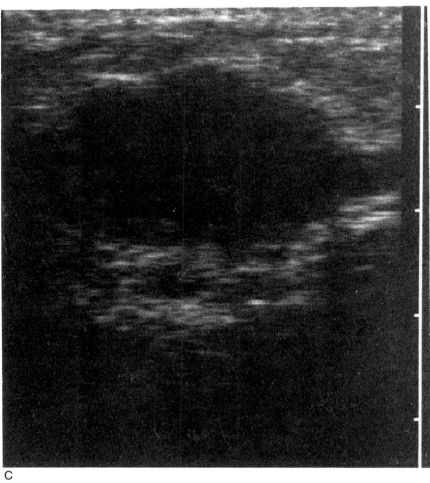

C

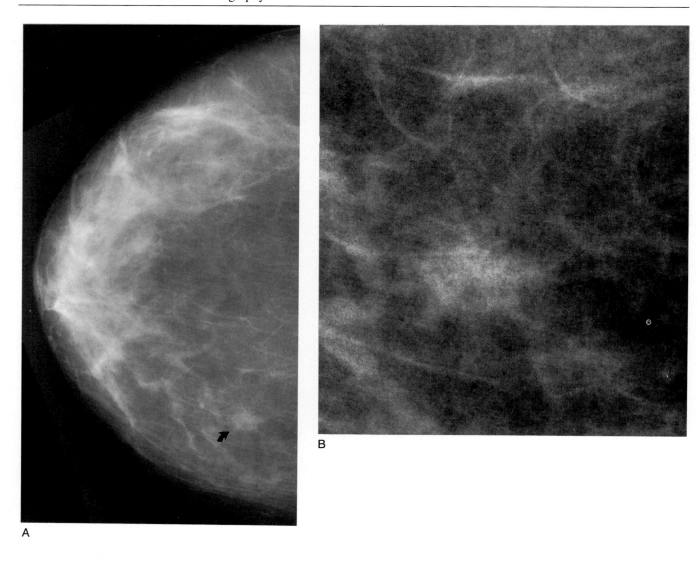

A

B

Figure 5.25.

Clinical: 47-year-old woman for screening.

Mammogram: Left craniocaudal view (**A**) and magnified image (**B**). There is an ill-defined low-density nodule *(arrow)* in the inner aspect of the left breast (**A**). This nodule had developed since a mammogram 2 years earlier. A magnified view of the nodule shows the poor definition of the margins.

Impression: Developing nodule of mild to moderate suspicion for malignancy.

Histopathology: Granular cell tumor.

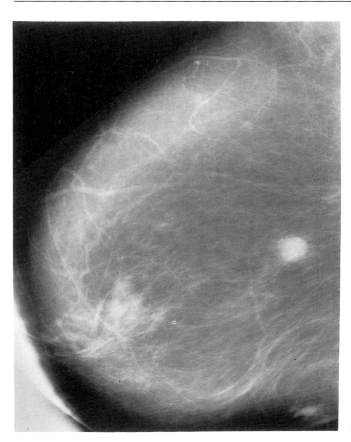

A

Figure 5.26.

Clinical: 39-year-old woman with a palpable nodule laterally in the left breast.

Mammogram: Left oblique (**A**) and craniocaudal (**B**) views. There is a slightly irregular, medium- to high-density mass in the left middle outer quadrant located in the subcutaneous area *(arrow)* (**B**). Lesions that most frequently occupy the subcutaneous region are sebaceous cysts and metastatic deposits. Another unusual lesion that may occur here is the granular cell myoblastoma, a benign tumor of the tongue and subcutaneous tissues.

Histopathology: Granular cell myoblastoma. (Case courtesy of Dr. Stephen Edge, Charlottesville, VA.)

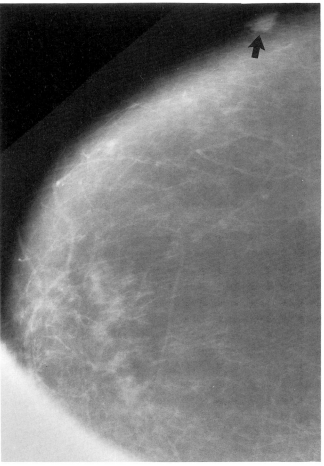

B

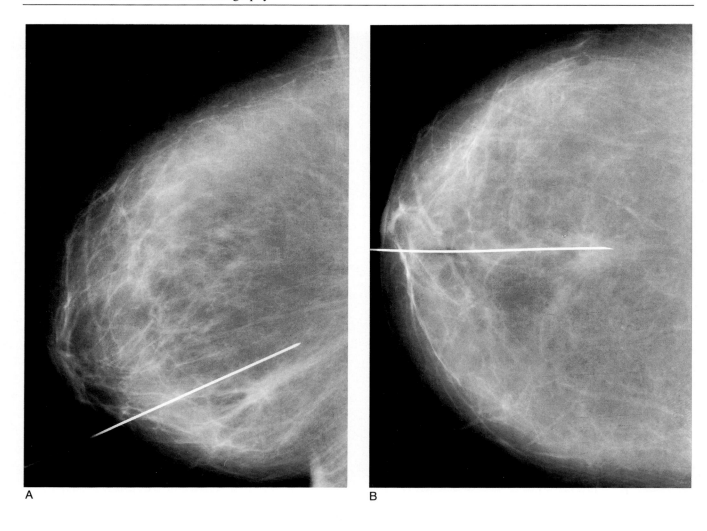

A   B

Figure 5.27.

Clinical: Screening mammogram.

Mammogram: Left mediolateral (**A**) and craniocaudal (**B**) views from a needle localization procedure. There is an ill-defined, somewhat-spiculated mass of medium density in the deep central portion of the left breast. The lesion is of moderate suspicion for malignancy.

Histopathology: Fibromatosis.

Note: Fibromatosis is a fibroblastic lesion that is nonmetastasizing but locally invasive. This lesion can occur in the soft tissues of the trunk and limbs as a "desmoid tumor." In the breast the lesion usually represents an extension from the pectoralis fascia. (Case courtesy of Dr. Gary Lichtenstein, South Boston, VA.)

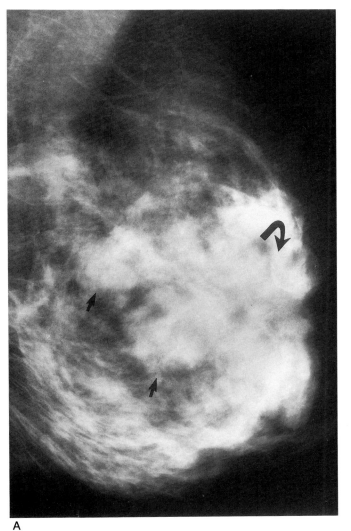

A

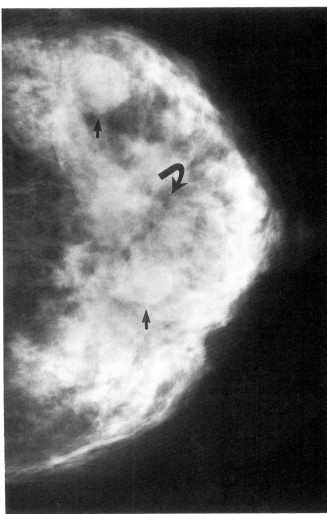

B

Figure 5.28.

Clinical: 55-year-old G2, P2 woman with a history of multiple cysts, for routine screening.

Mammogram: Right oblique (**A**) and craniocaudal (**B**) views. The breast is very dense for the patient's age. There are multiple circumscribed nodules *(arrows)* that were shown to be cystic by ultrasound. Scattered microcalcifications are present. There is a focal area of architectural distortion *(curved arrow)* in the 12 o'clock position. This area is spiculated, al-

though there is no high-density center to suggest a tumor. The area had developed since a prior mammogram 18 months earlier and was, therefore, regarded with a moderate degree of suspicion for malignancy. The differential includes a radial scar versus a carcinoma.

Histopathology: Intraductal carcinoma, extensive papillary and cribriform patterns.

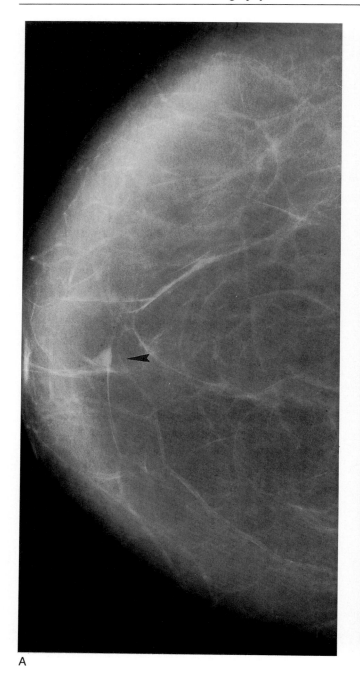

A

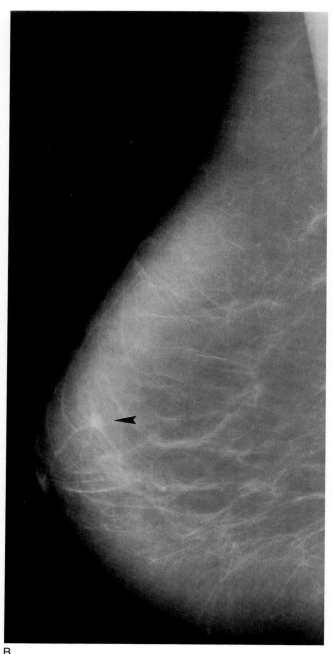

B

Figure 5.29.

Clinical: 62-year-old woman with a family history of breast cancer, for screening mammography.

Mammogram: Left craniocaudal (**A**) and oblique (**B**) views. There is a 5-mm nodule *(arrows)* in the supra-areolar area of the left breast. Slight poor definition of the borders is present, and the lesion is of moderately high density. The nodule had

appeared since a previous mammogram 2 years previously.

Impression: Nodule suspicious for carcinoma.

Histopathology: Intraductal carcinoma with microinvasion.

Note: Even if no previous mammogram had been available, the lesion would have been considered suspicious because of its poor definition.

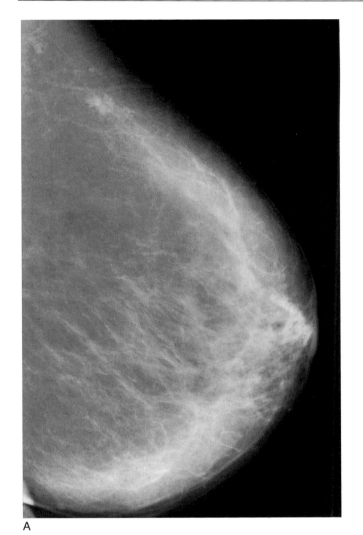

A

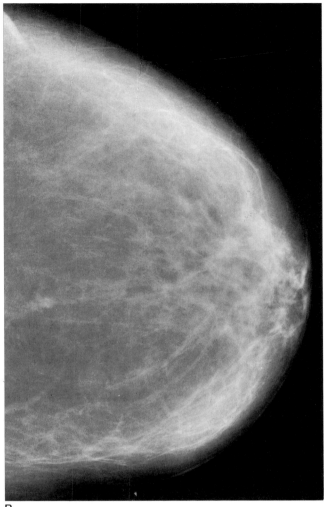

B

Figure 5.30.

Clinical: 75-year-old woman who had a left mastectomy in 1972 for adenocarcinoma, for routine follow-up of the right breast.

Mammogram: Right mediolateral (**A**), craniocaudal (**B**), and magnified (**C**) views. There is a 1-cm irregular, moderately dense nodule in the 12 o'clock position of the right breast. The nodular irregular margins of this lesion are well demonstrated on the magnified view; the mammogram 1 year earlier was normal.

Impression: Ill-defined nodule suspicious for carcinoma.

Histopathology: Intraductal carcinoma.

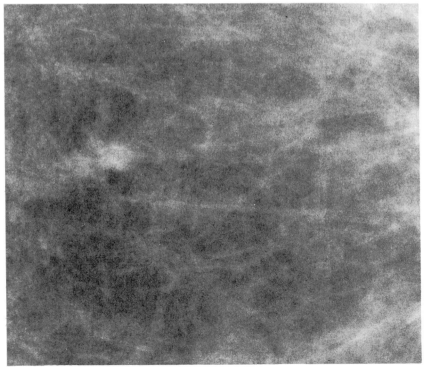

C

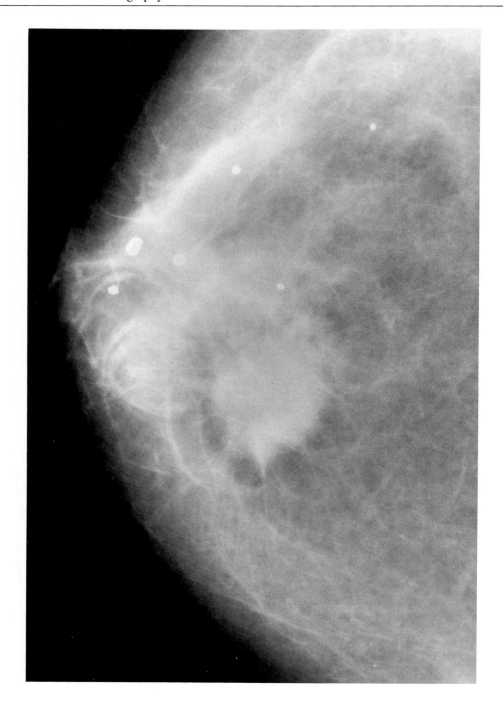

Figure 5.31.

Clinical: 67-year-old woman with a history of ovarian cancer who has developed a palpable 3.5-cm mass in the left breast.

Mammogram: Left craniocaudal view. There is a 2.5-cm mass of moderately high density in the inner aspect of the breast. Fine spicules extend around the circumference of the lesion. Note that on palpation the lesion seems larger than it ap-pears on mammography, which is typical of cancers, pre-sumably because of the surrounding fibrotic response.

Impression: Carcinoma.

Histopathology: Infiltrating ductal carcinoma, with 1 of 22 nodes positive for malignancy.

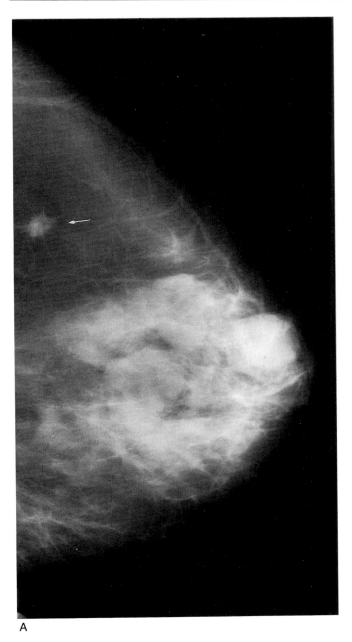

A

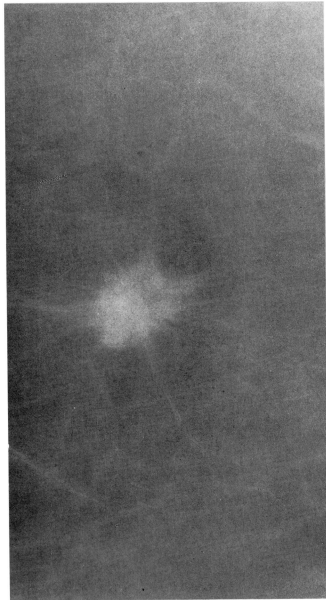

B

Figure 5.32.

Clinical: 48-year-old woman with a history of cysts and multiple palpable masses.

Mammogram: Right mediolateral view (**A**) and magnified image (**B**). There are multiple well-defined masses in the retroareolar area, suggesting the presence of multiple cysts. In the upper aspect of the breast, situated posteriorly, there is a 1-cm irregular nodule *(arrow)* (**A**). The coned-down view (**B**) shows the fine spicules surrounding this moderately dense lesion.

Impression: Cystic changes; probable upper outer quadrant carcinoma.

Histopathology: Infiltrating ductal carcinoma.

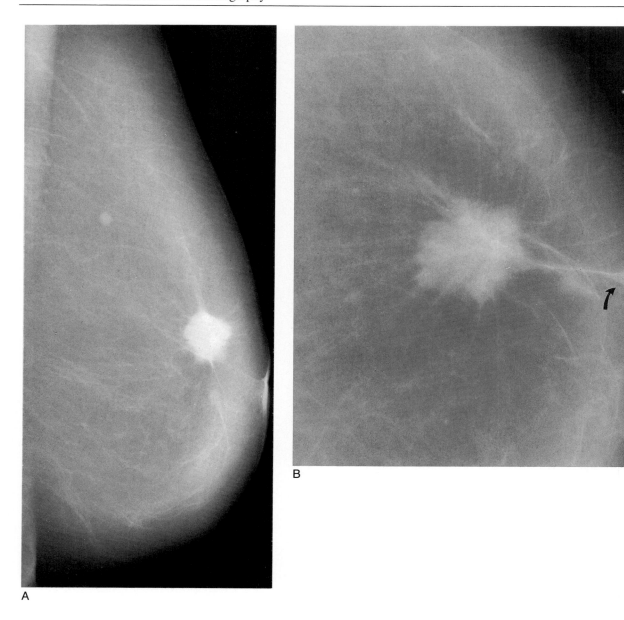

A

B

Figure 5.33.

Clinical: 69-year-old woman with lymphoma and induration around the right nipple.

Mammogram: Right oblique view (**A**) and magnified image (**B**). There is a high-density irregular mass beneath the nipple. On the coned-down view (**B**) the lesion is shown to have fine spicules surrounding it, nodular margins, linear extensions that retract the nipple slightly *(arrow),* and fine microcalcifications.

Impression: Primary carcinoma of the breast.

Histopathology: Infiltrating ductal carcinoma.

Note: The features of this lesion are typical of breast cancer. Lymphomatous involvement of the breast could appear as increased-density well-defined masses, poorly defined masses, or adenopathy.

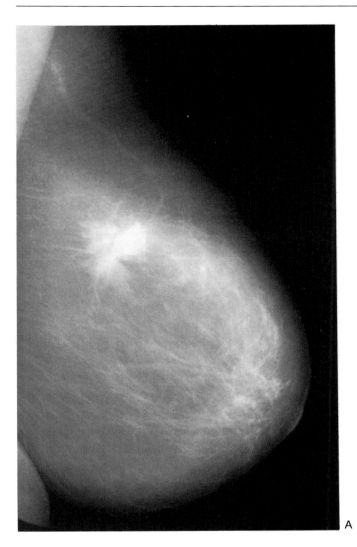

A

Figure 5.34.

Clinical: 65-year-old woman with a firm palpable mass in the right upper outer quadrant.

Mammogram: Right oblique view (**A**) and magnified cranio-caudal image (**B**). There is a high-density irregular mass in the upper outer quadrant. This lesion has a dense center and nodular and spiculated borders characteristic of malignancy.

Impression: Carcinoma.

Histopathology: Infiltrating ductal carcinoma, with positive axillary nodes.

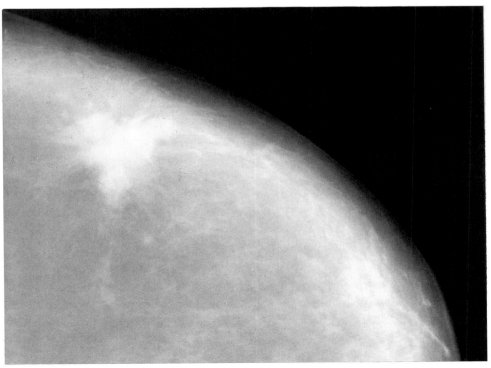

B

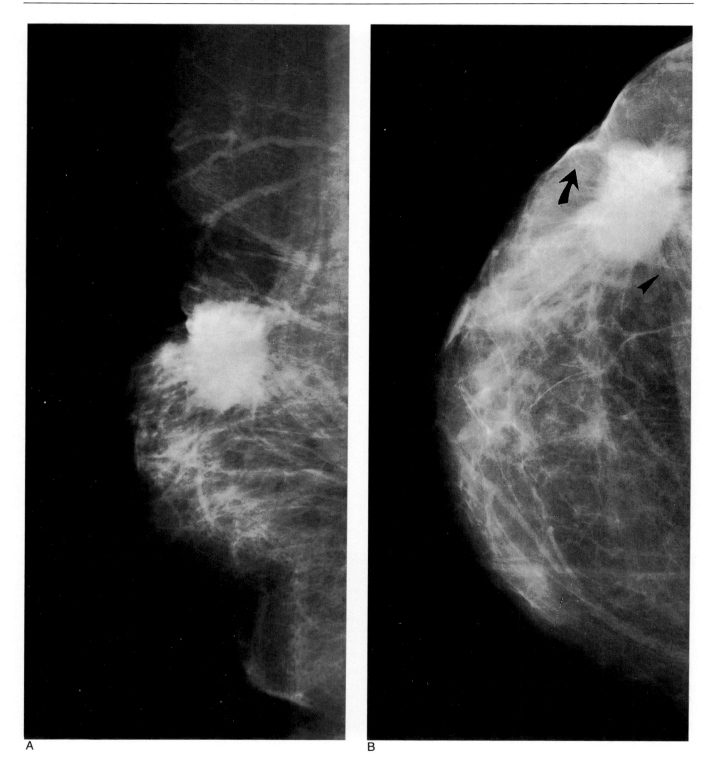

A

B

Figure 5.35.

Clinical: 70-year-old woman with a large left breast mass.

Mammogram: Left oblique (**A**) and craniocaudal (**B**) views. There is a high-density spiculated mass containing a few microcalcifications in the upper outer quadrant. The lesion has secondary signs of breast cancer, including linear extension to the nipple and the skin with skin thickening and retraction

(arrow) and tethering of the pectoralis major muscle *(arrowhead).*

Impression: Breast carcinoma with skin and possible muscle involvement.

Histopathology: Infiltrating ductal carcinoma, with negative axillary nodes.

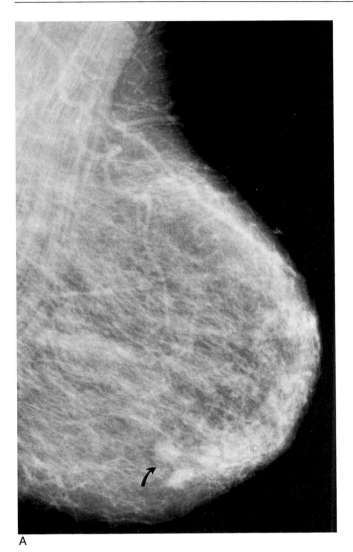

A

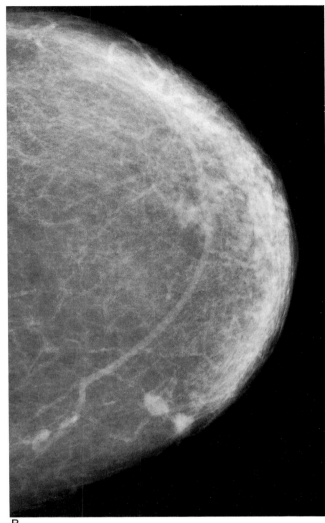

B

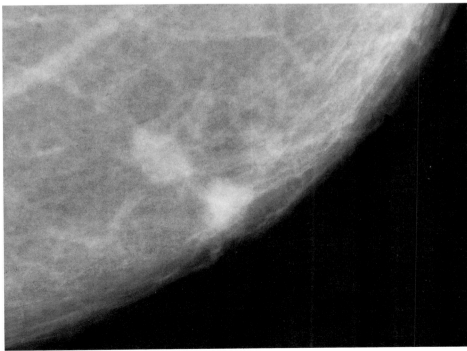

C

Figure 5.36.

Clinical: 82-year-old woman with a history of lobular neoplasia on biopsy of the right inner quadrant 1 year previously.

Mammogram: Right oblique (**A**) and craniocaudal (**B**) views. There are two irregular high-density nodules in close proximity in the right lower inner quadrant. On close inspection (**C**) the lesions are noted to have spiculated margins and an appearance highly suspicious for malignancy.

Impression: Highly suspicious for two foci of carcinoma.

Histopathology: Infiltrating ductal carcinoma.

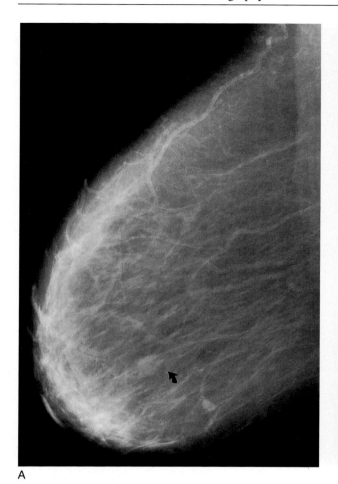

A

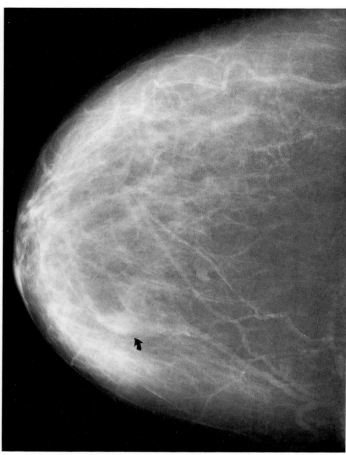

B

Figure 5.37.

Clinical: 80-year-old woman for screening mammography; a mammogram 2 years earlier *was* normal.

Mammogram: Left oblique view (**A**), craniocaudal view (**B**), and magnified image (**C**). There is an ill-defined round mass *(arrows)* in the left lower inner quadrant. The lesion is of moderate density. A magnified image (**C**) shows that the borders are irregular but not with radiating spicules more typical of carcinoma. Sonography was performed but failed to demonstrate the nodule. The nodule had developed since a previous mammogram and, because of the interval change and its characteristics, was biopsied.

Impression: Slightly irregular nodule suspicious for carcinoma.

Histopathology: Intracystic papillary carcinoma.

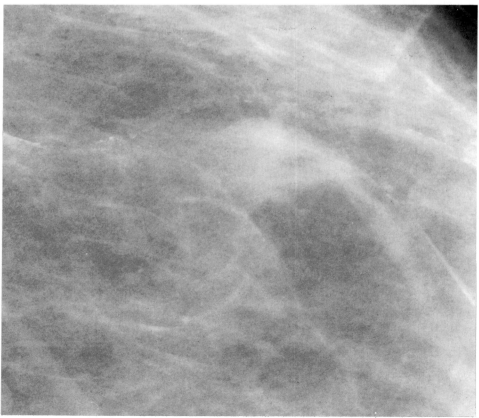

C

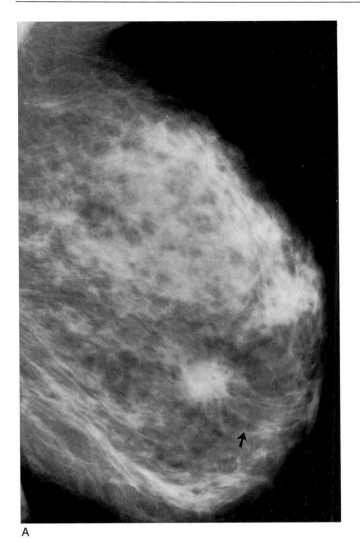

A

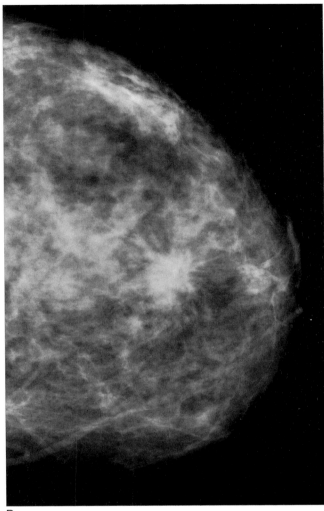

B

Figure 5.38.

Clinical: 59-year-old G2, P2 woman with fibrocystic breasts and no focal mass, considered suspicious by the referring clinician.

Mammogram: Left oblique (**A**) and craniocaudal (**B**) views. There is a moderately high density irregular mass in the retroareolar area. Fine microcalcifications are present within the mass, and there are linear extensions *(arrow)* (**A**) from the mass toward the nipple, suggesting extension in the subareolar ducts. These features are characteristic of carcinoma.

Histopathology: Infiltrating ductal carcinoma.

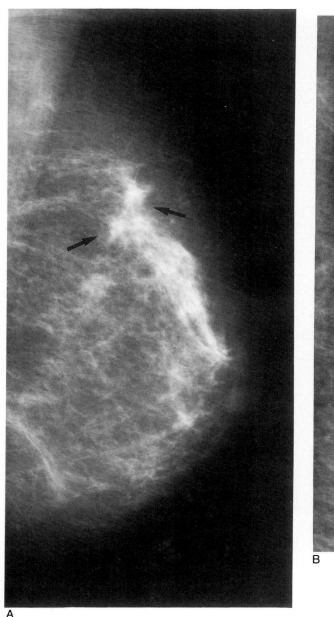

A

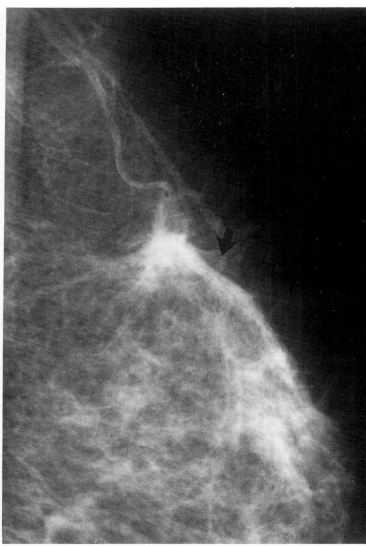

B

Figure 5.39.

Clinical: 70-year-old G5, P4 woman for screening.

Mammogram: Right oblique (**A**) and enlarged (2×) cranio-caudal (**B**) views. There is minimal residual glandularity present. In the upper outer quadrant, there is an irregular area of increased density that is producing architectural distortion *(arrows)* (**A**). Fine spicules surround this high-density lesion, and linear stranding appears to pucker *(arrow)* (**B**) the nor-

mal fibroglandular tissue inferiorly. The high density of the lesion and its secondary features are consistent with carcinoma.

Impression: Carcinoma.

Histopathology: Infiltrating ductal carcinoma, with 18 nodes negative.

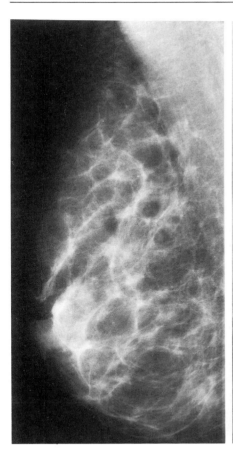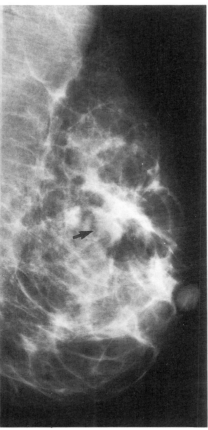

A

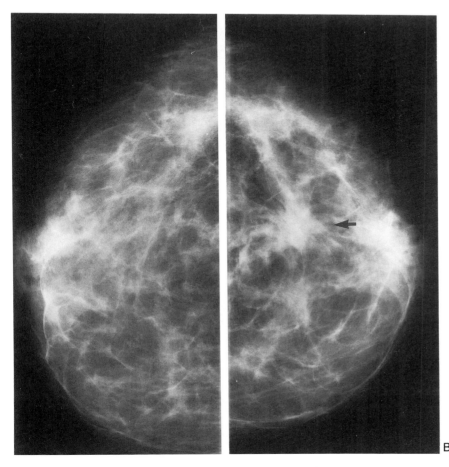

B

Figure 5.40.

Clinical: 70-year-old woman with a palpable mass in the right upper outer quadrant.

Mammogram: Right oblique (**A**) and craniocaudal (**B**) views. The breasts are moderately dense. In the upper outer quadrant of the right breast, there is a medium- to high-density spiculated mass *(arrows)*. This lesion has a similar shape and density on the two views and, even if it were nonpalpable, would be highly suspicious for malignancy.

Impression: Spiculated mass in the right breast, highly suspicious for carcinoma.

Histopathology: Poorly differentiated infiltrating ductal carcinoma, with metastases in 5 of 5 axillary nodes.

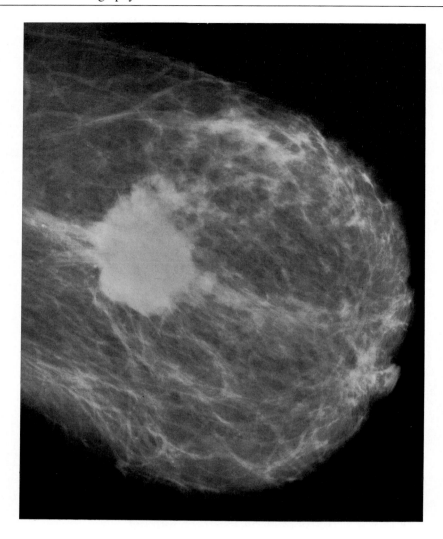

Figure 5.41.

Clinical: 78-year-old woman with a 4-cm mass in the right upper inner quadrant.

Mammogram: Right oblique view. There is a very high density spiculated mass in the upper aspect of the right breast.

The borders are nodular, and there are fine spicules that surround the mass. The findings are typical of carcinoma.

Histopathology: Infiltrating ductal carcinoma, with 3 of 18 nodes positive.

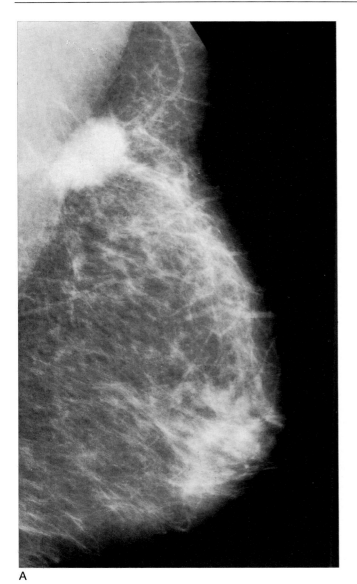

A

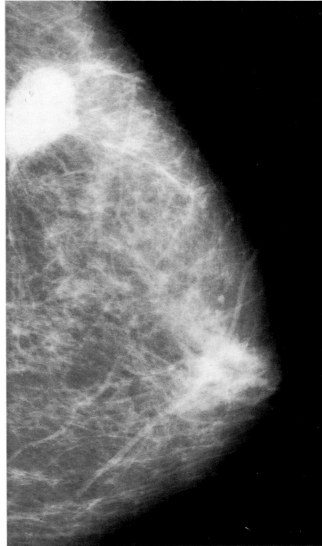

B

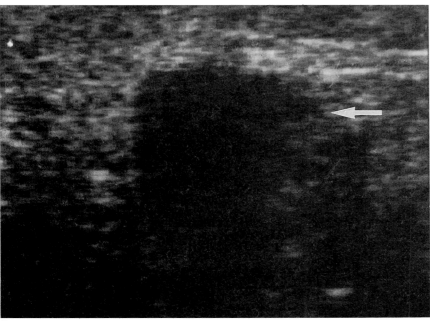

C

Figure 5.42.

Clinical: 55-year-old woman with a 4-month history of a mass in the right axillary tail.

Mammogram: Right oblique (**A**) and exaggerated lateral craniocaudal (**B**) views and ultrasound (**C**). There is a high-density ovoid mass deep in the upper outer quadrant. By rotating the patient for the craniocaudal view with the lateral aspect of the breast brought forward (**B**), the mass can be visualized. Fine spiculation surrounds the borders of the lesion, typical of carcinoma. On the real-time sonogram (**C**) the typical ultrasound features of carcinoma are noted: an ill-defined, hypoechoic mass with posterior shadowing *(arrow)*.

Impression: Carcinoma.

Histopathology: Infiltrating ductal carcinoma.

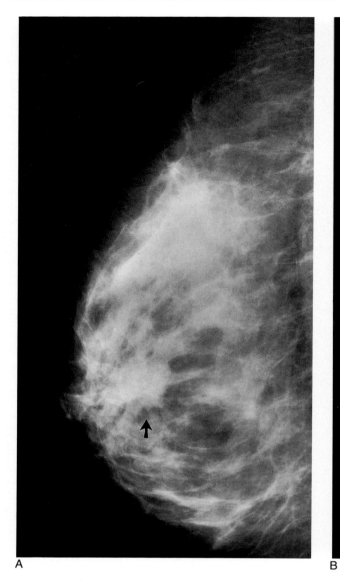

A

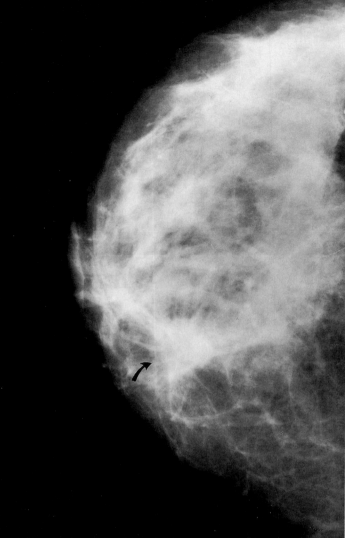

B

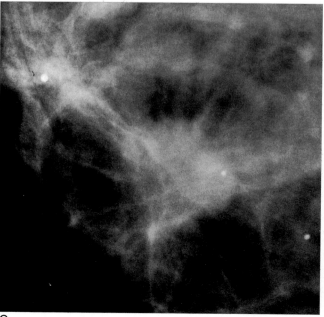

C

Figure 5.43.

Clinical: 52-year-old asymptomatic woman.

Mammogram: Left mediolateral view (**A**), craniocaudal view (**B**), and magnified craniocaudal image (**C**). The breast is dense, and there are diffusely scattered benign macrocalcifications. Medial to the nipple, there is a high-density spiculated mass *(arrow)* (**A** and **B**) distorting the architecture. The high-density center of the lesion and the fine surrounding spicules are highly suspicious of malignancy.

Impression: Probable carcinoma, left breast.

Histopathology: Infiltrating ductal and lobular carcinoma, with 1 of 19 nodes positive.

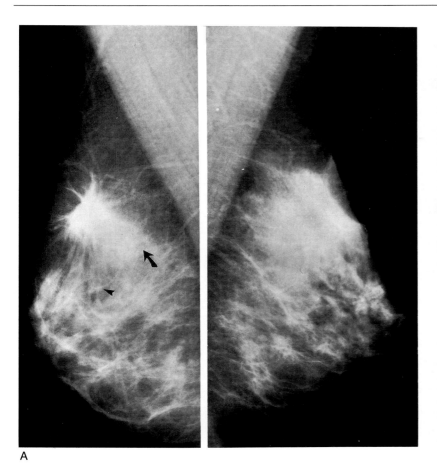

A

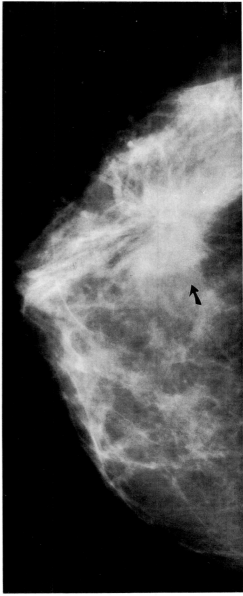

B

Figure 5.44.

Clinical: 40-year-old woman with a 2 × 3-cm mass in the left breast.

Mammogram: Bilateral oblique views (**A**) and left craniocaudal view (**B**). There is a high-density ill-defined mass producing distortion of the normal architecture in the left upper outer quadrant *(arrows)*. There are linear extensions around the mass, extending toward the nipple *(arrowhead)* (**A**).

Impression: Mass highly suspicious for carcinoma, left breast.

Histopathology: Infiltrating ductal carcinoma.

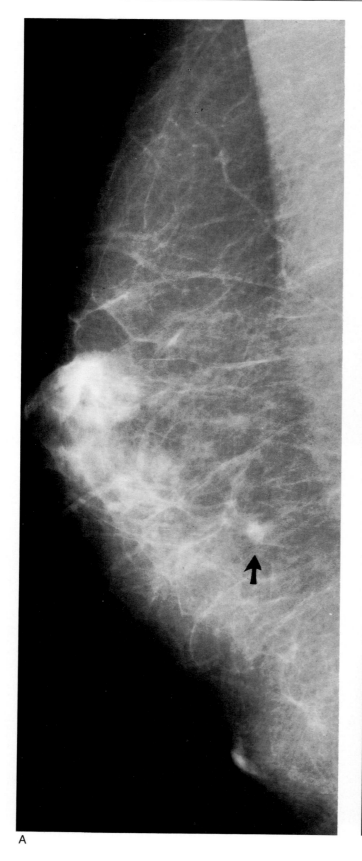

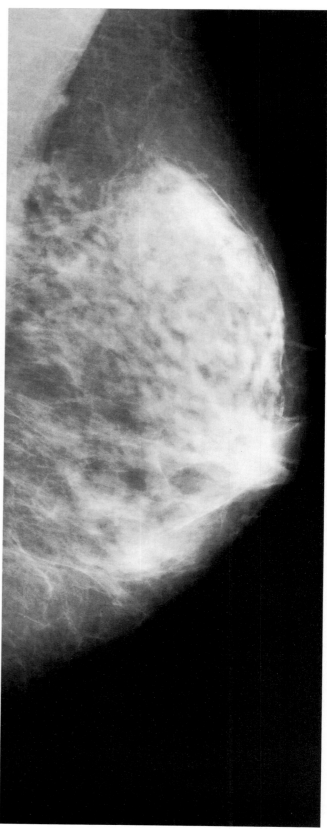

A

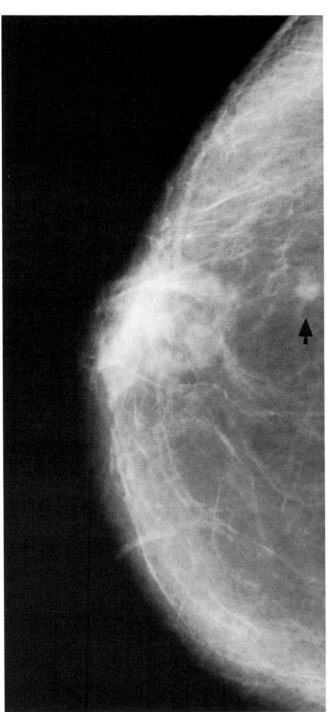

B

Figure 5.45.

Clinical: 77-year-old G0 woman with a history of left breast biopsy, for screening mammography.

Mammogram: Bilateral oblique views (**A**) and left craniocaudal view (**B**). Marked asymmetry in the glandularity is noted because of the previous left biopsy and removal of a large amount of glandular tissue. There is a small high-density irregular nodule in the lower outer aspect of the left breast *(arrows)*. This lesion is of higher density than the glandular tissue and is situated posteriorly, apart from the remainder of parenchyma. The characteristics of this lesion are highly suspicious for malignancy.

Histopathology: Infiltrating ductal carcinoma.

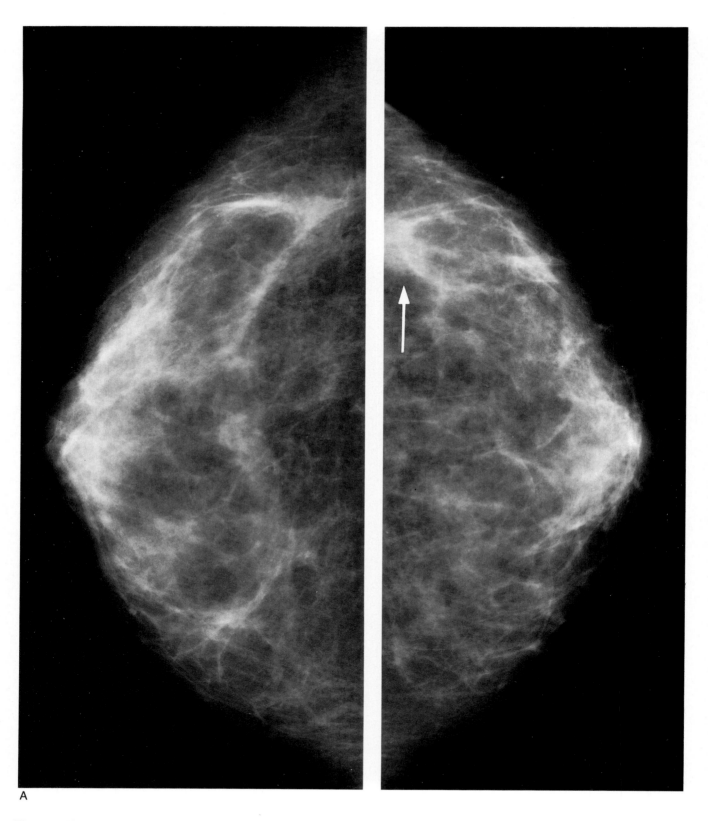

A

Figure 5.46.

Clinical: 65-year-old G0 woman with a hard mass in the right lower outer quadrant.

Mammogram: Bilateral craniocaudal (**A**), right oblique (**B**), and mediolateral (**C**) views. There is moderate glandularity in both breasts (**A**) with an ill-defined area of asymmetric increased density in the right outer quadrant *(arrow)*. The oblique view (**B**) shows the anterior margin of the lesion *(arrow)*. The

additional mediolateral view (**C**) shows a greater part of the lesion that is associated with skin retraction *(curved arrow)*.

Impression: Highly suspicious for malignancy.

Histopathology: Infiltrating ductal carcinoma, with 11 of 17 nodes positive.

Note: The mediolateral view may be particularly useful for demonstrating a deep lesion located inferiorly in the breast.

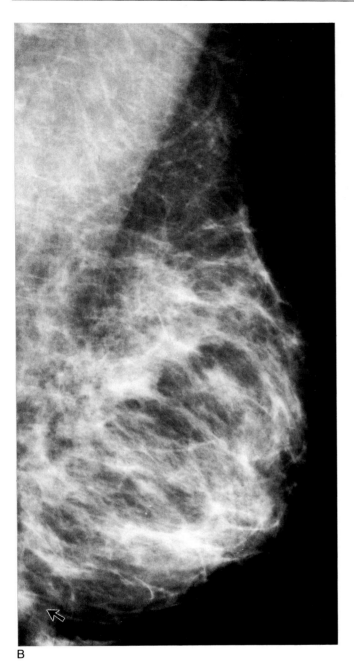

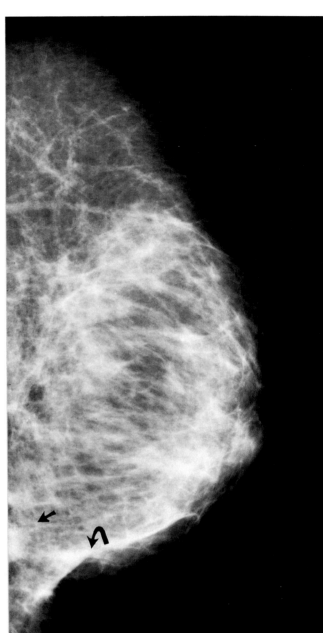

B

C

Figure 5.47.

Clinical: 79-year-old G8, P8 woman with a hard mass in the left breast.

Mammogram: Left oblique view. There is a spiculated mass of moderately high density in the left supra-areolar area. A few ductal calcifications are within the lesion. Long spicules surround the mass and tether the nipple-areolar complex, which is retracted and thickened *(arrow)*.

Impression: Carcinoma.

Histopathology: Infiltrating ductal carcinoma, with nodes negative.

Note: When the breast is compressed for the mammogram, the skin or nipple retraction may be accentuated because the tumor is tethering the superficial structures and not allowing them to be as easily flattened.

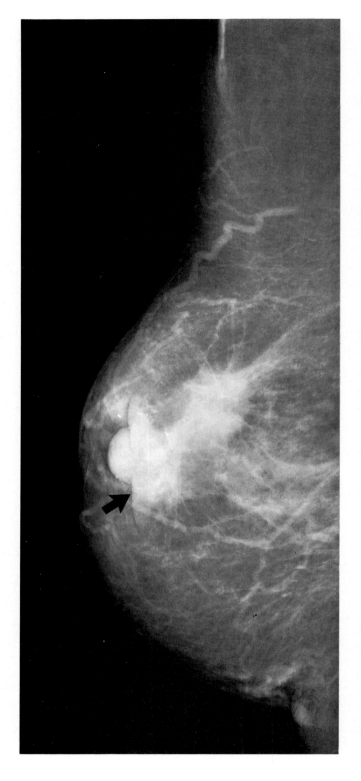

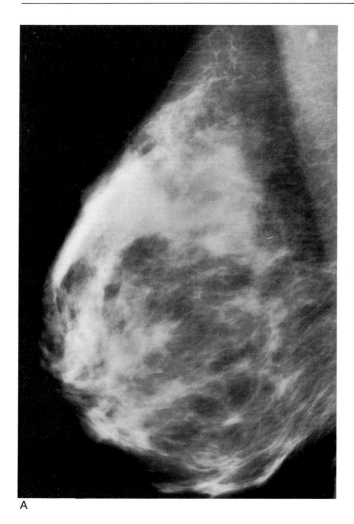
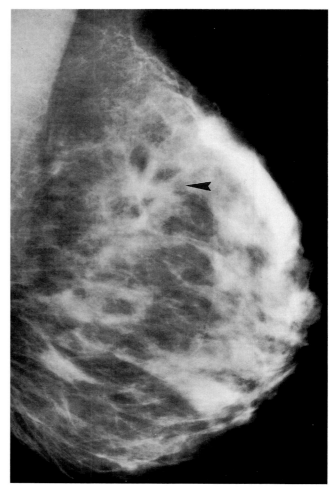

A

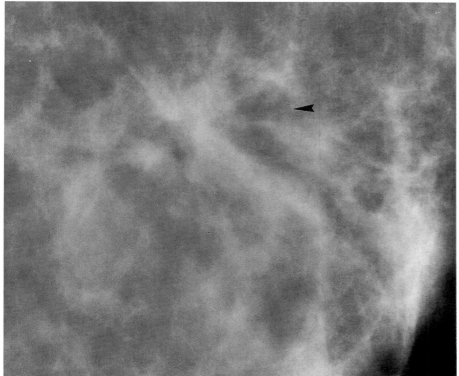

B

Figure 5.48.

Clinical: 43-year-old woman for screening mammography.

Mammogram: Bilateral oblique (**A**) and spot magnification (**B**) views. There is a moderate amount of glandular tissue present. In the right upper quadrant, there is a spiculated area of asymmetry *(arrowhead)* with disturbance of normal architecture. The spot magnification view (**B**) shows the lesion to be of moderately high density and to be surrounded by long spicules *(arrowhead)*. Of note is some lucency within the center of the lesion, a feature not typical of malignancy. This appearance is seen in tubular carcinoma, radial scar, or sclerosing adenosis.

Impression: Spiculated mass suspicious for carcinoma.

Histopathology: Tubular carcinoma.

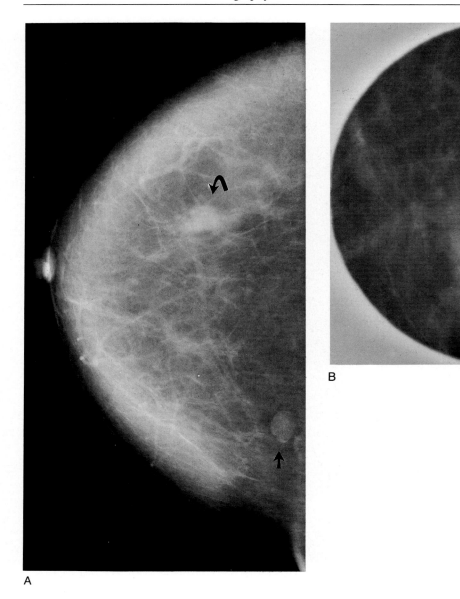

A

B

Figure 5.49.

Clinical: 75-year-old woman with no palpable masses, for screening mammography.

Mammogram: Left craniocaudal (**A**) and spot magnification (**B**) views. There are two masses present. In the inner aspect of the left breast, there is an extremely well-defined lesion of low density *(straight arrow)* with a lucent halo suggesting a benign skin lesion. In the outer aspect, there is a high-density irregular mass *(curved arrow)*. A magnification spot view

(**B**) of the lateral lesion demonstrates the ill-defined margins. Note that the spicules do not surround it in a radiating pattern, as is seen in many infiltrating carcinomas.

Impression: Lateral: irregular high-density mass highly suspicious for carcinoma. Medial: skin lesion.

Histopathology: Medullary carcinoma (lateral), benign nevus (medial).

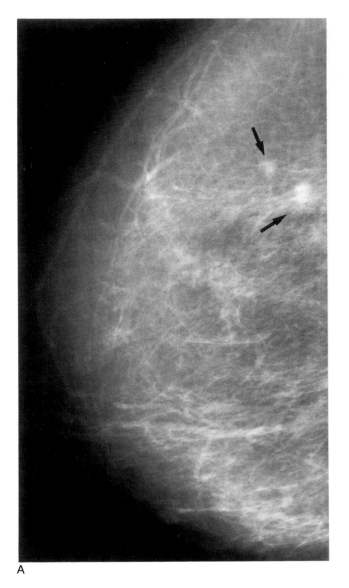

A

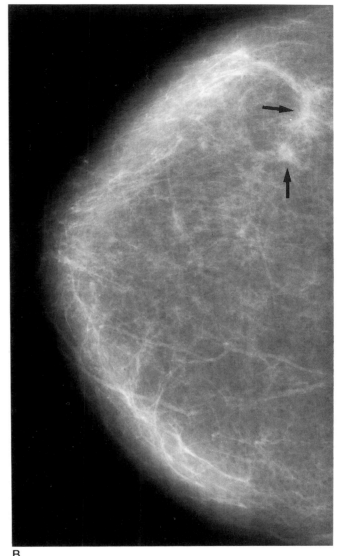

B

Figure 5.50.

Clinical: 66-year-old G8, P6, Ab2 patient for screening mammography.

Mammogram: Left mediolateral (**A**) and craniocaudal (**B**) views. There are two ill-defined densities *(arrows)* in close proximity in the upper outer quadrant of the left breast. The nodules are of relatively high density for their small size and in comparison with the background parenchymal density. There is a slight difference in the shape of each nodule on the two views; nonetheless, the densities remain very focal and irregular.

Impression: Two ill-defined nodules highly suspicious for multifocal carcinoma.

Histopathology: Infiltrating lobular carcinoma, intraductal carcinoma, lobular carcinoma in situ, no evidence of carcinoma in 21 axillary nodes.

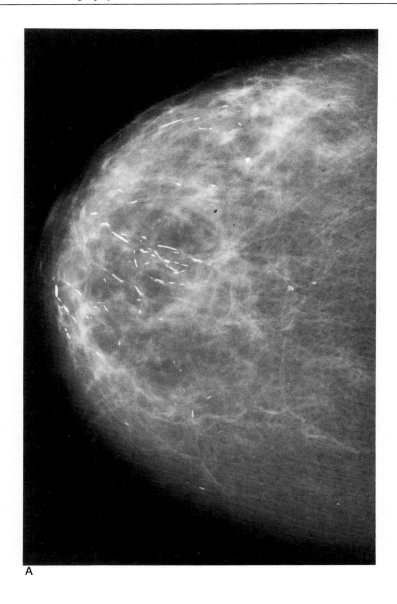

A

Figure 5.51.

Clinical: 80-year-old G0 woman with a 4-cm palpable right breast mass.

Mammogram: Left (**A**) and right (**B**) craniocaudal and right oblique (**C**) views. There are bilateral smooth linear calcifications present, consistent with secretory disease. In the right upper inner quadrant, there is a large high-density spicu-lated mass highly suspicious for carcinoma. Incidental note is made of a normal-sized intramammary node in the upper outer quadrant.

Histopathology: Infiltrating lobular carcinoma, with a large component of mucinous carcinoma. No evidence of carcinoma in 14 nodes.

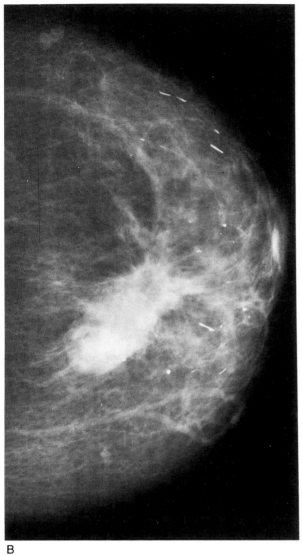

B

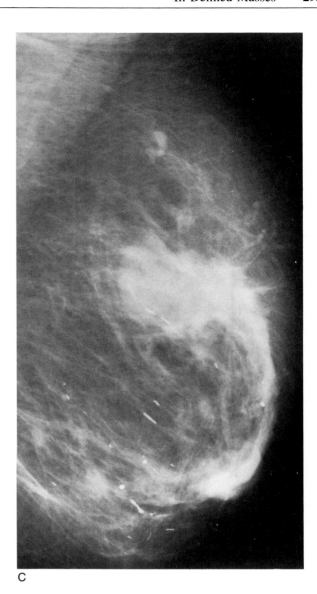

C

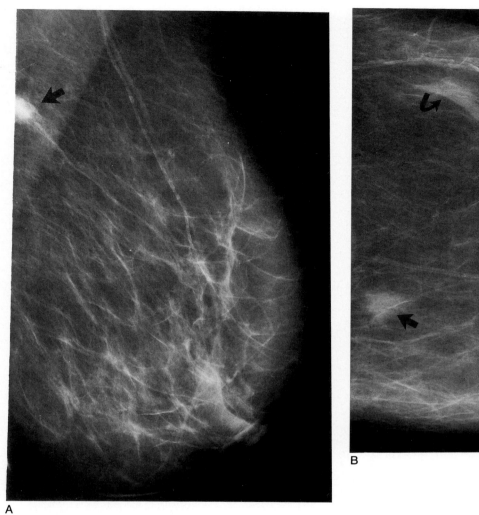

A

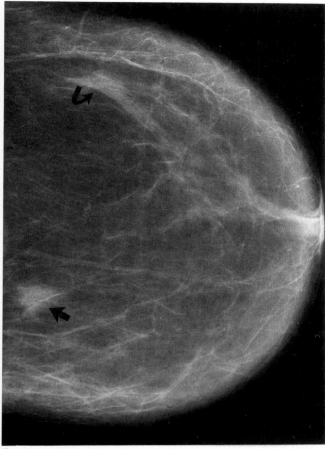

B

Figure 5.52.

Clinical: 75-year-old woman with history of lymphoma, for routine screening mammography.

Mammogram: Right oblique (**A**) and craniocaudal (**B**) views. There is a medium-density irregular mass located in the deep upper aspect of the right breast *(arrow)* on the oblique view (**A**). On the craniocaudal view (**B**) the lesion is located medially *(arrow)*. A second smaller irregular lesion is also pres-

ent laterally *(curved arrow)*. Although these lesions could represent lymphoma, the favored diagnosis is a primary breast carcinoma, because of the poorly defined margins.

Impression: Two irregular lesions, probably neoplastic: primary carcinoma versus lymphoma.

Histopathology (both sites): Malignant lymphoma, mixed small and large cell type.

References

1. Gold RH, Montgomery CK, Rambo ON. Significance of margination of benign and malignant infiltrative mammary lesions: roentgenographic-pathological correlation. AJR 1973;118:881–893.
2. Tabar L, Dean PB. Teaching atlas of mammography. Stuttgart: Georg Thieme Verlag, 1983.
3. Urban JA, Adair FE. Sclerosing adenosis. Cancer 1949;2:625–634.
4. Nielsen NSM, Nielsen BB. Mammographic features of sclerosing adenosis presenting as a tumour. Clin Radiol 1986;37:371–373.
5. Cotron RS, Kumar V, Robbins SL. Robbins pathologic basis of disease. Philadelphia: WB Saunders, 1989:1188.
6. Heimann G, Schwartz IS. Focal fibrous disease of the breast: mammographic detection of an unappreciated condition. AJR 1983;140:1245–1246.
7. Andersen JA, Gram JB. Radial scar in the female breast: a long-term follow-up study of 32 cases. Cancer 1984;53:2557–2560.
8. Fenoglic C, Lattes R. Sclerosing papillary proliferations in the female breast. Cancer 1974;33:691–700.
9. Tremblay G, Buell RH, Seemayer TA. Elastosis in benign sclerosing ductal proliferation of the female breast. Am J Surg Pathol 1977;1:155–159.
10. Fisher ER, Palekar AS, Kotwal N, Lipana N. A nonencapsulated sclerosing lesion of the breast. Am J Clin Pathol 1979;71:240–246.
11. Rickert RR, Kalisher L, Hutter RVP. Indurative mastopathy: a benign sclerosing lesion of breast with elastosis which may simulate carcinoma. Cancer 1981;47:561–571.
12. Cohen MI, Matthies HJ, Mintzer RA, et al. Indurative mastopathy: a cause of false positive mammograms. Radiology 1985;155:69–71.
13. Andersson I. Mammography in clinical practice. Med Radiogr Photogr 1986:62.
14. Mitnick JS, Vazquez MF, Harris MN, Roses DF. Differentiation of radial scar from scirrhous carcinoma of the breast: mammographic-pathologic correlation. Radiology 1989;173:697–700.
15. Bassett LW, Gold RH, Cove HC. Mammographic spectrum of traumatic fat necrosis: the fallibility of "pathognomonic" signs of carcinoma. AJR 1978;130:119–122.
16. Stigers KB, King JG, Davey DD, Stelling CB. Abnormalities of the breast caused by biopsy: spectrum of mammographic findings. AJR 1991;156:287–291.
17. Sickles EA, Herzog KA. Mammography of the postsurgical breast. AJR 1981;136:585–588.
18. Clarke D, Curtis JL, Martinez A, et al. Fat necrosis of the breast simulating recurrent carcinoma after primary radiotherapy in the management of early stage breast carcinoma. Cancer 1983;52:442–445.
19. Dershaw DD, McCormick R, Cox L, Osborne MP. Differentiation of benign and malignant local tumor recurrence after lumpectomy. AJR 1990;155:35–38.
20. Mendelson EB. Imaging the post surgical breast. Semin Ultrasound CT MR 1989;10(2):154–170.
21. D'Orsi CJ, Feldhaus L, Sonnenfeld M. Unusual lesions of the breast. Radiol Clin North Am 1983;21:67–79.
22. Bassett LW, Cove HC. Myoblastoma of the breast. AJR 1979;132:122–123.
23. Ali M, Fayemi AO, Braun EV, Remy R. Fibromatosis of the breast. Am J Surg Pathol 1979;3:501–505.
24. Kalisher L, Long JA, Peyster RG. Extra-abdominal desmoid of the axillary tail mimicking breast carcinoma. AJR 1976;126:903–906.
25. Leborgne R. Diagnosis of tumors of the breast by simple roentgenography: calcifications in carcinoma. AJR 1951;65:1–11.
26. Lundgren B. Malignant features of breast tumours at radiography. Acta Radiol (Diagn) 1978;19:623–633.
27. Sadowsky N, Kopans DB. Breast cancer. Radiol Clin North Am 1983;21:51–65.
28. Rosen PP. The pathology of breast carcinoma. In: Harris JR, Hellman S, Henderson IC, Kinne DW, eds. Breast diseases. Philadelphia: JB Lippincott, 1987, chap 7.
29. Gold RH, Main G, Zippin C, et al. Infiltration of mammary carcinoma as an indicator of axillary metastases: a preliminary report. Cancer 1972;29:35–40.
30. Feig SA, Shaber GS, Patchefsky AS, et al. Tubular carcinoma of the breast: mammographic appearance and pathological correlation. Radiology 1978;129:311–314.
31. Jao W, Recant W, Swerdlow MA. Comparative ultrastructure of tubular carcinoma and sclerosing adenosis of the breast. Cancer 1976;38:180–186.
32. Linell F, Ljungberg O. Breast carcinoma: progression of tubular carcinoma and a new classification. Acta Pathol Microbiol Scand (A) 1980;88:59–60.
33. Wellings SR, Alpers CE. Subgross pathologic features and incidence of radial scars in the breast. Hum Pathol 1984;15:475–479.
34. Lesser ML, Rosen PP, Kinne DW. Multicentricity and bilaterality in invasive breast carcinoma. Surgery 1982;91:234–240.
35. Mendelson EB, Harris KM, Doshi N, Tobon H. Infiltrating lobular carcinoma: mammographic patterns with pathologic correlation. AJR 1989;153:265–271.
36. Sickles EA. Mammographic features of "early" breast cancer. AJR 1984;143:461–464.
37. Sickles EA. Microfocal spot magnification mammography using xeroradiographic and screenfilm recording systems. Radiology 1979;131:599–607.
38. Meyer JE, Kopans DB. Xeromammographic appearance of lymphoma of the breast. Radiology 1980;135:623–626.
39. Ciatto S, Cataliotti L, Distante V. Nonpalpable lesions detected with mammography: review of 512 consecutive cases. Radiology 1987;165:99–102.

6

CALCIFICATIONS

Early work by Leborgne in 1951 (1) described the presence of calcifications associated with breast cancer on mammography. Gershon-Cohen et al. (2) further described the appearance of the malignant calcifications as clustered, irregular in size and shape, and ranging from minute to 3 mm in diameter (3). About 50% of all breast cancers (4) are associated with calcifications, and occult lesions may present more frequently as calcifications only or as a mass with calcifications. If microcalcifications are present without a mass, benign and malignant disease may be more difficult to differentiate. With improvements in mammography technology and better resolution, we are faced with dealing with various types of calcification every day. Often, one can differentiate from the great numbers of calcifications those that are clearly benign, such as fibroadenomas, fat necrosis, and vascular and secretory calcifications, from those that are clearly malignant (5). Between these two groups are the clustered indeterminate microcalcifications that are usually biopsied to be certain of their etiology. Features that are characteristic of some types of benign and malignant calcifications are described in this chapter, and the differential diagnosis for the indeterminate forms of calcium deposits are shown.

Fibroadenomas

Fibroadenomas are generally palpated as firm, well-defined breast masses in women under 30 years. The lesions tend to involute after menopause, with mucoid degeneration and calcification occurring later in their natural history. The masses may be large, are generally well defined, and may contain large bizarre irregular calcifications that should not be confused with carcinoma.

Early in the stages of calcification, a few punctate peripheral microcalcifications may develop and may occasionally be suspicious enough in appearance to be biopsied (Figs. 6.1–6.5). Occasionally, degenerating fibroadenomas may contain somewhat-irregular, mixed morphology microcalcifications that are indistinguishable from a ductal lesion, and biopsy is necessary. Later, the calcifications become more dense and coarse (6) and are easily differentiated from malignancy. In the latest stages, the soft tissue masses are no longer apparent and are totally replaced by typical large coarse "popcorn-like" calcifications (Figs. 6.6–6.13).

Fat Necrosis

Fat necrosis may appear in a variety of ways mammographically, from an irregular mass with overlying skin retraction, to an oil cyst, to a spectrum of forms of calcifications (7). Fat necrosis occurs after trauma and hemorrhage, such as after biopsy, aspiration, or blunt trauma with hematoma formation. Clinically, the patient may be asymptomatic or may appear with an indurated firm mass with or without overlying skin thickening and retraction. On histology, fat necrosis is characterized by anuclear fat cells with giant cells and phagocytic histiocytes. There may be central necrosis and liquefaction with formation of an oil cyst; aspiration of these lesions yields a clear oily fluid.

The calcifications that occur in fat necrosis may be small, smooth, and ringlike (liponecrosis microcystica calcificans) (8) and may be single or multiple (Figs. 6.14 and 6.15). Occasionally, these small calcifications may, over time, become amorphous and disappear (9), presumably related to the presence of phagocytes. Parker et al. (10) found that the disappearance of breast calcifications is uncommon; the most common form of calcification that did disappear was a round or oval macrocalcification. Other forms of calcification seen in fat necrosis include irregular microcalcifications that may look suspicious enough to be biopsied (Figs. 6.16 and 6.17) or large circumlinear calcifications seen in the walls of oil cysts (liponecrosis macrocystica calcificans) that are characteristically benign (7) (Figs. 6.18–6.22).

Secretory Disease

Plasma cell mastitis, or secretory disease, is an aseptic inflammation of the breast thought to be the result of extravasation of intraductal secretions into the periductal connective tissue. As a late phenomenon of secretory disease, calcifications may occur (11).

The calcifications associated with this condition may be intraductal, in the wall of the duct, or periductal, and the morphology depends on the location. Secretory calcifications are large (up to 5 mm in diameter), smooth bordered, and round, ovoid, linear, or needle-like in shape (11–14). The centers may be solid or hollow (if periductal). Typically, the disease is bilateral and the calcifications are in an orderly array, oriented toward the nipples along the direction of the lactiferous ducts. The appearance of these calcifications is characteristic, and they generally should not be confused with malignant calcifications (Figs. 6.23–6.28).

Vascular Calcifications

Most commonly, arterial calcifications occur as a result of atherosclerosis in elderly women or in patients with renal failure (15). A weak correlation exists between the presence of diabetes mellitus and arterial calcifications (16). Linear parallel streaks of calcium that follow a tortuous course along the path of the vessel are typical of arterial calcifications. Uncommonly, very early arterial calcifications in a dense breast may appear as a group of fine microcalcifications and may be confused with suspicious ductal calcifications (17). If calcifications are thought to be vascular, it is important to identify a vessel passing into the area and corresponding to the pattern of calcification (Figs. 6.29–6.31). Spot magnification views may be helpful in this situation to evaluate the orientation and morphology of the calcifications, and the vessel passing through may be identified on the magnified image (Fig. 6.32).

Skin Calcifications

The radiologist should suspect that a group of calcifications are in the skin, not the parenchyma, if they are located peripherally, are very well demarcated, and are ringlike, spheroidal, or polygonal (18). Dermal calcifications are usually related to a chronic inflammatory process such as folliculitis and are often located in sebaceous glands (19). Typically, dermal calcifications have very well defined margins and a central lucency (Figs. 6.33–6.37).

Although skin calcifications may occur in any location, the characteristic distribution is over the medial aspect of the breast near the chest wall (12). Because of the conical shape of the breast, skin calcifications may superimpose over the parenchyma on both craniocaudal and lateral views with compression and may appear to be intraparenchymal (18). Obtaining tangential views to the area of concern will prove that a cluster of dermal calcifications is actually within the skin.

Lesions, other than sebaceous glands, that may calcify are nevi (Fig. 6.38), hemangiomas, and skin tags. Another appearance of calcifications in the skin is that of dystrophic calcifications associated with scarring. These calcifications are generally quite coarse, are dense, may be irregular or ringlike, and are usually larger than the calcifications associated with malignancies. This type of dystrophic skin calcification is usually associated with thick scarring, such as after reduction mammoplasty, or with burns and keloid formation (Fig. 6.39).

Other Benign Lesions That Calcify

Lipomas may calcify uncommonly, presumably from infarction or fat necrosis. The calcifications may be ringlike, typical of fat necrosis (19) (Figs. 6.40 and 6.41), or may be larger and coarse. Regardless, a well-circumscribed radiolucent mass with associated calcification should not be confused with malignancy.

Solitary intraductal papillomas are often not visualized on the mammogram and are demonstrated with galactography. Because these are polypoid lesions, on a stalk within the duct, the blood supply may be tenuous (20). There is a tendency for papillomas to become fibrotic or to infarct, which may be followed by the development of calcifications. The appearances of the calcification vary from a few to a cluster of stippled calcifications simulating malignancy, to a larger, more dense, rounded calcification conforming to the walls of the duct (19) (Fig. 6.42).

Patients who have had silicone or paraffin injections for augmentation of the breasts are found to have very dense breasts with multiple small nodules (21). Imaging may be quite limited because of the density and incompressibility of the breast. These patients may develop extensive round or ringlike calcifications (22), which may be related to fat necrosis and foreign body reaction as well as to the presence of silicone itself. The calcifications have an appearance similar to those of fat necrosis and are typically benign (Fig. 6.43). If a breast implant containing silicone ruptures, similar-appearing ringlike calcifications form around the dense globules of silicone. Uncommonly, the silicone can extend into the lactiferous ducts, creating a "silicone cast" of the duct lumen (23).

A systemic cause of calcification formation in the breast, as in other areas of soft tissue, is secondary hyperparathyroidism and renal failure. Patients with hypercalcemia may develop deposition of coarse amorphous areas of calcium in the breasts (15, 24, 25). This process is usually bilateral, since it is of systemic origin (Fig. 6.44).

Fibrocystic Disease

Fibrocystic disease comprises pathologically a group of benign proliferative disorders of the breast, including fibrosis, cysts, adenosis, sclerosing adenosis, epithelial hyperplasia, papillomatosis, atypical hyperplasia, apocrine metaplasia, and chronic inflammation. Clinically, the patients are most commonly in the 30–50-year-old age group and present with lumpy tender breasts that are cyclically symptomatic. Microcalcifications occur frequently in patients who have fibrocystic disease. The differentiation between ductal calcifications of fibrocystic origin and intraductal carcinoma is often not possible (26, 27), and many of these clusters will need to be biopsied. About 15–30% of microcalcifications that are biopsied in asymptomatic patients are malignant (28–

30), and the remainder are benign, mostly representing some form of fibrocystic disease (31). Epithelial cells have the potential to secrete calcium actively, and indistinguishable deposits on mammography may be found in benign and malignant conditions.

The analysis of microcalcifications can be divided into two basic types: lobular and ductal. Lobular microcalcifications tend to be smooth, round, and similar in size and density (19). Lobular calcifications can be found in conditions that involve increased activity in the ductules—including adenosis, sclerosing adenosis, cystic hyperplasia, atypical lobular hyperplasia, and lobular carcinoma in situ.

Sclerosing adenosis and adenosis often represent a diffuse process involving both breasts with increased density and fine nodularity. The calcifications tend to be fine and round, spherical, or globular (32); they are homogeneous and may be laminated (13). The microcalcifications in adenosis tend to involve both breasts diffusely (32) and symmetrically. If the process is localized, however, the calcifications may be clustered, and biopsy often is performed to confirm the histology (32). When the condition is diffuse and bilateral, the diagnosis may be suggested by mammography, and biopsy is not necessary (Figs. 6.45 and 6.46).

Microglandular adenosis is a benign disease in which small uniform glands grow haphazardly in the mammary parenchyma. Microscopically, the appearance is similar to that of a tubular carcinoma (33, 34). Microcalcifications may be present (33) and have a nonspecific lobular appearance (Figs. 6.47 and 6.48).

In cystic hyperplasia, milk of calcium may be secreted into the cyst fluid (35). When the breast is imaged in the upright projection with a lateral beam (i.e., on the mediolateral view), the calcium lies in the dependent aspect of the tiny cysts and appears as circumlinear or saucer-shaped microcalcifications. On the craniocaudal view (with a vertical beam), these calcifications are much less clearly seen and appear as poorly defined smudges (35) (Figs. 6.49–6.54). The importance of identifying this condition is that the linear calcifications identified on the upright film might be misinterpreted as ductal and therefore suspicious for carcinoma (35). The process may be extensive or focal (36), and it is important that one not overlook suspicious microcalcifications that may be located in the region of microcysts. Occasionally also, macrocysts may calcify, creating the appearance of a cluster of microcalcifications in the craniocaudal view and a layer of calcium on the mediolateral view (37). There may also be complete calcification in the walls of small cysts, creating the mammographic appearance of multiple ringlike calcifications (Fig. 6.55).

Papillomatosis, similarly, produces fine round microcalcifications that extend over a large area of the breast (12). A dense prominent ductal pattern may be present and is associated with the fine microcalcifications (Fig. 6.56).

In periductal fibrosis the calcifications occur in the stroma and may be diffuse or grouped. On histology, broad islands of fibrous tissue replace the normal fat of the breast. The calcifications of fibrosis may mimic intraductal calcifications found in carcinoma in situ because they may be clustered, with irregular borders, and variable in size, shape, and density, but they tend to be more coarse than is usually found in malignancy (Fig. 6.57).

Intraductal microcalcifications occur in epithelial hyperplasia, a proliferative disorder with the ducts. The work of Gallager and Martin (38, 39) with whole-organ specimens in patients with breast cancer showed that there is a spectrum of disease from epithelial hyperplasia to atypical hyperplasia to carcinoma in situ, which occurs as nonobligate phases in the development of breast cancer. Depending on the extent of the process, microcalcifications may be focal or extensive and may be present bilaterally. The calcifications are small (less than 1 mm in diameter) and may be irregular in form and variable in size and density, which are the same features found in intraductal carcinoma. Egan et al. (26) found the calcifications in epithelial hyperplasia to be indistinguishable from those of intraductal carcinoma (Figs. 6.58–6.63).

The presence of hyperplastic lesions of the breast places a patient at higher risk for the development of carcinoma (40–42). In particular, atypical lobular hyperplasia increases the risk of developing breast cancer by approximately 6 times (40), and atypical ductal hyperplasia is associated with a 4–5 times subsequent risk (41). Additionally, the combined factors of a family history of breast cancer and an atypical lesion on biopsy increase the risk of subsequent breast cancer by 11 times that of women with nonproliferative lesions and no family history (42).

Lobular Neoplasia

Lobular carcinoma in situ, or lobular neoplasia, was described by Foote and Stewart (43) as originating in the lobular terminal duct complex. The lesion is associated with other types of cancers and has a high propensity toward multicentricity and bilaterality (44). In a follow-up of 99 patients with lobular carcinoma in situ treated by lumpectomy only. Rosen et al. (45) found that there was an equal risk of developing invasive carcinoma in both the ipsilateral and the contralateral breast. Since about one third of patients with lobular carcinoma in situ treated with excision alone will develop invasive carcinoma in either breast, the choices for therapy are variable, ranging from lumpectomy only to bilateral mastectomies (45, 46). The trend toward management of these patients has been toward excision only. Because of the high-risk status of patients with this condition, very careful follow-up with mammography is necessary if the breast is not treated after excision of the lesion. The mammographic findings are variable, but grouped, rounded, lobular microcalcifications are one of the more common presentations (47). These calcifications are indistinguishable from those of lobular hyperplasia or focal sclerosing adenosis (Figs. 6.64–6.69); occasionally, in biopsies of lesions found on mammography in which the histology reveals lobular carcinoma in situ, the calcifications may be located in the abnormal lobules, or they may be in adjacent benign lobules or areas of stroma (48).

Malignant Calcifications

Breast cancers are associated with malignant calcifications in about 50% of cases (4), including both palpable and nonpalpable carcinomas (49). Hermann et al. (50) found that microcalcifications accounted for 43% and that microcalcifications with associated nodules accounted for an additional 18% of mammographically detected breast cancers.

Intraductal carcinoma (ductal carcinoma in situ (DCIS)) accounts for 15–20% of all breast cancers (51) and is most frequently found by mammography rather than by physical examination. Stomper et al. (52) found that in 100 cases of intraductal carcinoma, 72% presented as microcalcifications only and 12% presented as nodules with calcifications. Other less common mammographic features of DCIS include circumscribed nodules, asymmetry, dilated ducts, ill-defined nodules, and focal architectural distortion (53).

Ultrastructural analysis by Ahmed (54) of the calcifications that occur in breast cancers showed the deposits to be contained within glandlike lumina formed by clumps of intraductal tumor cells. The calcium was thought to be the result of active secretion by the epithelial cells. Calcific deposits may also occur as the result of calcification of necrotic debris, as in comedocarcinoma. These intraductal calcifications may develop in association not only with carcinoma but also with hyperplastic conditions (55) within the epithelium, thereby making radiographic differentiation often impossible.

The calcifications in ductal malignancy (Figs. 6.70–6.92) are usually small (0.1–0.3 mm), although they rarely may be larger in diameter (up to 2 mm). The shape and size of the calcifications are variable. Because the calcifications are deposited between crypts formed by irregular projections of epithelial cells, they form casts of the lumina of the ducts and, similarly, have irregular borders (3). Combinations of forms including rod-shaped, punctate, comma-shaped, teardrop-shaped, Y or branching, and lacy calcifications, may be seen together and are considered of high suspicion for malignancy. Granular calcifications having a fine salt-and-pepper appearance may also be present in carcinomas; close examination of these with magnification views often shows the irregularity of their borders. Magnification mammography may also improve the detection of microcalcifications (56).

The greater the number of calcifications in an area, the more suspicious for malignancy (12, 57, 58). Egan et al.

(26) found that 84% of breast cancers containing microcalcifications had more than 10 calcifications in a group. Millis et al. (4) found that in 33 cancers, 6 had less than 5 calcifications in a cluster.

Malignant calcifications tend to occur in clusters of 1 cm² or less. However, it is important that one not exclude malignant-appearing calcifications as being suspicious if they are not tightly clustered or numerous. Malignant calcifications can involve a large area, even an entire quadrant or more of the breast, particularly in the case of comedocarcinoma, where the tumor may occur extensively throughout the ductal system. Also, multicentric foci of carcinoma may present with multiple separate clusters of microcalcifications in different areas of the breast.

The morphology of ductal calcifications is classically described as linear, irregular, and branching, yet the majority of calcifications of DCIS are not this type. Stomper et al. (52) found that 35% of cases of DCIS presented as casting calcifications, 52% had granular calcifications, and 13% were composed of mixed forms. Even diffusely scattered, profuse unilateral calcifications having spherical or hollow shapes, usually associated with benign lesions, have been described (59) in ductal malignancies with apocrine features. Also in cases of intraductal carcinoma in which there is retrograde involvement of the lobule (cancerization of the lobule), the form of calcification may be founded (60).

The identification of an extensive intraductal component (EIC) associated with an infiltrating cancer may be a predictor of a high risk of finding residual carcinoma on reexcision (61) and a higher local recurrence rate after breast conservation therapy (lumpectomy and breast irradiation) (62). An EIC is defined (63) as the presence of DCIS occupying an area of ≧25% of the area occupied by the infiltrating cancer and the presence of DCIS in areas beyond the edge of the infiltrating tumor. Tumors detected only by mammography or tumors presenting as microcalcifications are more likely to be EIC positive, but this preoperative analysis is not absolute (64).

The finding of clustered microcalcifications on mammography is often nonspecific (3, 26), and histologic examination is necessary to differentiate benign fibrocystic disease or hyperplastic conditions from carcinoma in situ.

Postradiation Therapy Changes

After lumpectomy and radiation treatment to the breast, follow-up mammograms may reveal the development of calcifications. The coarse round or ringlike calcifications represent calcified lipid-filled cysts and are of dystrophic origin (65) (Figs. 6.93 and 6.94). These calcifications are identical with those of fat necrosis from trauma or biopsy, and they should not be confused with the lacy, linear irregular microcalcifications indicating recurrence of carcinoma (66) (Figs. 6.95 and 6.96). The dystrophic calcifications that occur after conservative therapy for breast cancer may be present at the biopsy site or may occur elsewhere in the breast. It has been suggested (67) that 25% of patients who are treated with lumpectomy and radiation therapy for breast cancer will develop dystrophic calcifications as a normal effect of treatment.

Pseudocalcifications

Several types of foreign substances may calcify or create an artifactual appearance of calcifications. Patients who have undergone intramuscular gold therapy for rheumatoid arthritis may develop gold deposits simulating microcalcifications in intramammary (68) and axillary (69) lymph nodes. The appearance and location of the node and the appropriate clinical history should suggest this as an etiology of the "calcifications" (Fig 6.97).

Sutures placed in the breast during biopsy, lumpectomy, or reduction procedures may calcify (70). The appearances include smooth linear or curvilinear calcifications or knot-shaped calcifications (Fig 6.98). It is important to correlate the position of a surgical scar with the area of calcifications when one is suggesting this diagnosis.

A number of substances applied to the skin can look like calcium on the mammogram. These include deodorant (71), powders, creams, ointments (in particular, zinc oxide ointment), and adhesive tape (72) (Figs. 6.99–6.103). Many of these appear as very fine granular densities over the surface of the breasts. Deodorant produces larger, more clustered-appearing densities in the area of the axillary folds. If there is a suspicion that a calcific-like density on the mammogram may be artifactual, the film should be repeated after careful cleansing of the skin surface.

Figure 6.1.

Clinical: 61-year-old woman for screening.

Mammogram: Left craniocaudal view (**A**) and magnified image (**B**). There is a relatively well-defined lobulated mass in the left inner quadrant *(arrow)* (**A**). A magnified view of this area demonstrates the presence of several peripheral macrocalcifications. The finding suggests the appearance of a degenerating fibroadenoma with early calcification. The calcifications in this case are more coarse and more similar in appearance than is generally found in malignant calcification.

Impression: Degenerating fibroadenoma.

Histopathology: Fibroadenoma.

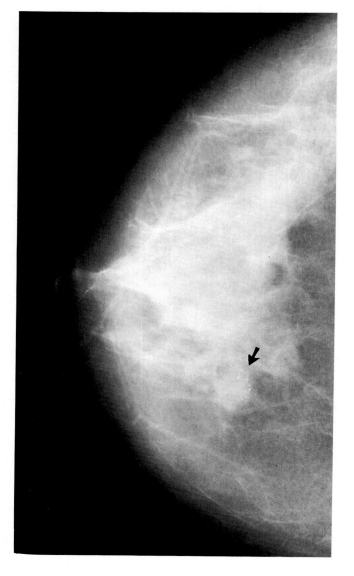

A

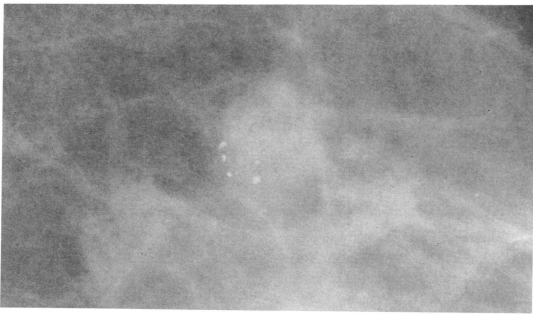

B

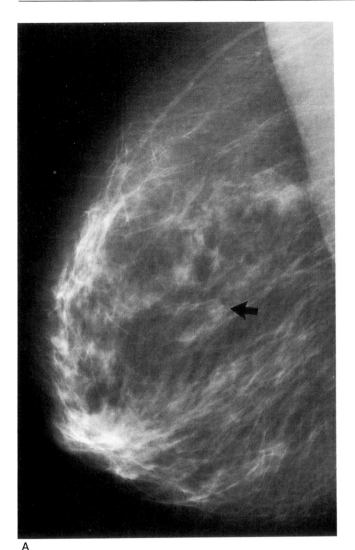

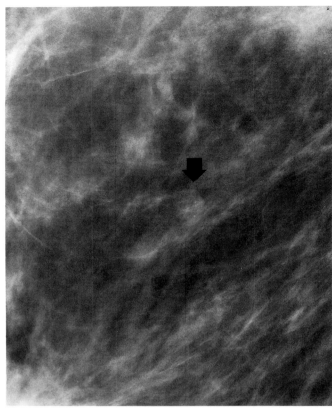

Figure 6.2.

Clinical: 63-year-old G2, P2 patient on estrogen replacement therapy, for routine screening.

Mammogram: Left oblique (**A**) and magnified (2×) cranio-caudal (**B**) views. The breast is mildly glandular with nodular densities present, unchanged from prior examination for 2½ years. One of these nodules *(arrows)* is of medium density, is very well circumscribed, and on the magnification view (**B**)

is noted to contain a few relatively smooth bordered, peripheral, punctate microcalcifications. This pattern of peripheral calcification is typical of that seen in early degeneration of a fibroadenoma.

Impression: Early calcifications in a degenerated fibroadenoma.

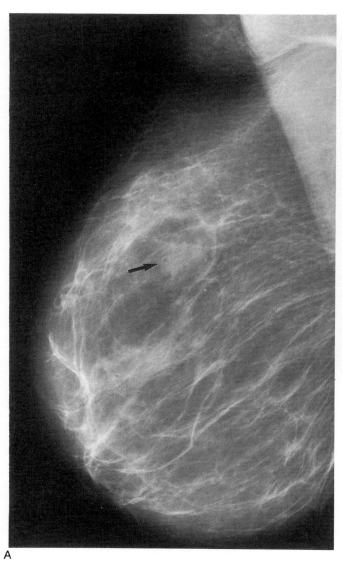

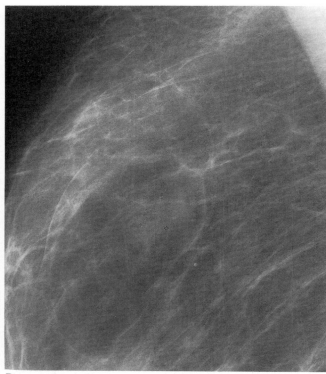

Figure 6.3.

Clinical: 72-year-old G2, P2 woman for screening mammography.

Mammogram: Left oblique (**A**) and enlarged (1.5×) (**B**) views. The breast is mildly glandular. In the upper outer quadrant, there is a low- to medium-density nodule with indistinct margins and associated microcalcifications *(arrow)* (**A**). The calcifications are rather smoothly marginated and round but vary in size (**B**). They are located peripherally in the soft tissue density. The peripheral calcification is consistent with a fibroadenoma; however, the indistinct margins of the mass are of concern. The lesion was considered moderately suspicious and was biopsied after needle localization.

Impression: Possible fibroadenoma with degeneration; neoplasm cannot be ruled out.

Histopathology: Fibroadenoma, fibrocystic changes with epithelial hyperplasia.

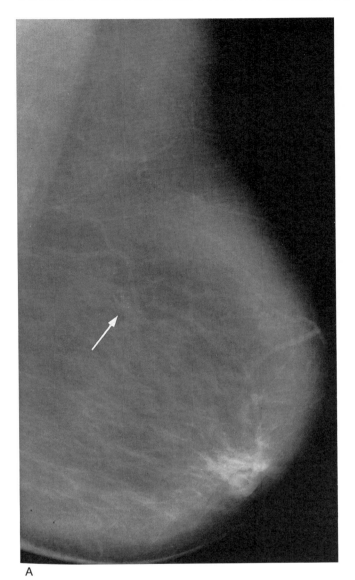

A

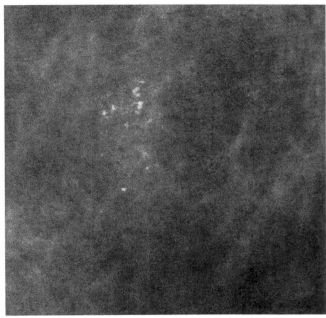

B

Figure 6.4.

Clinical: 68-year-old woman for screening mammography.

Mammogram: Right oblique view (**A**) and magnified image (**B**). In the upper outer quadrant of the right breast showing otherwise fatty replacement are clustered microcalcifications *(arrow)* in an area of low-density soft tissue (**A**). The magnified image shows the irregularity of borders of the calcifications, but no branching or linear forms are noted.

Impression: Cluster of calcifications of mild to moderate suspicion, favoring fibrocystic changes.

Histopathology: Fibroadenoma with calcifications.

Note: Occasionally, a small fibroadenoma may degenerate and the soft tissue mass decreases in size, leaving only calcifications visible. Although calcifications in fibroadenomas are generally coarse, microcalcifications may be seen, particularly early in the degenerative process.

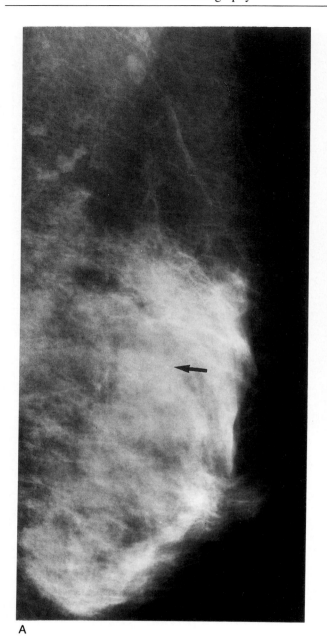

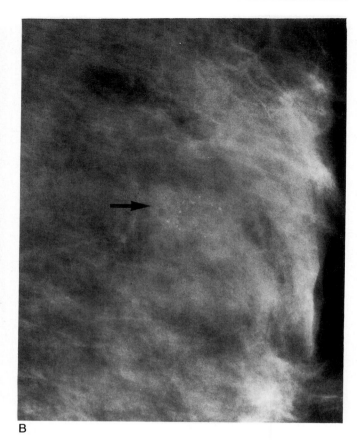

Figure 6.5.

Clinical: 42-year-old G0 woman with a history of Hodgkin's lymphoma, for baseline screening mammography.

Mammogram: Right oblique (**A**) and magnified (2×) craniocaudal (**B**) views. The breast is composed of dense glandular tissue. Lymph nodes in the low axillary area are nonenlarged. In the upper aspect of the right breast (**A**), there are clustered microcalcifications *(arrow),* which on magnification (**B**) are noted to be of mixed morphology with irregular mar-

gins. The calcifications are moderately suspicious for ductal malignancy.

Histopathology: Hyalinized fibroadenoma, focal epithelial hyperplasia.

Note: The calcification that typically occurs in degenerating fibroadenomas is located peripherally in the nodule and is less irregular than the calcifications in this case.

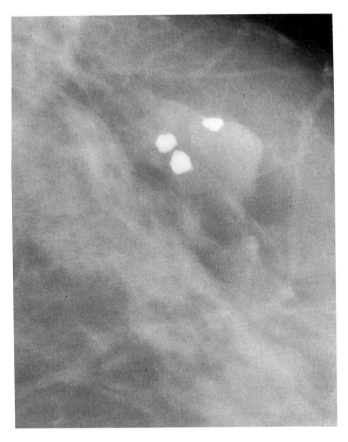

Figure 6.6.

Clinical: 64-year-old asymptomatic woman.

Mammogram: Right magnification view. There is a 1.5-cm well-defined ovoid mass in the right outer quadrant. This lesion contains coarse peripheral macrocalcifications typical of a degenerating fibroadenoma.

Impression: Degenerated calcified fibroadenoma.

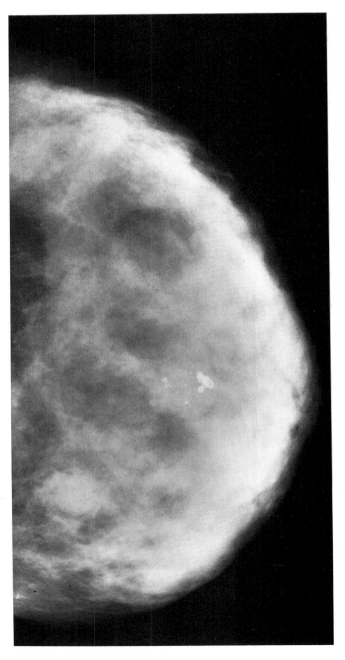

Figure 6.7.

Clinical: 51-year-old woman who has had a 1-cm palpable mass in the 6 o'clock position of the right breast for many years.

Mammogram: Right craniocaudal view. The breast is very dense and glandular. In the midportion of the breast, there is a very well defined nodule with a fatty halo around most of its margins. Dense popcorn-like calcifications are present in the mass and are typical of a degenerated fibroadenoma.

Impression: Degenerated calcified fibroadenoma.

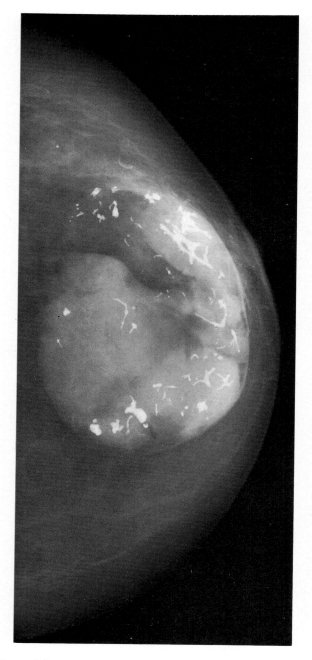

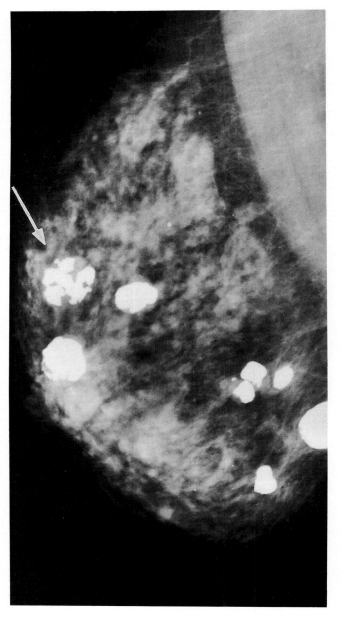

Figure 6.8.

Clinical: 72-year-old woman with a long history of a right breast mass unchanged in size.

Mammogram: Right craniocaudal view. There is a large well-defined mass in the subareolar area that contains coarse bizarre macrocalcifications. Smooth lobulated margins are present. The findings are typical of a fibroadenoma with coarse calcifications.

Impression: Fibroadenoma.

Figure 6.9.

Clinical: 76-year-old woman who has had multiple palpable breast masses for many years.

Mammogram: Bilateral oblique views. The breasts are rather glandular for the age of the patient. There are multiple, popcorn-like, very coarse, dense calcifications in both breasts. These have almost totally replaced the soft tissue masses from which they originated, except for a few partially calcified nodules *(arrows)*. The appearance of these lesions is characteristic of degenerated fibroadenomas.

Impression: Degenerated fibroadenomas.

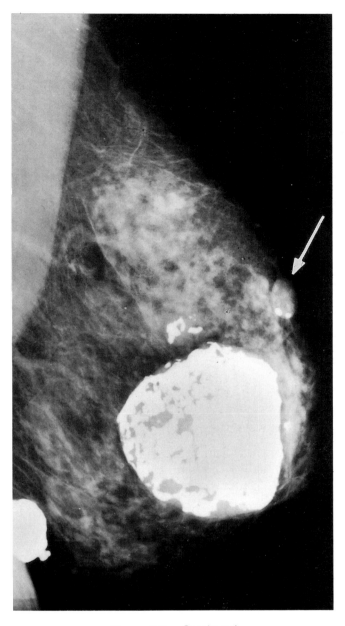

Figure 6.9. *Continued*

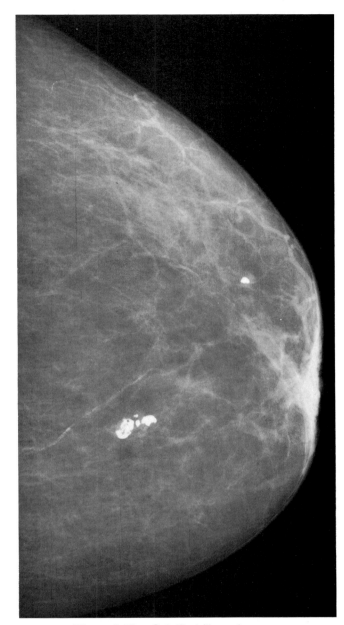

Figure 6.10. Calcified fibroadenoma.

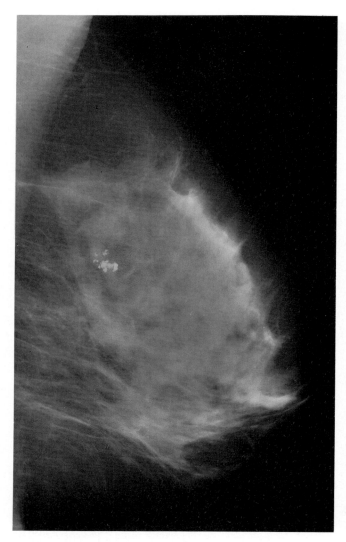

Figure 6.11.   Degenerated fibroadenoma.

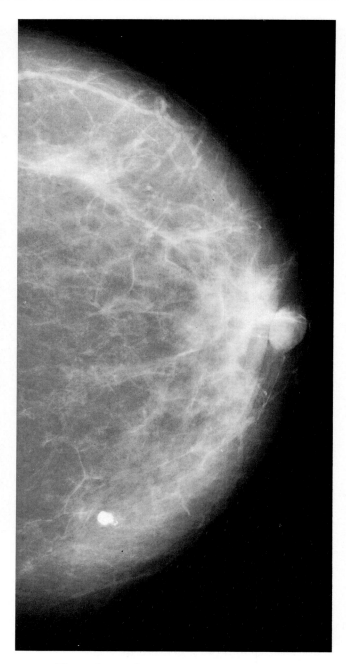

Figure 6.12.   Degenerated fibroadenoma.

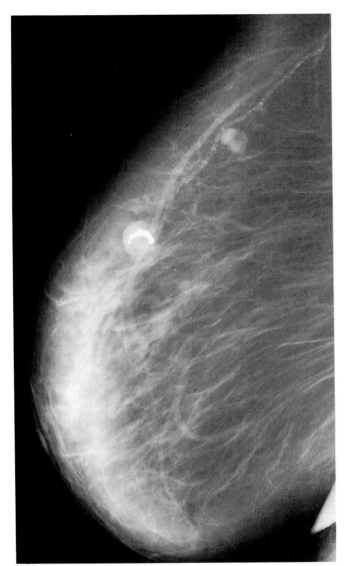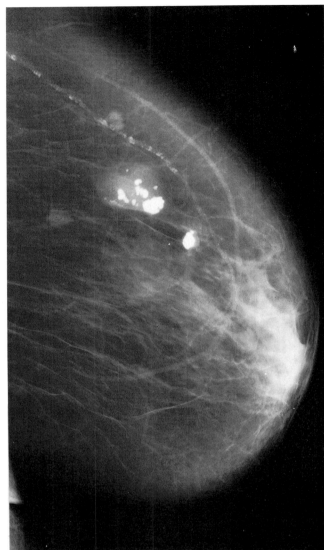

Figure 6.13.

Clinical: Screening mammogram.

Mammogram: Bilateral oblique views. There are multiple, bilateral, well-defined soft tissue masses associated with dense coarse macrocalcifications. These findings are characteristic of degenerating fibroadenomas. Incidental note is made of bilateral intramammary lymph nodes in the axillary tails.

Impression: Bilateral calcified fibroadenomas.

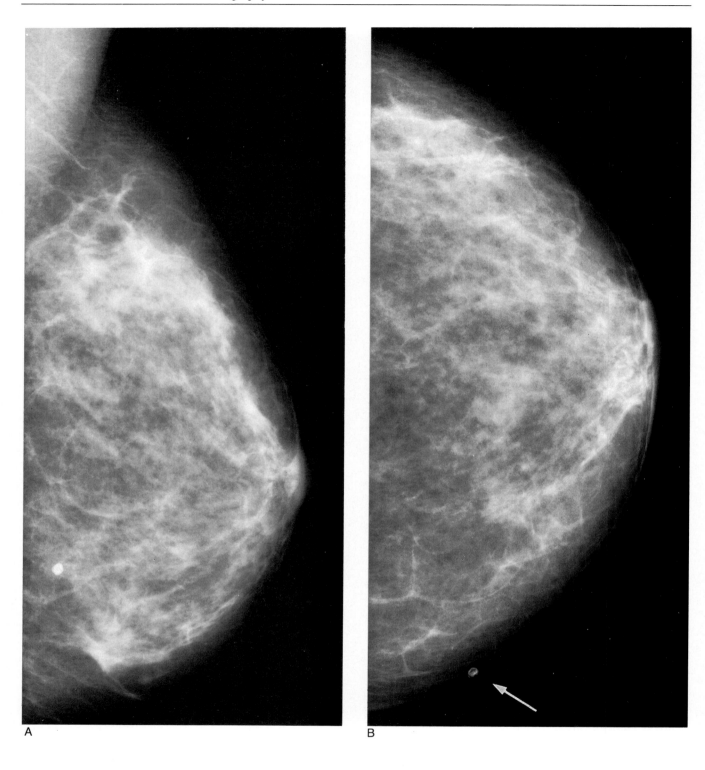

A

B

Figure 6.14.

Clinical: 64-year-old woman with a history of previous aspirations in both breasts, for screening mammography.

Mammogram: Right oblique (**A**) and (**B**) views. There is a single calcification that is coarse and partially ringlike. On the craniocaudal view it is located just beneath the skin me-

dially *(arrow)*. The appearance of the calcification and the location are typical of fat necrosis, presumably related to previous aspirations.

Impression: Fat necrosis.

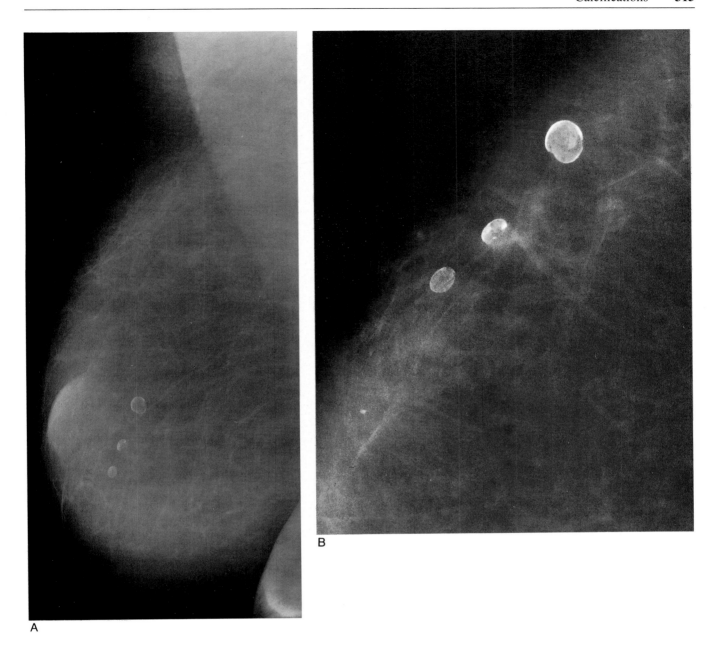

A

B

Figure 6.15.

Clinical: 33-year-old G1, P1 woman who has had bilateral reduction mammoplasties.

Mammogram: Left oblique views (**A**) and magnified image (**B**). The breast shows fatty replacement. There are three ringlike calcifications laterally in the area of surgical scar (**A**). These calcified nodules have relatively lucent centers, typical of oil cysts secondary to reduction mammoplasties (**B**).

Impression: Fat necrosis.

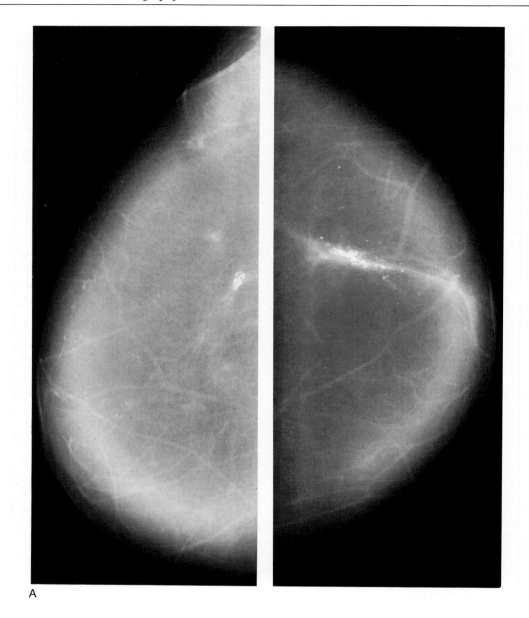

A

Figure 6.16.

Clinical: 65-year-old G1, P1 woman after bilateral reduction mammoplasties, referred for screening mammography.

Mammogram: Bilateral oblique craniocaudal views (**A**) and magnified image (**B**). There are numerous coarse irregular calcifications that are oriented in a linear arrangement and that were situated directly beneath the surgical scars. A magnified view (**B**) shows a variable morphology of circular calcifications associated with punctate and irregular patterns. The findings are typical of fat necrosis, and the extent and distribution are seen after reduction mammoplasty.

Impression: Fat necrosis.

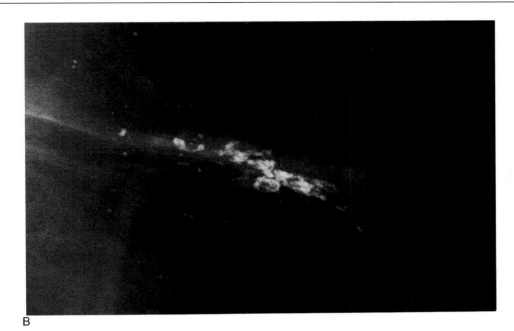

B

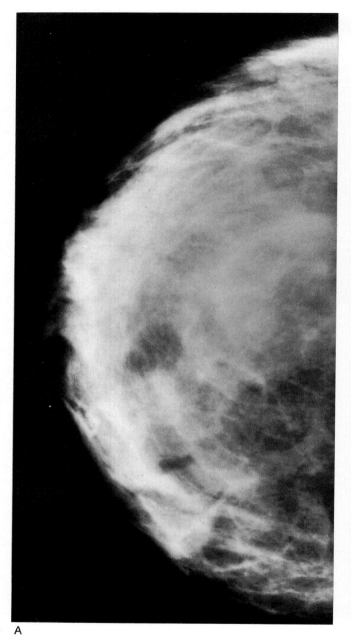
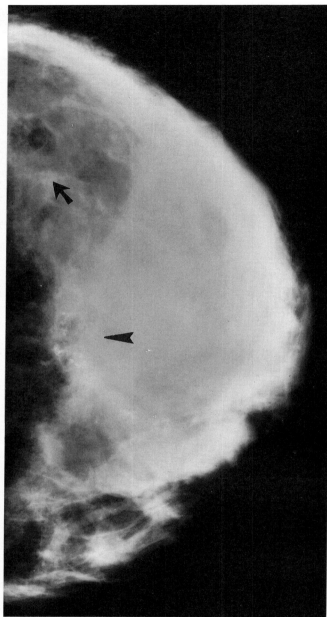

A

Figure 6.17.

Clinical: 25-year-old woman after bilateral reduction mammoplasties. Clinical examination showed multiple lumpy areas in both breasts.

Mammogram: Bilateral craniocaudal views (**A**), right mediolateral view (**B**), and magnified image (**C**). There is architectural distortion in both breasts that is compatible with postoperative changes. There are two areas of calcification in the right breast. In the upper aspect, there is a radiolucent nod-

ule with ringlike calcification *(arrow),* consistent with an oil cyst. In the deeper aspect of the breast, there is a long segment of irregular macrocalcifications *(arrowheads).* A coneddown view (**C**) shows the irregular lacy nature of these calcifications. The distribution of these corresponded to the scar, and these calcifications also represent fat necrosis.

Impression: Postoperative changes, multiple areas of fat necrosis in the right breast.

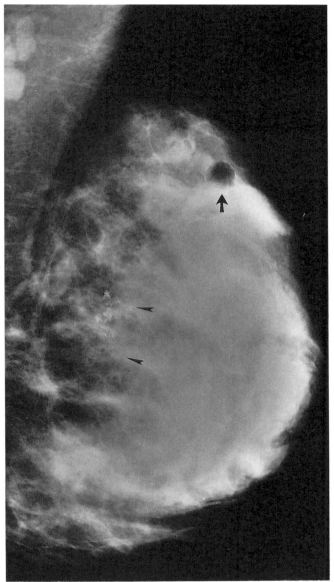

B

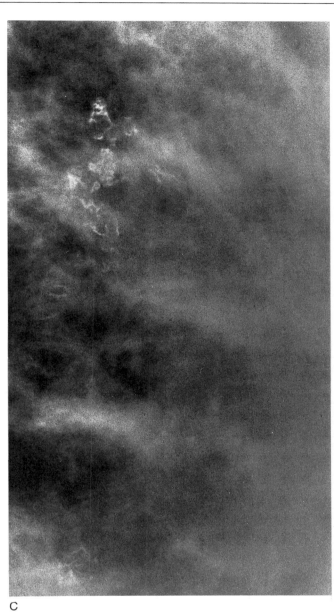

C

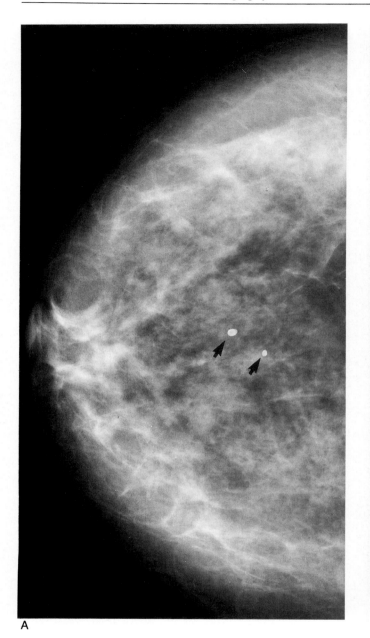

A

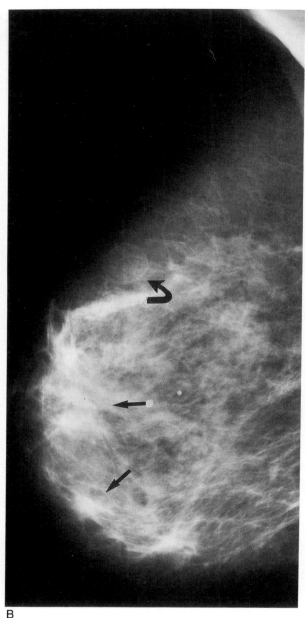

B

Figure 6.18.

Clinical: 65-year-old woman who sustained blunt trauma to the left breast in a motor vehicle accident.

Mammogram: Left craniocaudal baseline view prior to trauma (**A**), left oblique (**B**) and craniocaudal (**C**) views 12 months after trauma, and left oblique (**D**) and craniocaudal (**E**) views 18 months after trauma. On the baseline mammogram (**A**), the breast is moderately glandular, and two calcifications of fat necrosis are noted centrally *(arrows)*. After trauma (**B** and **C**), there has been interval development of a lucent mass with ringlike calcification, consistent with an oil cyst *(curved*

arrow). There are also two new irregular areas of increased density *(arrows)* that most likely represent residual hematoma and fat necrosis. Six months later (**D** and **E**), the irregular densities have resolved, and there has been interval development of coarse irregular calcifications associated with a second oil cyst *(arrow)* at the site of the medial area of fat necrosis.

Impression: Interval changes related to breast trauma, with development of various manifestations of fat necrosis. (Case courtesy of Dr. Cherie Scheer, Richmond, VA.)

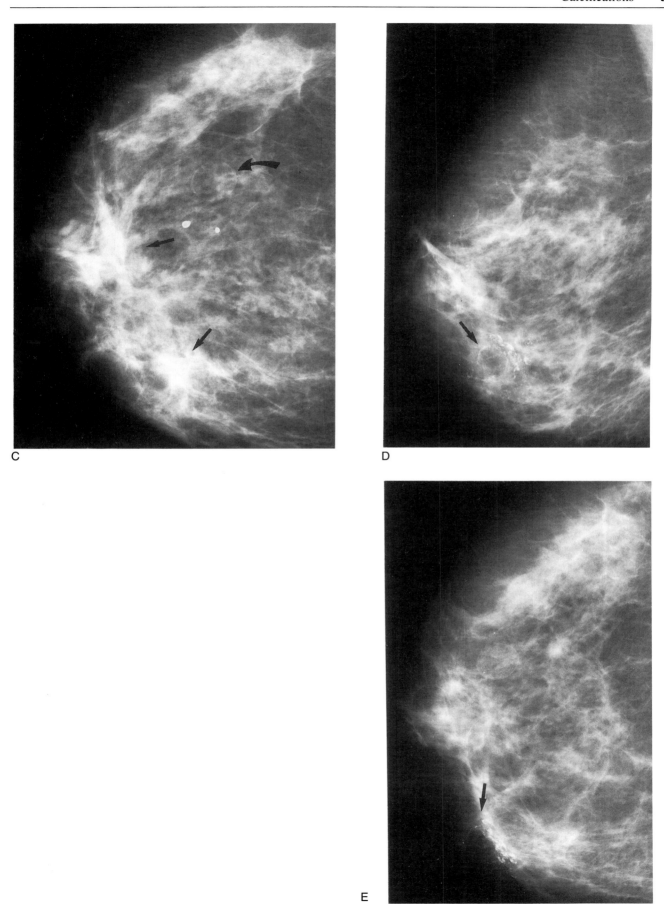

C

D

E

Figure 6.19.

Clinical: 37-year-old woman for screening mammography.

Mammogram: Oblique view (**A**) and magnified image (**B**). In a breast showing otherwise relatively fatty replacement (**A**), there is a ringlike calcification in the upper quadrant *(arrow)*. The coned-down view of this area (**B**) shows the lucent fatty center surrounded by a circumlinear calcification. This finding is typical of a benign calcification and represents an oil cyst from fat necrosis.

Impression: Fat necrosis, oil cyst.

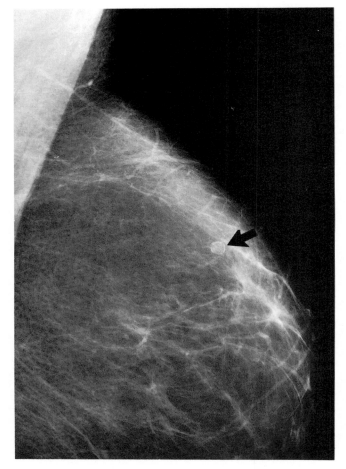

A

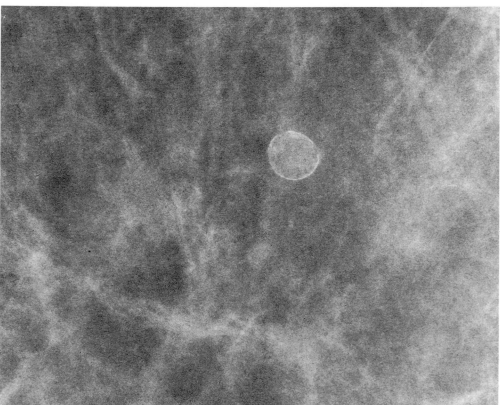

B

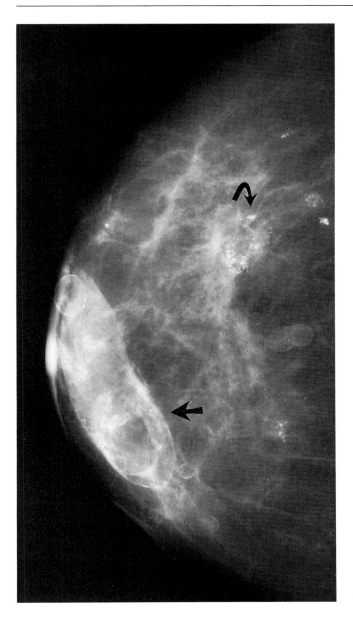

A

Figure 6.20.

Clinical: 54-year-old woman with a history of severe trauma to the upper torso and extremities from farm machinery 1 year previously, presenting with multiple palpable masses in the left breast.

Mammogram: Left craniocaudal view (**A**) and specimen radiograph (**B**). There are multiple, relatively lucent, well-defined masses *(straight arrow)* with calcific rims typical of posttraumatic oil cysts and fat necrosis. Clustered irregular microcalcifications are present *(curved arrow)* and had developed since the mammogram 1 year previously.

Impression: Oil cysts with new clustered calcifications, favoring fat necrosis and fibrosis.

Histopathology (of microcalcifications): Fibrosis, fat necrosis.

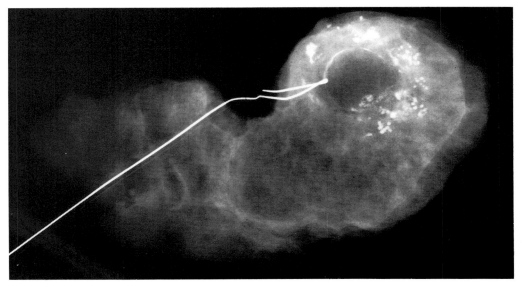

B

Figure 6.21.

Clinical: 70-year-old woman after bilateral reduction mammoplasties.

Mammogram: Right craniocaudal view. There is distortion of architecture in the subareolar area corresponding to the surgical scars. In the subareolar area, there is an ovoid radiolucent mass with a ringlike calcification *(arrow)* representing an oil cyst. It is not uncommon to see evidence for fat necrosis on mammography in patients who have undergone surgery, particularly reduction procedures.

Impression: Oil cyst. (Case courtesy of Dr. Bernard Savage, Richmond, VA.)

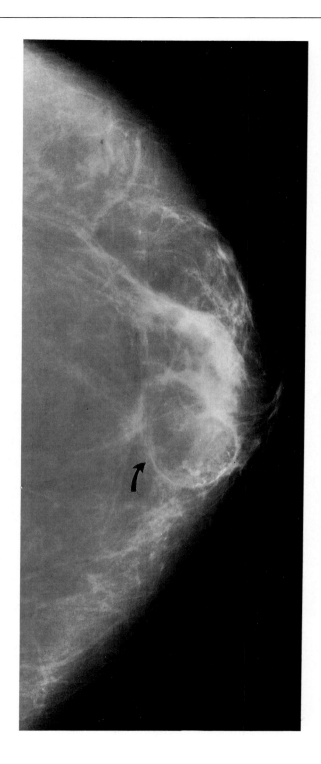

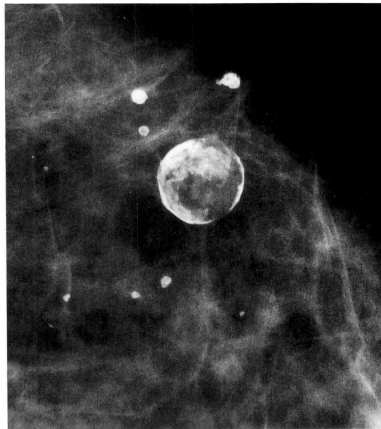

B

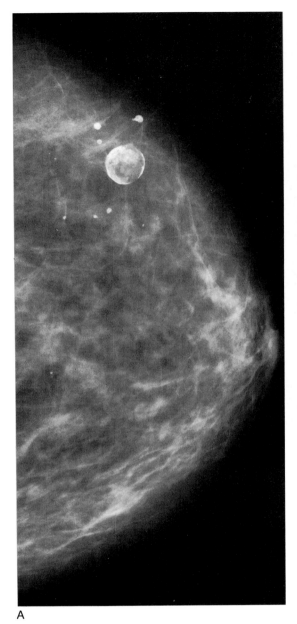

A

Figure 6.22.

Clinical: 44-year-old woman who had had a previous biopsy of a benign lesion in the right outer quadrant, presenting with a 1-cm smooth nodule at the edge of the surgical scar.

Mammogram: Right craniocaudal view (**A**) and magnified image (**B**). There is a well-defined, 1-cm, ringlike calcification in the periphery of a radiolucent mass, characteristic of a calcified oil cyst. Other smaller, dense, round, and circular calcifications of fat necrosis (liponecrosis microcystica) are seen. The changes are presumably related to the previous surgery.

Impression: Fat necrosis: liponecrosis macrocystica and microcystica.

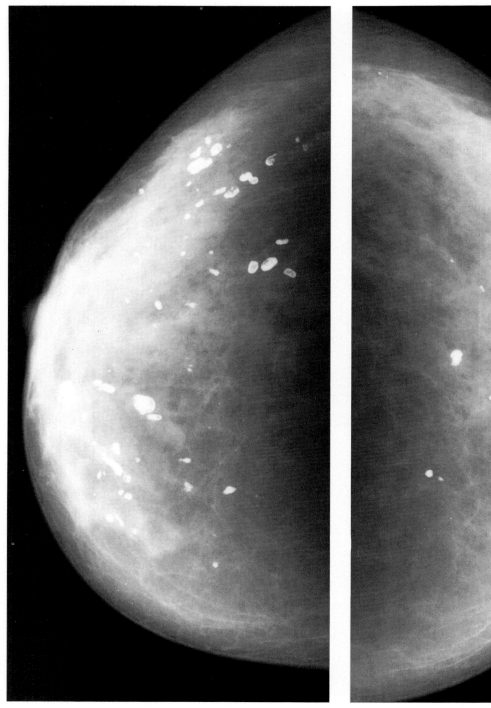
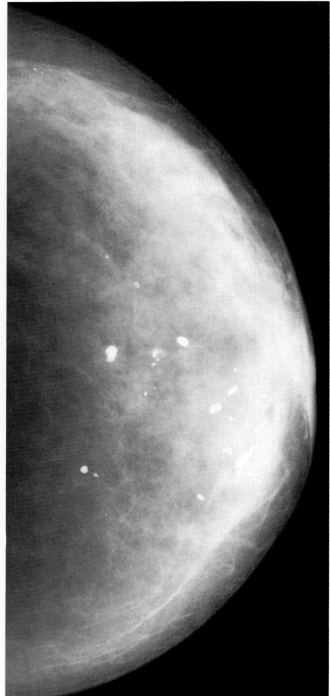

Figure 6.23.

Clinical: 74-year-old woman for screening mammography.

Mammogram: Bilateral craniocaudal views. In both breasts there are coarse and oval microcalcifications arranged in linear patterns radiating to the nipples. Many of these have hollow centers. These are characteristic of secretory disease or plasma cell mastitis and are benign.

Impression: Benign secretory calcifications.

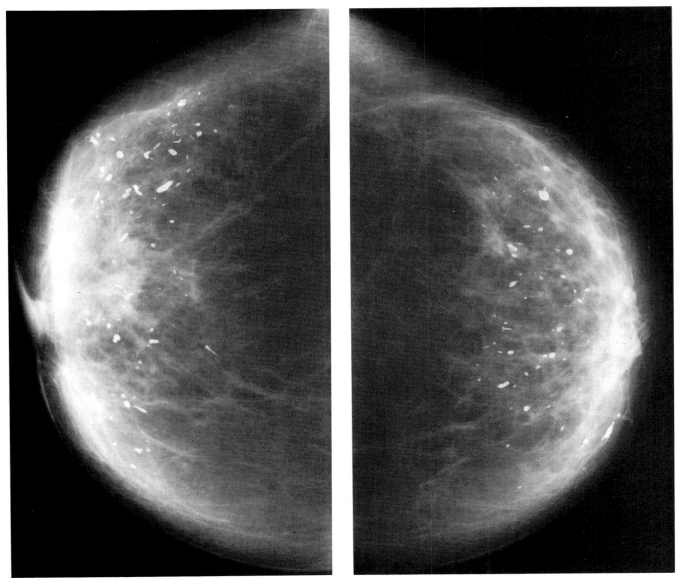

Figure 6.24.   Secretory calcifications.

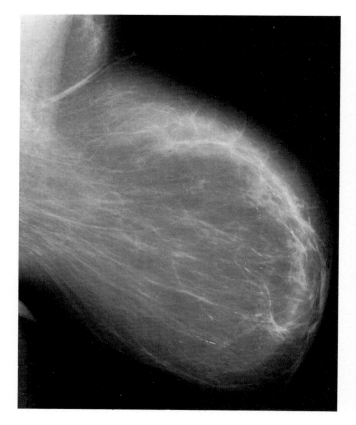

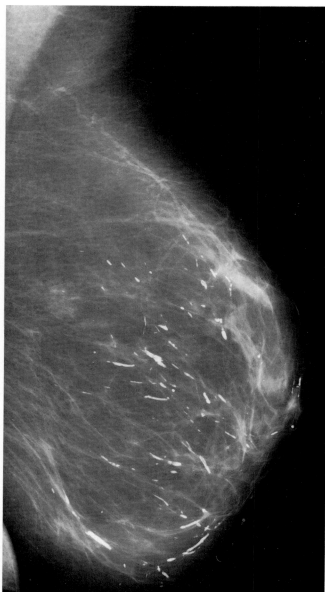

Figure 6.26. Coarse, needle-like and tubular linear calcifications.

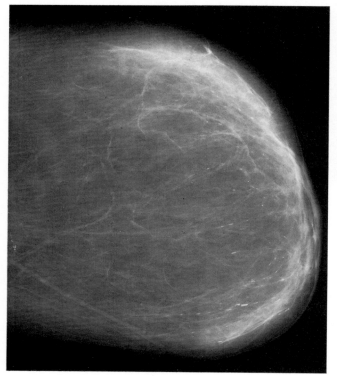

Figure 6.25. Fine, needle-like smooth ductal calcifications oriented toward the nipple.

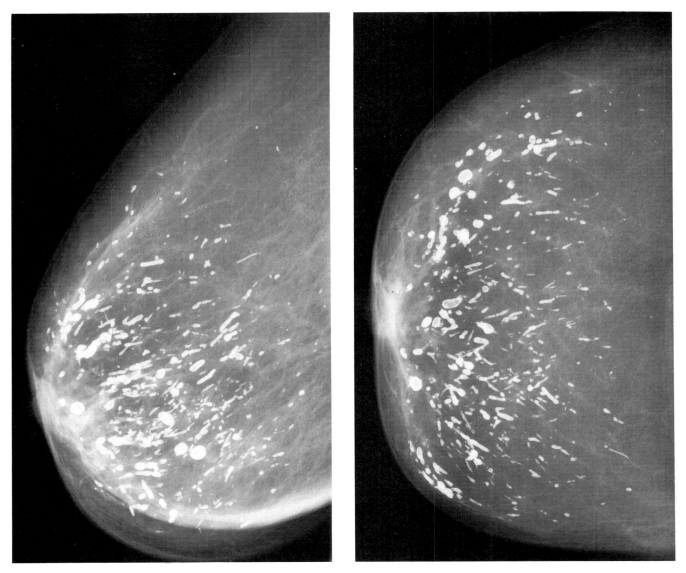

Figure 6.27.   Coarse tubular, round, circular calcifications radiating along the pattern of ducts.

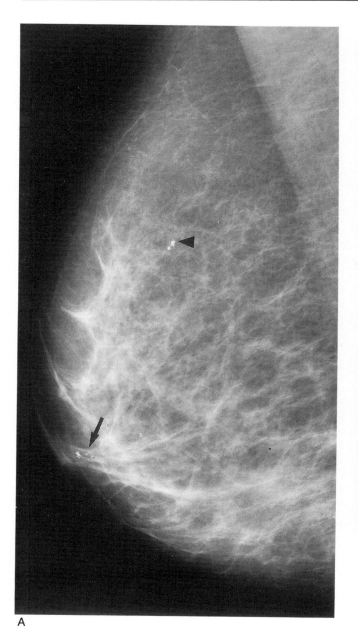

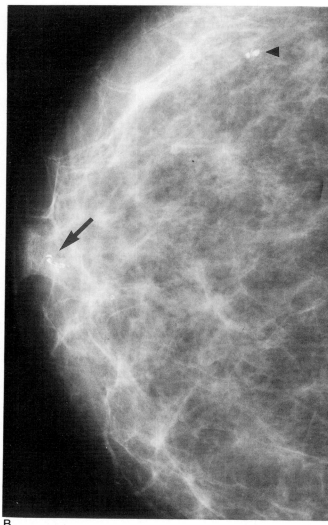

Figure 6.28.

Clinical: 67-year-old G3, P3 woman for screening mammography.

Mammogram: Left oblique (**A**) and craniocaudal (**B**) views. There are small calcifications in the subareolar area just beneath the nipple *(arrows)*. These calcifications are linear, oriented along the path of the lactiferous ducts, and somewhat irregular in contour (**A** and **B**). The finding is consistent with a ductal origin and could represent plasma cell mastitis with focal calcification, duct hyperplasia, or intraductal carcinoma. Since secretory calcifications are typically bilateral, the lack of other secretory calcifications in this patient was of concern, and biopsy was recommended. Incidental note is also made of a small degenerated fibroadenoma in the upper outer quadrant *(arrowhead)* (**A** and **B**).

Histopathology: Periductal mastitis with focal calcification.

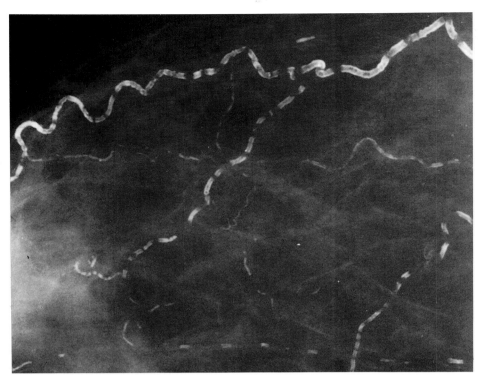

Figure 6.29.
Clinical: 65-year-old woman for screening.
Mammogram: Magnified image of left breast. Circuitous vessels are associated with calcification in the walls typical of arterial calcification.
Impression: Arterial calcification.

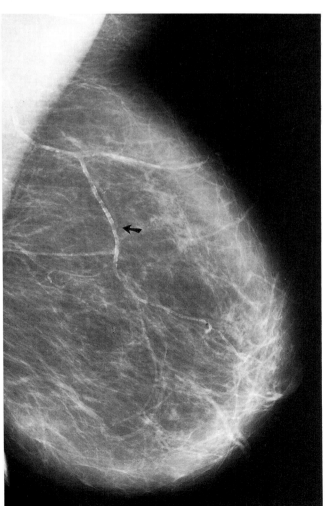

Figure 6.30.
Clinical: 65-year-old woman for screening mammography.
Mammogram: Right oblique view. The breast has a normal appearance. "Tramline" calcifications are present within arteries throughout the breast and extending into the axilla *(arrow)*.
Impression: Vascular calcification.

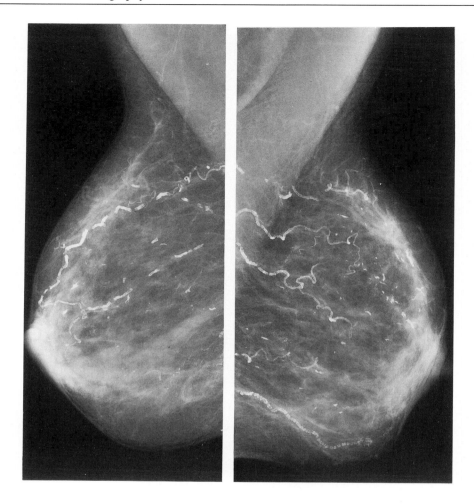

Figure 6.31.
Clinical: 67-year-old woman for screening mammography.
Mammogram: Bilateral oblique views. There are extensive linear calcifications bilaterally. These calcifications are serpiginous and in tramlines, typical of arterial calcifications.

Vascular calcifications are most commonly seen in older patients and are part of the spectrum of diffuse atherosclerotic disease.
Impression: Arterial calcifications.

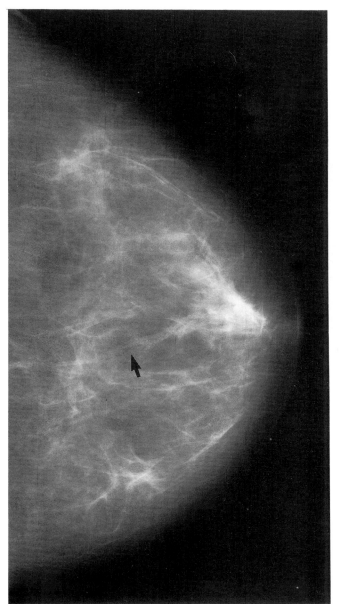

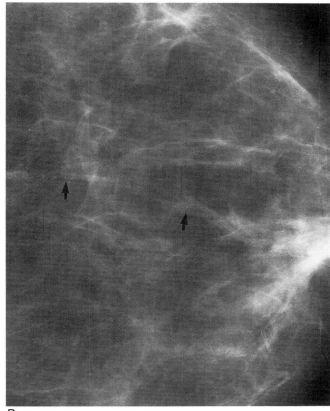

Figure 6.32.

Clinical: 67-year-old G3, P3 woman with a history of colon cancer, for screening mammography.

Mammogram: Right craniocaudal (**A**) and enlarged (2×) craniocaudal (**B**) views. The breast is mildly glandular, compatible with the patient's age and parity. Extending over the central aspect of the breast is an artery *(arrow)* (**A**) that contains early calcification. The enlarged view (**B**) demonstrates the fine granular microcalcifications *(arrows)* that lie in the wall of the vessel.

Impression: Early arterial calcification.

Note: It is important to verify that a vessel passes directly through an area of granular microcalcifications before one assumes that they are of vascular origin.

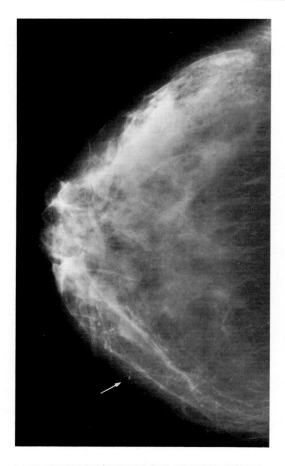

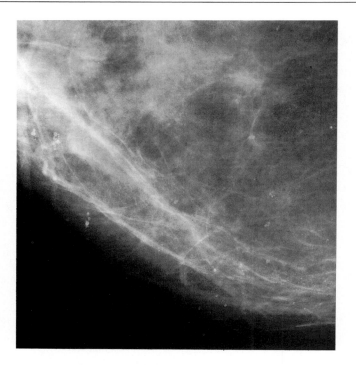

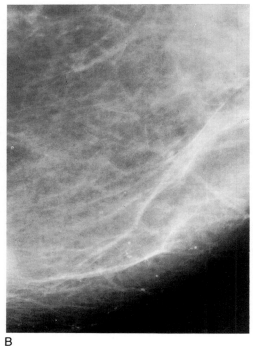

B

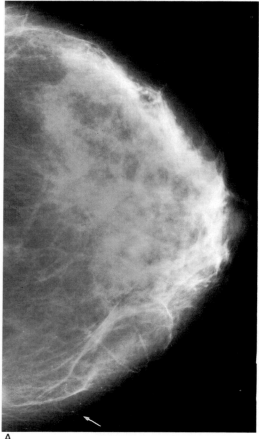

A

Figure 6.33.

Clinical: Screening mammogram.

Mammogram: Bilateral craniocaudal views (**A**) and magnified image (**B**). There are innumerable small calcifications scattered and in multiple clusters over the medial aspects of both breasts *(arrows)* (**A**). On close inspection (**B**), the well-defined round margins and central lucencies characteristic of skin calcifications are seen.

Impression: Benign skin calcifications.

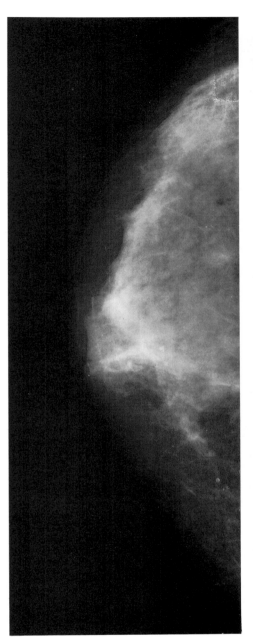
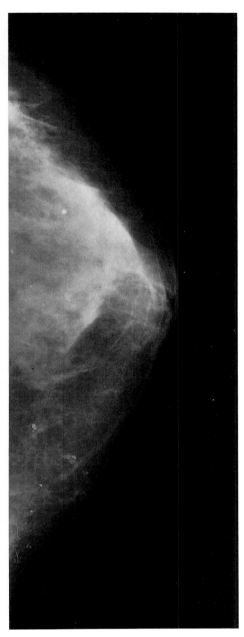

A

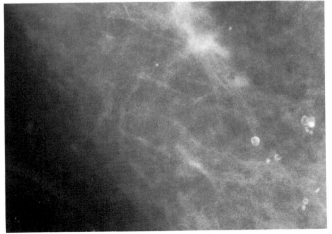
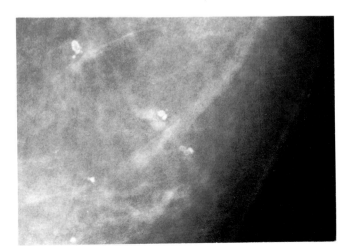

B

Figure 6.34.

Clinical: Screening mammography.

Mammogram: Bilateral craniocaudal views (**A**) and magnified images (**B**). On the medial aspects of both breasts, there are very well defined ringlike calcifications located superficially, typical of skin calcifications. These are usually located in sebaceous glands on the surface of the breast.

Impression: Benign skin calcifications.

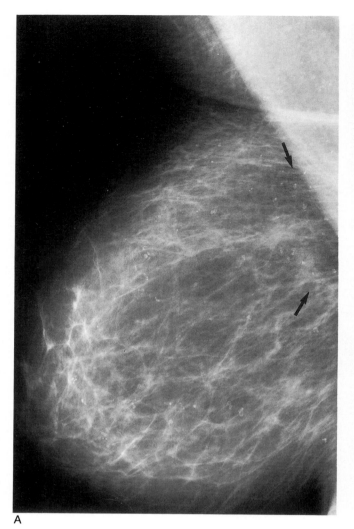

A

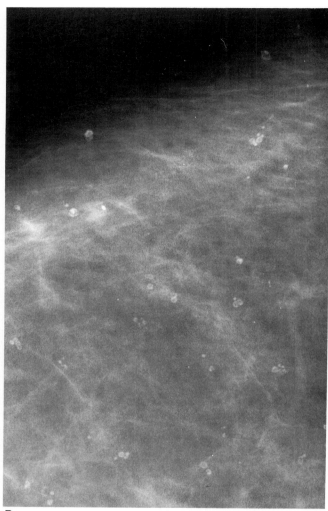

B

Figure 6.35.

Clinical: 53-year-old G4, P2 woman with a family history of breast cancer, for routine screening.

Mammogram: Left oblique (**A**) and enlarged (2×) cranio-caudal (**B**) views. The breast shows fatty replacement. There are extensive calcifications throughout the breast, located more over the deeper aspect of the breast *(arrows)* (**A**). On the enlarged view (**B**) these calcifications are noted to be very well circumscribed, circular and polygonal, with lucent centers. Many are clearly located very superficially. The appearance of these is characteristic of benign calcifications in the sebaceous glands of the skin.

Impression: Skin calcifications.

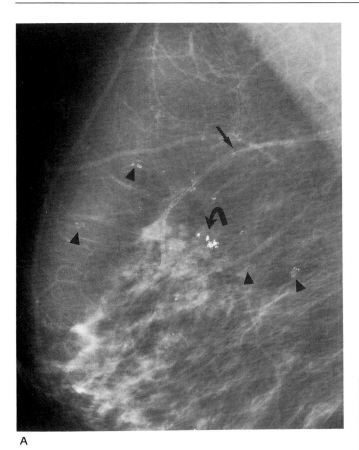

A

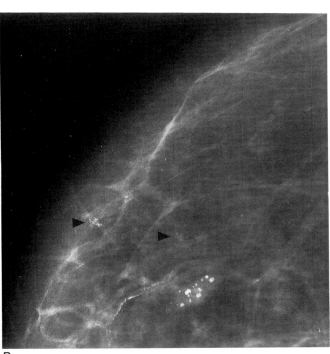

B

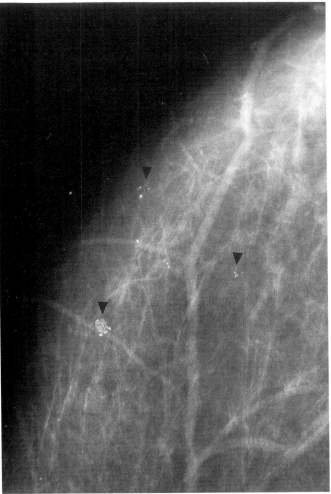

C

Figure 6.36.

Clinical: 70-year-old G4, P3, Ab1 woman with multiple nevi over both breasts, for screening.

Mammogram: Left oblique (**A**), craniocaudal (**B**), and enlarged craniocaudal (**C**) views. Three types of benign calcifications are present in the left breast. Tramline calcification in arteries is present *(arrow)* (**A**); coarse, popcorn calcification is noted in a degenerated fibroadenoma *(curved arrow)* (**A**); and multiple clusters of very clearly defined microcalcifications and macrocalcifications are located superficially *(arrowheads)* (**A–C**). Some of these clusters have a crenulated appearance, and others are ringlike. These features are typical of benign skin calcifications and are concurrent with the physical examination of the patient.

Impression: Multiple skin calcifications, fibroadenomas, and vascular calcifications.

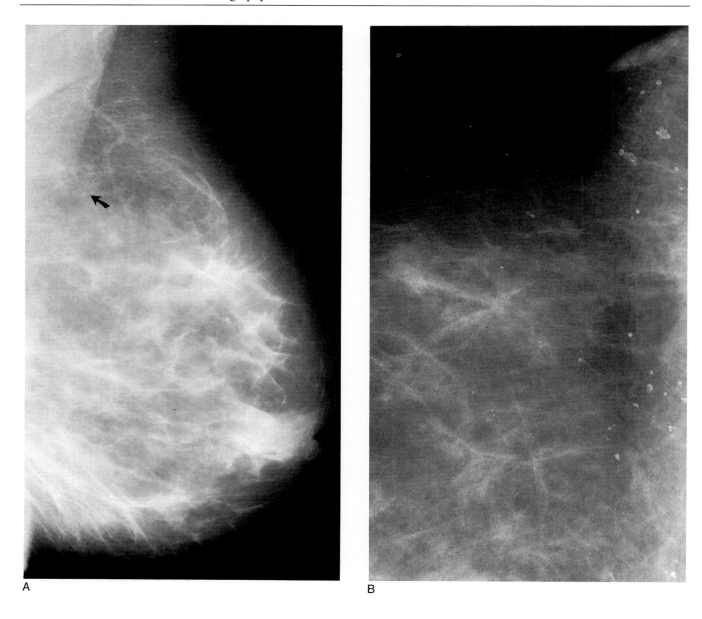

A

B

Figure 6.37.

Clinical: 72-year-old woman for screening mammography.

Mammogram: Right oblique (**A**) and magnification (**B**) views. Multiple small calcifications are superimposed over the deep upper aspect of the breast *(arrows)*. Magnification of these

shows the very well defined borders and central lucencies characteristic of skin calcifications.

Impression: Skin calcifications. (Case courtesy of Dr. Jay Levine, Richmond, VA.)

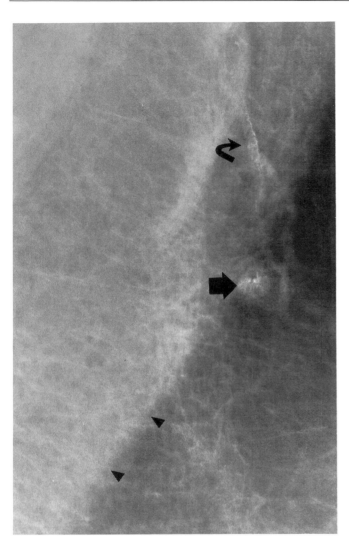

Figure 6.38.

Clinical: 60-year-old G2, P2 woman with a family history of breast cancer, for screening mammography.

Mammogram: Right oblique view (enlarged 2.5×). A very well circumscribed medium-density nodule *(arrow)* is present in the upper aspect of the breast, adjacent to the shadow of the pectoralis major muscle *(arrowheads)*. Punctate calcifications are present within the nodule. Examination of the skin revealed a raised nevus corresponding in exact location to the nodule noted on mammography. Although moles do not typically calcify, they may, or they may have a crenulated surface that traps deodorant or powder. Incidental note is also made of early arterial calcification *(curved arrow)* near the mole.

Impression: Calcification in a nevus.

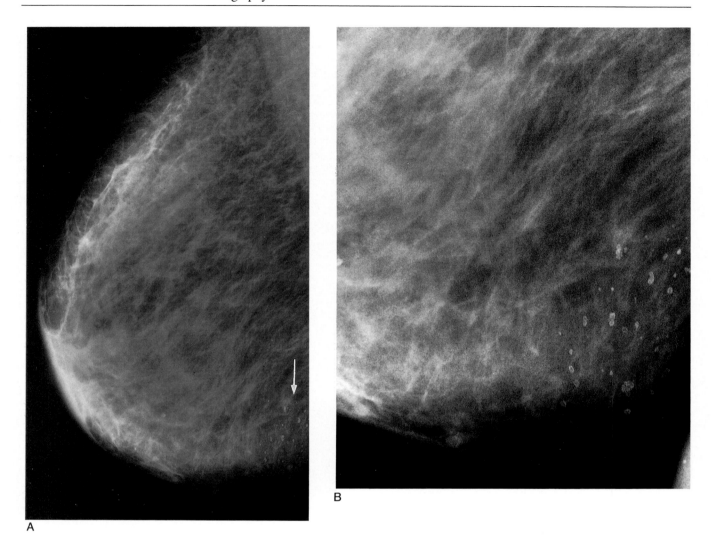

A

B

Figure 6.39.

Clinical: 50-year-old woman with a history of burns to the thorax, for screening mammography.

Mammogram: Left oblique (**A**) and magnification (**B**) views. There are extensive, well-defined circular calcifications over the lower aspect of the breast. These corresponded to the area of keloid and scar formation from the previous burn injury.

Impression: Dystrophic skin calcifications in scar tissue.

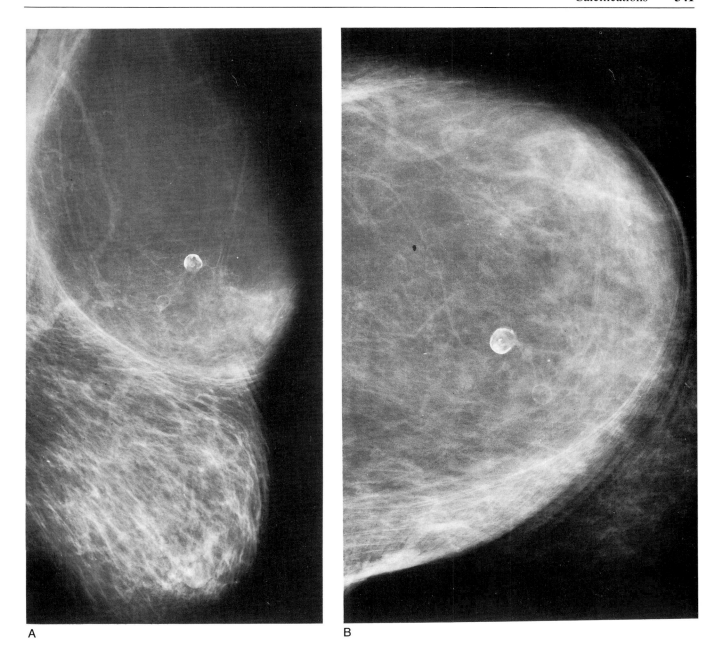

A   B

Figure 6.40.

Clinical: 54-year-old woman with a large soft mass in the right upper outer quadrant.

Mammogram: Right oblique (**A**) and craniocaudal (**B**) views. There is a 10-cm, well circumscribed, encapsulated, fat density mass in the right upper outer quadrant. The normal background parenchyma is draped around this lesion. There are coarse ringlike calcifications within this mass, typical of fat necrosis.

Impression: Large lipoma containing calcifications of fat necrosis. (Case courtesy of Dr. Ed Fallon, Reading, PA.)

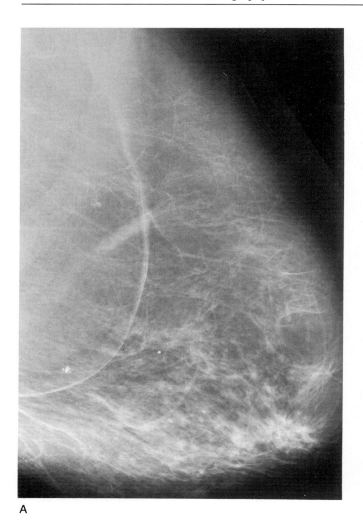

A

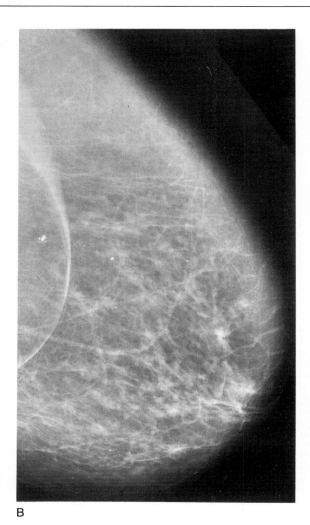

B

Figure 6.41.

Clinical: 62-year-old woman for screening mammography.

Mammogram: Right oblique (**A**) and lateral oblique cranio-caudal (**B**) views. There is a 12-cm, very well circumscribed, encapsulated radiolucent mass projecting anteriorly from the chest wall into the central aspect of the breast. Coarse cal-

cification is present within this mass and is consistent with the type of calcification that may occur in lipomas.

Impression: Large lipoma containing benign calcification. (Case courtesy of Ed Fallon, Reading, PA.)

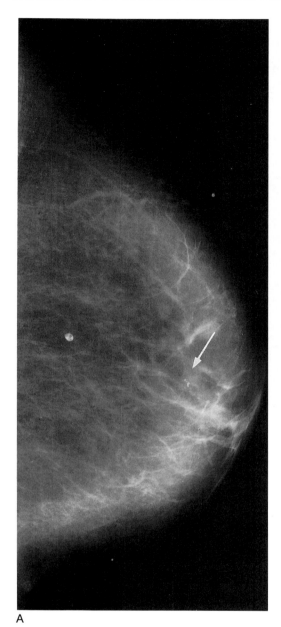

A

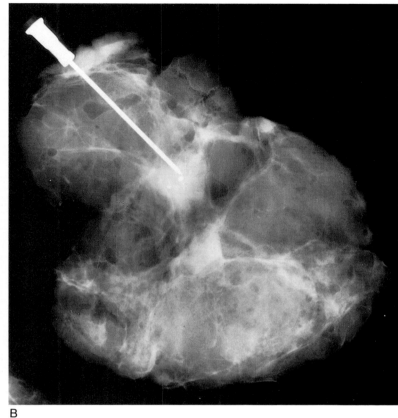

B

Figure 6.42.

Clinical: 62-year-old woman with a left breast cancer.

Mammogram: Right mediolateral view (**A**) and specimen radiograph (**B**). There is a cluster of rather coarse macrocalcifications associated with a soft tissue nodule *(arrow)* in the retroareolar area (**A**). The specimen film (**B**) shows the nodule to be fairly well defined and of medium density. The differential includes a fibroadenoma, focal fibrosis, and intraductal papilloma, with carcinoma less likely.

Histopathology: Infarcted papilloma with calcification.

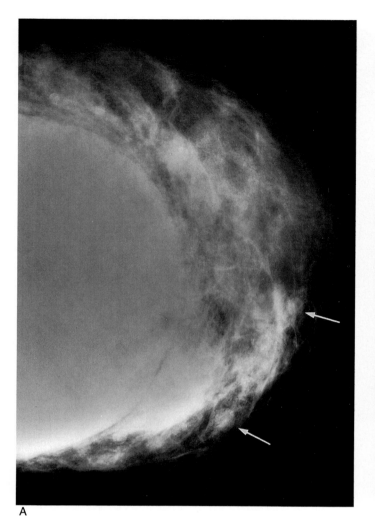

A

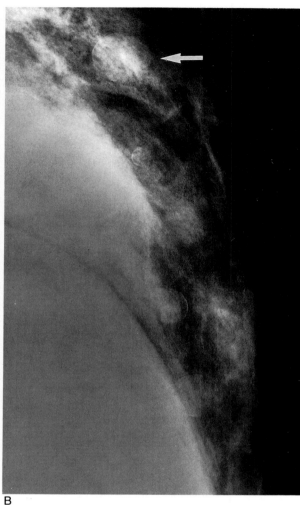

B

Figure 6.43.

Clinical: 35-year-old woman who has had augmentation mammoplasties with both silicone implants and silicone injections.

Mammogram: Left craniocaudal view (**A**) and magnified image (**B**). The implant is surrounded by very dense glandular tissue and focal areas of marked density, making imaging difficult. There are multiple ringlike calcific densities *(arrows)* of varying size up to 1 cm in diameter throughout the breast, better depicted on the magnified image (**B**). These calcifications may be secondary to the injected silicone or may represent oil cysts. The generalized increased density as well as the calcifications are typically seen after silicone injections, presumably from the marked foreign body reaction, fibrosis, and fat necrosis that occur.

Impression: Calcification secondary to silicone injection.

Figure 6.44.

Clinical: 76-year-old woman with chronic renal failure and hypercalcemia.

Mammogram: Bilateral oblique (**A**) and craniocaudal (**B**) views. The breasts are moderately dense. Extensive coarse calcifications are present bilaterally, mainly located in the upper outer quadrants. Incidental note is also made of arterial calcifications *(arrows)* bilaterally. If the coarse calcifications were focal, a degenerated fibroadenoma should be considered. However, because of the extensive bilateral nature, a more generalized process is likely. Given the clinical history, calcium deposition secondary to hypercalcemia is most likely.

Impression: Calcification secondary to hypercalcemia. (Case courtesy of Dr. Christine Llewellyn, Richmond, VA.)

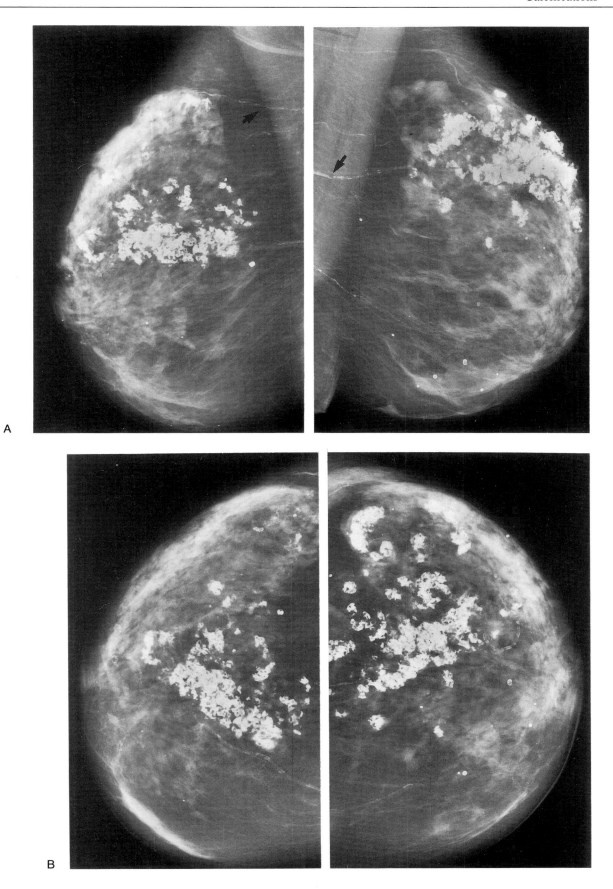

A

B

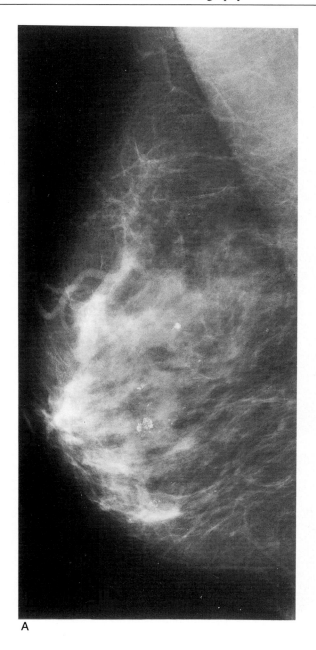

A

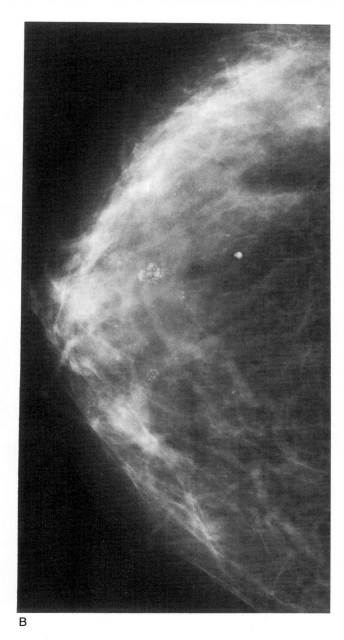

B

Figure 6.45.

Clinical: 53-year-old G1, P1 woman with a positive family history of breast cancer, for screening mammography.

Mammogram: Left oblique (**A**), and craniocaudal (**B**) views. The breasts are dense for the age of the patient. Macrocalcifications and microcalcifications are present (**A** and **B**). In the left breast centrally (**A** and **B**), there are several tight clusters of microcalcifications having a rather uniform appearance. A similar appearance was seen on the right. The appearance of these suggests most likely a lobular origin. The differential includes adenosis, sclerosing adenosis, cystic hyperplasia, lobular hyperplasia, and lobular carcinoma in situ.

Impression: Clusters of lobular microcalcifications of nonspecific nature.

Histopathology: Sclerosing adenosis, mild ductal hyperplasia.

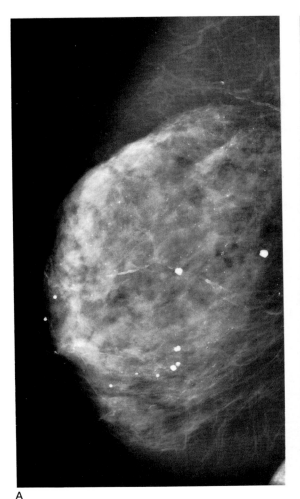
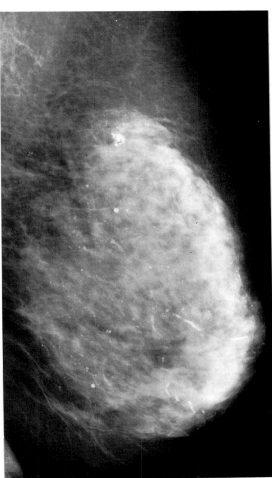

A

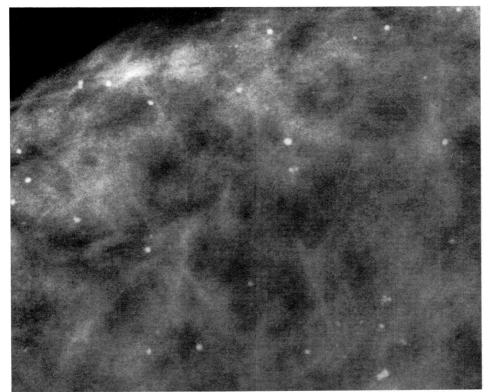

B

Figure 6.46.

Clinical: 83-year-old nulliparous woman with a pleural effusion and no palpable breast abnormalities.

Mammogram: Bilateral oblique views (**A**) and magnification image of the right breast (**B**). The breasts are dense and diffusely nodular, as may be seen in an elderly nulliparous woman. The "snowflake" pattern of nodularity suggests fibrocystic changes with adenosis. There are also innumerable round pearllike microcalcifications distributed evenly throughout both breasts. The smooth-bordered, rounded shapes of the microcalcifications and the similarity in appearance suggest a lobular origin and are consistent with adenosis.

Impression: Diffuse changes of adenosis.

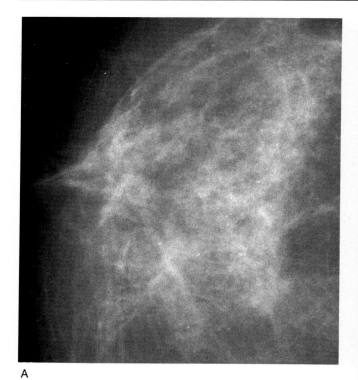

A

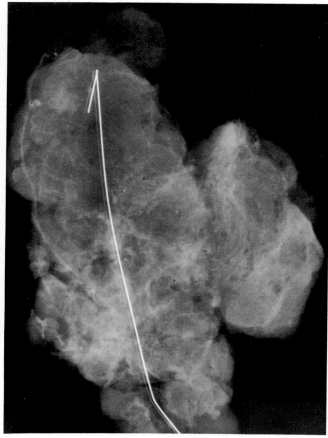

B

Figure 6.47.

Clinical: 71-year-old woman for screening mammography.

Mammogram: Left magnification view (**A**), specimen view (**B**), and histopathology (**C**). There are fine granular microcalcifications in the left breast. These are round and similar in size and shape, suggesting a lobular origin. The differential in-

cludes sclerosing adenosis, adenosis, lobular hyperplasia, and lobular carcinoma in situ.

Histopathology: Microglandular adenosis. Round lobular calcifications *(arrows)* are present in small glandular structures of microglandular adenosis (**C**).

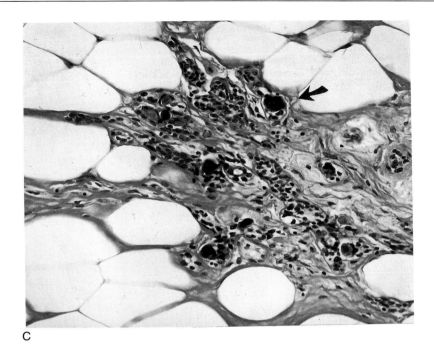

C

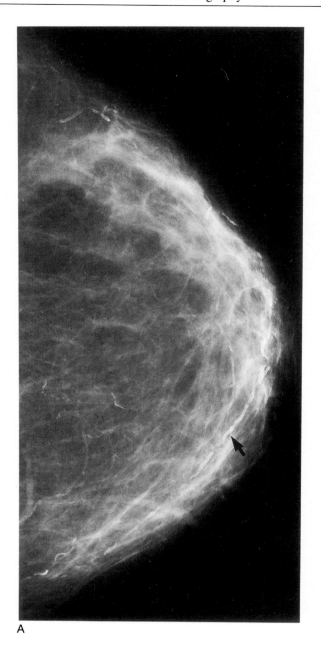

A

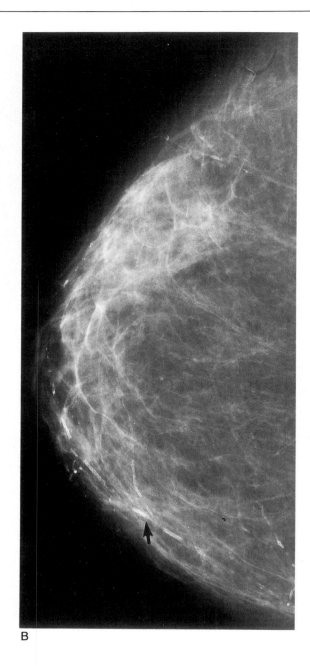

B

Figure 6.48.

Clinical: 68-year-old G9, P7 woman with a positive family history of breast cancer for routine screening.

Mammogram: Right (**A**) and left (**B**) craniocaudal views and enlarged (2×) view of the right outer quadrant (**C**). The breasts are mildly glandular. Extensive fine microcalcifications are present throughout both breasts but located primarily in the areas of glandular tissue. These calcifications are not clearly visible in the routine views (**A** and **B**) but can be seen in the right breast *(curved arrows)* on the enlargement (**C**). The calcifications are quite small and are of similar morphology, suggesting a lobular origin. Incidental note is also made of arterial calcification bilaterally *(arrow)* (**A** and **B**).

Impression: Extensive bilateral microcalcification of lobular origin, probable adenosis.

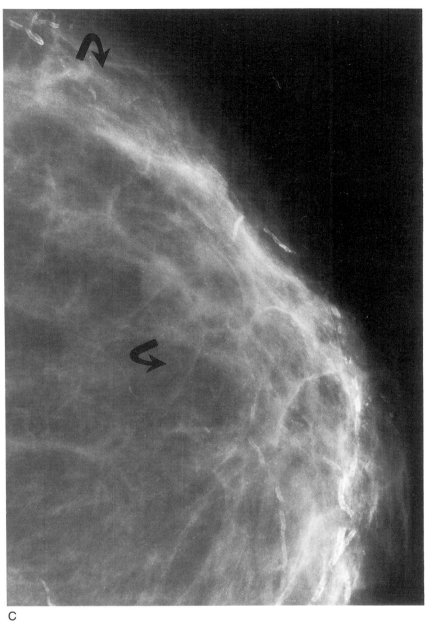

C

Figure 6.49.

Clinical: 45-year-old woman for screening mammography.

Mammogram: Left oblique (**A**), craniocaudal (**B**), and mediolateral (**C**) views. The breast is moderately dense. There are diffuse microcalcifications involving all quadrants, and a similar pattern was present in the contralateral breast. On the oblique view (**A**) some of the calcifications have a linear configuration *(arrows),* but on the craniocaudal view (**B**) the calcifications are rounded and smudged. With a horizontal beam (on the mediolateral view) (**C**), the calcifications are saucer shaped and dense. They are lying in the dependent aspects of microcysts on the upright view and are seen en face on the craniocaudal view.

Impression: Milk of calcium in microcysts.

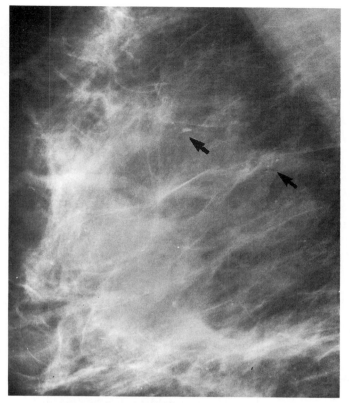

A

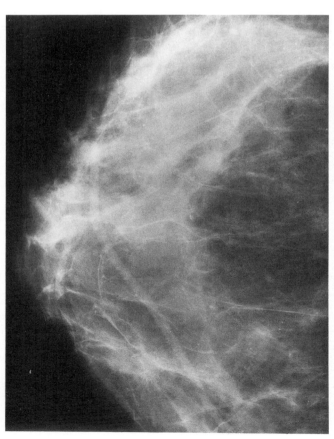

B

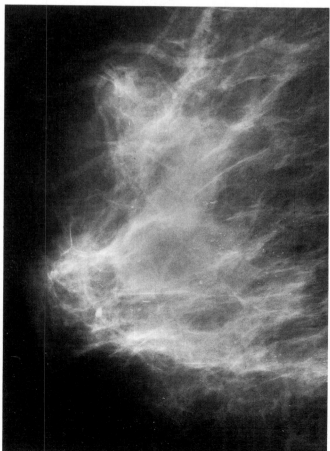

C

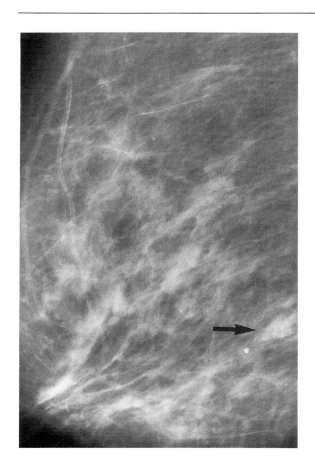

A

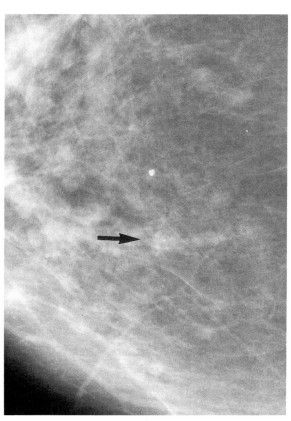

B

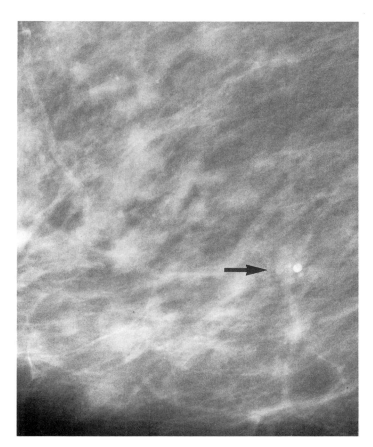

C

Figure 6.50.

Clinical: 84-year-old G3, P2, Ab1 woman with a positive family history of breast cancer and a personal history of cysts in the left breast.

Mammogram: Left oblique (**A**) and magnified (2×) craniocaudal (**B**) and mediolateral (**C**) views. The breast is dense for the age of the patient, and there are multiple small areas of nodularity consistent with fibrocystic changes. In the central portion of the breast, there is a cluster of microcalcifications associated with a soft tissue density *(arrows)*. These calcifications are round and faint on the craniocaudal view (**B**) but appear more dense and half-moon shaped on the upright mediolateral view (**C**). These findings are characteristic of cystic hyperplasia with milk of calcium. The calcifications were unchanged from previous mammograms.

Impression: Milk of calcium in tiny breast cysts.

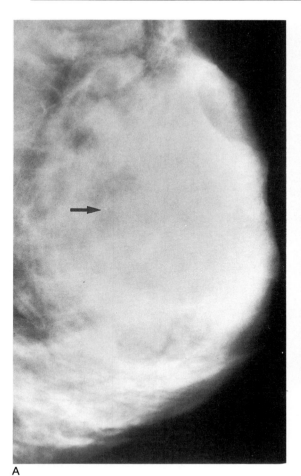

A

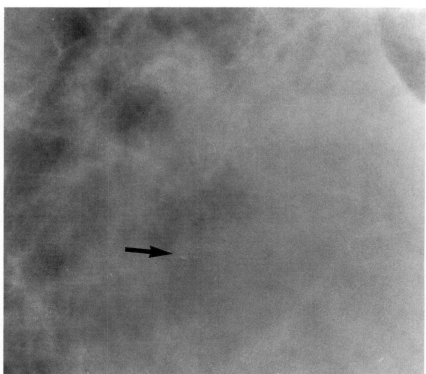

B

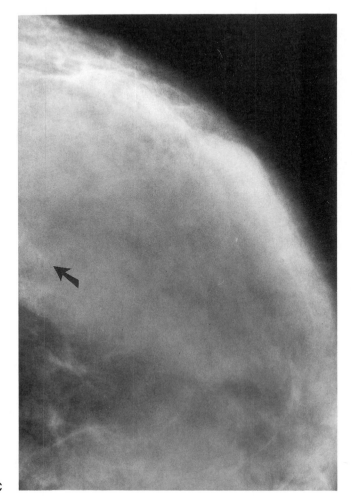

C

Figure 6.51.

Clinical: 51-year-old G2, P2 patient with a history of fibrocystic changes on previous biopsies, for routine mammography.

Mammogram: Right oblique (**A**) and magnified (2×) mediolateral (**B**) and craniocaudal (**C**) views. The breast is very dense for the age of the patient, consistent with fibrocystic changes. There are clustered microcalcifications *(arrow)* in the central aspect of the breast (**A**). On the upright mediolateral view (**B**) the calcifications are saucer shaped *(arrow),* but on the craniocaudal view (**C**) they appear smudged and rounded *(arrow).* This change in configuration of calcifications is typical of milk of calcium in tiny breast cysts and should not be considered suspicious for a malignant process.

Impression: Milk of calcium in tiny breast cysts.

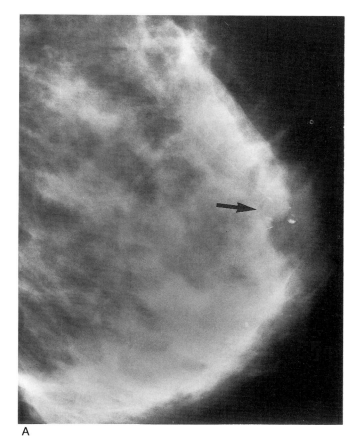

A

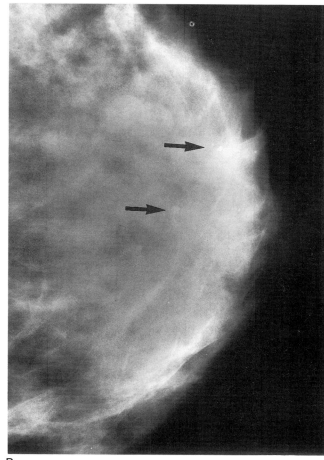

B

Figure 6.52.

Clinical: 43-year-old G4, P4 woman with a history of fibrocystic changes on previous biopsies, for routine follow-up.

Mammogram: Right magnified (1.5×) mediolateral (**A**) and craniocaudal (**B**) views. The breast is very dense, consistent with the previous histopathologic diagnosis of fibrocystic change. There are scattered microcalcifications as well as areas of clustered microcalcifications. In particular, in the supra-areolar area, there are clustered microcalcifications *(arrows)* associated with a small, circumscribed soft tissue nod-

ule. These calcifications are striking because they appear round and less distinct on the craniocaudal view (**B**) but linear or saucer shaped on the upright mediolateral view (**A**). This finding is characteristic of milk of calcium in breast cysts, which layers in the dependent aspect of the cyst on the upright view and is seen en face with the vertical beam. Ultrasound in this patient demonstrated the nodule to be cystic.

Impression: Milk of calcium in breast cysts.

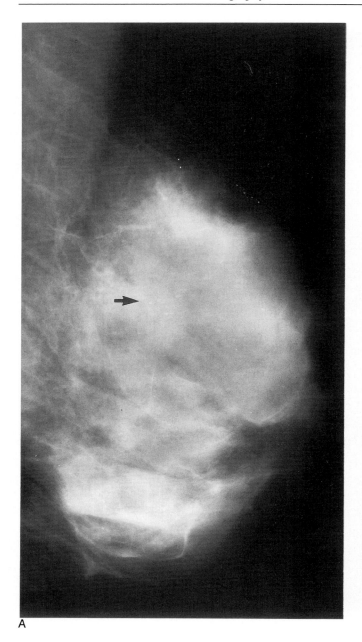

A

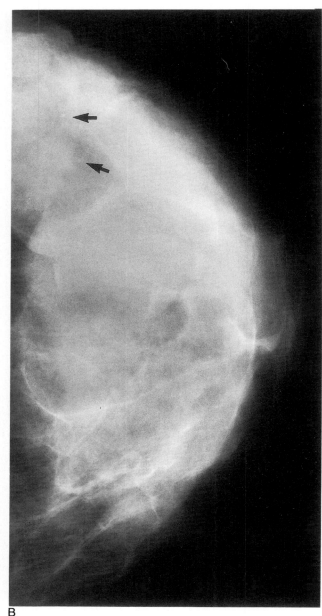

B

Figure 6.53.

Clinical: 42-year-old G2, P2 woman with multiple palpable nodules.

Mammogram: Right oblique (**A**), craniocaudal (**B**), and magnified (2×) mediolateral (**C**) and craniocaudal (**D**) views. The breast is extremely dense and glandular, suggesting fibrocystic changes. Ultrasound confirmed the presence of multiple cysts, which corresponded in location to the palpable nodularity. There are numerous microcalcifications scattered throughout the upper outer quadrant *(arrows)* of the right breast (**A** and **B**). These calcifications are saucer shaped on the upright mediolateral view (**C**) but appear less distinct and round on the craniocaudal view (**D**) *(arrows)*. This finding is typical of milk of calcium in tiny breast cysts, which layers in the dependent aspect of the cyst in the upright view and is seen en face on the craniocaudal view as a faintly visible round calcification.

Impression: Milk of calcium in tiny breast cysts.

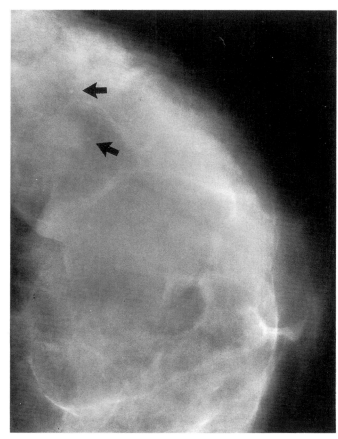

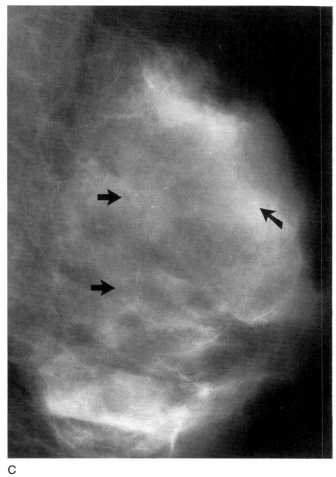

C

D

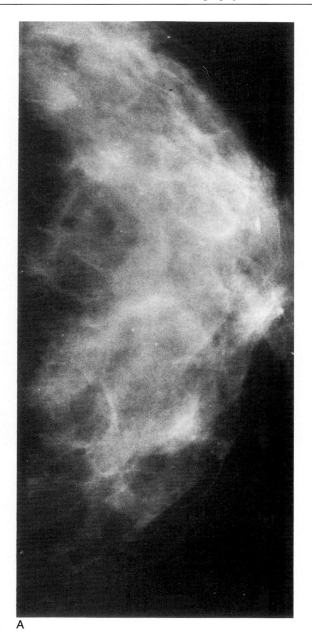

A

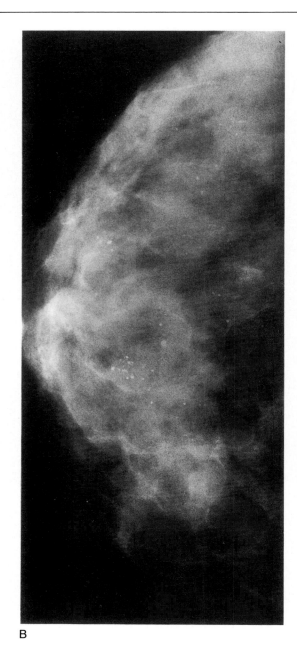

B

Figure 6.54.

Clinical: 48-year-old woman with a positive family history of breast cancer and a personal history of breast cysts.

Mammogram: Right craniocaudal (**A**), left craniocaudal (**B**), left oblique (**C**), and left magnification (2×) mediolateral (**D**) views. There are extensive round microcalcifications superimposed on dense parenchyma bilaterally (**A** and **B**). These calcifications involve all quadrants of both breasts and have a similar shape and size. These findings suggest a fibrocystic origin—adenosis or cystic hyperplasia. On the oblique view

(**C**) some of the calcifications have a linear or saucer shape *(arrow)*. On the true lateral magnification view (**D**) the saucer shapes are more clearly seen *(arrows)*. The difference in shape of calcifications on the vertical beam (craniocaudal) view versus the horizontal beam (mediolateral) view is characteristic of milk of calcium in tiny breast cysts. On the upright film the calcium layers and creates a meniscus, but on the craniocaudal view it is seen en face as a rounded shape.

Impression: Milk of calcium in cystic hyperplasia.

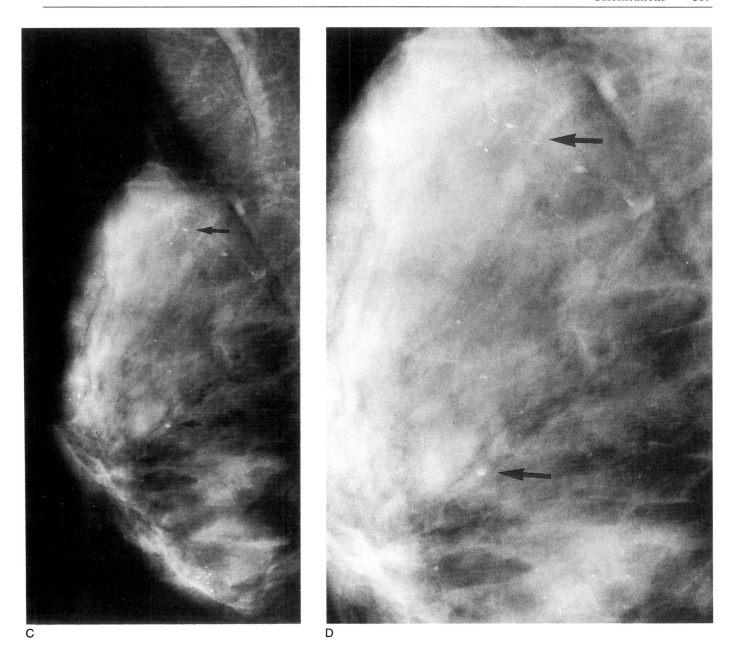

C

D

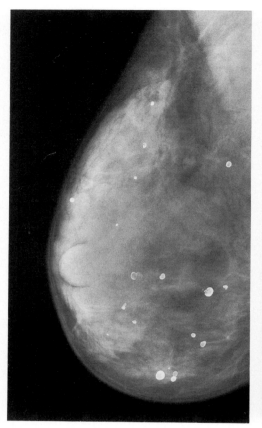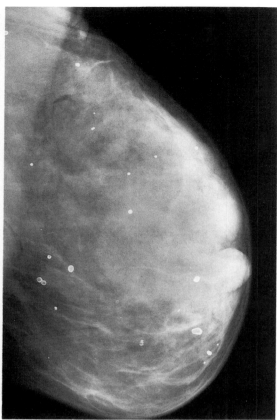

Figure 6.55.

Clinical: 64-year-old G4, P5 woman for screening.

Mammogram: Bilateral oblique views. The breasts are dense, related to a prominent amount of glandular tissue and a paucity of fat. Bilateral dense ringlike calcifications are present, scattered in all quadrants of both breasts. These are not lo-cated in the subcutaneous area, as is often seen with fat necrosis. These calcifications are thought to represent small calcified cysts of fibrocystic origin.

Impression: Cystic hyperplasia with calcified cysts.

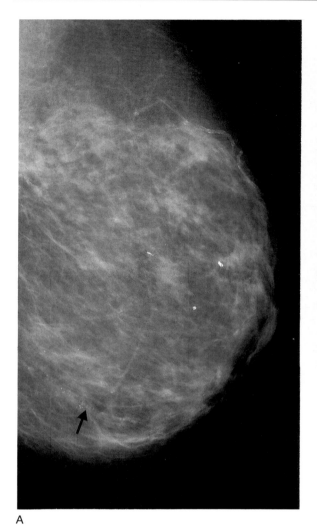

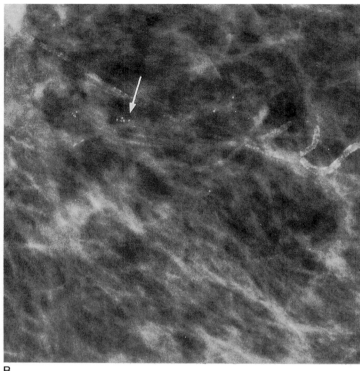

B

A

Figure 6.56.

Clinical: 69-year-old woman with nodularity in the right breast.

Mammogram: Right oblique (**A**) and craniocaudal (**B**) views. There are grouped microcalcifications in the 6 o'clock position of the right breast *(arrow)*. These calcifications are smooth and rounded, and they extend in a linear distribution along the orientation of the ducts. The findings suggest intraductal hyperplasia or papillomatosis as a likely possibility. Occa-

sionally, an intraductal carcinoma may produce similar-appearing calcifications. Biopsy after needle localization was performed.

Impression: Microcalcifications of indeterminate nature, most likely of fibrocystic origin.

Histopathology: Intraductal papillomatosis.

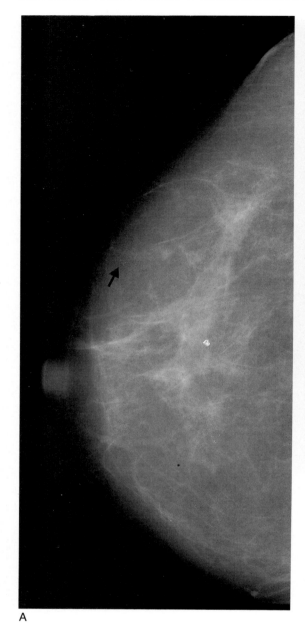

A

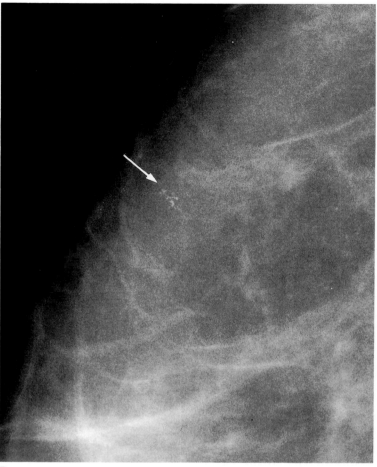

B

Figure 6.57.

Clinical: 58-year-old asymptomatic woman for screening mammography.

Mammogram: Left craniocaudal view (**A**) and magnified image (**B**). There is a cluster of fine microcalcifications *(arrows)* of varying size in the outer quadrant of the left breast. These are of indeterminate nature and are regarded with a moderate degree of suspicion.

Impression: Microcalcifications suspicious for carcinoma.

Histopathology: Fibrosis.

Note: The calcifications of fibrosis may be variable and may occasionally simulate those of intraductal carcinoma.

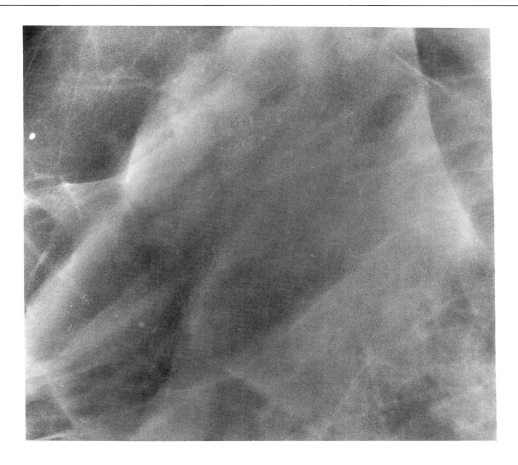

Figure 6.58.

Clinical: 41-year-old G3, P2, Ab1 woman with a history of biopsies showing fibrocystic changes with hyperplasia bilaterally. Comparison was made with a previous mammogram taken 1 year earlier.

Mammogram: Left magnified (2×) craniocaudal view of the retroareolar area. There are innumerable fine granular microcalcifications present, distributed in a ductal orientation. The borders of these are somewhat irregular, and there is a mix-

ture of sizes and shapes. The microcalcifications had developed since the prior examination, and because of the interval change as well as their morphology, the area was considered moderately suspicious for malignancy.

Histopathology: Atypical ductal hyperplasia.

Note: The microcalcifications associated with intraductal epithelial hyperplasia have a similar appearance to those of many intraductal carcinomas.

Figure 6.59.

Clinical: 64-year-old woman with a strong family history of breast cancer, for screening mammography.

Mammogram: Right mediolateral view (**A**) and magnified image (**B**). There are two clusters of calcification in the right breast *(arrows)* (**A**). On close inspection (**B**) these are shown to have irregular margins, but they are more coarse than the microcalcifications often found in malignancy.

Impression: Indeterminate microcalcifications, probably fibrocystic.

Histopathology: Epithelial hyperplasia with calcifications in ducts.

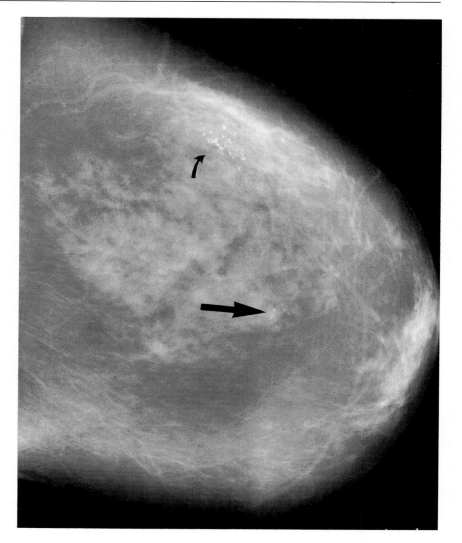

A

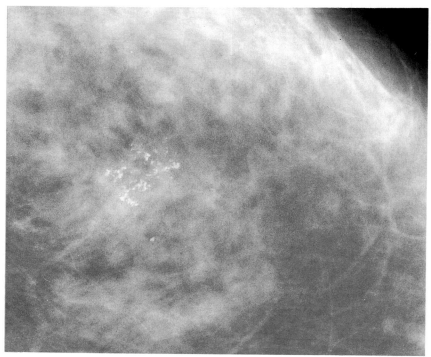

B

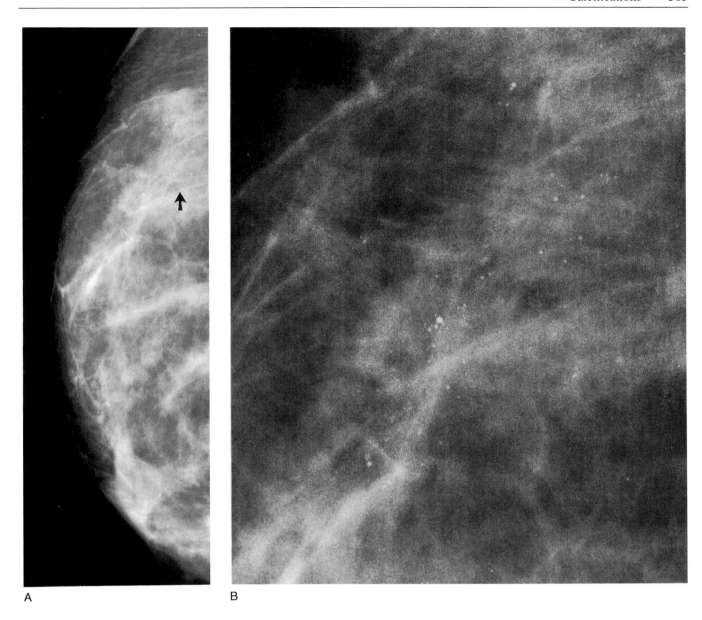

A

B

Figure 6.60.

Clinical: 49-year-old woman with a positive family history of breast cancer, for routine screening.

Mammogram: Left craniocaudal view (**A**) and enlarged image (**B**). There are grouped microcalcifications in the outer quadrant *(arrow)* (**A**). The morphology of the calcifications (**B**) is smooth and round with little variability, suggesting a lobular origin. The findings are nonspecific and may be seen in adenosis, lobular hyperplasia, and lobular carcinoma in situ. A needle localization-directed biopsy was performed.

Histopathology: Fibrocystic changes with epithelial hyperplasia.

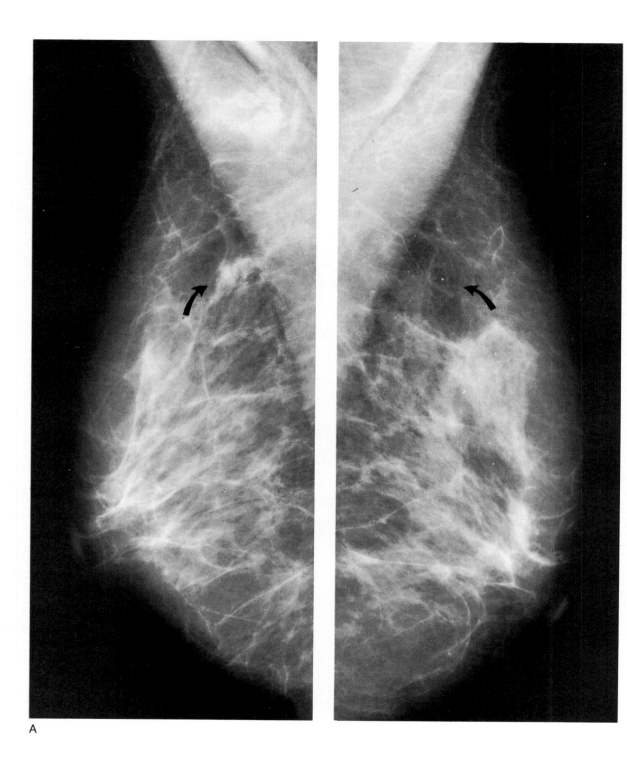

A

Figure 6.61.

Clinical: 58-year-old woman with a strong family history of breast cancer, for routine screening.

Mammogram: Bilateral oblique views (**A**), and magnification images of the left (**B**) and right (**C**) upper outer quadrants, and histopathology section (**D**). There are areas of focally clustered microcalcifications in the right upper outer quadrant (**A** and **C**) that are round, relatively smooth bordered, and similar in size and shape *(arrows)*. These have an appearance suggesting a lobular origin such as is found in adenosis or sclerosing adenosis. In the left upper outer quadrant, there is a cluster of irregularly bordered microcalcifications (**A** and **B**) associated with a soft tissue density.

Because of the jagged edges of these, they are of moderate suspicion for malignancy, particularly an intraductal lesion.

Impression: Right: lobular type of calcifications, favoring fibrocystic. Left: moderately suspicious calcifications, possible intraductal carcinoma.

Histopathology: Right: adenosis, fibrocystic changes.

Histopathology: Left: severely atypical intraductal hyperplasia. An enlarged duct (**D**) is filled with hyperplasia with architectural atypia, forming cribriform structures *(arrow)*. Irregular intraductal calcifications *(arrowhead)* are present in the adjacent ducts.

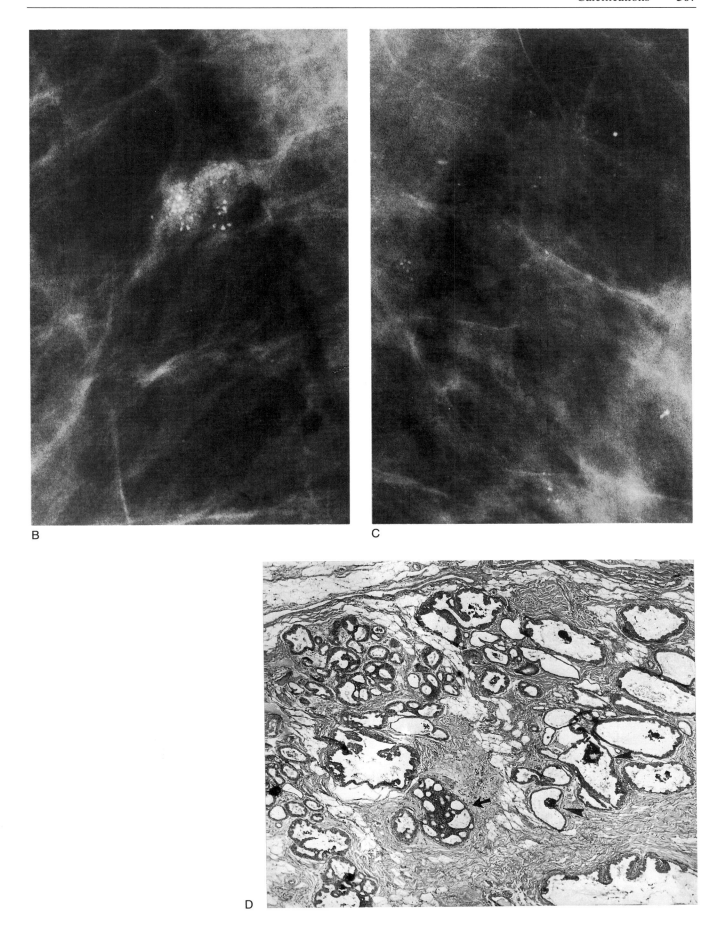

B

C

D

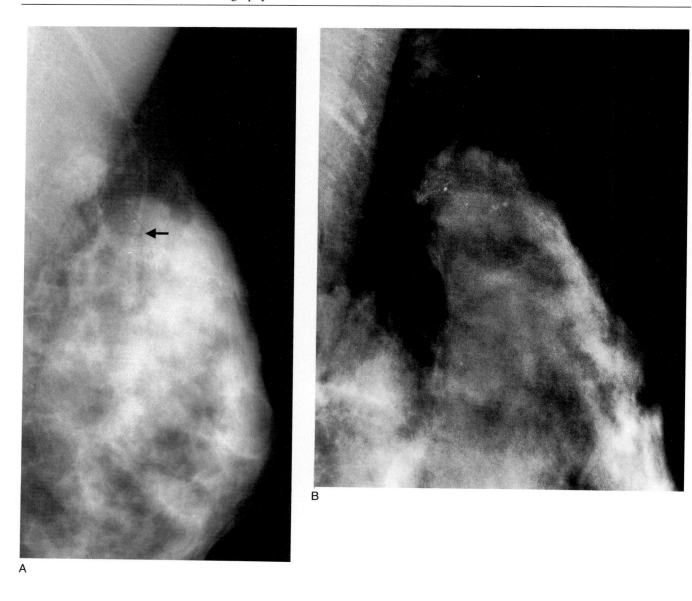

A

B

Figure 6.62.

Clinical: 47-year-old woman with a history of fibrocystic disease, for screening mammography.

Mammogram: Right mediolateral (**A**) and magnification (**B**) views. The breast is very dense, compatible with fibrocystic changes. There are clustered microcalcifications in the up-per outer quadrant *(arrow)* (**A**). Magnification of the calcifications demonstrates their mixed morphology and the presence of some linear forms, suggesting a ductal origin.

Impression: Microcalcifications suspicious for malignancy.

Histopathology: Atypical ductal hyperplasia.

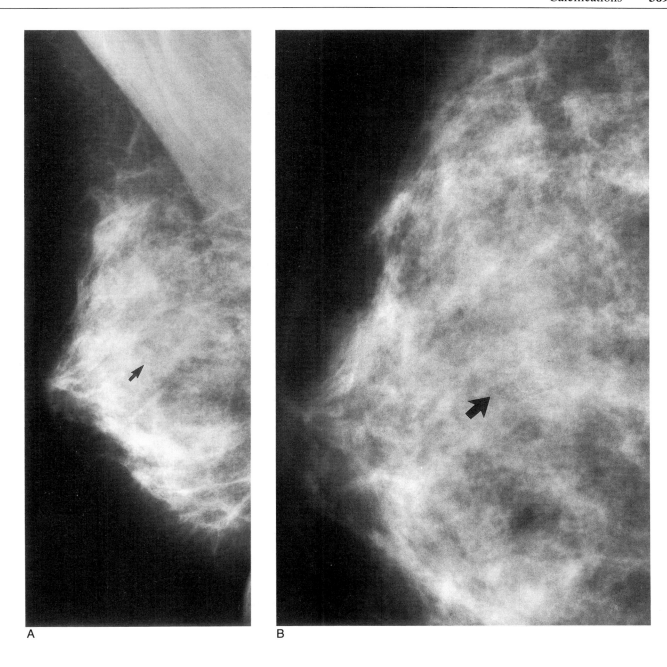

A   B

Figure 6.63.

Clinical: 52-year-old G0 woman with tender lumpy breasts, for routine mammography.

Mammogram: Left oblique (**A**) and magnified (1.5×) craniocaudal (**B**) views. The breast is dense and glandular for the age of the patient. There are clustered granular microcalcifications in the central aspect of the breast *(arrow)* (**A**).

On the magnification view (**B**), the irregular morphology of these calcifications *(arrow)* makes them moderately suspicious for a malignancy of ductal origin.

Histopathology: Severely atypical ductal and lobular hyperplasia.

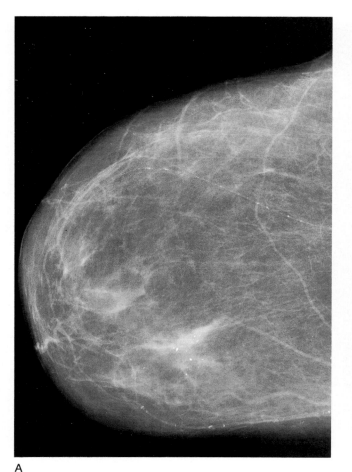

A

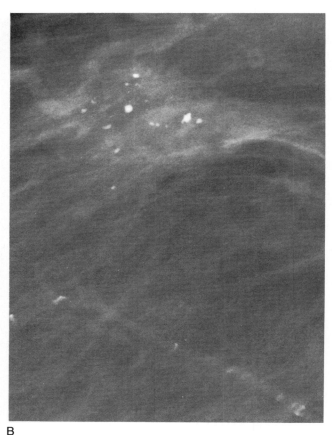

B

Figure 6.64.

Clinical: 80-year-old woman with lymphoma, for screening mammography.

Mammogram: Left mediolateral (**A**) and magnification (**B**) views and histopathology (**C**). There is an irregular high-density lesion in the lower inner quadrant, containing variably shaped microcalcifications and macrocalcifications. Many of these are smooth and round, suggesting a lobular origin, but histologic examination is necessary to confirm the diagnosis.

Impression: Sclerosing adenosis with focal lobular carcinoma in situ.

Histopathology: Distended lobules are filled by a monomorphic cell population diagnostic of lobular carcinoma in situ. Rounded microcalcifications are present within the lobules.

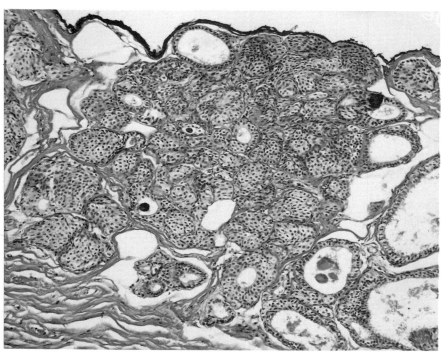

C

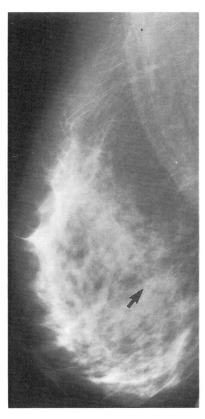 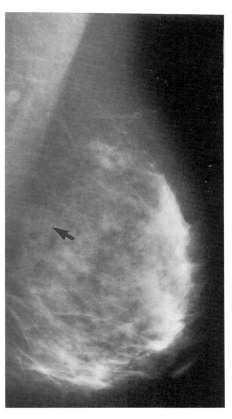

A

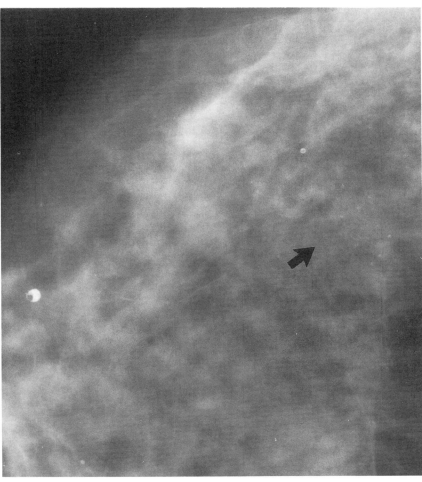

B

Figure 6.65.

Clinical: 56-year-old G4, P4 woman with a positive family history of breast cancer, for screening mammography.

Mammogram: Bilateral oblique (**A**) and left craniocaudal magnification (2×) (**B**) views. The breasts are moderately glandular. In both breasts, in the upper outer quadrants, there are loosely grouped micro-calcifications *(arrows)* (**A**). On magnification (**B**), these calcifications are relatively smooth and round, suggesting a lobular origin. Although they were bilateral, in a mirror image distribution, biopsy was recommended because of their clustered nature.

Histopathology: Bilateral lobular carcinoma in situ.

Note: The calcifications are nonspecific and of a lobular type. In this case, some occurred in the lobules involved with lobular neoplasia, and others were in adjacent lobules involved with hyperplastic epithelium.

Figure 6.66.

Clinical: 48-year-old woman with a history of right breast cancer treated with mastectomy 1 year earlier.

Mammogram: Left oblique view (**A**) and magnified image (**B**). The left breast is dense and nodular. There are scattered microcalcifications throughout the breast, as well as a clustered area of punctate microcalcifications *(arrow)* that had developed in the midportion of the breast since the mammogram 1 year earlier (**A**). On magnification (**B**) the calcifications are granular but not variable in size.

Impression: Dense fibrocystic breast, new clustered calcifications moderately suspicious for malignancy.

Histopathology: Lobular carcinoma in situ with microinvasion and pagetoid spread.

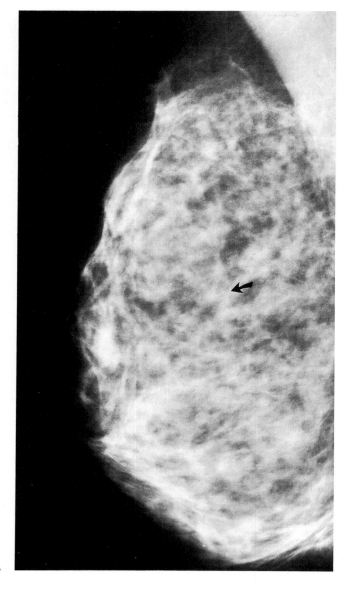

A

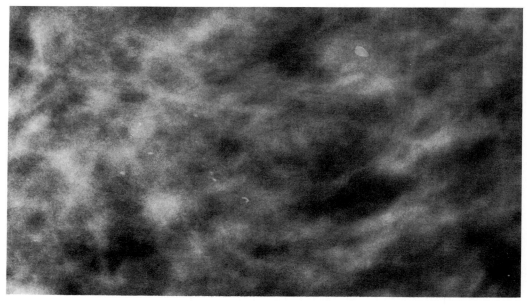

B

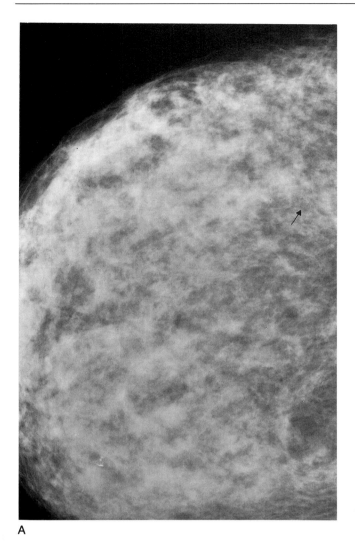

A

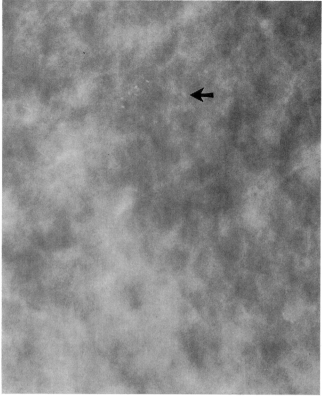

B

Figure 6.67.

Clinical: 73-year-old G9, P9 woman with multiple areas of palpable nodularity in both breasts.

Mammogram: Left craniocaudal (**A**) and magnification (**B**) views. The breast is more glandular than one would expect for the age and parity of the patient, suggesting fibrocystic changes. In the outer quadrant of the left breast is a cluster of fine microcalcifications *(arrow)*. A magnification of this area (**B**) shows the clustered nature of these rounded, lobular types of microcalcifications.

Impression: Moderately suspicious cluster of calcifications (adenosis versus hyperplasia versus lobular neoplasia).

Histopathology: Lobular carcinoma in situ.

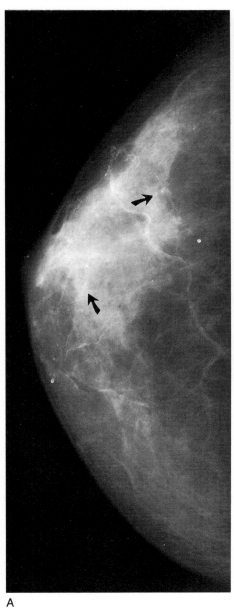

A

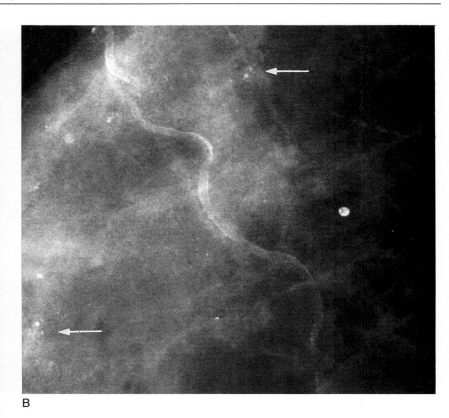

B

Figure 6.68.

Clinical: 71-year-old woman who had right breast cancer 1 year earlier.

Mammogram: Left craniocaudal (**A**) and magnification (**B**) views. Two clusters of microcalcifications *(arrows)* are present and had appeared from the mammogram 15 months earlier. A coned-down photograph (**B**) of these areas shows that there are about six round microcalcifications in each cluster, and there is some variability in their sizes. The areas are of indeterminate nature and could represent fibrocystic change, particularly sclerosing adenosis, or lobular hyperplasia or lobular carcinoma in situ. Incidental note is made of an artery with typical tramline calcifications.

Impression: Two clusters of moderately suspicious calcifications.

Histopathology: Lobular carcinoma in situ.

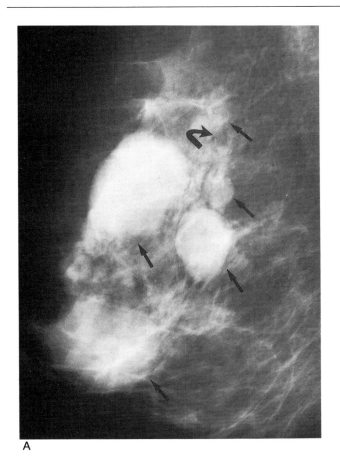

A

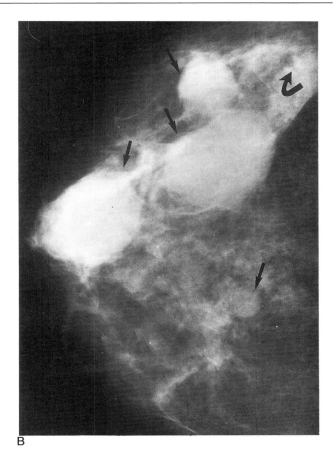

B

C

Figure 6.69.

Clinical: 50-year-old G1, P1 woman with a positive family history of breast cancer, presenting with a palpable mass in the left upper outer quadrant.

Mammogram: Left oblique (**A**), craniocaudal (**B**), and spot magnification (2×) (**C**) views. The breast is moderately dense, and there are multiple circumscribed masses *(arrows)* present (**A** and **B**). These masses are of medium density and relatively well circumscribed, with haloes on some margins. Ultrasound demonstrated all of these to be simple cysts. In the upper outer quadrant a group of microcalcifications *(curved arrow)* (**A–C**) had developed from the prior study. The spot magnification view (**C**) better demonstrates the morphology of these calcifications. Their size is similar, and most of the borders are smooth. The appearance of the calcifications and the associated cysts suggests most likely a lobular origin, including adenosis, sclerosing adenosis, cystic hyperplasia, lobular hyperplasia, and lobular carcinoma in situ. Because of their interval development and clustered nature they were biopsied.

Impression: Multiple cysts, new microcalcifications of moderate suspicion.

Histopathology: Lobular carcinoma in situ.

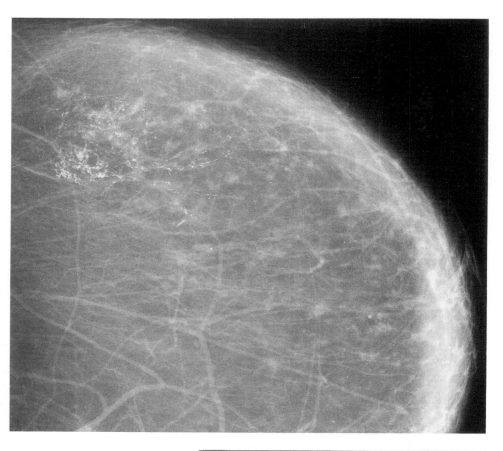

A

Figure 6.70.

Clinical: 65-year-old G3, P3 woman for baseline mammography.

Mammogram: Right craniocaudal (**A**) and mediolateral (**B**) views from a fine-needle aspiration procedure. There are extensive, irregular microcalcifications in a segmental distribution in the upper outer quadrant of the right breast. The morphology of these calcifications is highly malignant, being composed of a mixture of linear, punctate, and jagged forms of various sizes. Fine-needle aspiration was performed under standard mammographic guidance and yielded cells highly suggestive of carcinoma.

Histopathology: Comedocarcinoma.

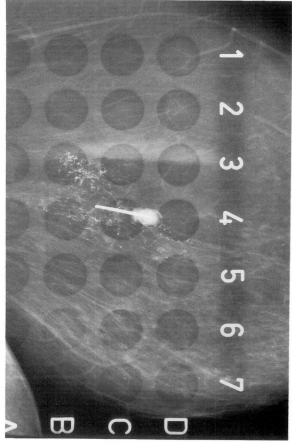

B

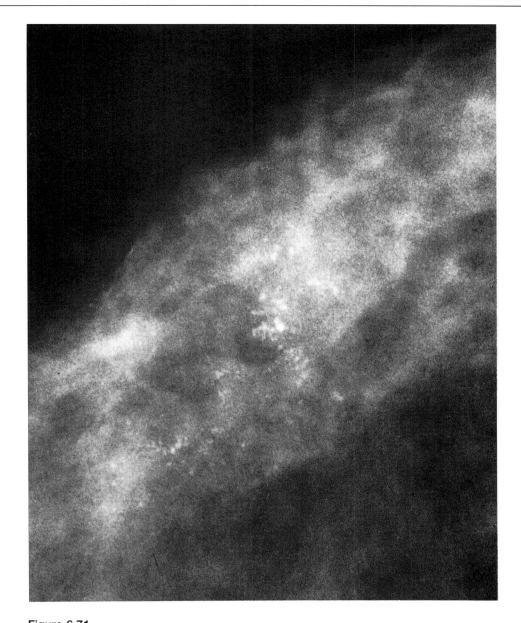

Figure 6.71.

Clinical: 55-year-old woman with a palpable mass in the right lower outer quadrant.

Mammogram: Right magnification view. There is a cluster of highly visible, fine microcalcifications within an area of dense tissue, typical of ductal carcinoma.

Histopathology: Comedocarcinoma with infiltrating ductal carcinoma, numerous macrometastases in axillary modes.

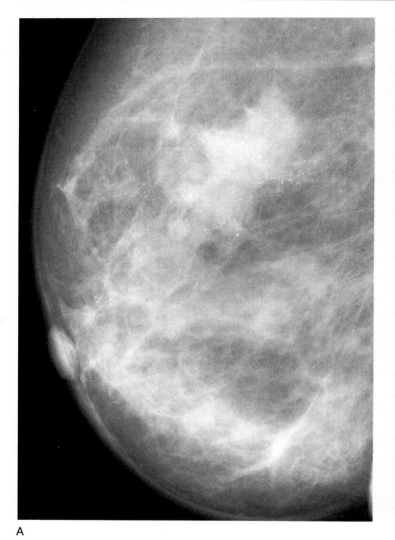

A

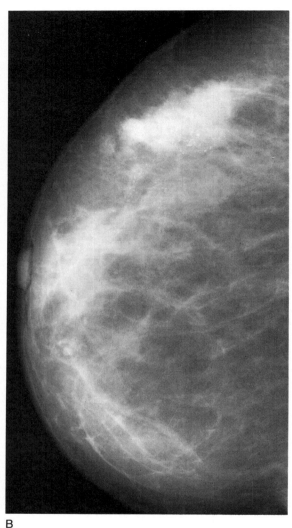

B

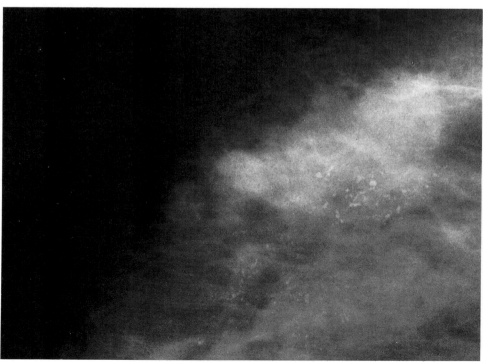

C

Figure 6.72.

Clinical: 68-year-old woman with a palpable left breast mass.

Mammogram: Left mediolateral (**A**), craniocaudal (**B**), and enlarged craniocaudal (**C**) views. There are innumerable microcalcifications associated with a high-density nodular tumor mass in the upper outer quadrant (**A** and **B**). Overlying skin thickening is present. A coned-down image (**C**) shows the irregular, long, jagged linear shapes of the calcifications, characteristic of malignant ductal calcifications.

Impression: Carcinoma with malignant calcifications.

Histopathology: Infiltrating ductal carcinoma with involvement of lymphatics.

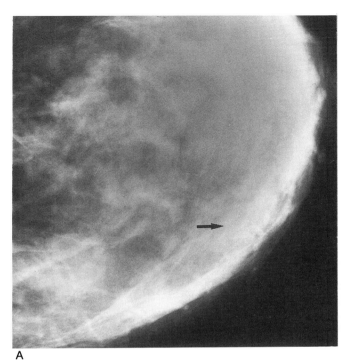

A

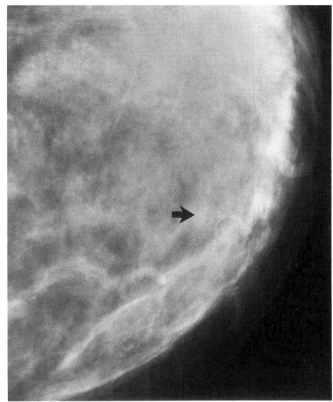

B

Figure 6.73.

Clinical: 46-year-old G4, P4 woman with a history of fibrocystic changes on biopsies of the left breast, for routine screening.

Mammogram: Right enlarged craniocaudal (**A**) and magnification (2×) mediolateral view (**B**). The breast parenchyma is dense for the age of the patient, consistent with the history of fibrocystic changes. There are clustered microcalcifications *(arrow)* (**A**) in the lower inner quadrant. These are variable in size, shape, and density on the magnification view (**B**) *(arrow)*. Their appearance is of moderate suspicion for a malignant process of ductal origin.

Impression: Moderately suspicious microcalcifications.

Histopathology: Comedocarcinoma.

Figure 6.74.

Clinical: 43-year-old G2, P2 woman for screening mammography.

Mammogram: Right oblique (**A**), craniocaudal (**B**), and magnified (2×) craniocaudal (**C**) views. The breast is dense for the age of the patient. There are innumerable microcalcifications throughout the upper outer quadrant of the right breast; none were present on the left. Some of the calcifications *(arrow)* have a linear shape on the upright film (**A**), suggesting milk of calcium in areas of cystic hyperplasia. Others *(curved arrow)* (**A–C**) are tightly clustered, with irregular margins, and are regarded, therefore, with moderate suspicion for malignancy. Needle localization was performed prior to biopsy.

Impression: Moderately suspicious microcalcifications in the right upper outer quadrant.

Histopathology: Focal area of intraductal carcinoma, extensive fibrocystic changes.

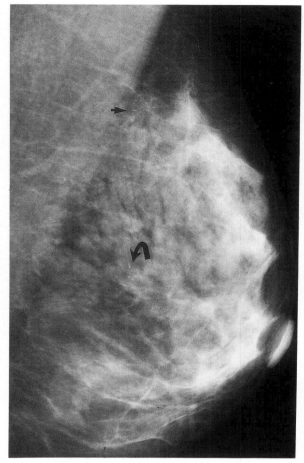

A

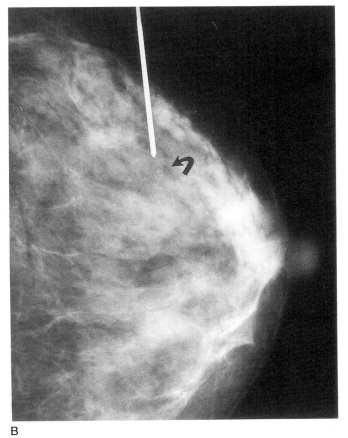

B

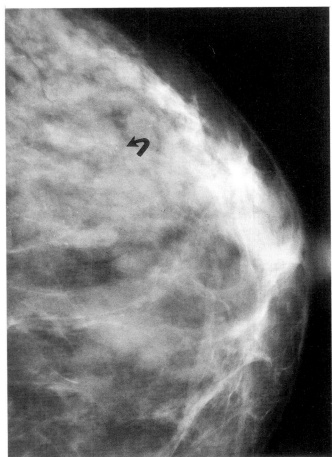

C

Figure 6.75.

Clinical: 50-year-old G2, P1, Ab1 woman with a firm 2-cm mass in the right upper outer quadrant.

Mammogram: Exaggerated lateral craniocaudal view (**A**), magnification view (**B**), and histology (**C**). There is a high-density spiculated mass in the outer quadrant, with micro-calcifications extending from the mass to the nipple. A magnification of this area (**B**) shows the typically malignant features of the calcifications: linear shapes, irregular margins, variability in size and shape, extension throughout the ductal system.

Impression: Ductal carcinoma.

Histopathology: Infiltrating ductal carcinoma with large intraductal component. Irregular calcification form casts of the malignant ducts.

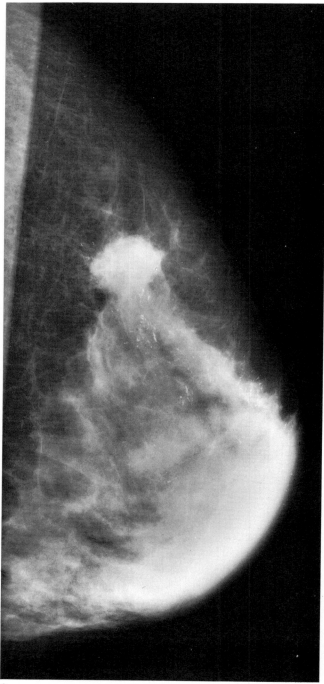

A

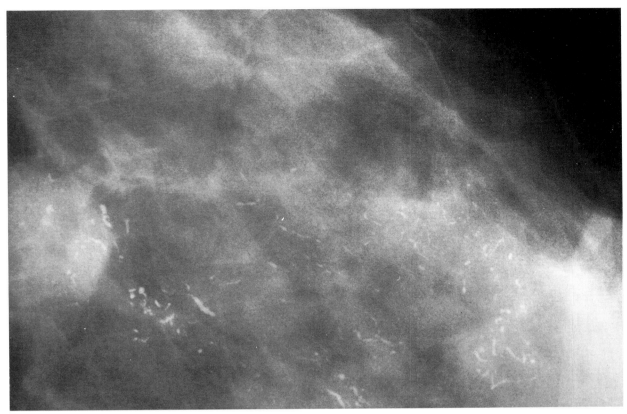

B

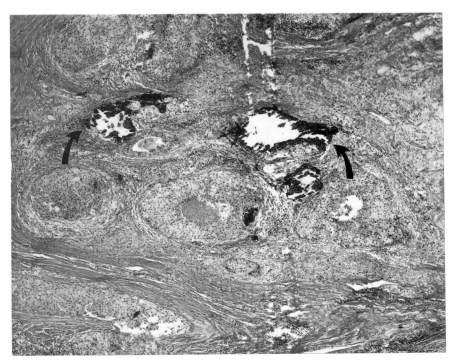

C

Figure 6.76.

Clinical: 61-year-old G8, P8 woman with ovarian cancer and a firm mass in the left breast.

Mammogram: Left craniocaudal (**A**) and spot magnification (**B**) views. There is a high-density spiculated mass that tethers the overlying skin of the left breast (**A**). Malignant microcalcifications are present and are much better demonstrated on the spot magnification view (**B**). The lacy irregular borders and linear shapes are characteristic of malignant calcifications.

Histopathology: Infiltrating ductal carcinoma.

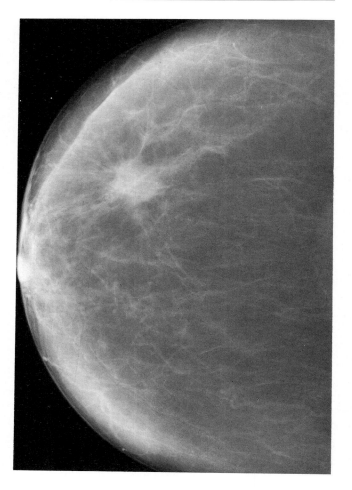

A

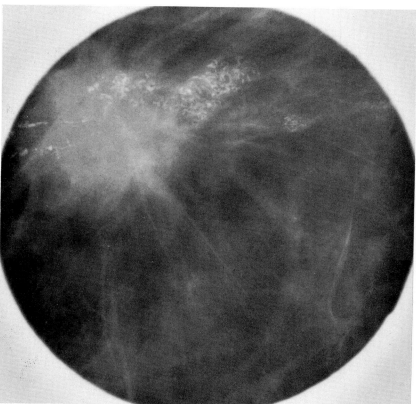

B

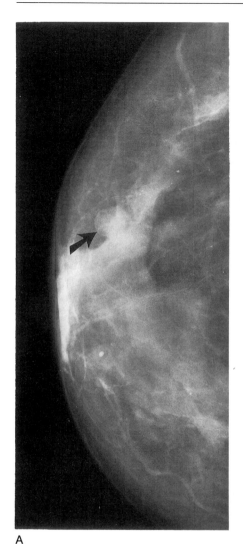

A

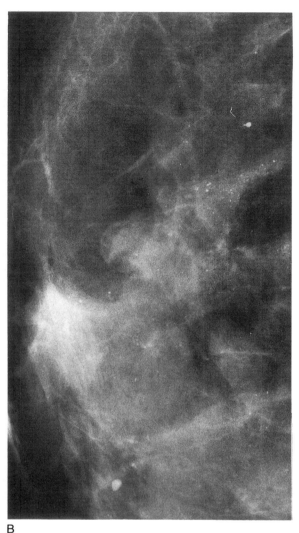

B

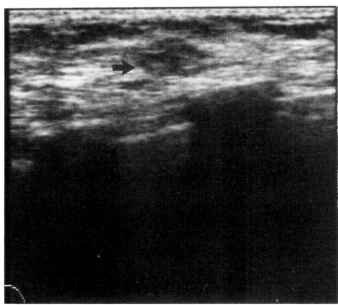

C

Figure 6.77.

Clinical: 59-year-old woman after right mastectomy, with a small palpable nodule at the 3 o'clock position in the left breast.

Mammogram: Left craniocaudal (**A**) enlarged mediolateral views (**B**) and ultrasound (**C**). There are diffuse, relatively round microcalcifications distributed extensively throughout the central aspect of the left breast (**A** and **B**). There is also a relatively well circumscribed nodule in the outer aspect at the 3 o'clock position *(arrow)* (**A**) corresponding to the palpable nodule. Sonography (**C**) reveals this mass to be solid and somewhat irregular in contour *(arrow)*, features suspicious for malignancy.

Impression: Microcalcifications and solid nodule highly suspicious for extensive carcinoma.

Histopathology: Infiltrating ductal and intraductal carcinoma.

Note: Even though microcalcifications are extensive, one should not exclude the possibility of malignancy. Calcifications in a ductal distribution, with any irregularity in their margins, should alert one to the possibility of a malignant process.

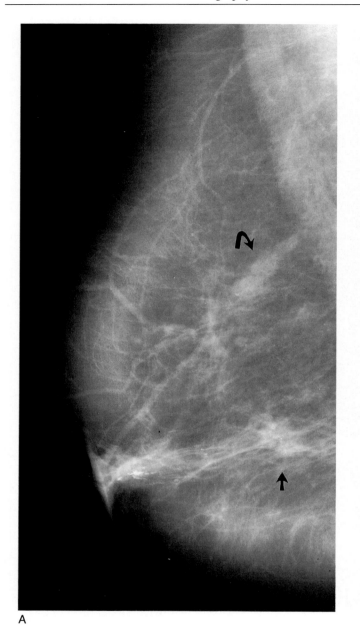

A

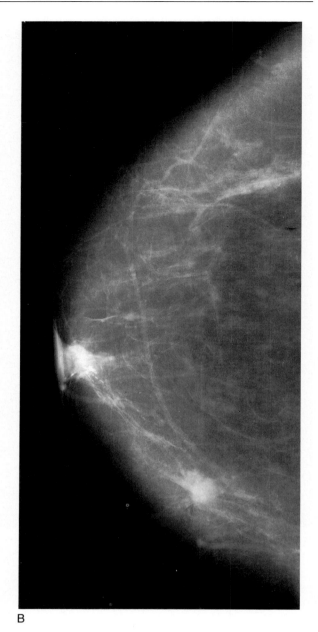

B

Figure 6.78.

Clinical: 61-year-old woman with a palpable mass in the left subareolar area.

Mammogram: Left oblique (**A**) and craniocaudal (**B**) views and magnified image (**C**). There are linear ductal calcifications of varying sizes extending back from a retracted nipple-aerolar complex to a spiculated mass *(straight arrow)*. A second nodular mass *(curved arrow)* is present in the upper outer quadrant (**A**). A magnified image (**C**) of the subareolar area shows the variability and irregularity of the casting calcifications that have a highly malignant appearance.

Impression: Multicentric carcinoma with ductal extension to the nipple.

Histopathology: Infiltrating ductal and intraductal carcinoma in two sites, with 2 of 25 lymph nodes positive for tumor.

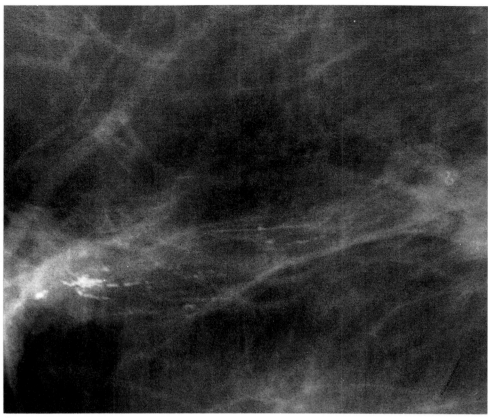

C

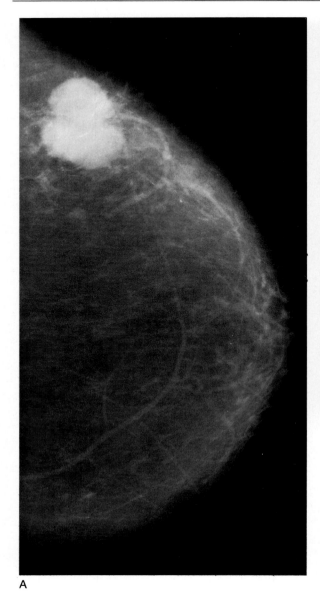

A

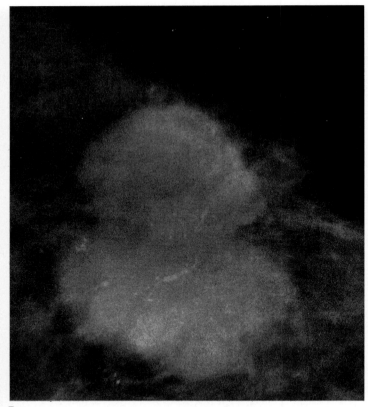

B

Figure 6.79.

Clinical: 57-year-old woman with 4 × 4-cm mass in the right upper outer quadrant.

Mammogram: Right craniocaudal view (**A**) and magnified image (**B**). There is a high-density irregular mass in the outer aspect of the breast. Within this area are irregular microcalcifications, some of which are forming linear casts of the ducts. The features of the calcifications as well as the mass are characteristic of carcinoma.

Impression: Carcinoma.

Histopathology: Infiltrating ductal carcinoma.

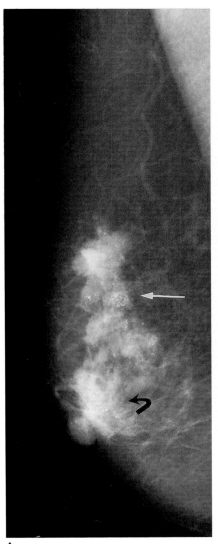
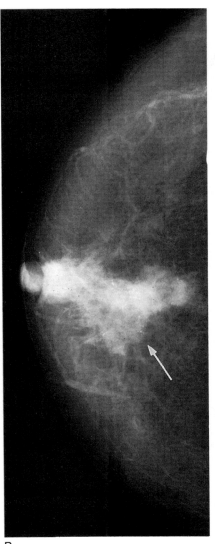

A

B

Figure 6.80.

Clinical: 63-year-old woman with a left breast mass suspicious for cancer.

Mammogram: Left oblique view (**A**), craniocaudal view (**B**), and magnification image (**C**). There is an irregular, moderately high density mass in the 12 o'clock position of the left breast. Associated with this are innumerable lacy, irregular-bordered microcalcifications *(arrow)* having a highly malignant appearance. There are additional clustered microcalcifications just beneath the nipple *(curved arrow),* suggesting extension of tumor into the subareolar ducts. It is important on mammography to identify extension of tumor or multicentric disease, particularly if the patient is being considered a possible candidate for lumpectomy and radiation therapy. In the evaluation of a suspicious palpable mass, the most important role of the mammogram is to evaluate the remainder of the breast for synchronous disease and the opposite breast for contralateral carcinoma.

Impression: Carcinoma with extension into subareolar ducts.

Histopathology: Infiltrating ductal adenocarcinoma, comedocarcinoma, intraductal papillary carcinoma; one positive axillary node.

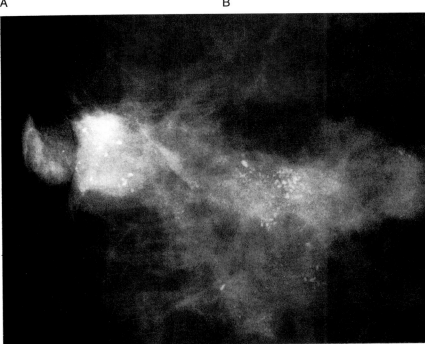

C

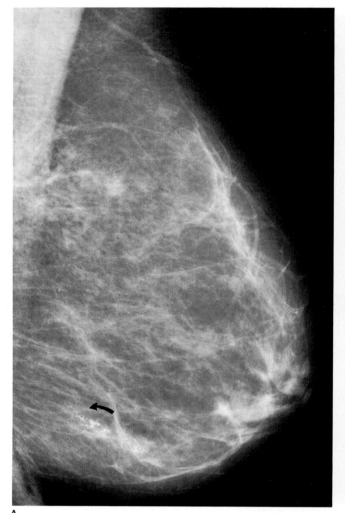

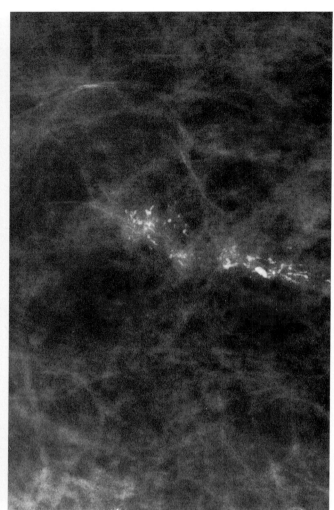

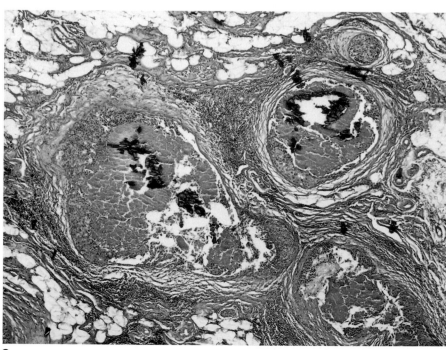

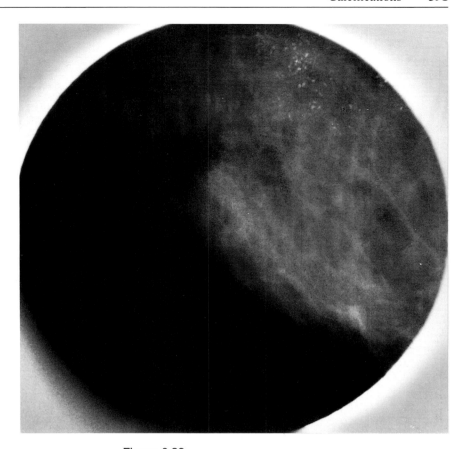

Figure 6.82.

Clinical: 43-year-old woman with a palpable mass in the left breast.

Mammogram: Spot magnification view. There are clustered irregular lacy microcalcifications present. The spot magnification view depicts well the mixed morphology of these deposits. Note the mixture of linear and punctate forms with jagged margins. These findings are characteristic of malignant calcifications.

Histopathology: Infiltrating ductal carcinoma.

Figure 6.81.

Clinical: 73-year-old woman for screening mammography.

Mammogram: Right oblique view (**A**), magnified image (**B**), and histopathology section (**C**). There is a cluster of innumerable irregular microcalcifications in the right breast at the 6 o'clock position *(arrow)*. These calcifications are of variable size and shape, are tightly clustered, and have jagged irregular margins and some linear shapes, all of which are suspicious features for malignancy.

Impression: Ductal carcinoma, possible comedocarcinoma.

Histopathology: Comedocarcinoma. Biopsy specimen with comedocarcinoma shows multiple distended ducts filled with intraductal carcinoma and prominent central necrosis. Irregular calcifications are present within the necrotic areas.

Note: In comedocarcinoma the tumor spreads along the ducts, and there is a thick material in the lumen that tends to calcify in the characteristic pattern shown here.

Figure 6.83.

Clinical: 80-year-old G11, P11 woman with a new palpable mass in the right breast.

Mammogram: Right oblique view (**A**), craniocaudal (**B**) view, and specimen film (**C**). The breast is mildly glandular, and there are extensive vascular calcifications present *(arrows)* (**A** and **B**). In the lower inner quadrant, there is a spiculated high-density mass *(curved arrow);* irregular microcalcifications are within the mass and extend in a linear distribution from it. On the specimen film (**C**), the irregular mixed morphology of the calcifications is seen, typical of a ductal malignancy.

Impression: Carcinoma with intraductal extension.

Histopathology: Infiltrating ductal carcinoma with an extensive intraductal component (solid and comedo variants).

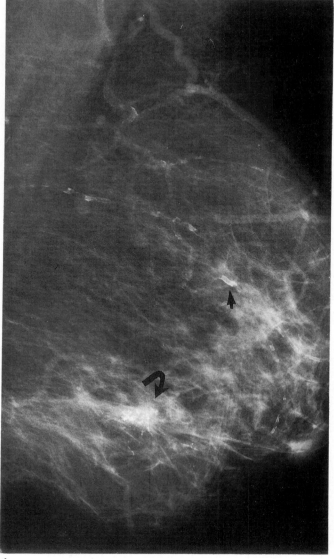

A

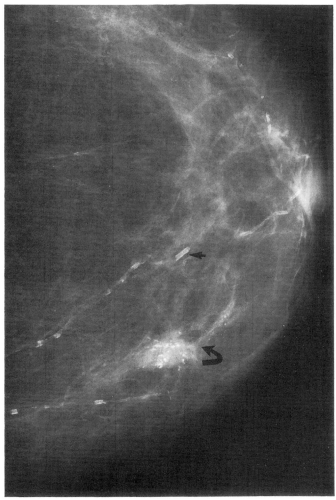

B

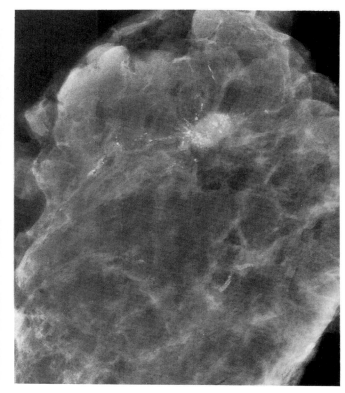

C

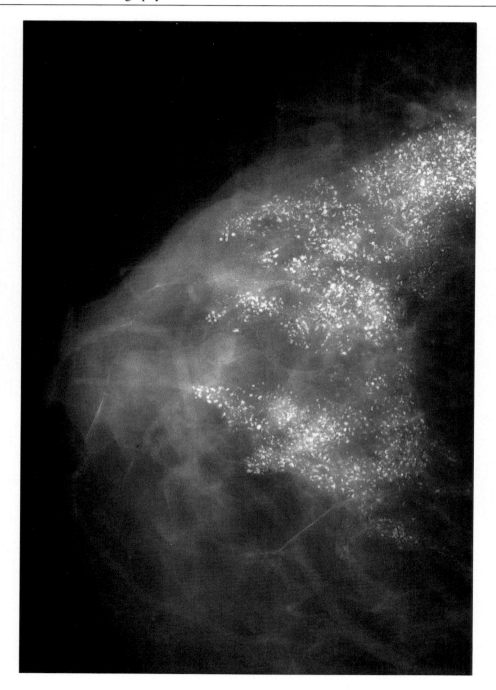

Figure 6.84.

Clinical: 63-year-old woman for screening mammography.

Mammogram: Left magnification view. The breast is noted to be very dense and nodular for the age of the patient. In the midportion there are clustered microcalcifications in a linear distribution. The contours are irregular and jagged, features that are suspicious for malignancy.

Impression: Highly suspicious for carcinoma—probable intraductal comedocarcinoma.

Histopathology: Comedocarcinoma.

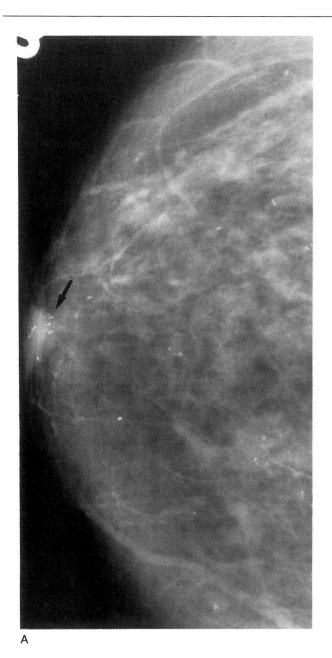

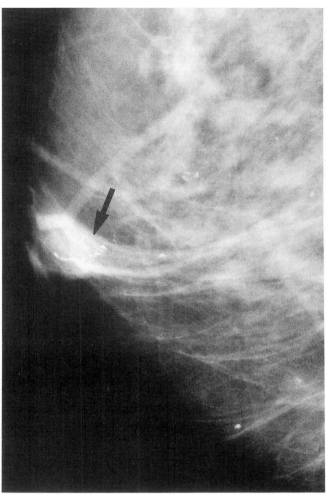

B

A

Figure 6.85.

Clinical: 85-year-old G2, P-0, Ab2 woman with a scaling left nipple.

Mammogram: Left craniocaudal (**A**) and enlarged (2×) mediolateral (**B**) views. The breast is moderately dense with scattered benign-appearing calcifications. In the subareolar area, extending into the nipple (**A** and **B**), there are linear, slightly irregular microcalcifications *(arrows)*. The distribution and the morphology of these calcifications suggest a ductal origin. The differential includes intraductal hyperplasia, intraductal carcinoma, and secretory disease. Particularly in light of the clinical findings, the presence of the calcifications suggests Paget's disease with intraductal extension.

Impression: Paget's disease with intraductal extension.

Histopathology: Paget's disease with underlying intraductal carcinoma.

Figure 6.86.

Clinical: 36-year-old woman with an enlarged lymph node in the right supraclavicular area and no palpable breast mass.

Mammogram: Right mediolateral (**A**) and magnification (**B**) views. There are innumerable round microcalcifications of varying size in the lower outer quadrant (**A**), extending from the retroareolar area posteriorly to near the chest wall. Magnification (**B**) of this area shows the rounded appearance of these calcifications without the linear branching forms often associated with ductal carcinomas.

Impression: Highly suspicious for carcinoma.

Histopathology: Comedocarcinoma and infiltrating ductal carcinoma, positive axillary and supraclavicular nodes.

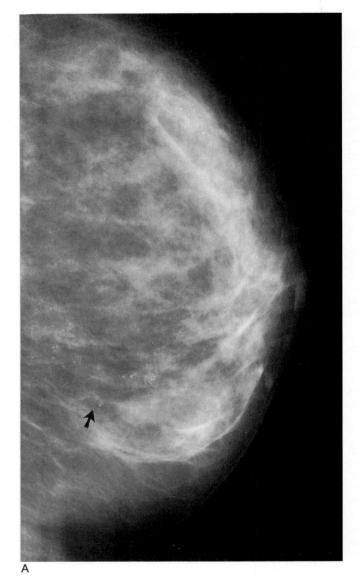

A

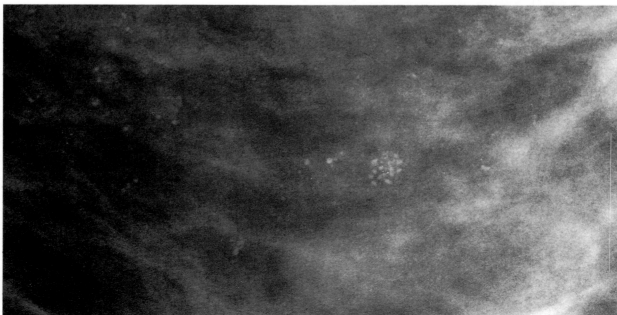

B

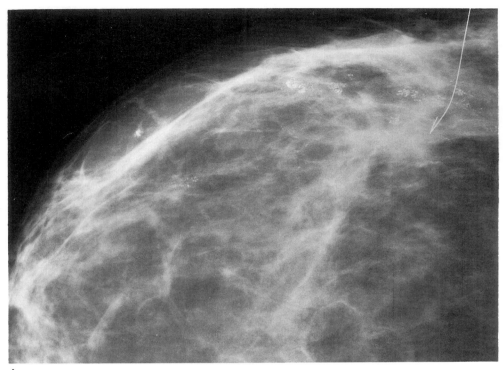

A

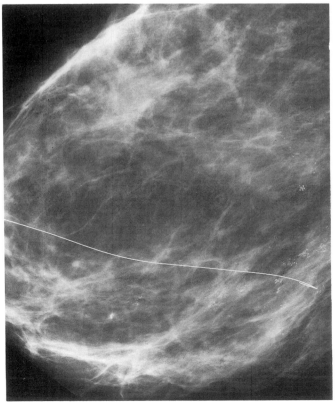

B

Figure 6.87.

Clinical: 41-year-old G3, P3 woman for screening.

Mammogram: Left enlarged craniocaudal (**A**) and mediolateral (**B**) views from a needle localization procedure. There are innumerable, irregular, round clustered microcalcifications extending in a linear distribution in the left lower outer quadrant. This appearance is characteristic of comedocarcinoma.

Histopathology: Comedocarcinoma with micrometastases in 2 of 30 axillary nodes.

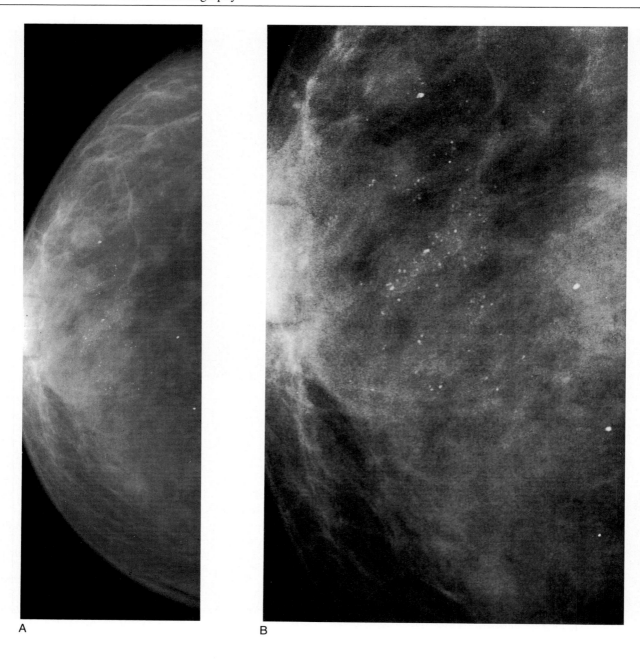

A

B

Figure 6.88.

Clinical: 76-year-old woman with a palpable carcinoma in the right breast.

Mammogram: Left craniocaudal (**A**) and magnification (**B**) views. There are fine granular microcalcifications extending throughout the subareolar ducts of the left breast. These are of variable morphology, suggesting a suspicious etiology.

Impression: Microcalcifications suspicious for ductal carcinoma.

Histopathology: Left breast: extensive intraductal carcinoma.

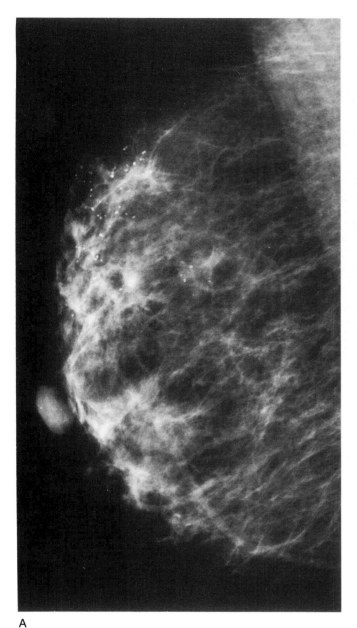

A

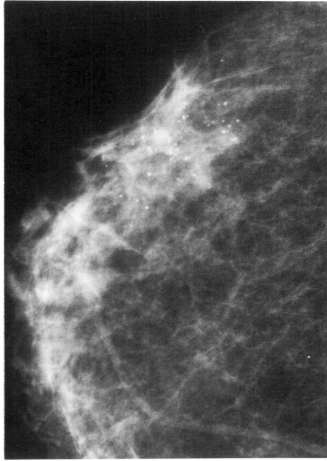

B

Figure 6.89.

Clinical: 58-year-old G6, P6 woman with a positive family history of breast cancer, for routine screening.

Mammogram: Left oblique (**A**) and enlarged (1.5×) craniocaudal (**B**) views. The breast is moderately dense. Extending throughout the upper outer quadrant are coarse microcalcifications of similar size, shape, and density. These calcifications are smooth and rounded, which is more in favor of a benign than a malignant origin. However, the calcifications were biopsied because they had increased in number from a previous outside study, indicating activity in the area.

Impression: Rounded microcalcifications of indeterminate nature, moderately suspicious.

Histopathology: Intraductal carcinoma of comedo and cribriform forms.

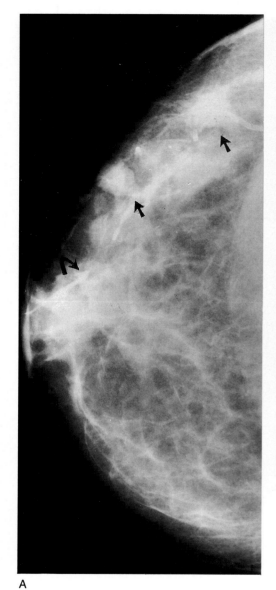

A

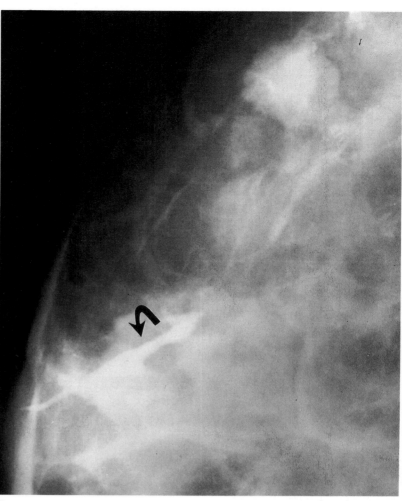

B

Figure 6.90.

Clinical: 48-year-old woman with a left breast mass.

Mammogram: Left craniocaudal view (**A**) and magnified image (**B**). There are several irregular nodules in the outer quadrant *(arrows)* (**A**). Calcifications extend away from the masses toward the nipple and coalesce to form casts of the ductal lumens *(curved arrows),* typical of malignant ductal calcifications (**A** and **B**).

Impression: Carcinoma with intraductal extension.

Histopathology: Multifocal infiltrating and intraductal carcinoma, medullary carcinoma. (Case courtesy of Dr. Ed Fallon, Reading, PA.)

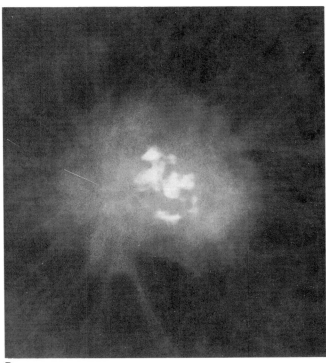

B

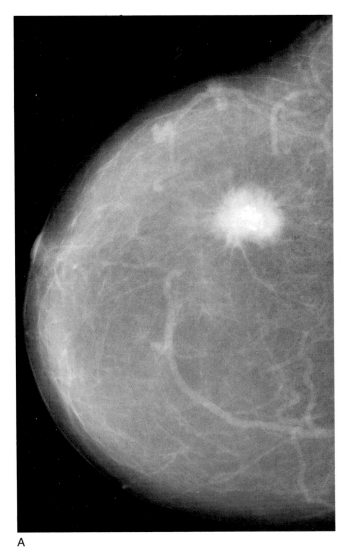

A

Figure 6.91.

Clinical: 64-year-old woman with a firm palpable mass in the left breast.

Mammogram: Left craniocaudal view (**A**) and magnified image (**B**). There is a high-density spiculated mass typical of malignancy. There are relatively coarse dense calcifications, 3–4 mm in diameter, within the mass (**B**) larger than are generally considered to be associated with malignancies. Occasionally, malignancies may contain larger calcifications, and their presence should not alter a diagnosis of carcinoma.

Impression: Carcinoma, left breast.

Histopathology: Infiltrating ductal carcinoma.

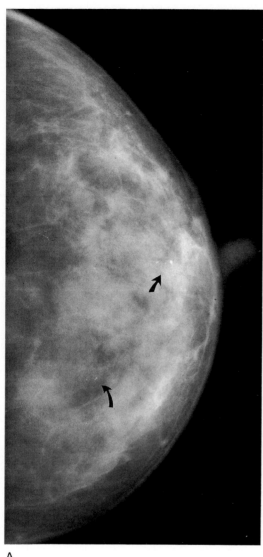

A

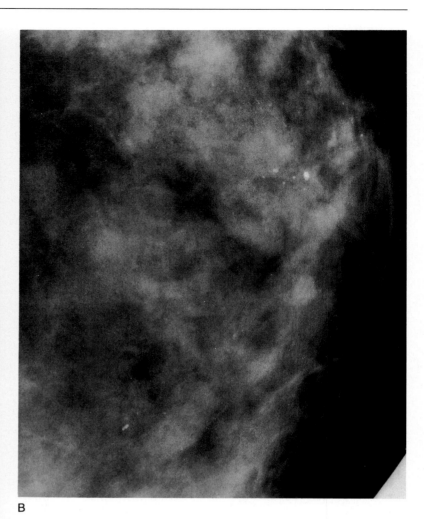

B

Figure 6.92.

Clinical: 69-year-old woman for screening mammography.

Mammogram: Right craniocaudal view (**A**) and magnified craniocaudal view (**B**). There is a cluster of microcalcifications in the retroareolar area *(straight arrow)* and an additional microcalcification medially *(curved arrow)* (**A**). On the magnification view the retroareolar cluster has variability in size and shape of the calcifications, but no linear or branching forms are present. On the magnification film the area me-

dially is shown to be a second cluster rather than a single calcification. The importance of identifying the second lesion is that, assuming biopsy shows malignancy, the patient has multicentric disease and might not be a good candidate for lumpectomy and radiation therapy.

Impression: Two clusters of calcifications suspicious for multicentric carcinoma.

Histopathology: Both sites: intraductal carcinoma.

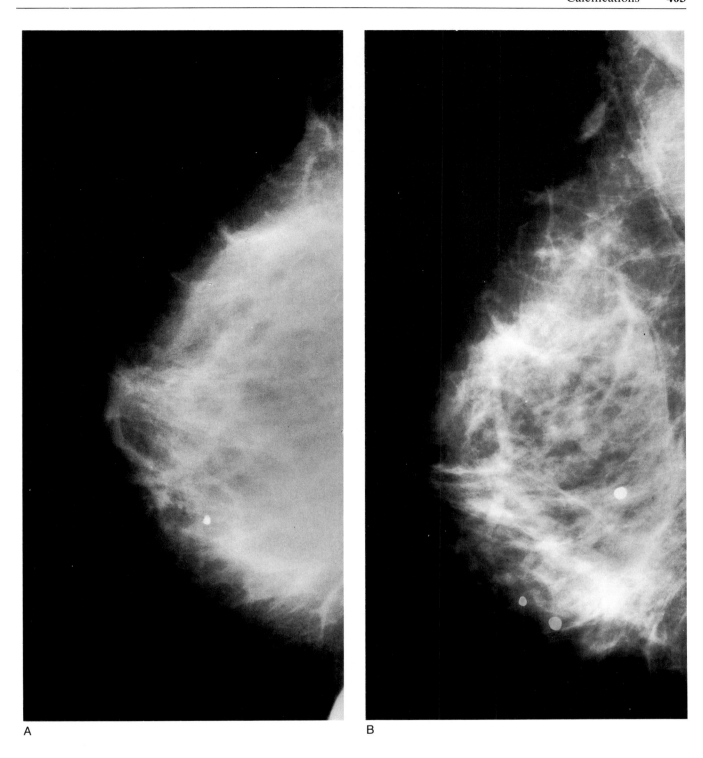

A

B

Figure 6.93.

Clinical: 61-year-old woman who in 1980 underwent lumpectomy and radiation therapy to the left breast for carcinoma.

Mammogram: Left mediolateral view taken in 1981 (**A**) and left oblique view taken in 1987 (**B**). In the left mediolateral view, the breast is very dense and there is diffuse skin thickening and edema as is expected 1 year after radiation therapy. A single coarse calcification is present. In the left oblique

view taken in 1987, the density has decreased, approaching a more normal appearance. There are several new coarse round calcifications typical of the dystrophic changes after radiation therapy.

Impression: Dystrophic calcifications secondary to radiation therapy.

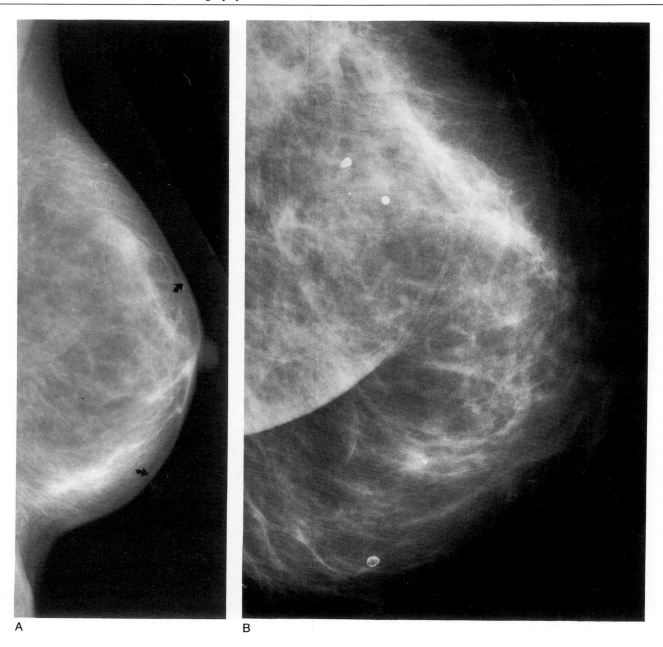

A

B

Figure 6.94.

Clinical: 59-year-old woman who in 1983 had a firm palpable mass in the inner quadrant of the right breast. This was biopsied and found malignant; she was treated with lumpectomy and radiation therapy.

Mammogram: Right oblique view in 1984 (**A**) and right oblique view in 1989 (**B**). There has been a lumpectomy deep in the inner quadrant. Diffuse skin thickening and increased density is present *(arrows),* as would be expected after radiation therapy to the breast. Five years after treatment (**B**), there has been development of coarse calcifications typical of the dystrophic changes secondary to lumpectomy and radiation therapy. These should not be confused with developing calcifications indicating recurrent carcinoma.

Impression: Dystrophic calcifications secondary to radiation therapy.

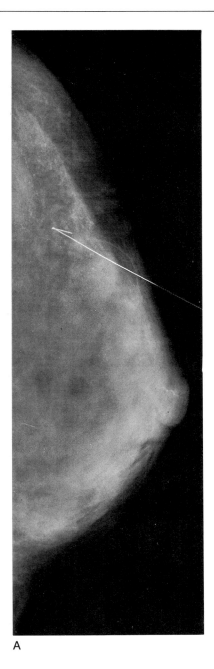

A

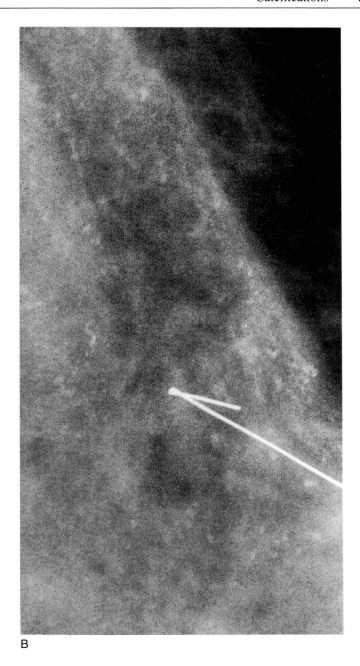

B

Figure 6.95.

Clinical: 26-year-old woman 6 months after lumpectomy and radiation therapy to the right breast for comedocarcinoma.

Mammogram: Right mediolateral view (**A**) and magnified image (**B**). A view from the needle localization shows the breast to be very dense with diffuse skin thickening, as expected soon after radiation therapy. There are innumerable microcalcifications in the upper half of the breast, which on the magnified image are shown to be lacy, casting ductal calcifications typical of malignancy.

Impression: Recurrent carcinoma.

Histopathology: Intraductal and infiltrating ductal carcinoma.

Note: The development of ductal calcifications in the postirradiated breast should alert one to the probable development of recurrent carcinoma.

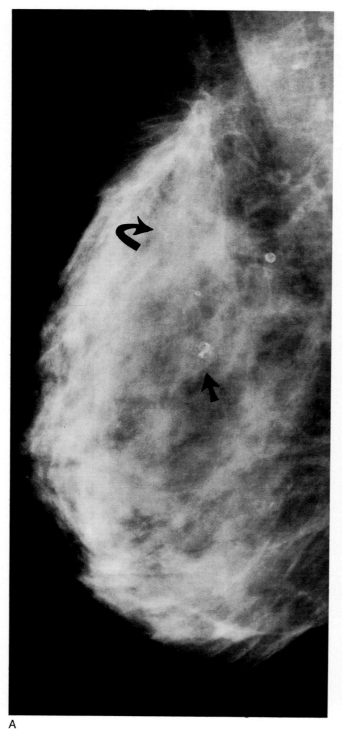
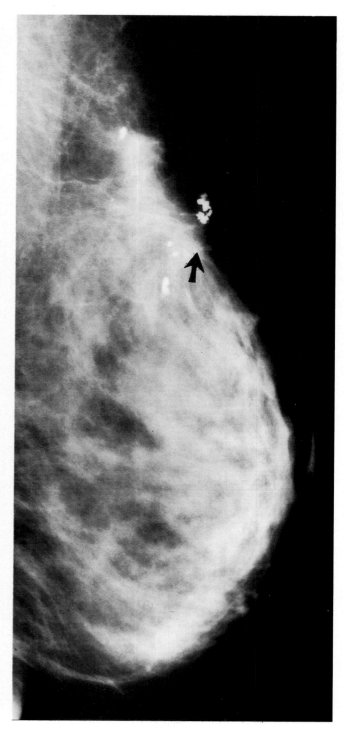

A

Figure 6.96.

Clinical: 54-year-old woman after lumpectomy and radiation therapy to both breasts for infiltrating carcinomas 3 years earlier.

Mammogram: Bilateral oblique views (**A**) and magnified images of the left breast (**B** and **C**). Architectural distortion related to surgery is present in the upper aspects of both breasts. There are coarse dystrophic calcifications of fat necrosis secondary to lumpectomy and radiation therapy bilaterally *(straight arrows)*. On the left, there are also fine micro-

calcifications in the tumor bed *(curved arrow)* (**A**). A magnified image of the left breast (**B**) better demonstrates the malignant ductal calcifications. The dystrophic calcifications (**C**), which occurred bilaterally, are an expected benign change after treatment, but the malignant calcifications on the left (**B**) indicate recurrence of tumor.

Impression: Right breast postradiation calcifications; left breast recurrent carcinoma.

Histopathology: Left breast: infiltrating ductal carcinoma.

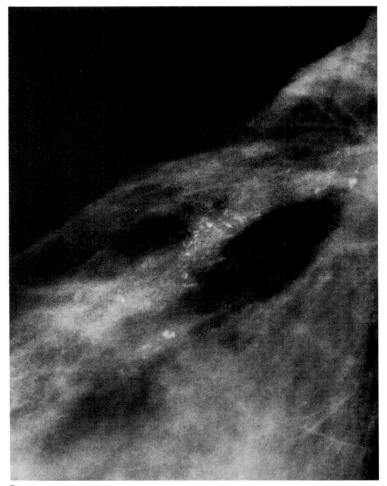

B

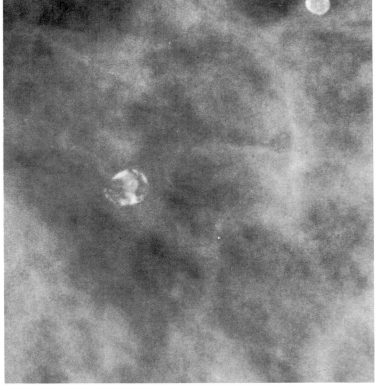

C

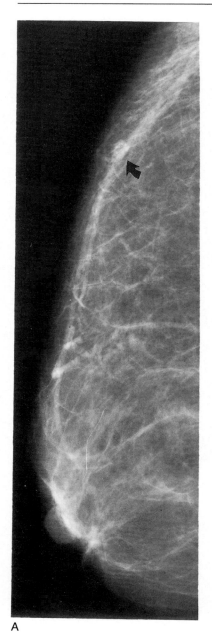

A

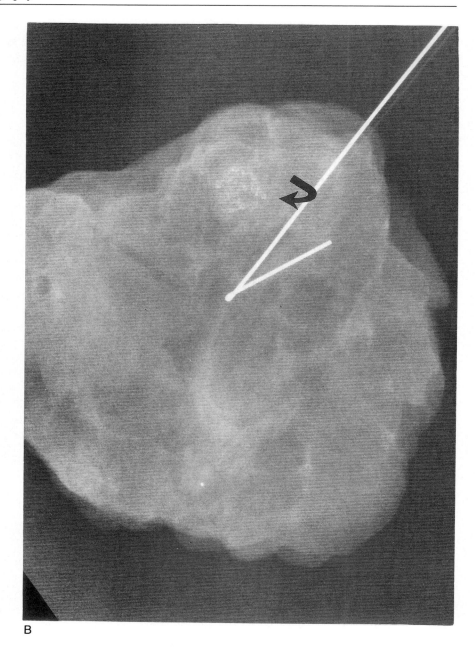

B

Figure 6.97.

Clinical: 50-year-old G3, P3 woman with a history of rheumatoid arthritis, for routine screening mammography.

Mammogram: Left oblique craniocaudal (**A**) view and specimen film (**B**). There is a small superficial circumscribed nodule *(arrow)* in the outer aspect of the breast (**A**). Faint calcific densities are present within this lesion. The specimen film (**B**) better demonstrates these irregular calcific densities. The shape and location of the nodule are suggestive of an intramammary node, although the calcifications are unusual. Microcalcifications within a node are an uncommon finding of metastatic breast carcinoma, but in this case the node is quite small, and there is no evidence for carcinoma elsewhere in the breast. Patients who have been treated with intramuscular gold injections for rheumatoid arthritis may develop intranodal gold deposits that simulate microcalcifications.

Impression: Probable gold deposits in an intramammary node.

Histopathology: Intramammary node containing gold.

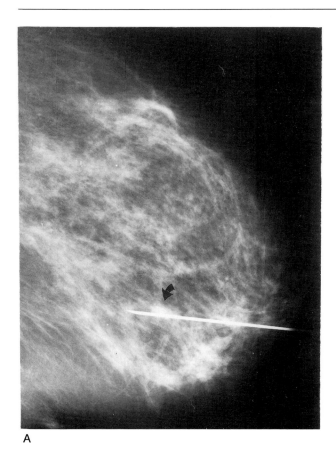

A

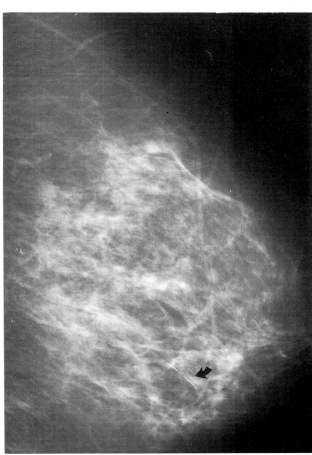

B

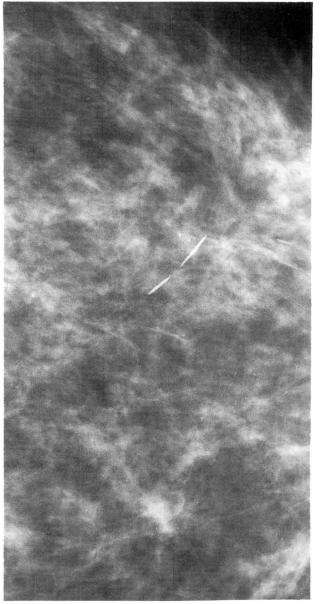

C

Figure 6.98.

Clinical: 48-year-old woman for routine mammography 1 year after right breast biopsy for a benign lesion.

Mammogram: Right mediolateral view from the needle localization 1 year earlier (**A**), and current right mediolateral (**B**) and magnified (2×) mediolateral (**C**) views. On the initial mammogram (**A**) the localization needle has been placed through the soft tissue nodule *(arrow)*. One year later (**B** and **C**) the nodule has been removed, and in the biopsy area there are two new smooth linear calcifications *(arrow)*. These calcifications are not oriented toward the nipple, as would be expected for a ductal origin. The coarse curvilinear appearance is typical of dystrophic calcification in sutures at the biopsy site. Impression: sutural calcification. (Case courtesy of Dr. Arch Wagner, Warrenton, VA.)

Figure 6.99.

Clinical: 36-year-old woman for screening mammography.

Mammogram: Left oblique view. There are calcific-like densities *(arrow)* superimposed over the axillary folds, consistent with pseudocalcifications from deodorant artifact.

Impression: Pseudocalcifications.

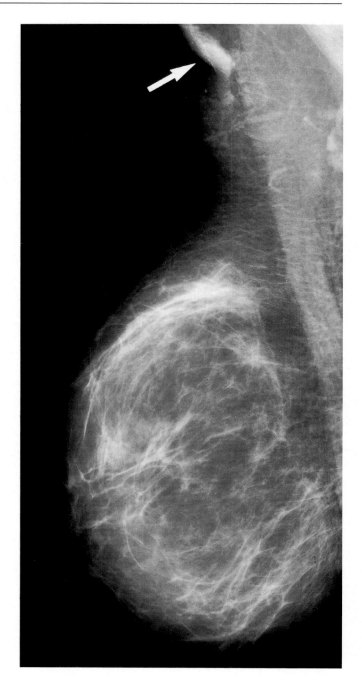

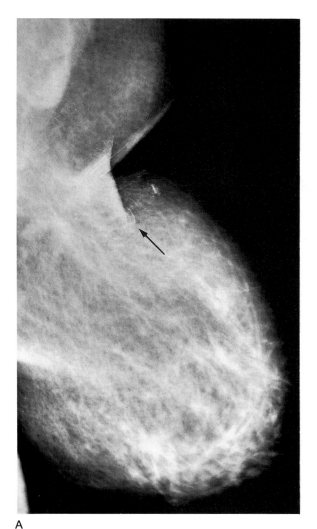

A

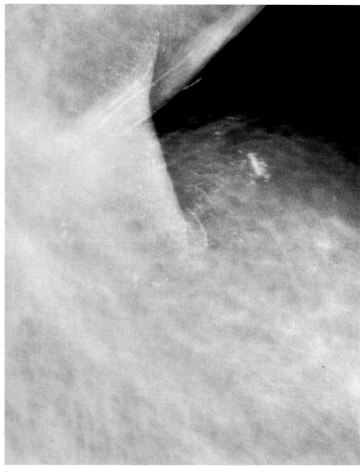

B

Figure 6.100.

Clinical: 73-year-old patient who had a biopsy in the left axillary tail 6 months previously for fibrocystic disease and who had a residual sinus tract in the area of biopsy.

Mammogram: Right oblique view (**A**) and magnified image (**B**). There is increased density and deformity in the area of surgical defect. There are fine linear and punctate calcific-like densities in the area of the biopsy *(arrow)* (**A**), superfi-

cially located and corresponding to the folds of skin. These represent pseudocalcifications from surgical tape adhesive on the patient's skin. It is important for the technologist to note any substances on the patient's skin and to cleanse the skin surface if an artifact-producing substance (cream, ointment, powder, deodorant, tape) is present.

Impression: Pseudocalcification.

Figure 6.101.

Clinical: Screening mammogram.

Mammogram: Bilateral oblique view—upper aspects. There are bilateral calcific-like densities superimposed over both axillary areas *(arrows)*, representing an artifact from deodorant.

Impression: Pseudocalcification.

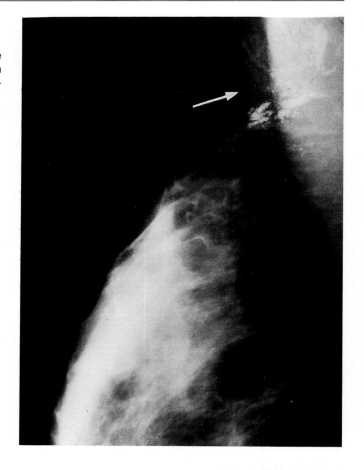

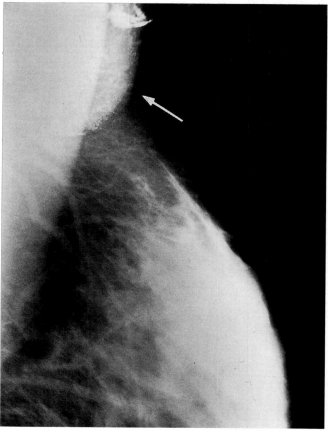

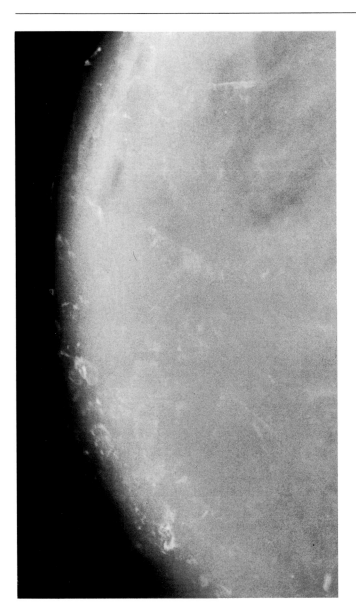

Figure 6.102.

Clinical: 75-year-old woman with Stevens-Johnson syndrome, multiple superficial ulcerations on the skin of the left breast, and a markedly dense, tender left breast. The skin lesions were being treated with zinc oxide ointment.

Mammogram: Left magnified mediolateral view. The breast is very dense, and there is marked skin thickening diffusely. There are also multiple lacy "calcifications" located superficially. The calcificlike densities represent the zinc oxide ointment on the skin surface. The skin thickening was related to an acute mastitis secondary to the skin infection and resolved on antibiotic therapy.

Impression: Pseudocalcifications from zinc oxide ointment.

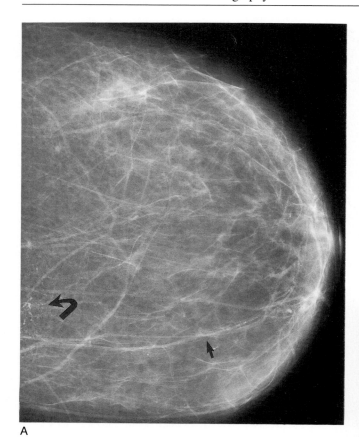

A

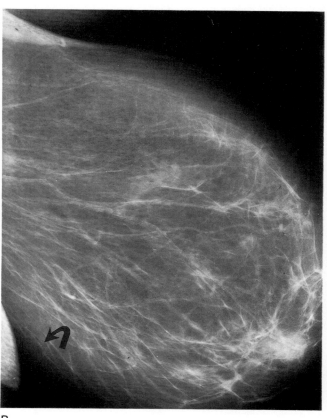

B

Figure 6.103.

Clinical: 42-year-old woman with large breasts difficult to examine, for routine mammography.

Mammogram: Right craniocaudal (**A**), oblique (**B**), and enlarged (2×) craniocaudal (**C**) views. The breast shows primarily fatty replacement. Early arterial calcifications are noted medially *(arrow)* (**A**). Deep near the chest wall in the inner quadrant *(curved arrow)* are irregular calcific densities grouped in a bizarre orientation (**A**). These are faintly seen inferiorly *(curved arrow)* on the oblique (**B**) view. On the enlargement (**C**) these densities are both globular and linear, following skin creases, a finding typical of powder or cream on the skin. Powder was cleansed from the inframammary crease, and these densities disappeared.

Impression: Pseudocalcifications from powder.

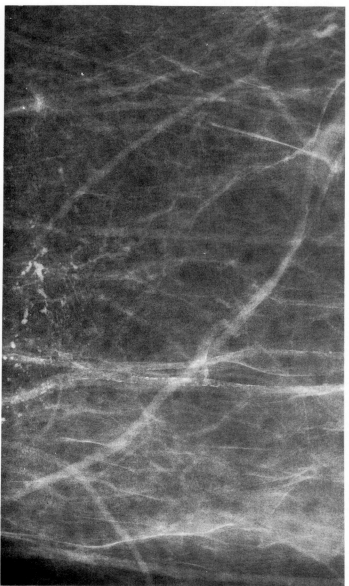

C

References

1. Leborgne R. Diagnosis of tumors of the breast by simple roentgenography: calcifications in carcinoma. AJR 1951;65:1–11.
2. Gershon-Cohen J, Yiu LS, Berger SM. The diagnostic importance of calcareous patterns in roentgenography of breast cancer. AJR 1962;88:1117–1125.
3. Gershon-Cohen J, Berger SM, Curcio BM. Breast cancer with microcalcifications: diagnostic difficulties. Radiology 1966; 87:613–622.
4. Millis RR, Davis R, Stacey AJ. The detection and significance of calcifications in the breast. A radiological and pathological study. Br J Radiol 1976;49:12–26.
5. Sickles EA. Breast calcifications: mammographic evaluation. Radiology 1986;160:289–293.
6. Gershon-Cohen J, Ingleby H. Roentgenography of fibroadenomas of the breast. Radiology 1952;59:77–87.
7. Bassett LW, Gold RH, Cove HC. Mammographic spectrum of traumatic fat necrosis: the fallibility of ''pathognomonic'' signs of carcinoma. AJR 1978;130:119–122.
8. Leborgne R. Esteatonecrosis quistica calcificata de la mama. Torace 1967;16:172.
9. Fewins HE, Whitehouse GH, Leinster SJ. The spontaneous disappearance or breast calcification. Clin Radiol 1988;39:257–261.
10. Parker MD, Clark RL, McLelland R, Daughtery K. Disappearing breast calcifications. Radiology 1989;172:677–680.
11. Gershon-Cohen J, Ingleby H, Hermel MB. Calcification in secretory disease of the breast. AJR 1956;76:132–135.
12. Wolfe JN. Xeroradiography: breast calcifications. Springfield, Illinois: Charles C Thomas, 1977.
13. Levitan LH, Witten DM, Harrison EG. Calcification in breast disease mammographic-pathologic correlation. AJR 1964;92:29–39.
14. Asch T, Fry C. Radiographic appearance of mammary duct ectasia with calcification. N Engl J Med 1962;266:86–87.
15. Sommer G. Kopsa H, Zazgornik J, Salomonowitz E. Breast calcifications in renal hyperparathyroidism. AJR 1987;148:855–857.
16. Sickles EA, Galvin HB. Breast arterial calcification in association with diabetes mellitus: too weak a correlation to have clinical utility. Radiology 1985;155:577–579.
17. Meybehm M, Pfeifer U. Vascular calcifications mimicking grouped microcalcifications on mammography. Breast Dis 1900;3:81–86.
18. Kopans DB, Meyer JE, Homer MJ, Grabbe J. Dermal deposits mistaken for breast calcifications. Radiology 1983;149:592–594.
19. Tabar L, Dean PB. Teaching atlas of mammography. Stuttgart: Georg Thieme Verlag, 1985.
20. Haagensen CD. Diseases of the breast. Philadelphia: WB Saunders, 1986.
21. Minagi H, Youker JE, Knudson HW. The roentgen appearance of injected silicone in the breast. Radiology 1968;90:57–61.
22. Koide T, Katayama H. Calcification in augmentation mammoplasty. Radiology 1979;130:337–340.
23. Shermis RB, Adler DD, Smith DJ, Hall JD. Intraductal silicone secondary to breast implant rupture. Breast Dis 1990;3:17–20.
24. Cooper RA, Berman S. Extensive breast calcification in renal failure. J Thorac Imaging 1988;3(2):81–82.
25. Han SY, Witten DM. Diffuse calcification of the breast in chronic renal failure. AJR 1977;129:341–342.
26. Egan RL, McSweeney MB, Swell CW. Intramammary calcifications without an associated mass in benign and malignant diseases. Radiology 1980;137:1–7.
27. Shaw de Paredes E, Abbitt PL, Tabbarah S, et al. Mammographic and histologic correlations of microcalcifications. RadioGraphics 1900;10:577–589.
28. Powell RW, McSweeney MB, Wilson CE. X-ray calcifications as the only basis for breast biopsy. Ann Surg 1983; 197:555–559.
29. Wilhelm MC, Shaw de Paredes E, Pope TL, Wanebo HJ. The changing mammogram: a primary indication for needle localization biopsy. Arch Surg 1986;121:1311–1314.
30. Feig SA, Shaber GS, Patchefsky A, et al. Analysis of clinically occult and mammographically occult breast tumors. AJR 1977;128:403–408.
31. Homer MJ. Nonpalpable breast abnormalities: a realistic view of the accuracy of mammography in detecting malignancies. Radiology 1984;153:831–832.
32. MacErlean DP, Nathan BE. Case reports: calcification in sclerosing adenosis simulating malignant breast calcification. Br J Radiol 1972;45:944–945.
33. Rosen PP. Microglandular adenosis: a benign lesion simulating invasive mammary calcification. Am J Surg Pathol 1983;8:137–144.
34. Clement PB, Azzopardi JG. Microglandular adenosis of the breast—a lesion simulating tubular carcinoma. Histopathology 1983;7:169–180.
35. Sickles EA, Abele JS. Milk of calcium within tiny benign breast cysts. Radiology 1981;141:655–658.
36. Homer MJ, et al. Milk of calcium in breast microcysts: manifestation as a solitary focal disease. AJR 1988;150:789–790.
37. Pennes DR, Rebner M. Layering granular calcifications in macroscopic breast cysts. Breast Dis 1988;1:109–112.
38. Gallager HS, Martin JE. Early phases in the development of breast cancer. Cancer 1969;24:1170–1178.
39. Gallager HS, Martin JE. The study of mammary carcinoma by mammography and whole organ sectioning: early observations. Cancer 1969;23:855–873.
40. Page DL, Zwaag RV, Rogers LW, Williams LT, Walker WE, Hartmann WH. Relation between component parts of fibrocystic disease complex and breast cancer. JNCI 1978;61:1055–1063.
41. Page DL, Dupont WD, Rogers LW, Rados MS. Atypical hyperplastic lesions of the female breast: A long-term follow-up study. Cancer 1985;55:2698–2708.
42. Dupont WD, Page DL. Risk factors for breast cancer in women with proliferative breast disease. N Engl J Med 1985;312:146–151.

43. Foote FW, Stewart FW. Lobular carcinoma in situ: a rare form of mammary cancer. Am J Pathol 1941;17:491–495.

44. Urban JA. Bilaterality of cancer of the breast—biopsy of the opposite breast. Cancer 1967;20:1867–1870.

45. Rosen PP, Lieberman PH, Braun DW. Lobular carcinoma in situ of breast: detailed analysis of 99 patients with average follow-up of 24 years. Am J Surg Pathol 1978;2:225–251.

46. Hutter RV. The management of patients with lobular carcinoma in situ of the breast. Cancer 1984;53:798–802.

47. Synder RE. Mammography and lobular carcinoma in situ. Surg Obstet Gynecol 1966;122:255–260.

48. Pope TL, Jr, Fechner RE, Wilhelm MC, et al. Lobular carcinoma in situ of the breast: mammographic features. Radiology 1988;168:63–66.

49. Stamp GWH, Whitehouse GH, McDicken IW, Leinster SJ, George WD. Mammographic and pathological correlations in a breast screening programme. Clin Radiol 1983;34:529–542.

50. Hermann G, Janus C, Schwartz IS, et al. Occult malignant breast lesions in 114 patients: relationship to age and the presence of microcalcifications. Radiology 1988;169:321–324.

51. Rosner D, Bedwani RM, Vana J, et al. Noninvasive breast carcinoma: results of a national survey by the American College of Surgeons. Ann Surg 1980;192:139–147.

52. Stomper PC, Connolly JL, Meyer JE, Harris JR. Clinically occult ductal carcinoma in situ detected with mammography: analysis of 100 cases with radiologic-pathologic correlation. Radiology 1989;172:235–241.

53. Ikeda DM, Andersson I. Ductal carcinoma in situ: atypical mammographic appearances. Radiology 1989;172:661–666.

54. Ahmed A. Calcification in human breast carcinoma: ultrastructural observations. J Pathol 1975;117:247–251.

55. Price JL, Gibbs NM. The relationship between microcalcification and in situ carcinoma of the breast. Clin Radiol 1978;29:447–452.

56. Sickles EA. Mammographic detectability of breast microcalcifications. AJR 1982;139:913–918.

57. Hassler O. Microradiographic investigations of calcifications of the female breast. Cancer 1969;23:1103–1109.

58. Muir BB, Lamb J, Anderson TJ, Kirkpatrick AE. Microcalcification and its relationship to cancer of the breast: experience in a screening clinic. Clin Radiol 1983;34:193–200.

59. Kopans DB, Nguyen PL, Koerner FC, et al. Mixed form, diffusely scattered calcifications in breast cancer with apocrine features. Radiology 1990;177:807–811.

60. Homer MJ, Safaii H. Cancerization of the lobule: implication

61. Schnitt SJ, Connolly JL, Khettry U, et al. Pathologic findings on re-excision of the primary site in breast cancer patients considered for treatment by primary radiation therapy. Cancer 1987;59:675–681.

62. Harris JR, Connolly JL, Schnitt SJ, et al. The use of pathologic features in selecting the extent of surgical resection necessary for breast cancer patients treated by primary radiation therapy. Ann Surg 1985;201:164–169.

63. Osteen RT, Connolly JL, Recht A, et al. Identification of patients at high risk for local recurrence after conservative surgery and radiation therapy for stage I or II breast cancer. Arch Surg 1987;122:1248–1252.

64. Wazer DE, Schmidt-Ullrich R, Homer MJ, et al. The utility of preoperative physical examination and mammography for detecting an extensive intraductal component in early stage breast carcinoma. Breast Dis 1990;3:181–185.

65. Bassett LW, Gold RH, Mirra JM. Nonneoplastic breast calcifications in lipid cysts: development after excision and primary irradiation. AJR 1982;138:335–338.

66. Stomper PC, Recht A, Berenberg AL, Jochelson MS, Harris JR. Mammographic detection of recurrent cancer in the irradiated breast. AJR 1987;148:39–43.

67. Dershaw DD, Shank B, Reisinger S. Mammographic findings after breast cancer treatment with local excision and definitive irradiation. Radiology 1987;164:455–461.

68. Bolen JW, Jr, Shaw de Paredes E, Carter T. Mammographic determination of gold deposits simulating malignant calcifications in an intramammary lymph node. Breast Dis 1988;1:105–107.

69. Bruwer A, Nelson GW, Spark RP. Punctate intranodal gold deposits simulating microcalcifications on mammograms. Radiology 1987;163:87–88.

70. Davis SP, Stomper PC, Weidner N, Meyer JE. Suture calcification mimicking recurrence in the irradiated breast: a potential pitfall in mammographic evaluation. Radiology 1989;172:247–248.

71. Barton JW, Kornguth PJ. Mammographic deodorant and powder artifact: is there confusion with malignant microcalcifications? Breast Dis 1990;3:121–126.

72. Pamilo M, Soiva M, Suramo I. New artifacts simulating malignant microcalcifications in mammography. Breast Dis 1989;1:321–327.

regarding analysis of microcalcification shape. Breast Dis 1990;3:131–133.

PROMINENT DUCTAL PATTERNS

Linear densities on the mammogram may represent arteries, veins, and lactiferous ducts. There should be no confusion between vascular shadows and ducts.

Lactiferous ducts are linear, slightly nodular densities that radiate back from the nipple into the breast. The normal lactiferous ducts are thin, measuring 1–2 mm in diameter, and often are not evident as separate structures on mammography. Enlarged ducts may occur in benign and malignant conditions (Fig. 7.1). When ducts are enlarged, correlation with clinical examination as to the presence of discharge is important. Galactography is of help in providing further information in the evaluation of a nipple discharge, with or without dilated ducts being seen on mammography.

A diffusely prominent ductal pattern bilaterally (Fig. 7.2), associated with small nodular densities, has been described by Wolfe et al. (1, 2) as placing the patient at higher-than-average risk for developing breast cancer. Because of surrounding collagen, individual ducts may not be identified; instead, a dense triangular fan-shaped density is present beneath the areola (3). The association between a prominent ductal pattern and breast cancer incidence has been debated, with some authors (4, 5) agreeing with the association and others (6–8), finding no reliable indicator of risk by mammographic pattern. Ernster et al. (9) suggested that nulliparous women and women with a family history of breast cancer are more likely to have dense breasts and a prominent ductal pattern and that breast parenchymal pattern may be related to other risk factors. Andersson et al. (10) also found an increased frequency of the dense ductal patterns with advancing age at first pregnancy and with nulliparity.

Duct Ectasia

Another cause of bilateral ductal prominence is duct ectasia (Figs. 7.3 and 7.4). Haagenson (11) described the condition as beginning with bilateral dilation of the main lactiferous ducts in postmenopausal women. Amorphous debris within the ducts is irritating and causes periductal inflammation and fibrosis without epithelial proliferation. Retraction of the nipple may occur with fibrosis. In a more recent study, Dixon et al. (12) found that periductal inflammation around non-dilated ducts occurred in younger patients and that older patients had duct dilatation as the main feature. Neither parity nor breast-feeding was found to be an important etiologic factor in this condition (12).

Papillomatosis

Intraductal papillomatosis is a benign lesion characterized by a papillary proliferation of the epithelium that may fill and distend the duct (13). This lesion is distinguished from a solitary intraductal papilloma. Papillomatosis tends to be scattered throughout the parenchyma. On mammography the finding of a prominent ductal pattern may be evident, and fine microcalcifications are sometimes seen (Figs. 7.5 and 7.6). On galactography an irregular filling defect or multiple filling defects are found (Fig. 7.6).

Papillary duct hyperplasia is an unusual lesion that occurs in children and young adults (14). Three patterns have been described: a solitary papilloma, papillomatosis, and sclerosing papillomatosis. The condition causes a distension of the duct or ducts.

Solitary or Focally Dilated Ducts

When asymmetrically dilated ducts or a solitary duct are found on mammography, the possibility of ductal malignancy must be considered. Other benign causes for this appearance include a solitary papilloma, multiple papillomas, papillomatosis, ductal hyperplasia, and ductal adenoma.

Intraductal Papilloma

A solitary intraductal papilloma often presents when small and nonpalpable with a serosanguineous or bloody nipple discharge. Depending on the size, the lesion may not be seen on mammography, and a galactogram may be necessary to identify the location of the lesion. When papillomas are identified on the mammogram, they appear as a dilated duct or as a well-defined mass (15) (Figs. 7.7–7.9). Papillomas are usually situated beneath the nipple in a major duct. The papilloma is connected to the duct by a thin connective tissue stalk that contains the blood supply. Because of the tenuous blood supply, these lesions tend to undergo infarction and sclerosis (15, 16).

Intraductal Carcinoma

Unilateral dilated ducts, with or without microcalcifications (17), or a solitary dilated duct (Figs. 7.10–7.19) (18, 19) may be the only mammographic indication of a malignancy. Usually, no mass is palpable (19). The solitary duct has a tubular, slightly nodular shape that tapers as it proceeds into the parenchyma (19). When the lesion is associated with microcalcifications, the level of suspicion is greater. Although the presentation of a nonpalpable cancer as a solitary dilated duct is not common (20, 21), this finding should not be overlooked. In a series of 73 women with intraductal carcinoma in whom no microcalcifications were present on mammography, Ikeda and Andersson (22) found that 12 presented with focal ductal-nodular patterns and 2 had dilated retroareolar ducts. An appreciation of the indirect and subtle signs of malignancy is key in making the diagnosis of breast cancer at an early stage.

Ductal Adenoma

Another cause of focally dilated ducts or a solitary dilated duct is ductal adenoma. These are benign glandular tumors that fill and distend the ductal lumen (23). The lesion may present as a palpable mass and is not associated with a nipple discharge. It can simulate malignancy both radiographically and macroscopically. Microcalcifications may occur and may be irregular, in a linear orientation (24). Pathologically, two forms have been described: a solitary adenomatous nodule within a ductal lumen, and a more complex form with apparent encroachment on the ductal wall (23) (Fig. 7.20).

Other Linear Densities

Vascular structures also appear as linear densities on mammography and should not be confused with a prominent ductal pattern. Vessels are smooth and undulating. Arteries are smaller than veins and may be seen extending into the upper aspect of the breast and the axillary area. Tramline calcifications occur often in the arteries of elderly women. Prominence of venous structures has been described as a secondary sign of malignancy (25), but this is not common and is nonspecific. Other causes of dilated veins include (a) obstruction of the subclavian vein with development of venous collaterals over the breast (26) (Figs. 7.21 and 7.22) and (b) Mondor's disease (Fig. 7.23) or superficial thrombophlebitis of the breast and upper abdominal wall (27).

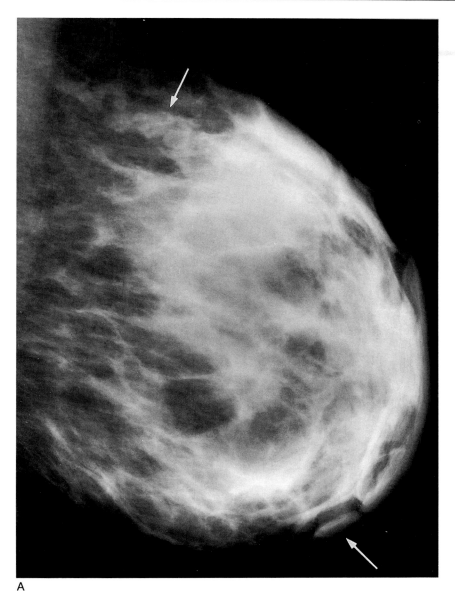

A

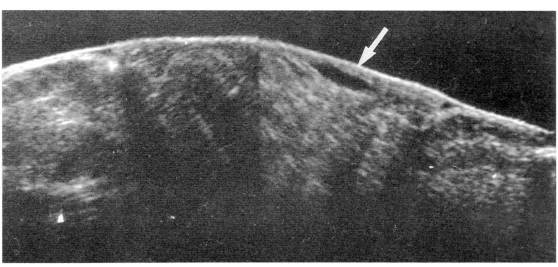

B

Figure 7.1.

Clinical: 24-year-old woman who is lactating and who had a negative biopsy of the right breast 6 months earlier. She now complains of tender nodularity bilaterally.

Mammogram: Right oblique view (**A**) and ultrasound (**B**). The breast is quite dense, as would be expected for a lactating woman (**A**). There are fusiform structures (**A**) near the nipple and in the upper outer quadrant that represents distended lactiferous ducts *(arrows)*. Sonography (**B**) shows the fluid-filled dilated ducts *(arrows)*.

Impression: Distended ducts consistent with a lactating breast.

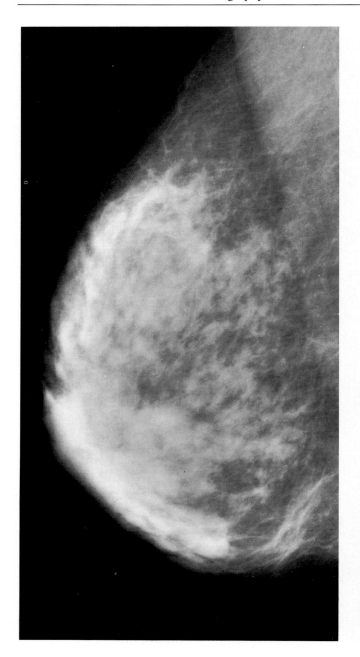
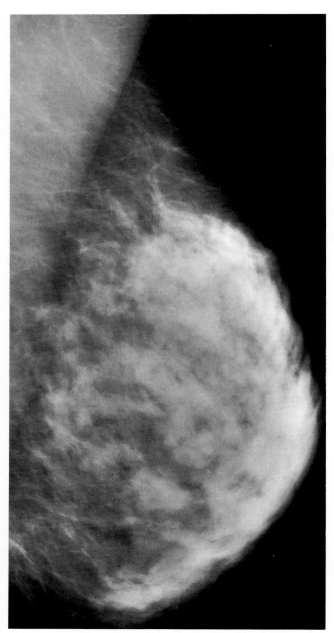

Figure 7.2.

Clinical: 75-year-old nulliparous woman with nodular breasts, for screening.

Mammogram: Bilateral oblique views. The breasts are dense, and there are linear nodular densities bilaterally, radiating from the nipples. These linear densities represent a prominent ductal pattern, but because the changes are diffuse and symmetrical, the finding is not suspicious.

Impression: Diffusely prominent ductal pattern.

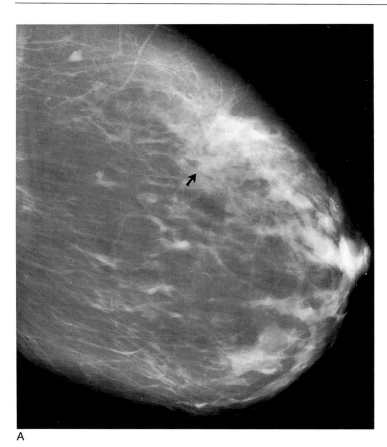

A

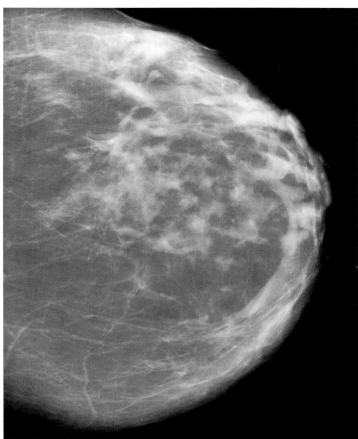

B

Figure 7.3.

Clinical: 64-year-old woman 3 years after right breast biopsy, for routine screening.

Mammogram: Right oblique (**A**) and craniocaudal (**B**) views. There are linear structures radiating back from the nipple, representing dilated ducts. Architectural distortion in the area of surgical scar is noted *(arrow)*. The ductal prominence was bilateral and unchanged from examination over a 10-year period.

Impression: Ductal ectasia.

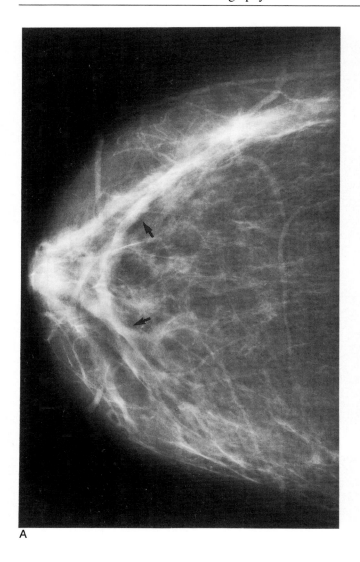

A

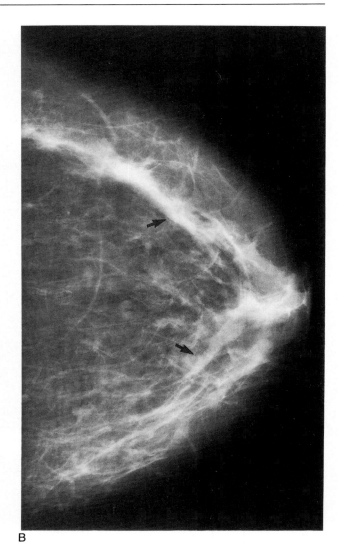

B

Figure 7.4.

Clinical: 58-year-old G8, P8 woman for screening mammography.

Mammogram: Left craniocaudal view (**A**), right craniocaudal view (**B**), and ultrasound (**C**). The breasts are moderately glandular. Bilateral prominent ducts are present *(arrows),* appearing as nodular tubular structures extending back from the nipples (**A** and **B**). The sonographic finding of duct ectasia is that of tubular, nearly anechoic structures. If seen in cross section, these will look like small cysts, but when viewed longitudinally, they can be identified as ducts (**C**).

Impression: Bilateral duct ectasia.

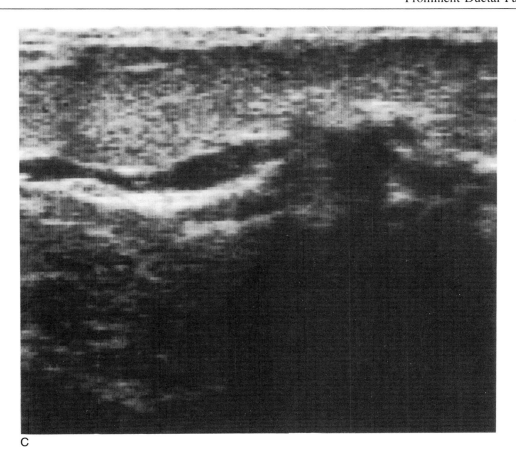

C

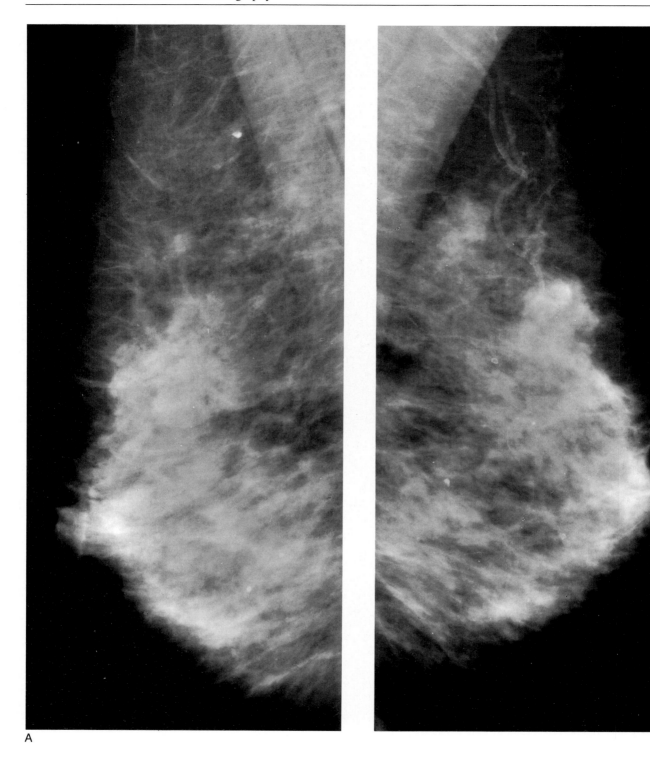

A

Figure 7.5.

Clinical: 63-year-old G2, P2 woman with a positive family history of breast cancer.

Mammogram: Bilateral oblique views (**A**) and left magnification view (**B**). The breasts are dense bilaterally, more so than would be expected for the age of the patient. There are linear and nodular densities consistent with a prominent ductal pattern. On biopsy this pattern often represents a form of fibrocystic disease—either papillomatosis or ductal hyperplasia. The patient had developed some fine microcalcifications in the left breast *(arrows)* (**B**), which are nonspecific, and a biopsy was performed.

Histopathology: Severely atypical lobular hyperplasia, fibrocystic changes, papillomatosis.

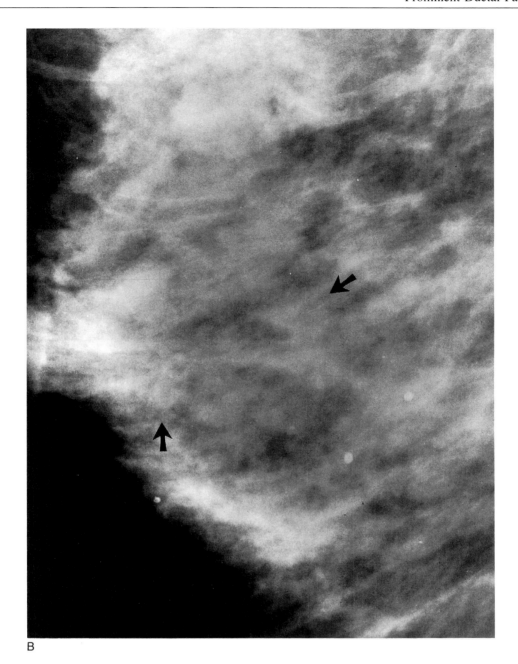

B

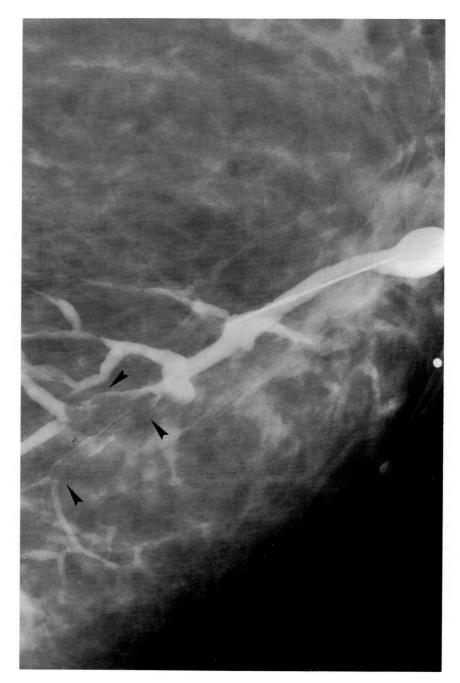

Figure 7.6.

Clinical: 46-year-old woman with a bloody left nipple discharge.

Mammogram: Left galactogram magnification view. The cannulated duct is dilated. There is a smooth filling defect *(arrowheads)* involving two branches of the lactiferous duct, without evidence for distortion of architecture or encasement of the ducts. The finding suggests intraductal papilloma or papillomatosis, although a papillary carcinoma cannot be excluded.

Histopathology: Intraductal papillomatosis. (Case courtesy of Dr. George Oliff, Richmond, VA.)

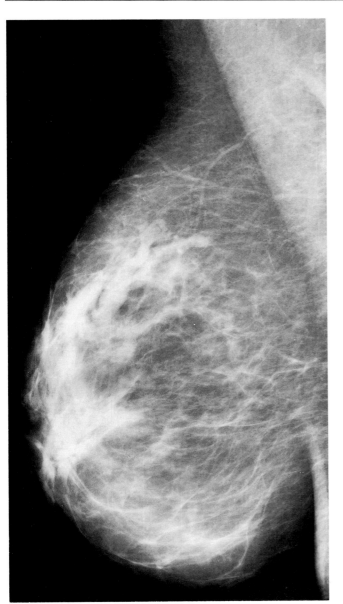

A

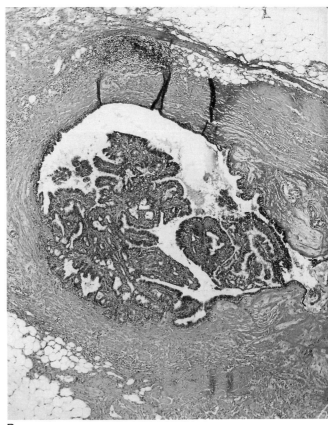

B

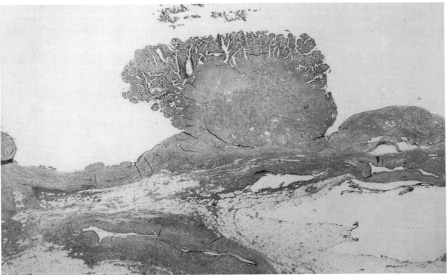

C

Figure 7.7.

Clinical: 47-year-old asymptomatic woman for screening mammography.

Mammogram: Left oblique view (**A**) and histopathology (**B** and **C**). There is moderate glandularity present. In the upper aspect of the breast, there is a linear, slightly nodular density representing a solitary duct. A solitary dilated duct is one of the least common signs of nonpalpable breast cancer. Other possible diagnoses in this case are a papilloma, papillomatosis, or duct ectasia.

Impression: Solitary dilated duct: intraductal carcinoma versus papilloma.

Histopathology: Intraductal papilloma.

Note: The papilloma projects into the ductal lumen; its dense central connective tissue core is covered by the papillary epithelium (12.5×) (**B**). A cross section through the duct (**C**) shows a less sclerotic portion of the papilloma with complex branching and prominent fibrovascular stalks (50×).

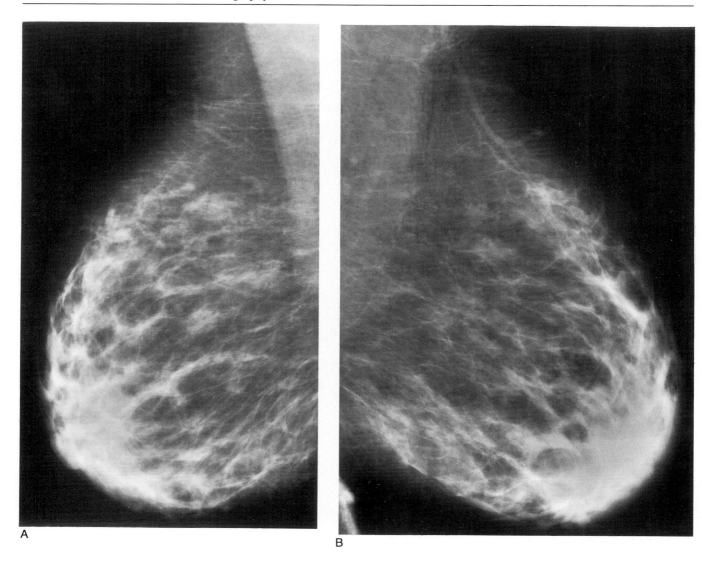

A   B

Figure 7.8.

Clinical: 49-year-old G5, P5 woman with a palpable nodular ridge in the left subareolar area.

Mammogram: Left (**A**) and right (**B**) oblique views and ultrasound (**C**). In the subareolar areas bilaterally, there are fan-shaped areas of increased density radiating back from the nipples. This appearance is typical of prominent or dilated ducts. Sonography (**C**) demonstrates cystic tubular struc-

tures *(arrows)* in the left breast that corresponds to the palpable nodule. This finding is nonspecific and could represent duct ectasia or dilated ducts secondary to benign or malignant intraductal lesions.

Histopathology: Multiple intraductal papillomas, focal epithelial hyperplasia.

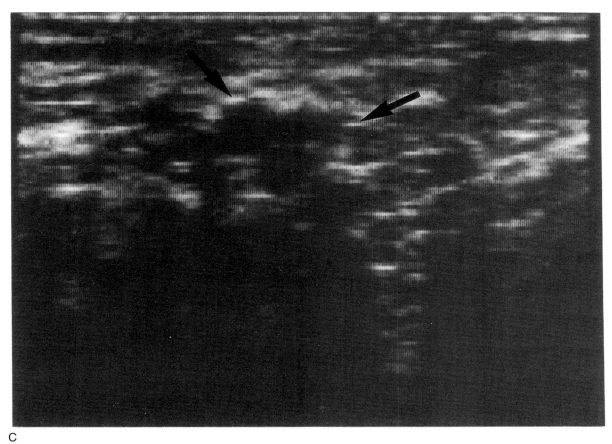

C

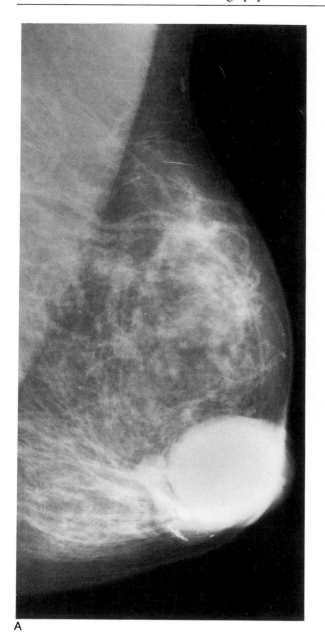

A

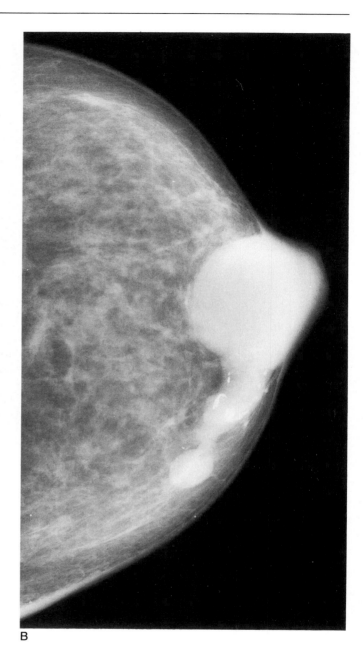

B

Figure 7.9.

Clinical: 65-year-old G3, P3 woman with a family history of breast cancer, presenting with a right nipple discharge and a subareolar mass of at least 10 years duration.

Mammogram: Right oblique (**A**) and craniocaudal (**B**) views and ultrasound (**C**). The breast is mildly glandular. There is a large, high-density circumscribed mass in the immediate subareolar area. The posterior margin of the lesion is contiguous with a tubular density containing coarse calcifications (**B**). Ultrasound (**C**) demonstrates the mass to be relatively

anechoic, suggesting that it is fluid filled. The shape of the lesion suggests that this is a dilated duct, obstructed and mostly fluid filled. The calcification may be related to chronic hemorrhage. The chronicity of findings is more consistent with a benign lesion, such as an intraductal papilloma, although a neoplasm cannot be entirely excluded.

Impression: Massive duct dilatation secondary to an obstructing lesion.

Histopathology: Intraductal papilloma, cystic dilatation of duct.

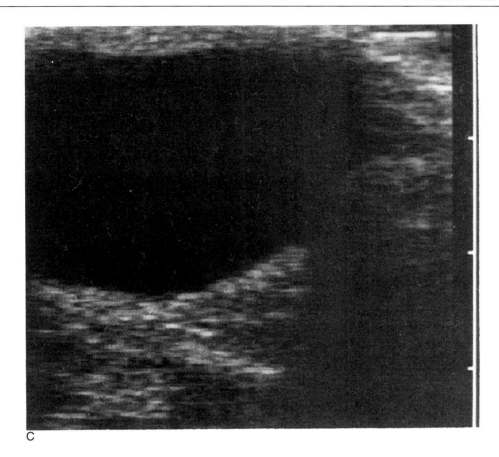

C

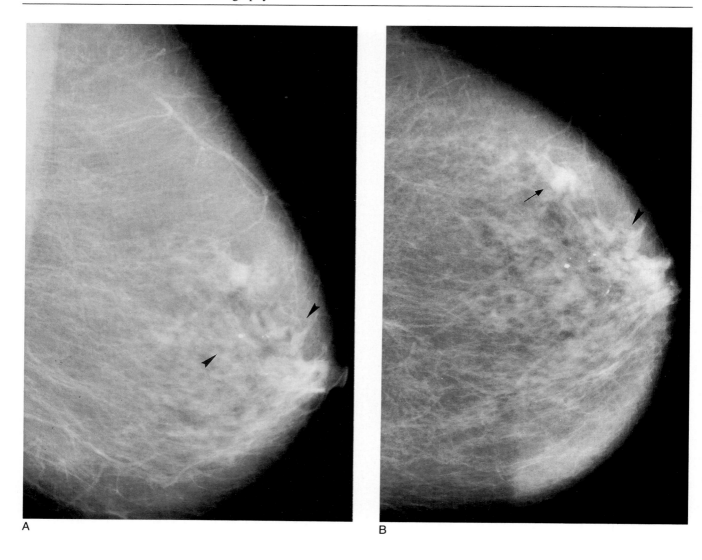

A

B

Figure 7.10.

Clinical: 82-year-old woman 10 years after left mastectomy, for screening mammography to the right breast.

Mammogram: Right oblique (**A**) and craniocaudal (**B**) views and magnified image (**C**). There are focally prominent, dilated ducts *(arrowheads)* extending from the nipple toward the upper outer quadrant. These ducts are associated with some irregular but fairly coarse calcifications. The ducts ex-

tend to a relatively well defined but high-density 1-cm nodule *(arrow),* which is suspicious for malignancy because of its density and margins. The ducts probably represent intraductal extension of tumor.

Impression: Carcinoma with intraductal extension.

Histopathology: Infiltrating ductal and intraductal carcinoma.

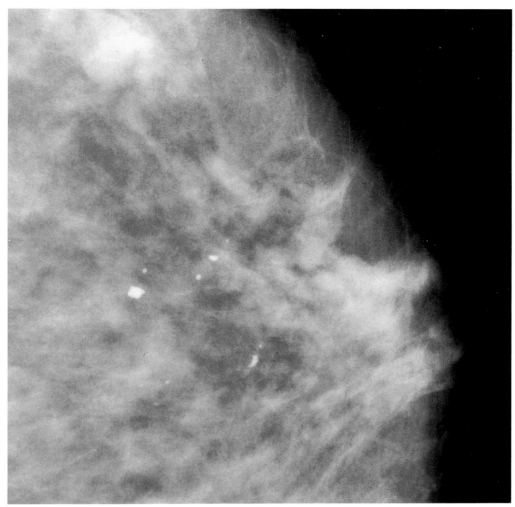

C

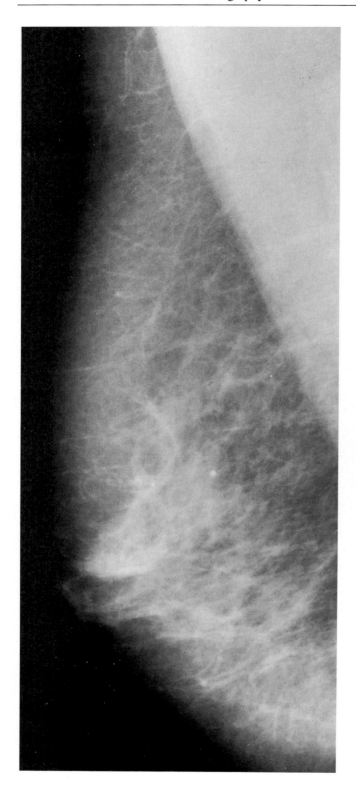
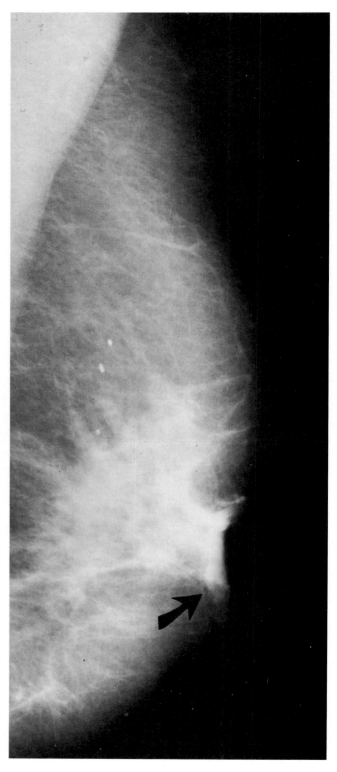

Figure 7.11.

Clinical: 71-year-old G1 woman with a history of right breast abscess who presents with right breast erythema and no palpable mass.

Mammogram: Bilateral oblique views. There is diffuse increase in the density of the right breast compared with the left breast, secondary to diffusely prominent ductal tissue.

Nipple thickening and retraction are present *(arrow)* and associated with the asymmetrically dilated ducts. Although a similar appearance may be seen in mastitis, because of the prominent ductal tissue in the retroareolar area, malignancy was considered as the primary diagnosis.

Histopathology: Intraductal and infiltrating ductal carcinoma.

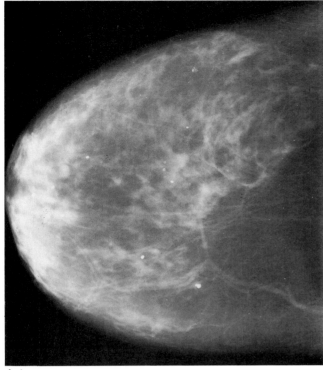

A-1

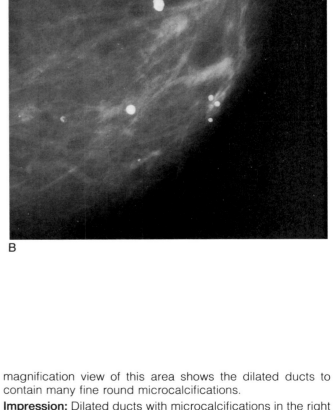

B

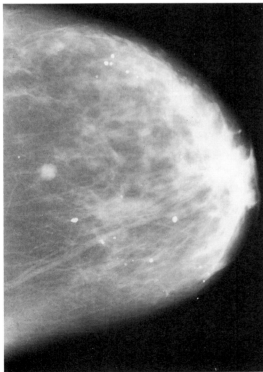

A-2

Figure 7.12.

Clinical: 79-year-old woman with right nipple retraction and no palpable mass.

Mammogram: Bilateral craniocaudal views (**A-1** and **A-2**) and magnification view (**B**). There is a prominent ductal pattern bilaterally. On the right, there is architectural distortion with asymmetrically dilated ducts and nipple retraction *(arrow)*. A

magnification view of this area shows the dilated ducts to contain many fine round microcalcifications.

Impression: Dilated ducts with microcalcifications in the right breast, highly suspicious for carcinoma.

Histopathology: Intraductal and infiltrating ductal carcinoma; negative axillary nodes.

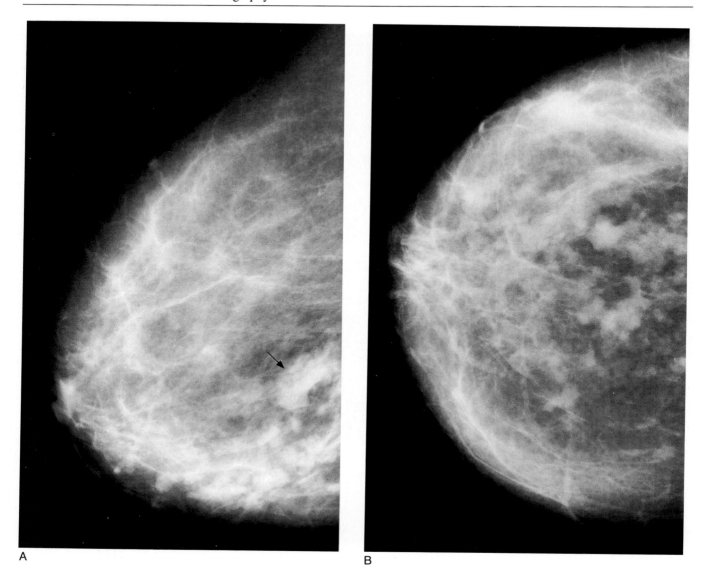

A

B

Figure 7.13.

Clinical: 65-year-old woman for screening mammography.

Mammogram: Left mediolateral (**A**) and craniocaudal (**B**) views. There is mild glandularity present. In the 6 o'clock position of the breast, there, are well-defined tubular nodular densities that represent focally dilated ducts. The focal nature of these ducts—particularly the location, apart from the main ducts at the nipple—suggest an area of localized in-traductal activity. The differential includes multiple papillomas, papillomatosis, intraductal carcinoma, and ductal hyperplasia.

Impression: Focally dilated ducts moderately suspicious for carcinoma.

Histopathology: Extensive multifocal intraductal carcinoma with papillomatosis.

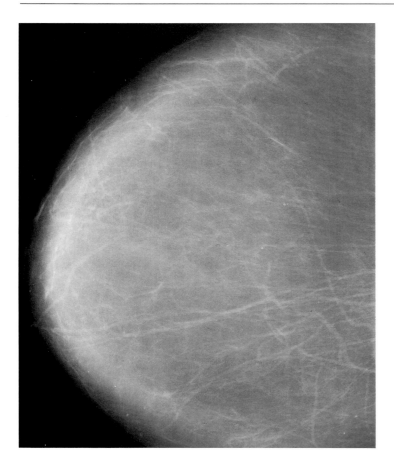

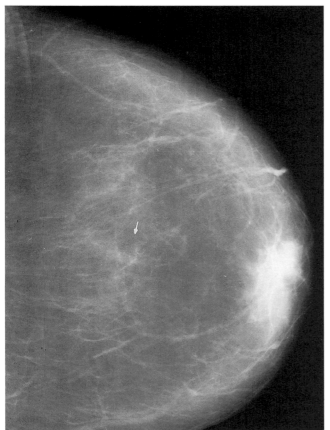

Figure 7.14.

Clinical: 65-year-old woman with a scaling, ulcerating lesion of the right nipple.

Mammogram: Bilateral craniocaudal views. The breasts show fatty replacement. There is a fan-shaped asymmetric density radiating back from the right nipple, corresponding to the location of the subareolar lactiferous ducts. The asymmetric ductal dilatation should be regarded with suspicion, and particularly with the nipple lesion, this finding is highly compatible with that of Paget's disease and intraductal carcinoma. There are also two groups of microcalcification deeper in the right breast that are suspicious for other foci of intraductal carcinoma *(arrow)*.

Impression: Paget's disease, ductal carcinoma.

Histopathology: Intraductal papillary small cell carcinoma and large cell carcinoma with pagetoid spread.

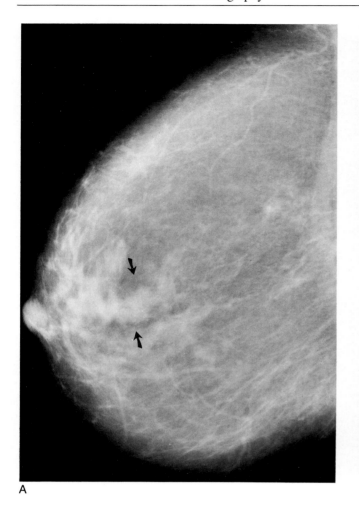

A

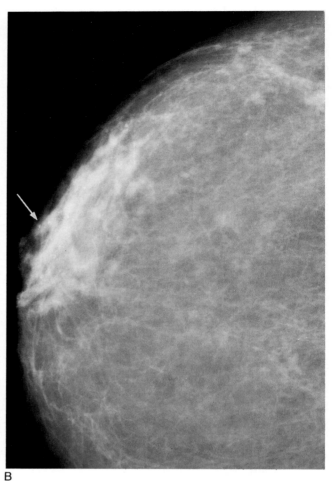

B

Figure 7.15.

Clinical: 70-year-old woman for screening mammography.

Mammogram: Left oblique (**A**) and craniocaudal magnification (**B**) views. There are several dilated ducts *(arrows)* in the left subareolar area (**A**). Within these ducts are linear and punctate microcalcifications *(arrow)* (**B**). No similar findings were noted in the opposite breast. Focal ductal dilatation is one of the less common signs of breast cancer. With the associated ductal calcifications in this case, the degree of suspicion that this was a malignant lesion was increased.

Impression: Ductal carcinoma.

Histopathology: Intraductal small cell carcinoma.

Figure 7.16.

Clinical: 78-year-old woman with family history of breast cancer, for screening mammography.

Mammogram: Left oblique view (**A**), magnified craniocaudal view (**B**), and histopathology (**C**). There is a relatively well defined high-density tubular structure *(arrow)* (**A**) in the lower aspect of the breast. The lobulated fusiform shape of the lesion is also demonstrated on the magnified image (**B**). Sonography of the lesion showed it to be solid and hypoechoic. The shape of the lesion suggests a dilated duct. The lesion had appeared since a previous mammogram 6 years earlier. Because of this, a fibroadenoma would not be likely, and primary considerations are carcinoma, possibly localized within a dilated duct, or focal fibrocystic disease.

Impression: Solitary dilated duct in the left breast, highly suspicious for carcinoma.

Histopathology: Intraductal carcinoma.

Note: The histopathologic section shows the dilated duct filled with intraductal carcinoma (**C**).

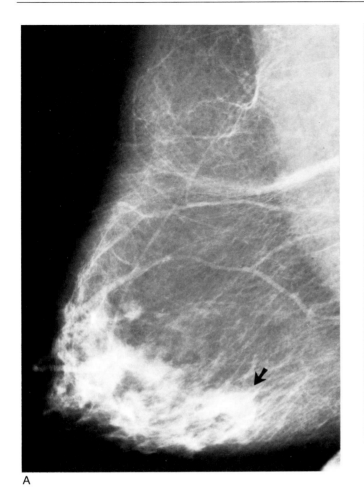

A

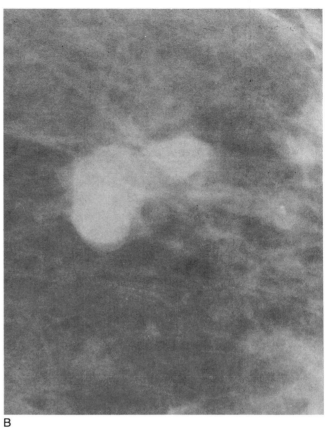

B

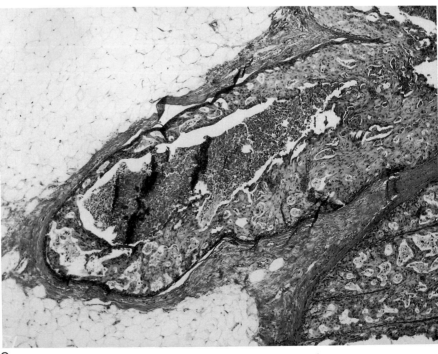

C

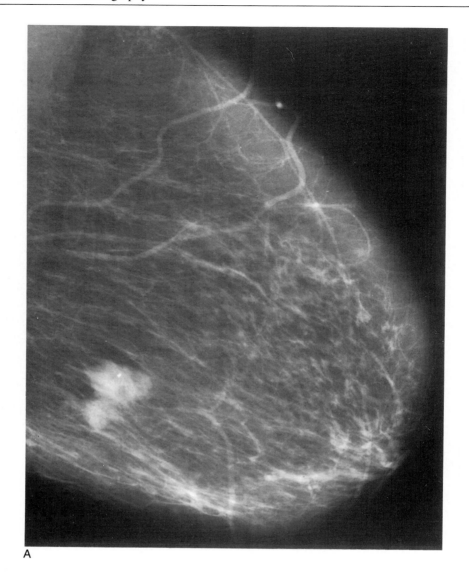

A

Figure 7.17.

Clinical: 78-year-old G3, P3 woman with a family history of breast cancer.

Mammogram: Right oblique (**A**) and enlarged craniocaudal (**B**) views. In an otherwise mildly glandular right breast, there is a focal irregular 2 × 1.5-cm area of increased density in the lower outer aspect of the breast. This lesion is multinodular and has areas that have a tubular configuration *(arrows)* (**B**). Two coarse calcifications are in the upper outer aspect of the lesion. The multinodular tubular appearance suggests that this is a focus of dilated ducts, and the differential diagnosis includes intraductal carcinoma, papillomatosis, and intraductal papilloma. Because of the deep location and high density, intraductal carcinoma is favored.

Impression: Focally dilated ducts suspicious for intraductal carcinoma.

Histopathology: Intraductal carcinoma, extensive intraductal papillomatosis.

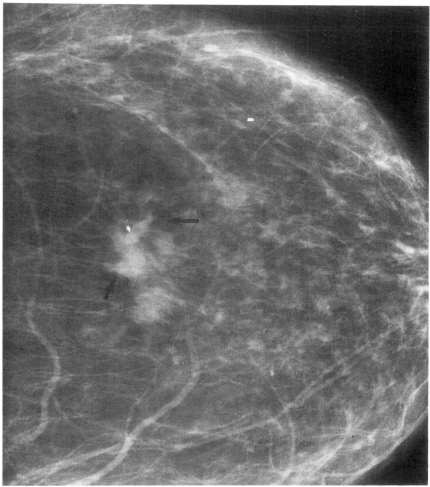

B

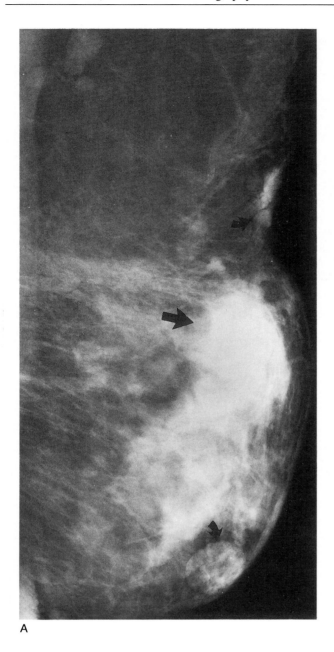

A

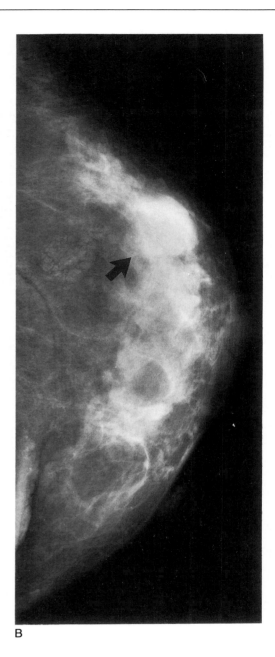

B

Figure 7.18.

Clinical: 88-year-old G3, P3 woman for routine screening mammography.

Mammogram: Right oblique (**A**) and craniocaudal (**B**) views, left oblique view (**C**), and ultrasound of the right breast (**D**). The breasts are asymmetrical in appearance (**A** and **C**), with the right breast being relatively more dense than the left. The subareolar density on the right suggests a prominent ductal pattern. In the right upper quadrant, there is a relatively circumscribed high-density mass (straight arrow) in the area of prominent ducts (**A** and **B**). Incidental note is made of two circumscribed nodules (curved arrows) on the oblique view (**A**), which represented seborrheic keratoses on the skin.

Sonography (**D**) of the right breast mass shows a thick-walled cystic structure, with irregularity of the back wall (arrow) adjacent to other cystic structures. This finding suggests either an intracystic lesion or cystically dilated ducts with an intraductal lesion.

Impression: Mass, right breast, with associated dilated ducts, suggesting an intracystic or intraductal lesion.

Histopathology: Dilated ducts with florid papillomatosis, atypical intraductal epithelial hyperplasia, intraductal epithelial hyperplasia, intraductal carcinoma, and lobular carcinoma in situ.

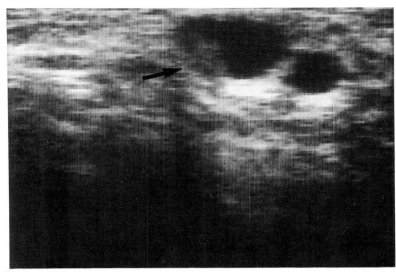

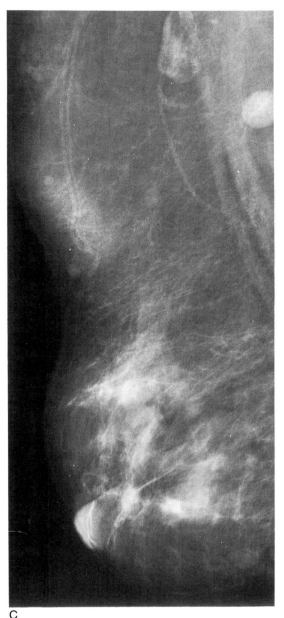

C

D

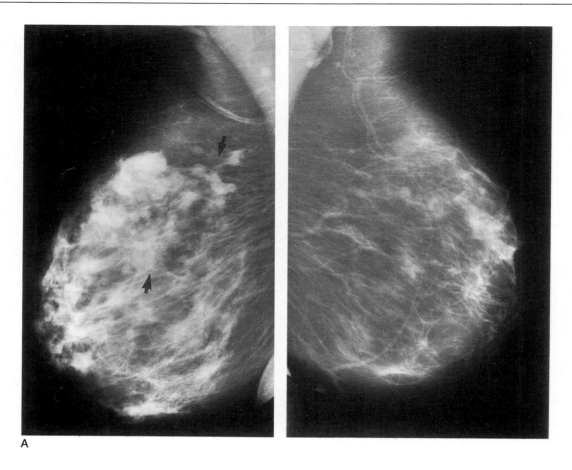

A

Figure 7.19.

Clinical: 44-year-old G4, P4 woman with a positive family history of breast cancer, presenting with a "heavy" sensation in the left breast. Clinical examination showed a thicker left breast, without a dominant palpable mass.

Mammogram: Bilateral oblique (**A**), craniocaudal (**B**), and enlarged (1.5×) left craniocaudal (**C**) views. There is marked asymmetry in the appearance of the breasts (**A** and **B**). In the left upper quadrant, there are numerous tubular and rounded densities *(arrows)* radiating back from the nipple.

This pattern of tubular structures represents markedly dilated ducts. In addition, within these ducts and extending more medially into the central aspect of the left breast (**C**) are extensive granular irregular microcalcifications *(arrows)*. This finding alone is highly suspicious for carcinoma and, in combination with the prominent duct pattern, is even more so.

Impression: Highly suspicious for extensive ductal carcinoma, left breast.

Histopathology: Intraductal and infiltrating ductal carcinoma.

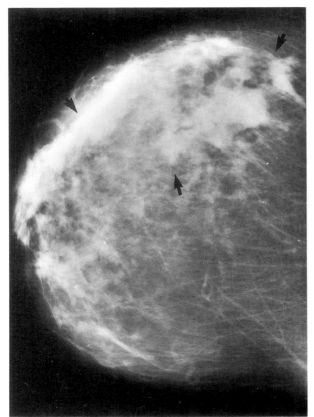
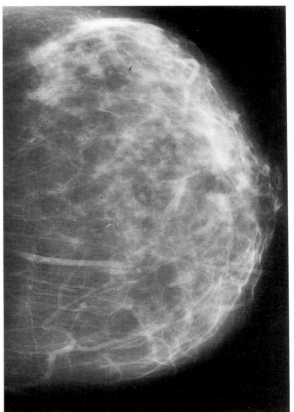

B

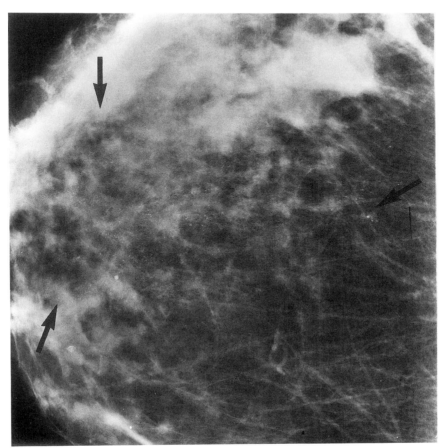

C

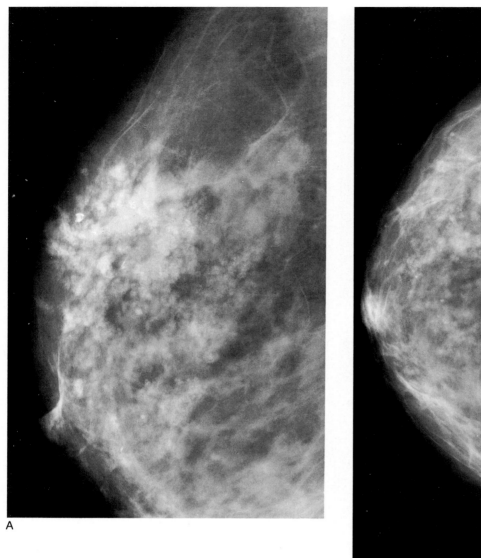

A

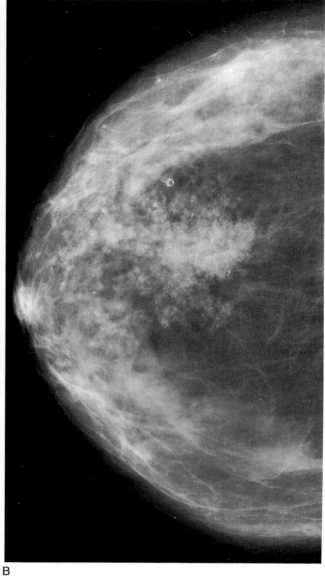

B

Figure 7.20.

Clinical: 52-year-old woman for screening mammography.

Mammogram: Left oblique (**A**) and craniocaudal (**B**) views. In the 12 o'clock position of the left breast, there is a 5-cm area of focal ductal dilatation and proliferation in a bizarre shape. Fine granular microcalcifications are associated with this lesion. The differential was thought to include ductal carcinoma, papillomatosis, or other epithelial proliferation.

Histopathology: Ductal adenoma, complex form. (Case courtesy of Dr. Alexander Girevendulis, Richmond VA.)

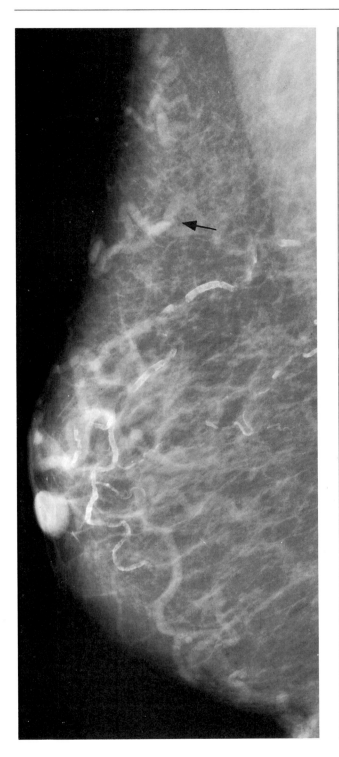
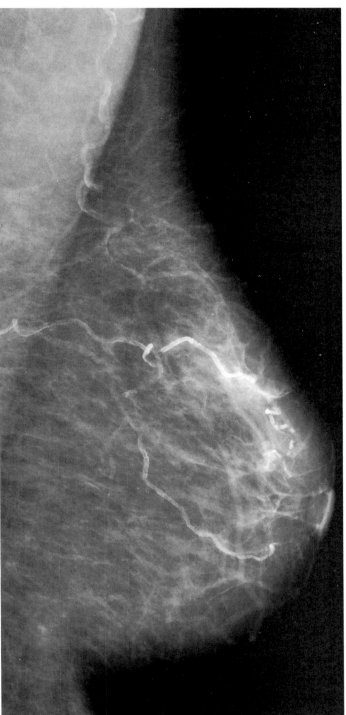

Figure 7.21.

Clinical: 67-year-old woman for screening. She had a past history of thrombosis in the left subclavian vein.

Mammogram: Bilateral oblique views. The underlying pattern is that of fatty replacement. Arterial calcifications are present bilaterally. In the left breast, there are tortuous vascular structures extending from the axilla, throughout the breast, to the anterior abdominal wall. These are dilated collateral veins secondary to venous obstruction.

Impression: Dilated collateral veins, left breast.

Note: Vascular structures, which are smooth and tortuous, should not be confused with ducts that are more irregular in caliber and radiate back from the nipples.

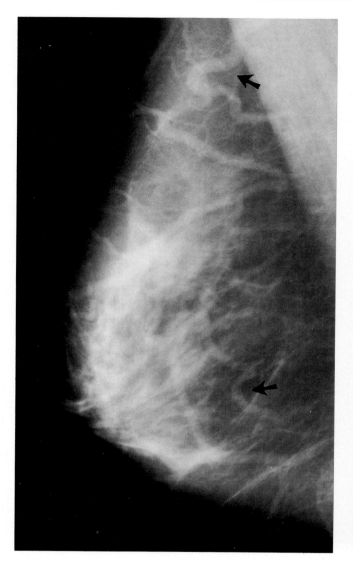
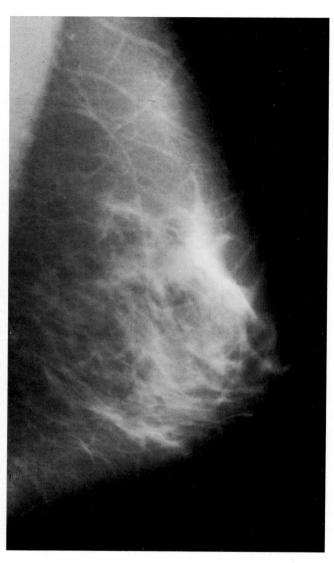

Figure 7.22.

Clinical: 38-year-old woman with a tender swollen left breast and axilla.

Mammogram: Bilateral oblique views. There are asymmetric circuitous linear densities *(arrows)* in the left breast, extending into the left axilla. These represent asymmetrically dilated veins. The patient was sent for venography of the left upper extremity, which showed thrombosis in the left subclavian vein and dilated venous collaterals over the left breast.

Impression: Dilated venous collaterals secondary to subclavian vein thrombosis.

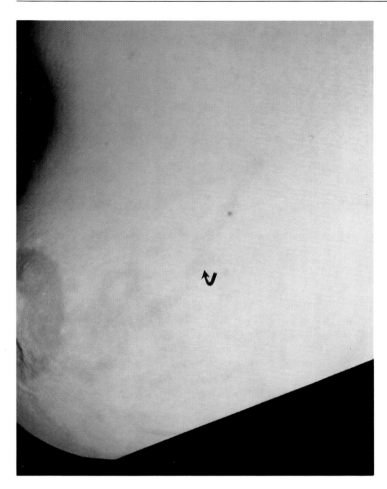

A

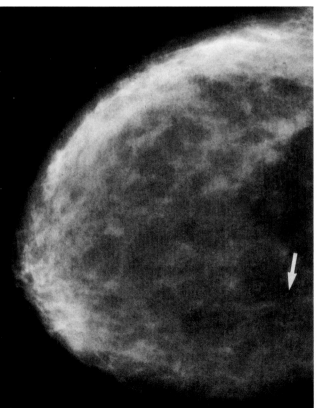

B

Figure 7.23.

Clinical: 35-year-old nurse whom, after excessive lifting, developed severe pain, tenderness, and swelling of the upper aspect of the left breast. A purplish palpable cord *(curved arrow)* extended from the nipple toward the upper outer quadrant (**A**).

Mammogram: Left craniocaudal view (**B**). The breast parenchyma appears normal. There is a single linear structure having a smooth undulating course from the nipple posteriorly *(straight arrow)*. This vein corresponded to the palpable abnormality.

Impression: Mondor's disease (superficial thrombophlebitis).

Note: On this mammogram the pertinent finding is the lack of abnormalities with the exception of the vein in the area of palpable thickening. This condition may occur after trauma or repeated exercise and regresses on anticoagulants and anti-inflammatory medications.

References

1. Wolfe JN. The prominent duct pattern as an indicator of cancer risk. Oncology 1968;23:149–158.
2. Wolfe JN, Albert S, Belle S, Salane M. Breast parenchymal patterns: analysis of 332 incident breast carcinomas. AJR 1982;138:113–118.
3. Wolfe JN, Albert S, Belle S, Salane M. Breast parenchymal patterns and their relationship to risk for having or developing carcinoma. Radiol Clin North Am 1983;21(1):127–136.
4. Janzon L, Andersson I, Petersson H. Mammographic patterns as indicators of risk of breast cancer. Radiology 1982;143:417–419.
5. Threatt B, Norbeck JM, Ullmann NS, et al. Association between mammographic parenchymal pattern classification and incidence of breast cancer. Cancer 1980;45:2250–2256.
6. Egan RL, McSweeney MB. Mammographic parenchymal patterns and risk of breast cancer. Radiology 1979;133:65–70.
7. Egan RL, Mosteller RC. Breast cancer mammography patterns. Cancer 1977;40:2087–2090.
8. Moskowitz M, Gartside P, McLaughlin C. Mammographic patterns as markers for high-risk benign breast disease and incident cancers. Radiology 1980;134:293–295.
9. Ernster VL, Sacks ST, Peterson CA, Schweitzer RJ. Mammographic parenchymal patterns for risk factors for breast cancer. Radiology 1980;134:617–620.
10. Andersson I, Janzon L, Pettersson H. Radiographic patterns of mammary parenchyma. Radiology 1981;138:59–62.
11. Haagenson CD. Mammary-duct ectasia: a disease that may simulate carcinoma. Cancer 1951;4:749–761.
12. Dixon JM, et al. Mammary duct ectasia. Br J Surg 1983;70:601–603.
13. Haagenson CD, Papillomatosis. In: Diseases of the breast. Philadelphia: WB Saunders, 1971.
14. Rosen PP. Papillary duct hyperplasia of the breast in children and young adults. Cancer 1985;56:1611–1617.
15. D'Orsi CJ, Weissman BNW, Berkowitz DM. Correlation of xeroradiography and histology of breast disease. CRC Crit Rev Diagn Imaging 1978;75–119.
16. Haagenson CD. Solitary intraductal papilloma. In: Diseases of the breast. Philadelphia: WB Saunders, 1971.
17. Wolfe JN. Mammography: ducts as a sole indicator of breast carcinoma. Radiology 1967;89:206–210.
18. Martin JE. Mammographic diagnosis of minimal breast cancer and treatment. In: Feig SA, McLelland R, eds. Breast carcinoma: current diagnosis. New York: Masson Publishing, 1983.
19. Sickles EA. Mammographic features of early breast cancer. AJR 1984;143:461–464.
20. Moskowitz M. The predictive value of certain mammographic signs in screening for breast cancer. Cancer 1983;51:1007–1011.
21. Sickles EA. Mammographic features of 300 consecutive nonpalpable breast cancers. AJR 1986;146:661–663.
22. Ikeda DM, Andersson I. Ductal carcinoma in situ: atypical mammographic appearance. Radiology 1989;172:661–666.
23. Azzopardi JG, Salm R. Ductal adenoma of the breast: a lesion which can mimic carcinoma. J Pathol 1984;144:15–23.
24. Moskovic E, Ramachandra S. Ductal adenoma of the breast: mammographic appearances and pathological correlation. Br J Radiol 1989;62:1021–1023.
25. Dodd GD, Wallace JD. The venous diameter ratio in the radiographic diagnosis of breast cancer. Radiology 1968;90:900–904.
26. Grow JL, Lewison EF. Superficial thrombophlebitis of the breast. Surg Gynecol Obstet 1963;53:180–182.
27. Carter MM, McCook BM, Shoff MI, et al. Case report: dilated mammary veins as a sign of superior vena cava obstruction. Appl Radiol 1987;16:100–102.

THE THICKENED SKIN PATTERN

Thickening of the skin over the surface of the breast may occur in primary inflammatory carcinoma, other malignancies, and several benign conditions. It is important for the radiologist to be aware of ranges for normal thickness and to evaluate the skin carefully on the mammogram in order to detect an alteration that may be associated with an underlying process.

Although the normal skin thickness of the breast has been described as generally less than 1.5 mm (1), a study by Wilson et al. (2) of 150 normal patients showed the range to vary from 0.8 to 3 mm in thickness. In 92% of patients, the medial skin thickness was greater than the lateral skin thickness, and in 91% of patients, the skin was thicker inferiorly than superiorly. The mean thickness of the skin was greater in smaller breasts. Table 8.1 shows the ranges of skin thickness for different sizes of breasts as determined by Wilson et al. (2).

Edema of the breast is characterized by an increase in skin thickness and prominence of the interstitial markings. An edema pattern may occur with primary breast cancers, with metastatic carcinoma to the breast, or in a number of benign conditions (3) (Table 8.2).

Breast cancer may extend locally into the subcutaneous fat and produce focal skin thickening and/or retraction, indicating locally advanced disease. Dunkley et al. (4) found skin thickening on mammography in 24% of breast cancer patients; in 68% of these patients the skin thickening seen on mammography was not evident on clinical examination. In these cases, invasion of the dermis and of dermal lymphatics may be seen on histologic examination (Figs. 8.1–8.3).

Inflammatory breast cancer was described in Bell's surgery text of 1816 (5, 6) as "a purple color on the skin over the tumor accompanied by shooting pains." Inflammatory breast cancer is a stage IIIB, locally advanced lesion and has a poor prognosis.

In inflammatory breast cancer the patient presents clinically with a tender, firm, heavy breast with purplish discoloration and a *peau d'orange* thickening of the skin. A focal mass may be palpable, or the entire breast may be hardened.

Table 8.1. Range of Normal Skin Thickness

Size of Breast	Skin Thickness (mm)
Small	
Medial	1.3–2.5
Lateral	1.0–2.2
Superior	1.0–2.0
Inferior	1.4–3.0
Medium	
Medial	1.2–2.7
Lateral	0.8–2.5
Superior	0.9–2.0
Inferior	1.1–3.0
Large	
Medial	1.0–2.8
Lateral	0.9–2.0
Superior	0.8–2.1
Inferior	1.0–3.0

Table 8.2. Causes of Skin Thickening

	Benign Causes
Common	Small breasts
	Postirradiated breast
	Mastitis—acute
	Obstruction to lymphatic drainage after axillary node dissection
	Hematoma and fat necrosis
	Cardiac failure
	Renal failure
	Hypoalbuminemia
Uncommon	Complication of Coumadin therapy
	Unintentional subcutaneous infusion of fluid (4)

	Malignant Causes
	Locally advanced primary breast cancer—focal thickening
	Inflammatory breast cancer—diffuse thickening
	Recurrent carcinoma after lumpectomy and radiation therapy
	Lymphatic obstruction secondary to metastatic axillary nodes
	Metastatic disease to the breast (to breast from nonbreast primaries)
	Lymphoma (secondary) of the breast

Mammographically, skin thickening and marked increase in the density of the breast are seen. The underlying tumor mass may be evident on mammography, or the density may be so great, because of the edema and the decreased compression of the thickened breast, that evaluation of the underlying parenchyma is unsatisfactory (Figs. 8.4–8.6).

The mammographic finding of diffuse skin thickening and increase in density of the breast may be present several weeks before the clinically inflammatory signs appear (7). Keller and Herman (8) found that patients with inflammatory cancers had an average skin thickness of 6 mm and diffuse increase in density on mammography, compared with a skin thickness of 9 mm and a prominent reticular pattern in patients with a benign cause of a breast edema pattern. Histologically, no specific dermal lesion is consistently present with inflammatory carcinoma. Three histologic lesions that have been found are: (a) carcinoma cells plugging the upper dermal lymphatics, (b) malignant cells in the dermal lymphatics associated with infiltrative carcinoma in the deeper dermis, and (c) edema of the dermis without demonstrable involvement with tumor (7).

Another malignant cause of diffuse skin edema is metastatic disease to the breast from a nonbreast primary carcinoma. Metastatic disease may manifest itself as skin thickening (9) by diffusely invading the dermal lymphatics or by producing impaired lymphatic drainage of the breast by involving the axillary nodes (Figs. 8.7 and 8.8). Lymphomas and pseudolymphomas (Fig. 8.9) may produce a similar appearance, secondary to either infiltration of the breast or lymphatic obstruction from malignant axillary nodes. Primary lymphoma of the breast tends to infiltrate the lobules, surrounding and compressing the ducts (10), and mammographically presents as a mass with minimal spiculation (11). Secondary lymphomatous involvement of the breast may produce a focal mass but more often presents as diffuse increase in density with skin thickening (11).

Pseudolymphoma is a benign pathologic process that resembles malignant lymphoma. In a series of five patients, the presentation of pseudolymphoma was of an enlarging breast mass that was composed of mature lymphoid cells on histologic examination (12).

After therapeutic irradiation of the breast, skin thickening and edema are generally seen (Figs. 8.10). The findings are most prominent during the first 6 months after treatment and gradually decline, approaching a normal appearance in a variable time period. Libshitz et al. (13) found that 60% of patients treated with tylectomy and radiation therapy had returned to a normal skin thickness by 2 years and that 80% had returned by 3 years. If a patient who has been treated with radiation develops a new onset of breast edema with skin thickening after the initial edema has resolved or decreased, the radiologist must be alerted to the possible development of recurrent carcinoma (Fig. 8.11). It is therefore very important in evaluating the mammogram of a treated

patient, to compare with the series of pretreatment and post-treatment films. The clinical examination of these patients may, at times, be difficult if the breast becomes firm and fibrotic, and therefore, the radiologist must be aware of any changes that may suggest recurrent disease.

Mastitis may produce focal or diffuse skin edema (Figs. 8.12–8.14). Typically, acute mastitis occurs in young women and is related to lactation. Other causes of mastitis are skin or nipple infections with extension into the breast or hematogenous spread of infection. The patient often has a fever and elevated white count. Diffuse mastitis may be associated with a breast abscess that appears as an ill-defined mass mammographically. Ultrasound may demonstrate a complex mass; aspiration of purulent fluid and positive cultures confirm the diagnosis. The dermal manifestations on biopsy in acute mastitis generally are prominent perivascular and periductal inflammation with or without dilated dermal lymphatics (1).

In patients with obstructed lymphatic drainage of the breast from node removal or nodal involvement with neoplasm, skin edema occurs (4). Prominence of the interstitium and thickening of the skin without an underlying mass are present mammographically. Enlarged axillary nodes may be present when neoplastic involvement obstructs lymphatic drainage. After node removal or dissection, edema of the breast may persist mammographically and may be less obvious clinically. If an axillary node dissection is performed for metastatic disease (i.e., melanoma) and skin thickening occurs, it is often impossible to determine on mammography if the finding represents metastatic involvement of the breast or impaired lymphatic drainage from surgery (Fig. 8.15).

Fat necrosis and interstitial hematoma of the breast may produce skin thickening. Generally, the edema is focal unless the trauma is severe or the hemorrhage is extensive. Clinical history is key in suggesting the diagnosis, since posttraumatic changes with skin involvement may have an identical appearance with that of locally advanced breast cancer (Figs. 8.16–8.18). Patients who have been treated with Coumadin for thromboembolic disorders may develop acute breast necrosis, appearing mammographically as an edema pattern. Burns to the chest area with scarring can also produce prominent skin thickening of a chronic nature, and this is usually not associated with interstitial thickening. There may be distortion of the normal breast contour because of contractures (Fig. 8.19).

Systemic conditions that produce a fluid overload state are manifested in the breast as bilateral diffuse skin thickening. Cardiac failure, renal failure, cirrhosis, and hypoalbuminemia are other benign causes of a thickened skin syndrome (4). The thickening occurs mostly in the dependent aspect of the breast. If the patient has been lying on one side, the edema is unilateral in the dependent breast (Figs. 8.20–8.22).

The range of normal skin thickness varies from patient to patient, with the inferior and medial aspects of the breasts being thicker. When skin thickening is present, whether focally, diffusely, or bilaterally, the correlation of clinical history and physical examination is important to the radiologist in suggesting the probable cause. In many cases, however, diffuse carcinoma cannot be excluded without biopsy.

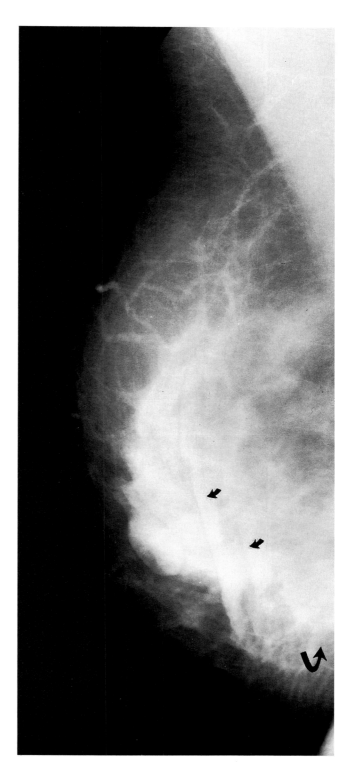

Figure 8.1.

Clinical: 62-year-old woman with 3 × 6-cm palpable mass in the left lower outer quadrant.

Mammogram: Left oblique view. There is a 3-cm high-density mass near the chest wall in the lower aspect of the breast *(curved arrow).* Overlying this are high-density linear shadows *(arrows)* corresponding to focal skin thickening and retraction.

Impression: Carcinoma with associated skin changes.

Histopathology: Infiltrating ductal carcinoma, negative nodes.

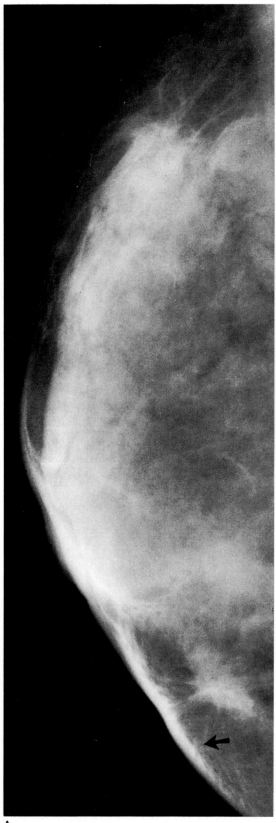

A

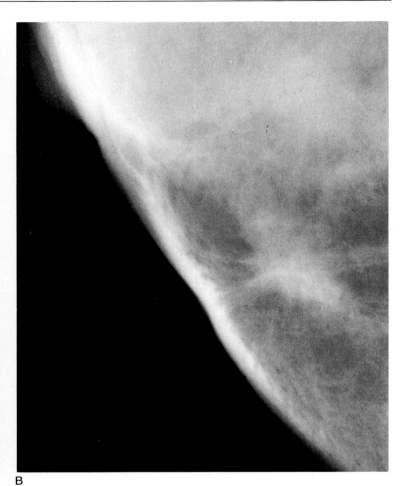

B

Figure 8.2.

Clinical: 46-year-old woman for screening.

Mammogram: Left oblique view (**A**) and magnified image (**B**). The breast is quite dense and glandular. There is focal skin thickening *(arrow)* on the lower aspect of the breast. Beneath the thickening is a 1-cm spiculated mass that is tethering the skin by fine spicules (**B**).

Impression: Focal skin thickening associated with underlying carcinoma.

Histopathology: Infiltrating ductal carcinoma.

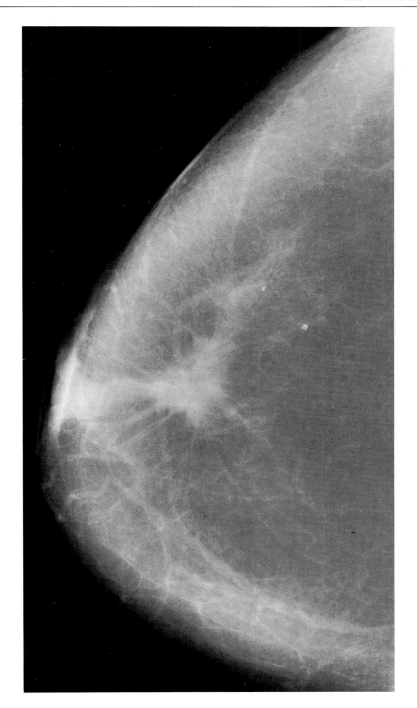

Figure 8.3.

Clinical: 64-year-old woman with a left breast mass and dimpling of the skin.

Mammogram: Left craniocaudal view. A high-density spiculated mass is present in the subareolar area. Long spicules surround the mass and extend anteriorly to the periareolar area, where they tether the skin. Focal prominent skin thickening is seen. The findings are typical of malignancy.

Histopathology: Infiltrating lobular carcinoma, with 1 of 16 nodes positive.

Note: Focal skin thickening is more commonly seen with a malignant or inflammatory process or with postsurgical changes.

Figure 8.4.

Clinical: 35-year-old woman with an ulcerating mass of the left breast.

Mammogram: Left craniocaudal view. There is markedly increased density, making imaging difficult. A large high-density mass involves the entire central portion of the breast. Marked skin thickening is present with multiple layers of retraction *(arrows)*.

Impression: Large carcinoma with diffuse skin involvement (inflammatory).

Histopathology: Poorly differentiated adenocarcinoma with dermal lymphatic involvement.

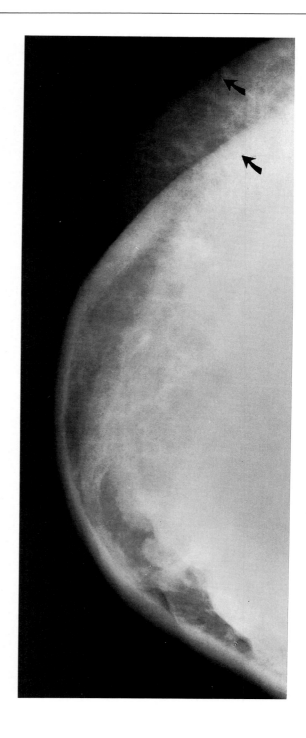

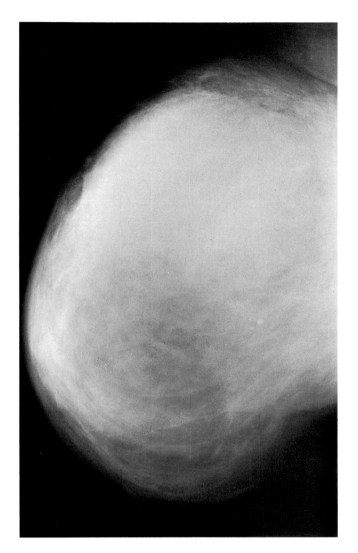
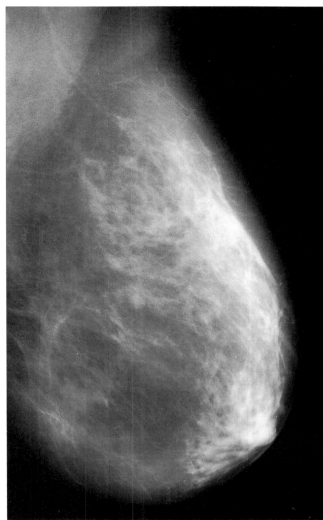

Figure 8.5.

Clinical: 60-year-old woman who presented with a red, tender, very firm left breast with a 15-cm palpable mass in the upper outer quadrant.

Mammogram: Bilateral oblique views. There is markedly increased density of the left breast relative to the right. Diffuse increase in density of the stroma is noted with marked thickening of the skin diffusely. A large rounded mass is noted in the left upper outer quadrant.

Impression: Inflammatory carcinoma.

Histopathology: Infiltrating ductal carcinoma, inflammatory.

Note: The concurrent finding of a mass with the marked skin thickening in older patient makes the level of suspicion for carcinoma extremely high.

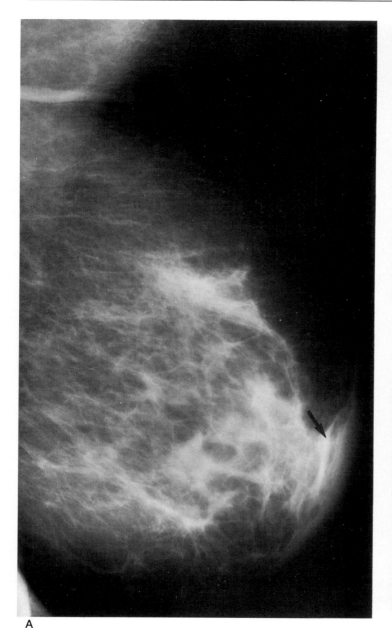

A

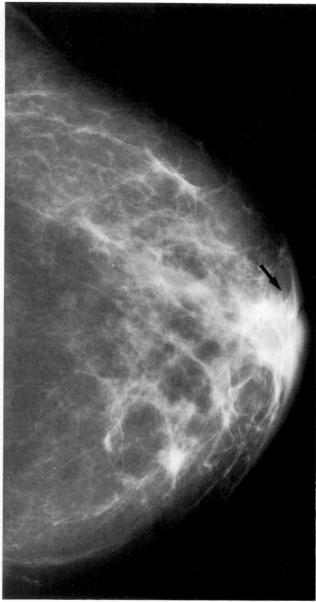

B

Figure 8.6.

Clinical: 66-year-old G7, P7 woman 10 years after left mastectomy, presenting with a painful, firm right breast.

Mammogram: Right oblique (**A**) and craniocaudal (B) views from August 1990 and right oblique (**C**) and craniocaudal (**D**) views from October 1989. There is generalized increased density in the right subareolar area, with prominent interstitial markings throughout the breast. Skin thickening is present in the periareolar area *(arrow)* (**A** and **B**) and had developed since the examination (**C** and **D**) 10 months earlier. The pattern of breast edema includes inflammatory carcinoma, metastatic disease, fluid overload, acute mastitis, and acute hemorrhage. Given the clinical history of this patient, primary or metastatic breast carcinomas are most likely.

Impression: New edema pattern suspicious for neoplasm.

Histopathology: Poorly differentiated adenocarcinoma, with 7 of 8 axillary nodes positive for metastatic disease.

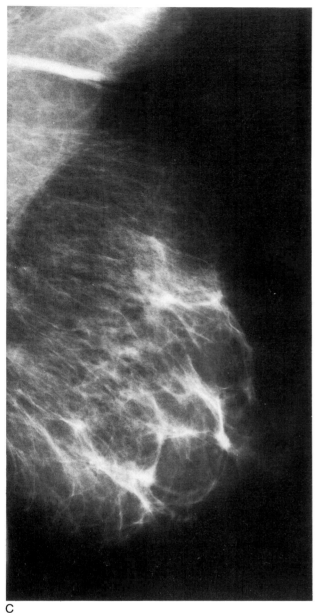

C

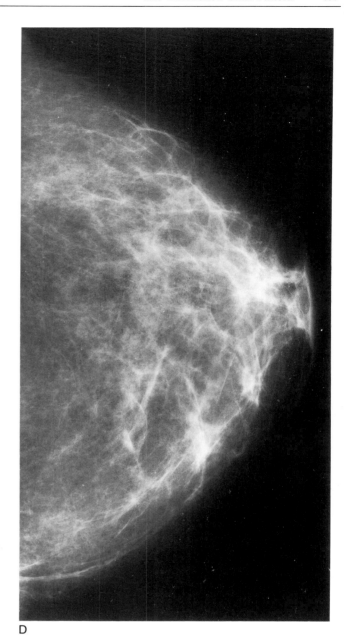

D

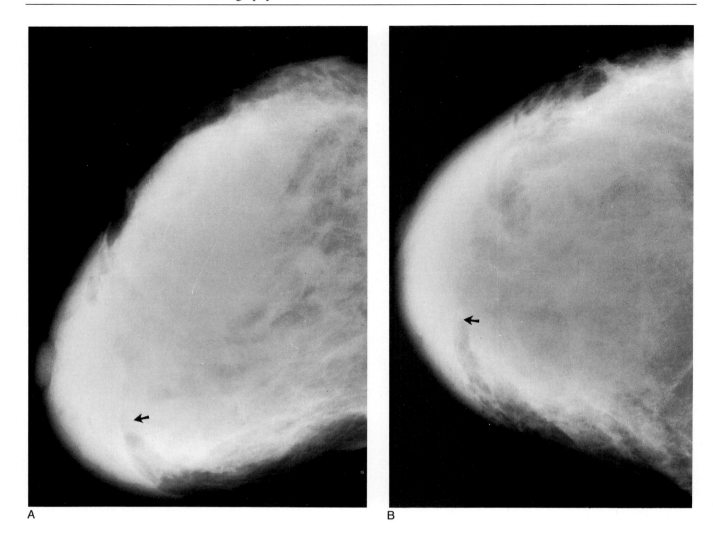

A

B

Figure 8.7.

Clinical: 70-year-old woman with a history of endometrial carcinoma, presenting with a painful swollen left breast.

Mammogram: Left mediolateral (**A**) and craniocaudal (**B**) views. The left breast is very dense. There is a diffuse edema pattern with an increase in skin thickness *(arrow)* and prominence of the interstitium. The primary differentials in this pa-

tient are metastatic carcinoma to the breast, inflammatory breast cancer, and edema secondary to axillary adenopathy.

Impression: Edema pattern, favoring metastases to the breast from endometrial cancer.

Histopathology: Endometrial cancer metastatic to the breast.

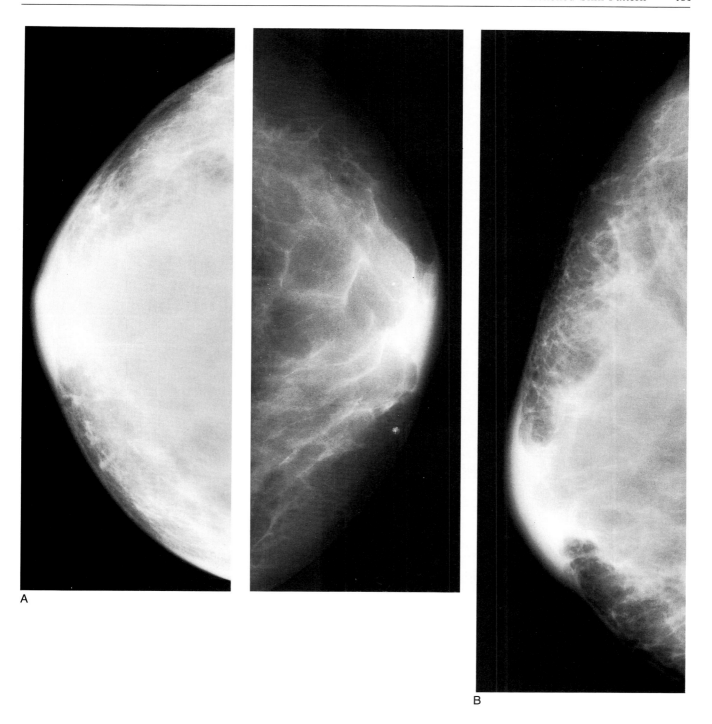

Figure 8.8.

Clinical: 49-year-old woman with a history of melanoma, presenting with new heaviness and thickening of the left breast.

Mammogram: Bilateral craniocaudal (**A**) and left mediolateral (**B**) views. There is marked asymmetry in the appearance of the breasts, with the left being diffusely more dense than the right. There is diffuse skin thickening over the left breast with prominence of the interstitial markings. Melanoma is a tumor that metastasizes to the breast and should be considered when this mammographic pattern occurs.

Impression: Metastatic melanoma to the left breast.

Histopathology: Metastatic melanoma involving breast, skin, and subcutaneous tissue.

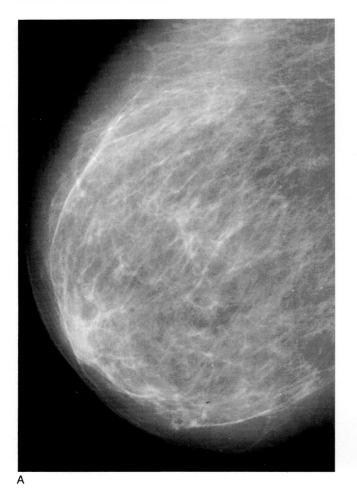

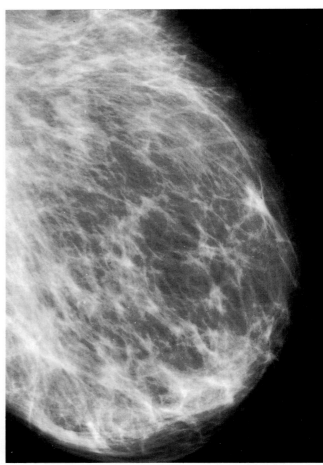

A

Figure 8.9.

Clinical: 81-year-old woman with a right parotid gland mass and a right breast mass.

Mammogram: Bilateral oblique (**A**) and craniocaudal (**B**) views. There is generalized asymmetry between the breasts. The right breast is more dense, and there is a prominence of interstitial markings. There is slight skin thickening inferi-

orly. With the history of a parotid gland tumor, one might consider metastatic disease to the breast or lymphoma or pseudolymphoma as high in the differential diagnosis.

Histopathology: Lymphocytic infiltration of the breast (lymphoma found in the parotid gland). (Case courtesy of Dr. Melvin Vink, Richmond, VA.)

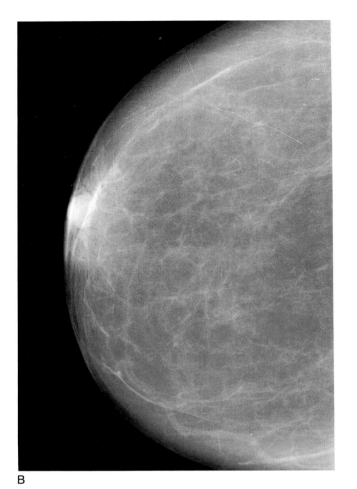
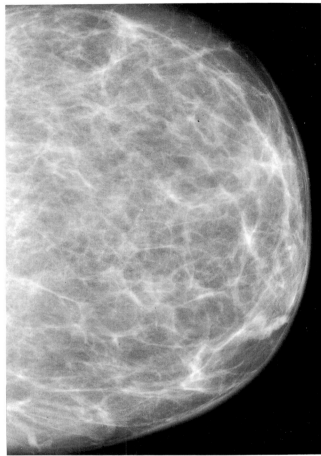

B

Figure 8.10.

Clinical: 65-year-old woman 6 months after lumpectomy and radiotherapy for intra-ductal carcinoma in the left upper outer quadrant.

Mammogram: Bilateral oblique views (**A**) and bilateral craniocaudal views (**B**). There is diffuse increased density with intersti-tial edema involving the left breast. Sur-gical clips in the upper outer quadrant mark the lumpectomy site. Skin thicken-ing is present *(arrows)* diffusely on the treated side. The diffuse changes are re-lated to radiotherapy and are maximum on this study. The edema will gradually decrease and approach a normal skin thickness and breast density.

Impression: Skin thickening and intersti-tial prominence secondary to radiother-apy.

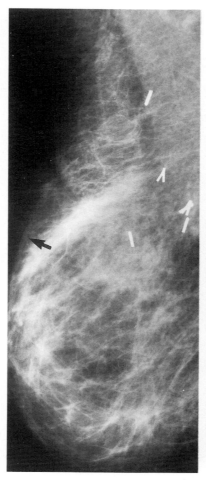
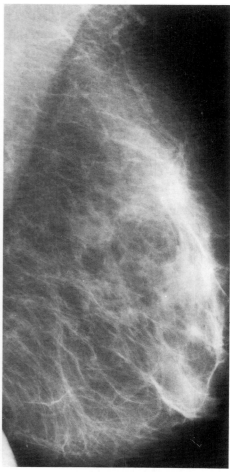

A

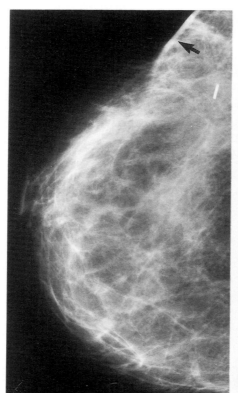
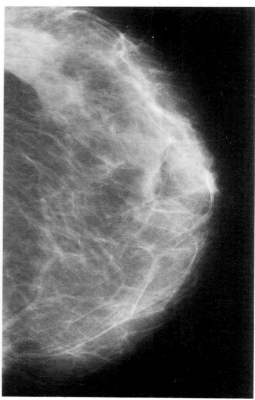

B

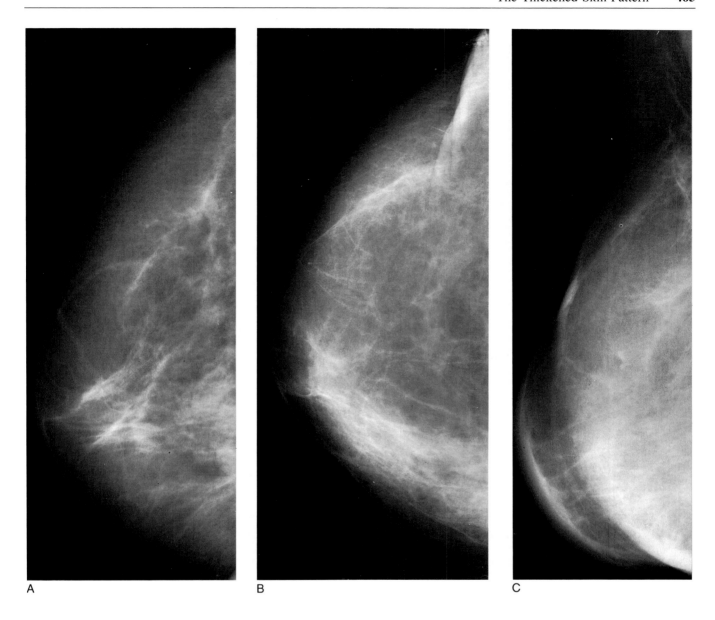

A   B   C

Figure 8.11.

Clinical: 55-year-old woman who, in March 1982, had lumpectomy and radiation therapy for a carcinoma in the lower inner quadrant of the left breast. In 1985, she returned with an increase in thickness of the left breast.

Mammogram: Left mediolateral (**A**) and craniocaudal (**B**) views in 1982 and left oblique view in 1985 (**C**). Three months after treatment, there is increased density of the breast with mild skin thickening. There is focal increased density remaining at the lumpectomy site, presumed to be related to resolving hematoma. Three years later, on the left oblique view (**C**), there is marked skin thickening with greater density of the breast diffusely near the chest wall.

Impression: Recurrent carcinoma after tylectomy and radiation therapy.

Histopathology: Infiltrating ductal carcinoma.

Note: The skin thickening and edema of the breast that occur after radiation therapy are greatest in the months immediately following treatment, and the changes gradually resolve over several years. The development of new skin thickening should alert the radiologist to the possible development of recurrent carcinoma. When the treated breast is being evaluated, it is very important to review the entire series of mammograms after treatment for subtle changes in skin thickness or parenchymal density.

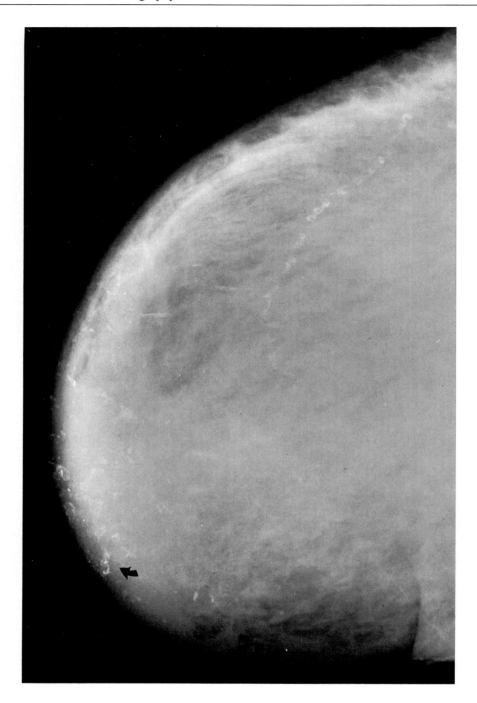

Figure 8.12.

Clinical: 75-year-old woman with Stevens-Johnson syndrome, multiple superficial ulcerations on the skin of the left breast, and a markedly dense, tender left breast. The skin lesions were being treated with zinc oxide ointment.

Mammogram: Left mediolateral view. The breast is very dense, and there is marked skin thickening diffusely. There are also multiple lacy "calcifications" located superficially, particularly in the periareolar area *(arrow)*. The findings are most suggestive of a diffuse mastitis secondary to a skin infection. The calcific-like densities represent the zinc oxide ointment on the skin surface. The patient was treated with antibiotics, and a follow-up mammogram was normal 3 months later.

Impression: Acute mastitis.

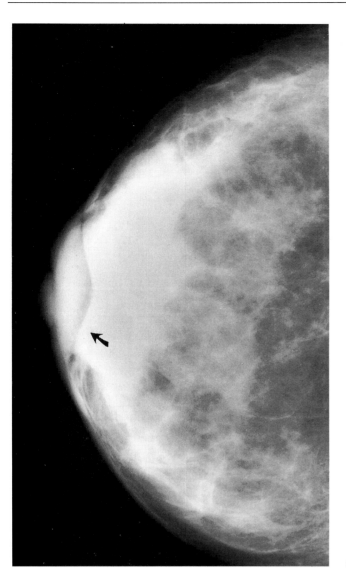

A

Figure 8.13.

Clinical: 33-year-old woman with history of breast abscess, presenting with induration around the left areolar area.

Mammogram: Left craniocaudal view (**A**) and ultrasound (**B**). There is prominent skin thickening over the areolar *(arrow)* area with diffuse skin thickening elsewhere (**A**). Increased density is present in the area of the subareolar lactiferous ducts. The whole-breast sonogram (**B**) shows an irregular, relatively sonolucent mass *(arrow)* beneath the nipple.

Impression: Mastitis with breast abscess.

Histopathology: Abscess

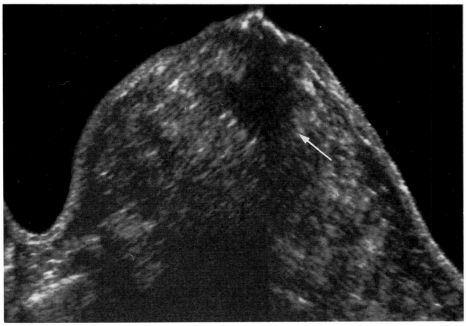

B

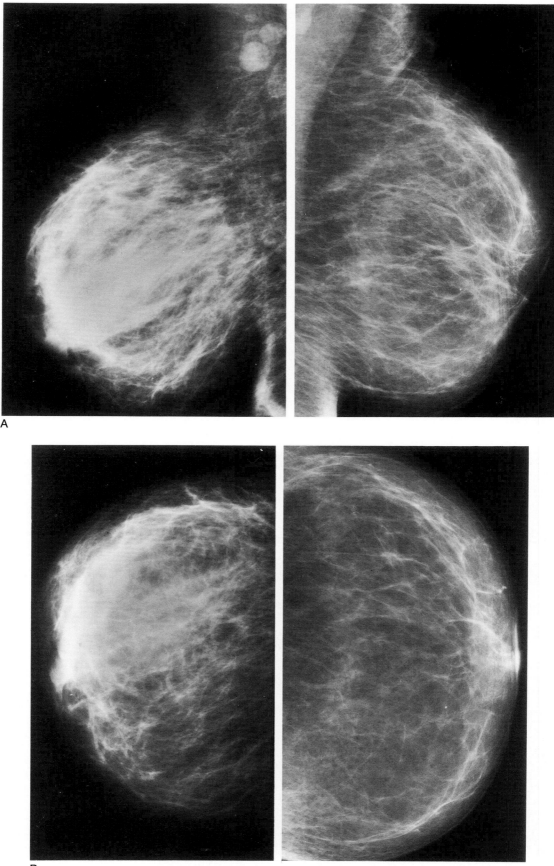

A

B

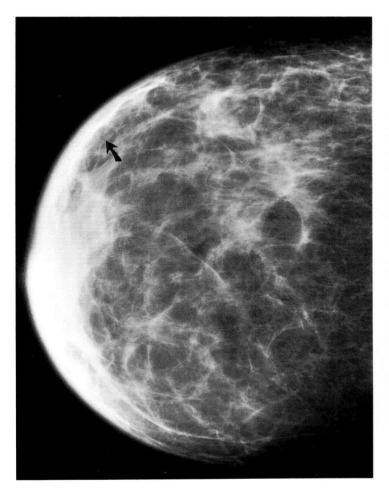
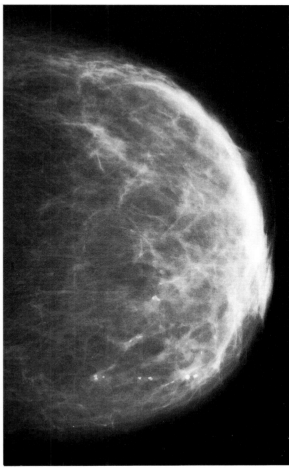

Figure 8.15.

Clinical: 82-year-old G1, P1 woman with a history of melanoma. Clinical examination showed enlarged tender lymph nodes in the axilla and firmness diffusely throughout the left breast.

Mammogram: Bilateral craniocaudal views. Marked asymmetry in the appearance of the breasts is noted. There is diffuse increase in the density of the interstitium of the left breast with marked skin thickening *(arrow)*. Skin thickening in a patient with a history of melanoma could represent diffuse metastatic involvement of the breast with melanoma or edema secondary to lymphatic obstruction from axillary adenopathy. (Biopsy of the breast and axillary dissection were performed.)

Histopathology: Metastatic melanoma in 38 of 40 lymph nodes with no involvement of the breast.

←

Figure 8.14.

Clinical: 52-year-old G4, P4 woman presenting with fever, chills, and a large hard mass in the left breast.

Mammogram: Bilateral oblique (**A**) and craniocaudal (**B**) views. There is marked asymmetry in the appearance. The left breast is diffusely dense with prominent interstitial markings. The left breast appears smaller than the right because of the thickening present and the lesser degree of compression. Enlarged nodes are present in the axilla. The differential diagnosis includes primarily acute mastitis versus inflammatory breast cancer. The extensive nature of the process is suspicious for neoplasm, but because of the patient's constitutional symptoms, mastitis is more likely.

Histopathology: Fat necrosis, acute inflammation, abscess.

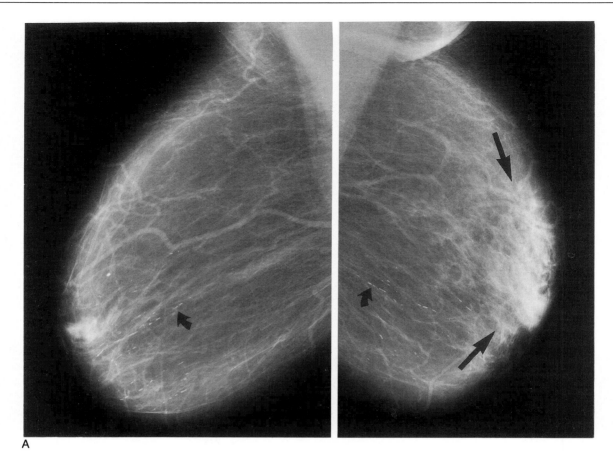

A

Figure 8.16.

Clinical: 81-year-old woman with a palpable right breast mass and a recent history of trauma to the breast.

Mammogram: Bilateral oblique views (**A**) and right cranio-caudal view (**B**) 6 months later. On the initial films (**A**), there is diffuse increased density *(straight arrows)* in the right sub-areolar area, associated with mild skin thickening. Inciden-tally noted are benign secretory calcifications bilaterally *(curved arrows)*. The findings were believed to represent an interstitial hematoma secondary to trauma, and the patient was followed clinically. On the mammogram 6 months later (**B**), the hematoma has resolved, and oil cysts *(arrows)* sec-ondary to fat necrosis are developing.

Impression: Interstitial hematoma resolving, with formation of oil cysts.

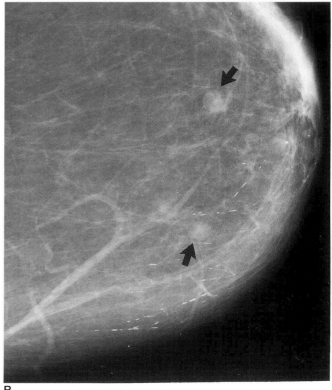

B

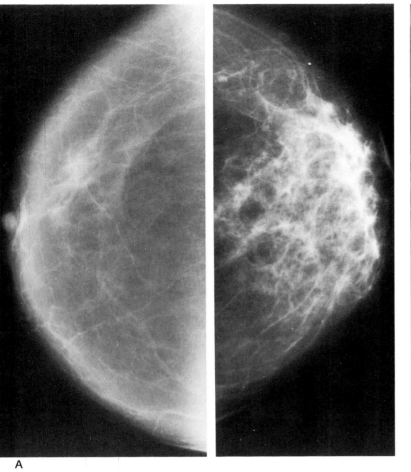

A

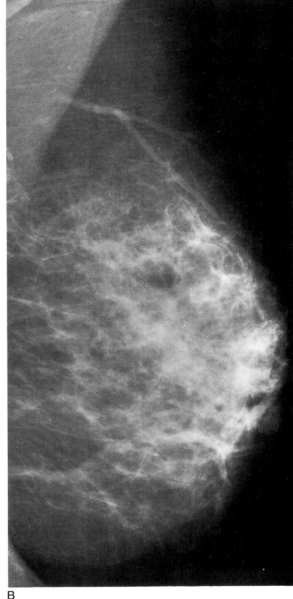

B

Figure 8.17.

Clinical: 82-year-old G5, P5 woman with severe breast trauma to the right breast 6 months earlier, presenting with a right breast mass, which was unchanged in size since the trauma.

Mammogram: Bilateral craniocaudal (**A**) and right oblique (**B**) views. There is marked asymmetry in the appearance of the breasts (**A**), with the right breast being diffusely more dense than the left. Prominence of the interstitium is present on the right (**A** and **B**), but no significant skin thickening is noted. Given the clinical history, this finding is most consistent with a diffuse interstitial hematoma with fat necrosis. The time for resolution of a hematoma is variable, and late changes of fat necrosis may be palpated as a firm mass.

Impression: Interstitial hematoma with fat necrosis.

Note: The breast was biopsied because of clinical concern about the palpable finding, and the biopsy showed fat necrosis.

Figure 8.18.

Clinical: 54-year-old woman who sustained severe blunt trauma to the upper torso and left breast 6 months earlier, now presenting with palpable masses and skin retraction.

Mammogram: Left mediolateral view. Multiple radiolucent masses with rimlike calcifications typical of fat necrosis and oil cysts are present. There is also increased density with skin thickening and retraction inferiorly *(arrow),* associated with the marked degree of fat necrosis.

Impression: Skin thickening secondary to fat necrosis.

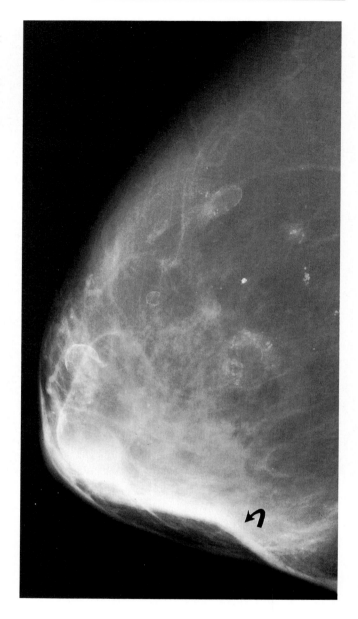

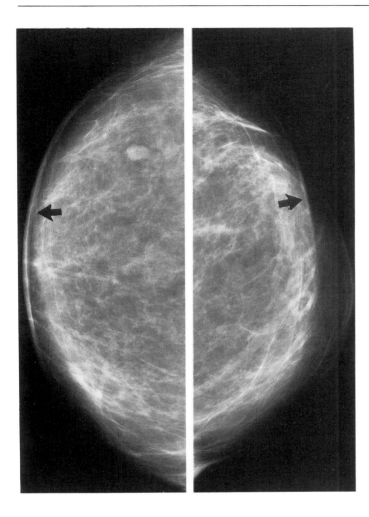

A

Figure 8.19.

Clinical: 36-year-old G4, P4 woman who had suffered burns to the anterior chest area years ago, for screening mammography.

Mammogram: Bilateral craniocaudal (**A**) and oblique (**B**) views. There is distortion of the contour of the breasts bilaterally, with retraction centrally. Skin thickening *(arrows)* (**A**) is present bilaterally, consistent with scarring from the burns. Coarse dystrophic skin calcification, probably secondary to the scarring, is present on the right *(arrowhead)* (**B**). Incidental note is made of a well-defined nodule in the left upper outer quadrant, which was found to be cystic on ultrasound.

Impression: Skin thickening secondary to a burn injury.

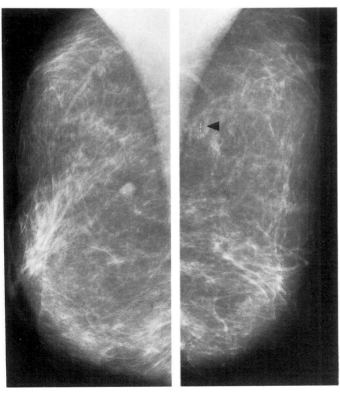

B

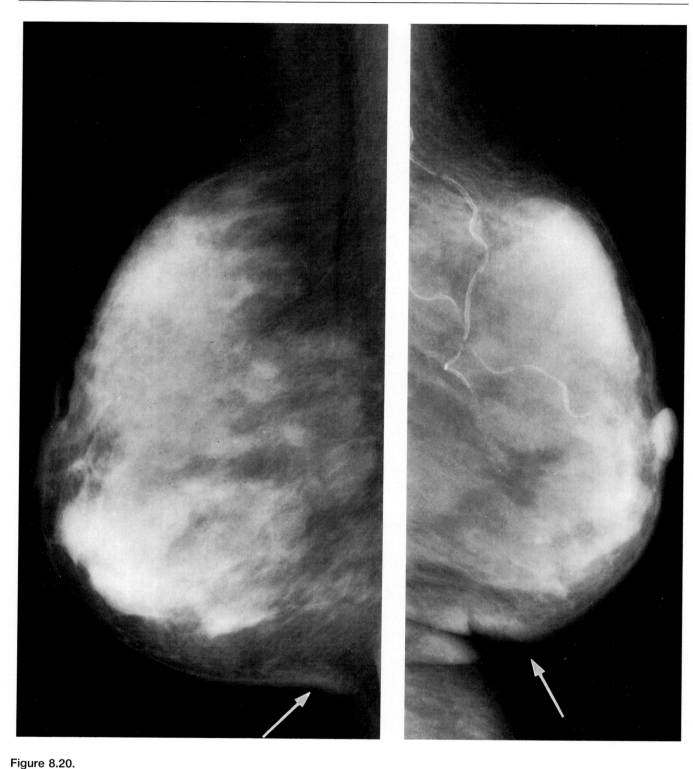

Figure 8.20.

Clinical: 46-year-old G3, P2, Ab1 woman with congestive heart failure and renal failure.

Mammogram: Bilateral mediolateral views. The breasts are dense and glandular. In the right breast, there are vascular calcifications that may be seen in young patients with renal failure and hypercalcemia. There is prominent skin thicken-

ing bilaterally, more so on the right than on the left and in the dependent aspects of the breasts *(arrows)*. This is seen in patients with anasarca or heart failure and may be unilateral if the patient has remained on one side for an extended time.

Impression: Diffuse skin thickening secondary to congestive heart failure.

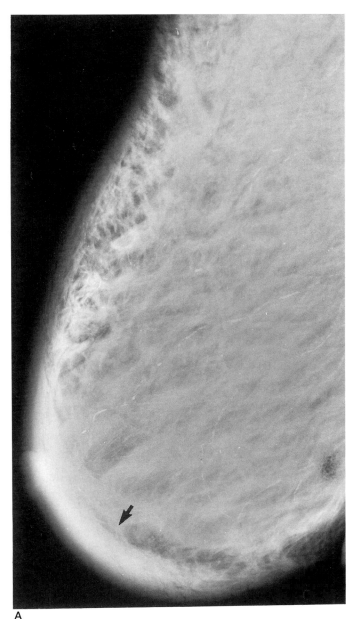

A

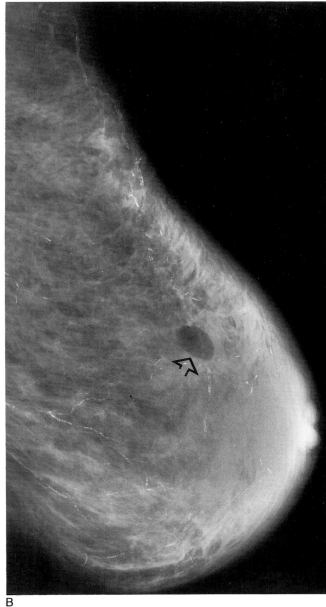

B

Figure 8.21.

Clinical: 81-year-old with thickening of the left breast and no focal palpable mass.

Mammogram: Left oblique (**A**) and right oblique (**B**) views. There is bilateral skin thickening, worse on the left (**A**) *(arrow)* than on the right (**B**). A diffuse edema pattern is noted with thickening of the interstitial markings of the breast. Incidental note is made of a small lipoma *(open arrow)* in the right breast. The differential diagnosis for bilateral asymmetric skin thick-

ening includes systemic causes such as fluid overload states, congestive heart failure, renal failure, metastatic disease to the breast, and hemorrhage secondary to anticoagulant therapy.

Impression: Congestive heart failure producing an edema pattern in the breasts.

Note: The patient had been lying on the left side, presumably accounting for the asymmetric edema on the left.

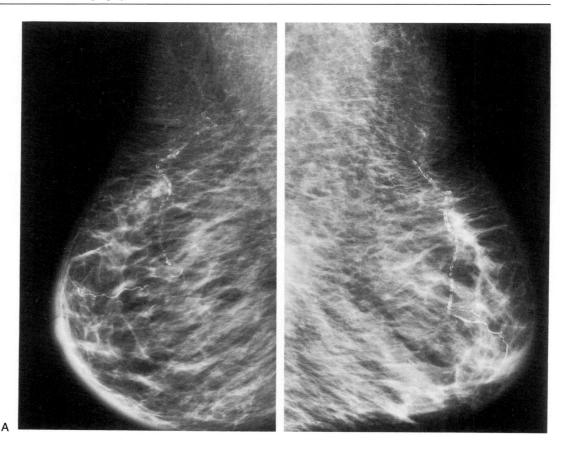

A

Figure 8.22.

Clinical: 75-year-old woman for screening mammography. She has a history of chronic renal failure secondary to an allergic reaction to penicillin.

Mammogram: Bilateral oblique views (**A**) and bilateral oblique views prior to the onset of renal failure (**B**). The breasts show a symmetrical edema pattern (**A**) characterized by increased interstitial markings and skin thickening. These findings were not present on the baseline mammogram (**B**). Diffuse bilateral edema suggests a systemic origin and in this case is secondary to renal failure. There is a fluid overload state and an increase in thickness of the interstitium by this fluid filling.

Impression: Edema pattern secondary to renal failure. (Case courtesy of Dr. Cherie Scheer, Richmond, VA.)

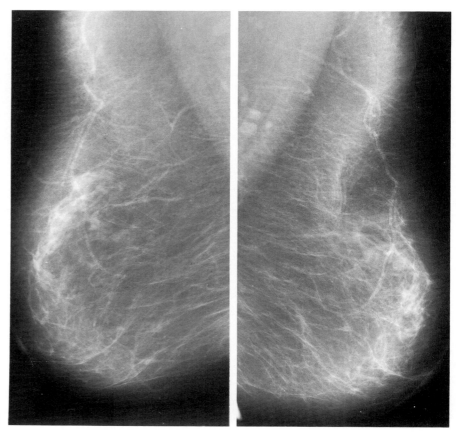

B

References

1. Gold RH, Montgomery CK, Minagi H, Annes GP. The significance of mammary skin thickening in disorders other than primary carcinoma: a roentgenologic-pathologic correlation. AJR 1971;112:613–621.

2. Wilson SA, Adam EJ, Tucker AK. Patterns of breast skin thickness in normal mammograms. Clin Radiol 1982;33:691–693.

3. Andersson I. Mammography in clinical practice. Med Radiogr Photogr 1986;62(2):1–41.

4. Dunkley B, Frankl G, Haile RWC, Bailey A. The importance of skin thickening in breast cancer. Breast Dis 1988;1:205–210.

5. Bell C. A system of operative surgery, vol 2. Hartford: Hale & Hasmer, 1816:136.

6. Parker LM, Sheldon TA, Cady B. Inflammatory breast cancer. In: Harris JR, Hellman S, Henderson IC, Kinne DW, eds. Breast Diseases. Philadelphia: JB Lippincott, 1987:570–577.

7. Droulias CA, Sewell CW, McSweeney MB, Powell RW. Inflammatory carcinoma of the breast: a correlation of clinical, radiologic and pathologic findings. Ann Surg 1976;184:217–222.

8. Keller RJ, Herman G. Unilateral edema simulating inflammatory carcinoma of the breast. Breast Dis 1990;3:61–74.

9. Bohman LG, Bassett LW, Gold RH, Voet R. Breast metastases from extramammary malignancies. Radiology 1982;144:309.

10. Mambo NC, Burke JS, Butler JJ. Primary malignant lymphomas of the breast. Cancer 1977;39:2033–2040.

11. Meyer JE, Kopans DB, Long JC. Mammographic appearance of malignant lymphomas of the breast. Radiology 1980;135:623–626.

12. Lin JJ, Farha GJ, Taylor RJ. Pseudolymphoma of the breast. I. In a study of 8,654 consecutive tylectomies and mastectomies. Cancer 1980;45:973–978.

13. Libshitz HI, Montague ED, Paulus DD. Skin thickness in the therapeutically irradiated breast. AJ 1978;130:345–347.

14. Anderssen F, Adler DD, Ljungberg O. Breast necrosis associated with thromboembolic disorders. Acta Radiol 1987;28:517–521.

CHAPTER
9

THE AXILLA

On routine mammography, the low axilla is visualized and a variety of findings may be identified. Physical examination is extremely important in the evaluation of the axilla, particularly in the assessment of adenopathy and fixation of nodes associated with breast carcinoma. In addition to lymph nodes, a breast lesion occurring in the axillary tail may be identified as a mass on mammography.

On the routine oblique view, lymph nodes in the low to middle axillary region can normally be identified (Figs. 9.1 and 9.2). An additional axillary view can yield more information about the upper axillary area, which may not be seen on the routine oblique projection. This is particularly important when a palpable mass is present and is not identified on mammography.

Normal axillary nodes are very well defined, medium- to low-density nodules that are less than 1.5 cm in diameter (1). Lymph nodes are round, ovoid, elliptical, or bean shaped. A lucent notch or center is often seen, representing fat in the hilum. This finding helps to confirm the diagnosis of a lymph node (Fig. 9.3).

Lipomatosis or fatty infiltration occurs in axillary nodes and is commonly seen in older patients. The fat distends the capsule and enlarges the node, and the surrounding lymphoid tissue atrophies (2) (Fig. 9.4).

In 1965, Leborgne et al. (2) described six patterns of fatty infiltration of nodes. The fatty replacement may occur centrally or eccentrically, producing densities of nodal tissue described as ring, sickle, or crescent in shape. As the fatty infiltration increases, the rim of the lymphoid tissue narrows, eventually leaving a distended capsule surrounding a fatty center (2). Fatty-replaced nodes may be as large as 3 cm in diameter (1) and benign. Large fatty-infiltrated nodes are more commonly seen in elderly obese women (1).

Inflammatory nodes are usually dense, enlarged, and with distended margins (1). Coarse calcification may occur, particularly with granulomatous infections (Figs. 9.5 and 9.6). In sarcoidosis (Fig. 9.7), enlarged axillary lymph nodes may occur as a manifestation of the generalized adenopathy that occurs in 23–50% of patients (3).

Axillary lymphadenopathy occurs in patients with rheumatoid arthritis (Figs. 9.8 and 9.9) (4, 5), along with the generalized lymphadenopathy that occurs in about 50% of patients with the disease. Abnormal axillary nodes in pa-

tients with rheumatoid arthritis are characterized by rounded shapes, higher density, little or no fatty replacement, and sizes of greater than 1 cm (5). Other arthritides associated with axillary adenopathy are psoriasis (Fig. 9.10), systemic lupus erythematosus, and scleroderma (5).

Malignant involvement of axillary nodes may occur as a result of primary lymphomatous tumors, metastatic disease from breast cancer, and metastatic disease from nonbreast primaries.

In lymphoma, the involved axillary nodes are enlarged (greater than 2.5 cm) and dense (Figs. 9.11–9.13). The pericapsular fat line bordering the nodes is not obliterated. This finding is important in differentiating a primary lymph node tumor from metastatic involvement. The nodes are dense but retain their shape and are well marginated (1). In lymphoid hyperplasia the adenopathy demonstrated on mammography cannot be distinguished from that found in lymphoma.

Metastatic nodes from breast carcinoma are generally enlarged (2–2.5 cm or more) (1), dense, and rounded (6) (Figs. 9.14–9.18). The normal architecture is lost, and the pericapsular fat line is obliterated as the borders of the node are infiltrated by tumor (1). Metastatic nodes may be multiple and matted together.

Although microcalcifications are uncommon in an axillary node, this finding is most consistent with metastatic involvement. Gold deposits can occur in axillary nodes of patients treated with chrysotherapy for rheumatoid arthritis and may simulate microcalcifications (7).

In a comparison of clinical examination and mammography with pathologic examination of axillary nodes, Kalisher et al. (8) found no significant difference in clinical examination and radiography in predicting metastatic involvement of nodes. When nodes were dense and greater than 2.0 cm in diameter, the true positive rate in predicting metastases was 85% and the false negative rate was 37%. When the criterion for abnormality was a nodal size of greater than 2.5 cm, the rates were 100% and 41%, respectively (8).

When metastatic carcinoma is found in axillary nodes, the primary breast cancer is usually seen, but occasionally it may not be identified (9). Metastases to the axillary nodes may also develop from nonbreast primaries and have a similar appearance to those from breast carcinoma, except for the lack of calcification.

Other lesions that may occur in the axillar or axillary tail and that must be differentiated from lymph nodes are sebaceous cysts, breast tumors (malignant and benign), cysts, lipomas, and ectopic breast tissue (Figs. 9.19–9.23). It may be impossible to differentiate a primary tumor from an enlarged lymph node when a solitary, relatively well defined mass in the axillary tail or axilla is present. Unless a patient has a reason to have generalized adenopathy, solid masses of greater than 1.5 cm in the axilla or smaller lesions without characteristic features of nodes should be regarded with suspicion.

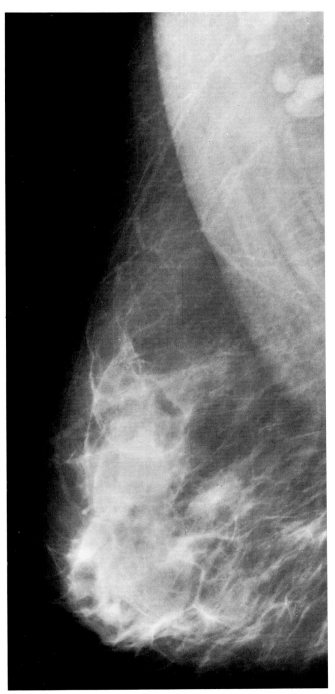

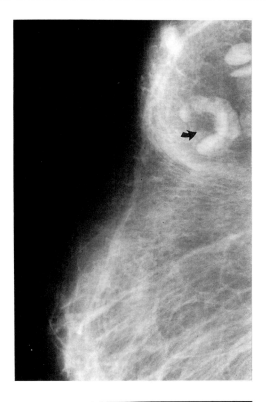

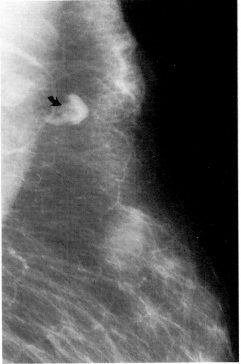

Figure 9.1.

Clinical: 45-year-old woman for screening mammography.

Mammogram: Left oblique view. The breast has a normal appearance. There are multiple well-defined round and ovoid nodules less than 1 cm in diameter in the left axilla. These nodules represent the appearance of normal axillary nodes.

Impression: Normal axillary nodes.

Figure 9.2.

Clinical: 58-year-old woman with chronic cutaneous infections over the breasts and upper extremities.

Mammogram: There are prominent nodes in both axillae. Fatty replacement is noted *(arrows)* in the central portions of several nodes, as is seen in postinflammatory adenopathy.

Impression: Postinflammatory adenopathy.

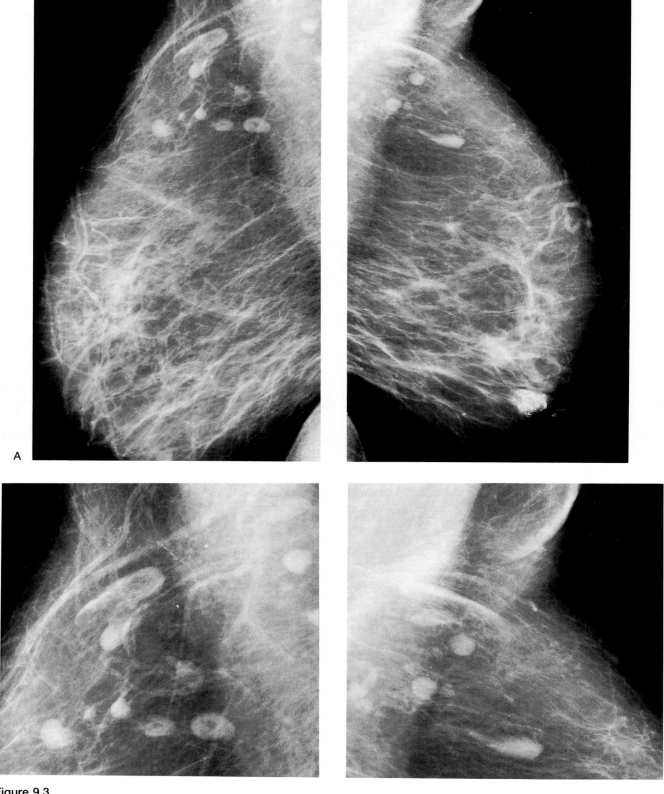

Figure 9.3.

Clinical: 75-year-old woman for screening.

Mammogram: Bilateral oblique views (**A**) and magnified image of the axillae (**B**). There are many small, very well defined, medium- to low-density nodules in the axillary areas bilaterally. These nodules have characteristic appearances of normal lymph nodes with fatty hila and notched ovoid shapes. Incidental note is made of a degenerated calcified fibroadenoma in the right breast.

Impression: Normal axillary nodes.

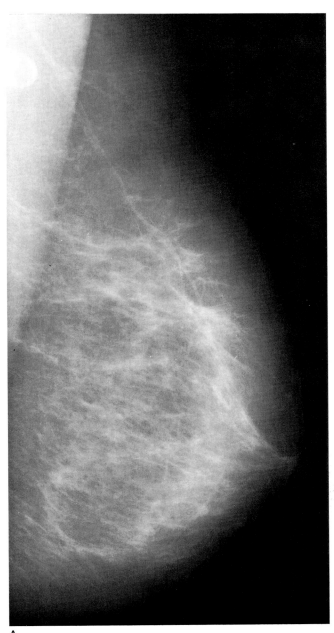

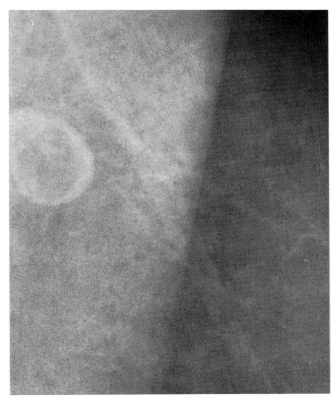

B

Figure 9.4.

Clinical: 63-year-old woman for screening.

Mammogram: Right oblique view (**A**) and magnification image (**B**). The breast has a normal appearance. There is a single fatty-replaced node in the right axilla. The thin rim of nodal tissue surrounding a fatty hilum is typical of benign adenopathy.

Impression: Benign fatty-replaced axillary node.

A

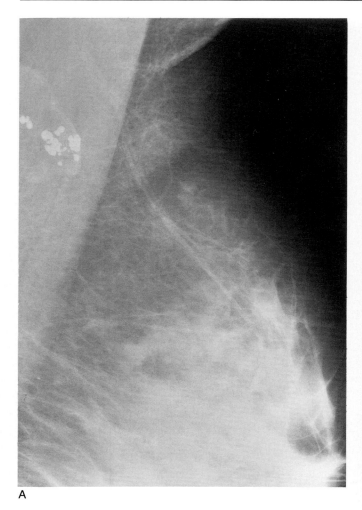

A

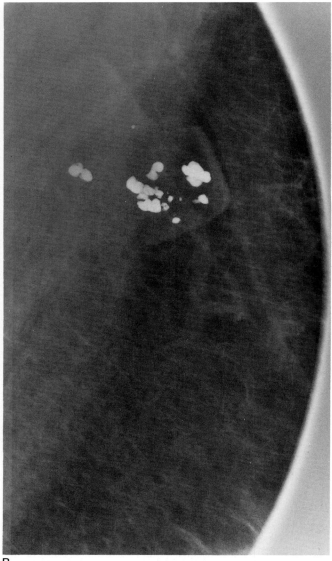

B

Figure 9.5.

Clinical: 71-year-old G2, P2 woman with a lump in the left breast.

Mammogram: Right oblique (**A**) and enlarged (1.5×) axillary (**B**) views. There is an enlarged, fatty-replaced lymph node in the right axilla. Coarse calcification is present, consistent with previous granulomatous infection.

Impression: Granulomatous calcification in an axillary node.

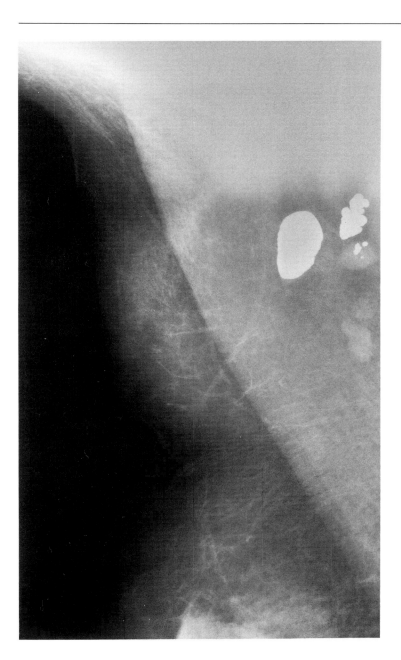

Figure 9.6.

Clinical: 61-year-old G0 woman for screening.

Mammogram: Left axillary view. There are three nodes in the left axilla that contain calcification. Two of the nodes are completely calcified, and the third contains dense round calcifications. The finding is most consistent with old granulomatous infection.

Impression: Calcified axillary nodes secondary to old granulomatous changes.

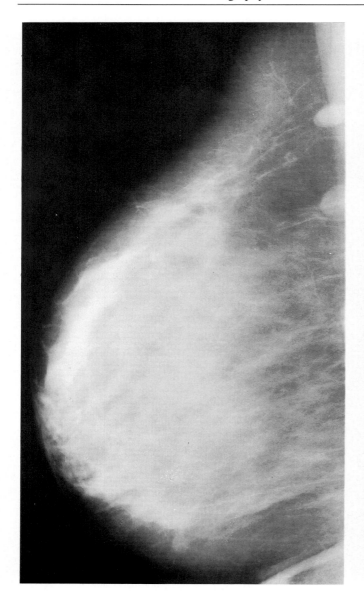
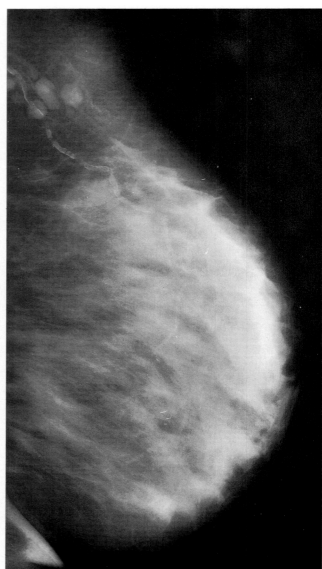

Figure 9.7.

Clinical: 40-year-old woman with a history of sarcoidosis whose breast examination is normal except for new palpable axillary nodes bilaterally.

Mammogram: Bilateral oblique views. There are prominent nodes in the right axilla and enlarged nodes (up to 2 cm) in the left axilla and tail of the breast. Benign adenopathy in the axilla and intramammary areas from involvement with non-caseating granulomas may be present in sarcoidosis or in conjunction with the generalized adenopathy present.

Impression: Axillary adenopathy secondary to sarcoidosis.

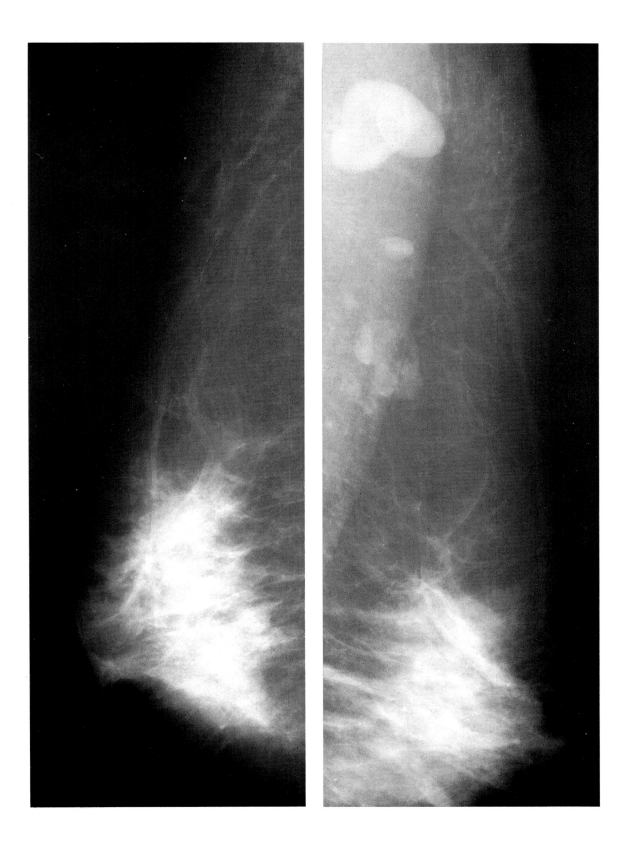

Figure 9.8.

Clinical: 58-year-old G0 woman with multiple areas of nodularity in both breasts and a history of rheumatoid arthritis.

Mammogram: Bilateral oblique views. The breasts are very dense for a postmenopausal patient, compatible with fibrocystic changes. Of note are prominent nodes in the right axilla, as might be seen in a patient with rheumatoid arthritis. The enlarged nodes in rheumatoid arthritis are solid and usually do not show fatty replacement, as is seen in postinflammatory nodes. In this patient, in addition, no pectoralis major muscle is seen on the left. One of the causes of this problem in positioning is a frozen shoulder (in this case because of arthritic involvement).

Impression: Mild adenopathy secondary to rheumatoid arthritis.

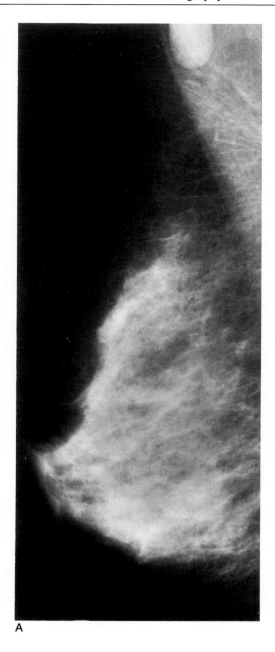

A

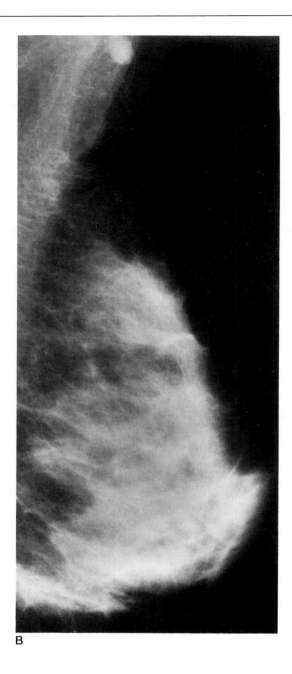

B

Figure 9.9.

Clinical: 46-year-old G3, P2, Ab1 woman with a history of rheumatoid arthritis, for screening mammography.

Mammogram: Left oblique (**A**) and right oblique (**B**) views. The breasts are dense for the age and parity of the patient. In the axillae bilaterally are non-fatty-replaced lymph nodes. The node on the right is not, by strict criteria, enlarged, but

the node on the left is clearly greater than 1.5 cm. The adenopathy is consistent with the patient's known history of rheumatoid arthritis and is not suspicious.

Impression: Bilateral adenopathy secondary to rheumatoid arthritis.

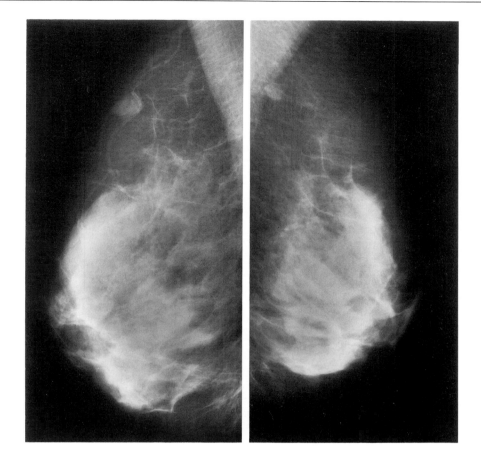

Figure 9.10.

Clinical: 67-year-old G4, P4 woman with a history of psoriasis, for screening mammography.

Mammogram: Bilateral oblique views. Dense parenchyma is present bilaterally, with the right breast being smaller than the left. There are enlarged lymph nodes in both low axillary areas, consistent with benign adenopathy related to the patient's known psoriasis.

Impression: Benign adenopathy secondary to psoriasis.

Figure 9.11.

Clinical: 84-year-old woman with a history of left breast cancer and malignant lymphoma, presenting with increasing adenopathy in the right axilla.

Mammogram: Right axillary view. There is massive solid adenopathy in the right axilla. Note the haloes that surround these large lobulated masses. Although one could not exclude involvement with metastatic breast cancer, this degree of adenopathy is more typical of lymphoma.

Impression: Lymphoma involving right axillary nodes.

Histopathology: Malignant lymphoma.

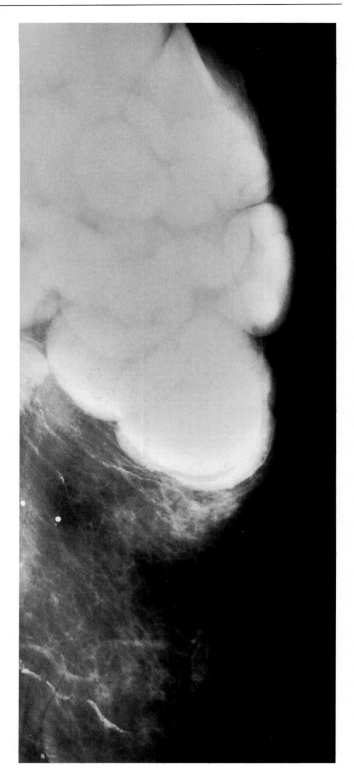

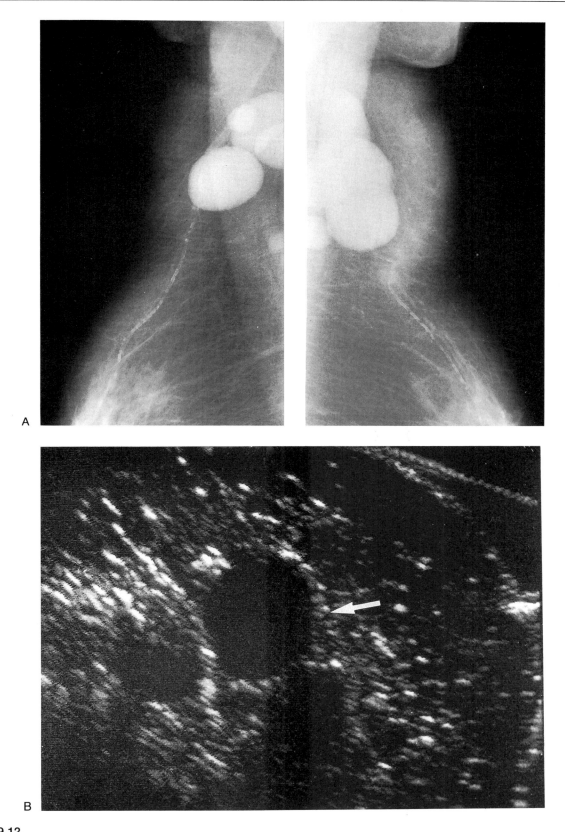

Figure 9.12.

Clinical: 63-year-old woman with a history of lymphoma.

Mammogram: bilateral axillary views (**A**) and ultrasound (**B**). There are bilateral, massively enlarged solid nodes in both axillae. Sonography (**B**) demonstrates the well-defined mar-gins and hypoechoic solid internal character of these lesions. The finding of bilateral adenopathy is one of the presentations of lymphoma on mammography.

Impression: Adenopathy secondary to lymphoma.

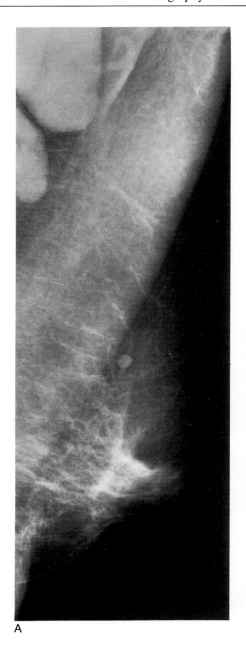

A

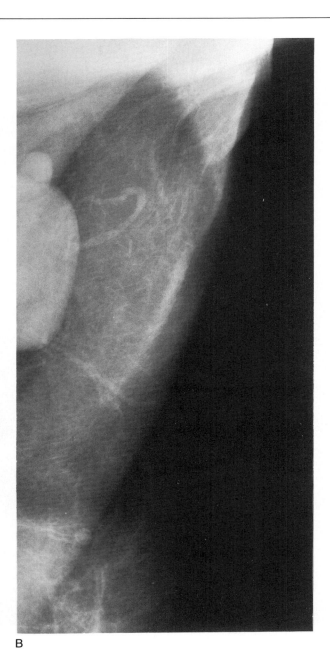

B

Figure 9.13.

Clinical: 63-year-old woman with a history of lymphoma, for screening.

Mammogram: Right oblique (**A**) and axillary (**B**) views. There are smoothly marginated, enlarged solid nodes in the axilla. An intramammary node is also present. The smoothly mar-

ginated, round enlarged nodes are more typical of lymphoma than of metastatic breast carcinoma. The findings are consistent with recurrence of lymphoma.

Impression: Recurrent lymphoma.

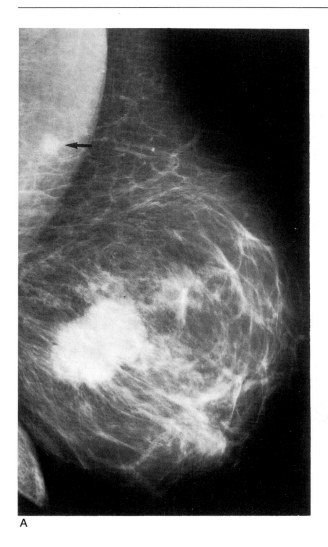

A

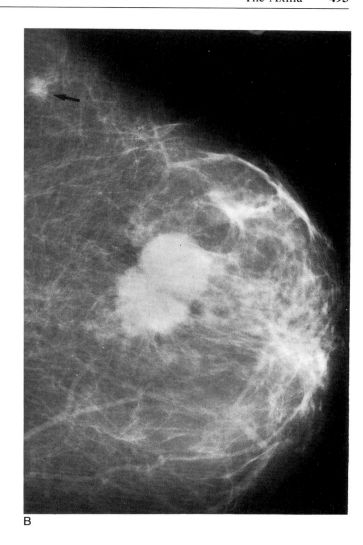

B

Figure 9.14.

Clinical: 45-year-old G4, P4 patient with a 3 × 3-cm mass in the right breast.

Mammogram: Right oblique (**A**) and craniocaudal (**B**) views. There is a large high-density spiculated mass with linear extension toward the nipple, having an appearance typical of carcinoma. Additionally, in the axillary tail there is a second smaller ill-defined nodule *(arrow)* (**A** and **B**). Although this could be a second primary lesion, because of its location and appearance, a metastatic node would be the more likely diagnosis.

Impression: Carcinoma with metastatic adenopathy in the low axilla.

Histopathology: Infiltrating ductal carcinoma, with 7 of 14 nodes with macroscopic foci of metastatic carcinoma.

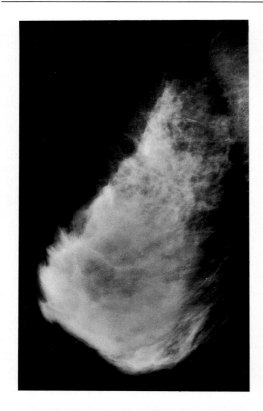

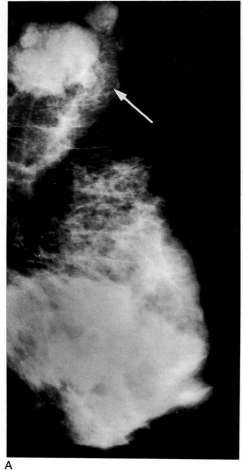

A

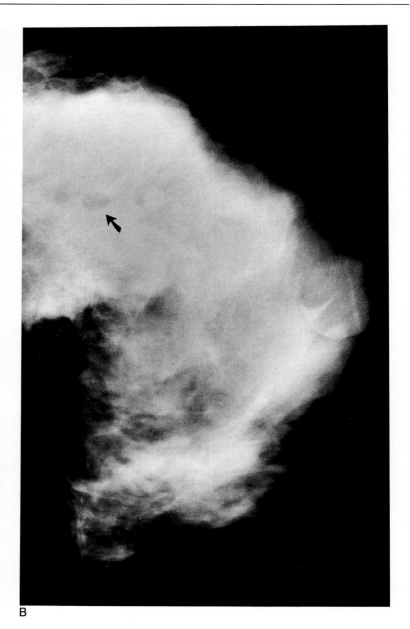

B

Figure 9.15.

Clinical: 63-year-old G0 woman with an ulcerating right breast mass.

Mammogram: Bilateral oblique (**A**) and right craniocaudal (**B**) views. The breasts are moderately dense. In the right middle outer quadrant, deep in the breast extending toward the chest wall, is a 7-cm high-density irregular mass consistent with a carcinoma. The lesion was ulcerating, and pockets of air are identified within it *(arrow)* (**B**). The right axilla (**A**) is filled with enlarged solid lymph nodes *(arrow),* indicating the presence of metastatic disease.

Histopathology: Infiltrating ductal carcinoma with positive nodes.

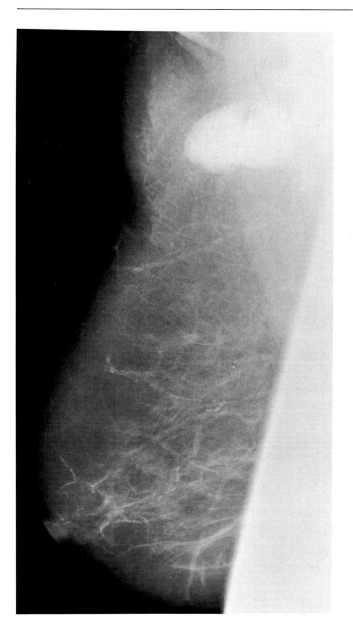

Figure 9.16.

Clinical: 73-year-old debilitated woman with a positive bone scan and no known primary carcinoma. The patient could cooperate only in a limited manner for mammography.

Mammogram: Left oblique view. In the left axillary area, there is a 4.5-cm lobulated high-density mass with relatively well circumscribed margins. The primary differentials include a neoplastic node versus a well-circumscribed carcinoma of breast origin. Because of the well-defined margin and the lobulated contours, the lesion was more likely thought to represent a node.

Impression: Left axillary mass, favoring neoplastic node.

Histopathology: Poorly differentiated adenocarcinoma in a left axillary node.

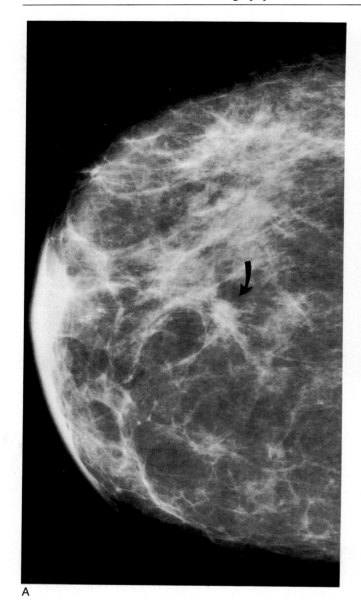

A

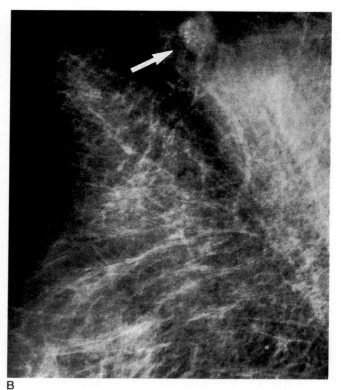

B

Figure 9.17.

Clinical: 70-year-old woman for screening mammography.

Mammogram: Left craniocaudal view (**A**) and oblique view (**B**). There is a 1-cm spiculated density in the midportion of the breast *(curved arrow)* (**A**), with associated malignant ductal calcifications in it and extending into the ducts around it. On the oblique view (**B**), there is an irregular nodule *(arrow)* in the axilla that contains similar malignant-appearing calcifications. The position of the axillary nodule and its lobulated shape suggest that it is more likely a lymph node involved with metastatic carcinoma (as evidenced by the malignant calcifications).

Impression: Carcinoma of the left breast with metastatic axillary adenopathy.

Histopathology: Infiltrating ductal carcinoma with positive nodes. (Case courtesy of Dr. A. C. Wagner, Culpeper, VA.)

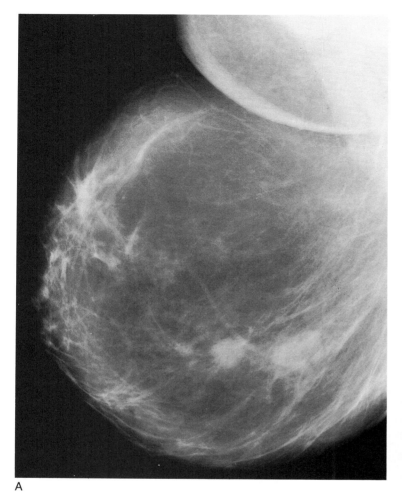

A

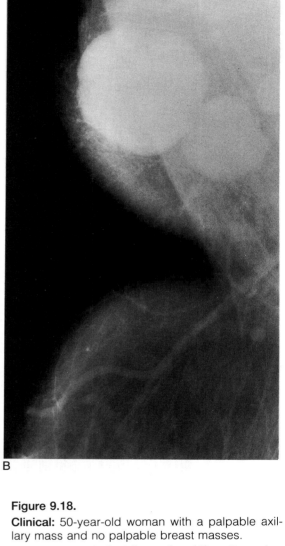

B

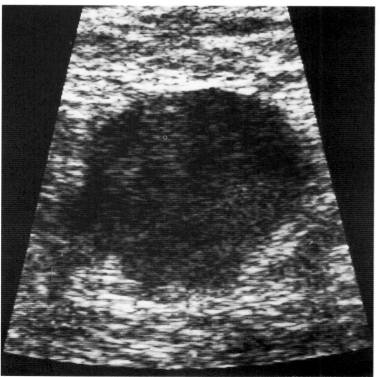

C

Figure 9.18.

Clinical: 50-year-old woman with a palpable axillary mass and no palpable breast masses.

Mammogram: Left oblique view (**A**), axillary view (**B**), and sonogram of the left axilla (**C**). There are two adjacent spiculated high-density masses in the lower aspect of the left breast, having an appearance typical of carcinoma. In the axilla, there are several large smooth lobulated masses. Sonography demonstrates the hypoechoic characteristics of these solid lesions.

Impression: Multicentric carcinoma with large metastatic axillary nodes.

Histopathology: Infiltrating ductal carcinoma with macrometastases in axillary nodes. (Case courtesy of Dr. Jay Levine, Richmond, VA.)

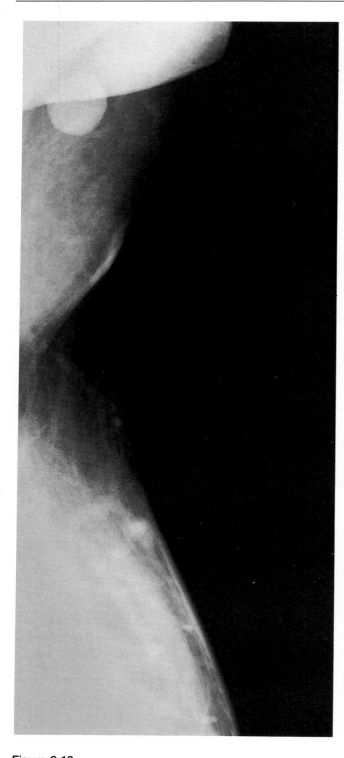

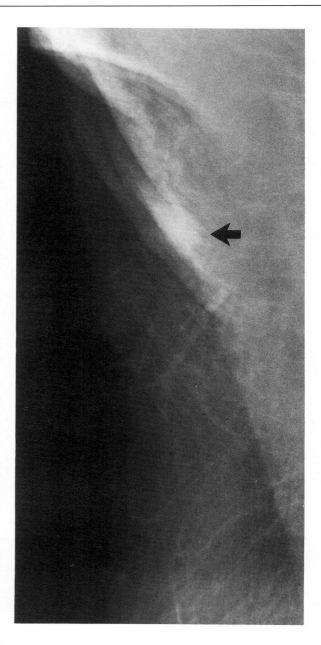

Figure 9.20.

Clinical: 72-year-old G0 woman for screening.

Mammogram: Left axillary view. There is a relatively well circumscribed nodule *(arrow)* in the left axilla. Although a non-fatty-replaced node would be the most likely etiology of this nodule, examination of the patient showed the nodule to correspond in location to a sebaceous cyst.

Impression: Sebaceous cyst, left axilla.

Figure 9.19.

Clinical: 52-year-old woman for screening mammography.

Mammogram: Right axillary view. There is an extremely well defined homogeneous mass in the area of the right axilla. Although this nodule could represent an enlarged node or other well-defined mass, the very well demarcated border suggested that the lesion was surrounded by air and was, therefore, on the skin. This was confirmed as a nevus on clinical examination of the patient.

Impression: Skin lesion: nevus.

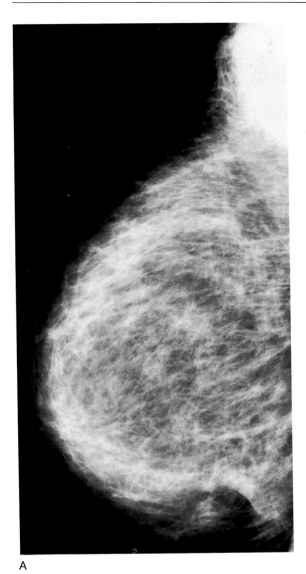

A

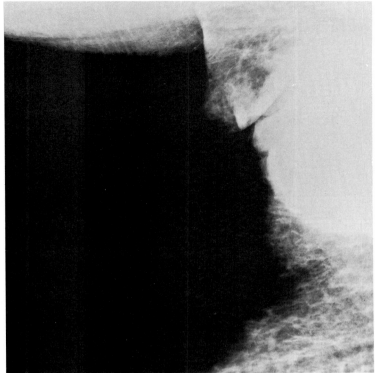

B

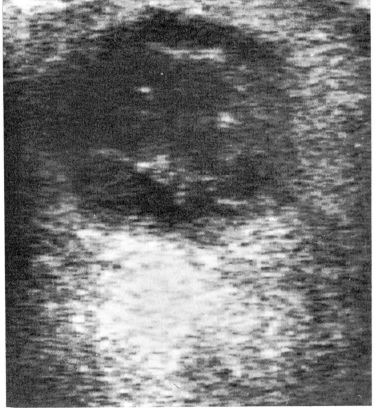

C

Figure 9.21.

Clinical: 68-year-old woman 3 weeks after an excisional biopsy for carcinoma of the left breast and a left axillary node dissection.

Mammogram: Left oblique view (**A**), axillary view (**B**), and ultrasound (**C**). There is a large high-density spiculated mass in the left axilla. The clinical history is critical to suggesting the correct diagnosis in this case. The appearance of the lesion may suggest carcinoma, but the recent surgery on the axilla should alert one to the possibility of a large hematoma. On ultrasound (**C**) the mass is complex, consistent with hematoma.

Impression: Axillary hematoma secondary to node dissection.

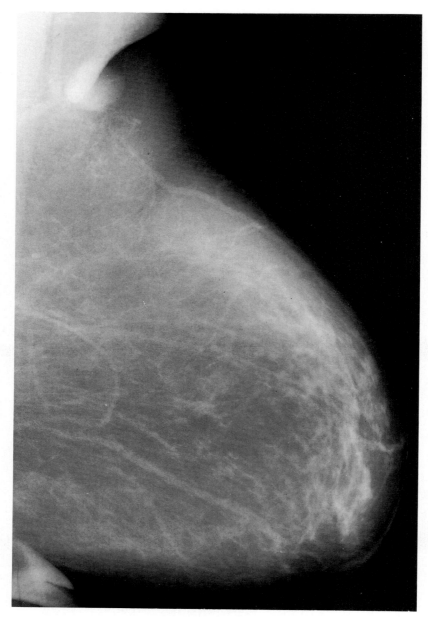

Figure 9.22.

Clinical: 52-year-old woman with a palpable right axillary mass.

Mammogram: Right oblique view. There is a very well defined, moderately dense round mass in the right axilla. This lesion could represent an enlarged lymph node involved with a neoplastic process or a well-circumscribed carcinoma.

Impression: Right axillary mass, favoring malignant node.

Histopathology: Signet ring cell carcinoma.

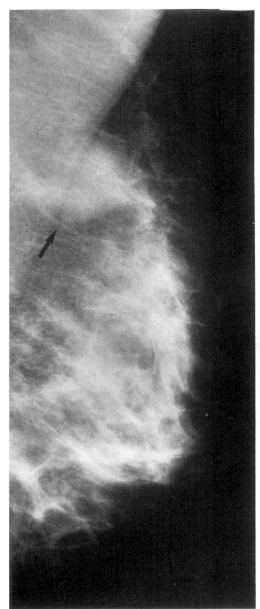

A

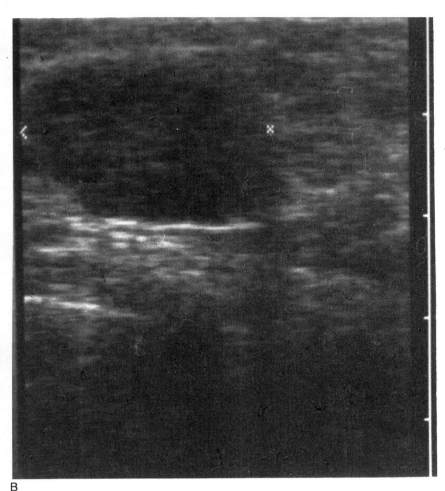

B

Figure 9.23.

Clinical: 43-year-old G5, P3 woman with a palpable mass in the right axillary tail.

Mammogram: Right oblique view (**A**) and ultrasound (**B**). The breast is dense and glandular. In the axillary tail (**A**), there is a focal area of tissue *(arrow)* that is partially circumscribed inferiorly and ill defined posterosuperiorly. This tissue is of medium density, having the same density as the background parenchyma. It did, however, correspond to the palpable finding, and therefore, ultrasound was performed to evaluate it further. On ultrasound (**B**) the lesion is partially circumscribed and uniformly hypoechoic, without shadowing. The lateral borders of the lesion on ultrasound are not well defined, a feature more suggestive of a malignancy than of a fibroadenoma. In addition, the partially ill defined margins on mammography are more suggestive of carcinoma than of a benign lesion.

Impression: Mass in the right breast, highly suspicious for carcinoma.

Histopathology: Infiltrating ductal carcinoma, with 16 nodes negative.

References

1. Kalisher L. Xeroradiography of axillary lymph node disease. Radiology 1975;114:67–71.
2. Leborgne R, Leborgne F, Leborgne JH. Soft-tissue radiography of axillary nodes with fatty infiltration. Radiology 1965;84:513–515.
3. Lazarus AA. Sarcoidosis. Otolaryngol Clin North Am 1982;15(3):621–633.
4. Weston WJ. Enlarged axillary glands in rheumatoid arthritis. Australas Radiol 1971;15(1):55–56.
5. Andersson I, Marshal L, et al. Abnormal axillary lymph nodes in rheumatoid arthritis. Acta Radiol (Diagn) 1980;21:645–649.
6. Leborgne R, Leborgne F, Leborgne JH. Soft tissue radiography of the axilla in cancer of the breast. Br J Radiol 1963;36:494–496.
7. Bruwer A, Nelson GW, Spark RP. Punctate intranodal gold deposits simulating microcalcifications on mammograms. Radiology 1987;163:87–88.
8. Kalisher L, Chu AM, Peyster RG. Clinicopathological correlation of xeroradiography in determining involvement of metastatic axillary nodes in female breast cancer. Radiology 1976;121:333–335.
9. Abrams RA, O'Connor T, May G, Homer MJ. Breast cancer presenting as an axillary mass: a case report and review of the literature. Breast Dis 1990;3:39–46.

CHAPTER 10

THE MALE BREAST

Benign and malignant conditions affect the male breast to a much lesser degree than the female breast, and mammography is of help in the differentiation of some of these lesions. Although mammography, and particularly the craniocaudal view, may be difficult to perform unless the breast is enlarged, the lateral oblique view can generally be quite satisfactorily obtained. Ultrasound may be a helpful modality in the evaluation of male breast enlargement (1), but it cannot replace mammography, particularly in the evaluation of a unilateral breast mass (2). The signs of male breast carcinoma are subtle on sonography, and mammography is necessary for complete evaluation.

Gynecomastia

Gynecomastia is the development of a male breast into the shape of a female breast and is clinically palpable as a firm breast mass in the subareolar area. Gynecomastia occurs most commonly in adolescent boys and in men older than 50 years, and the condition represents 85% of breast masses in men (3). The etiologies of gynecomastia include: (a) hormonal—related to an imbalance in estradiol-testosterone levels or to dysfunction of the adrenal, thyroid, or pituitary; (b) systemic—in cirrhosis, chronic renal failure with hemodialysis, chronic obstructive pulmonary disease, and tuberculosis; (c) drug induced—secondary to exogenous estrogens, digitalis, cimetidine, antihypertensives, ergotamine, tricyclic antidepressants, and marijuana; (d) tumors—particularly of testicular, pituitary, and adrenal origin or secondary to hepatomas or lung cancers; and (e) idiopathic.

The normal male breast contains subcutaneous adipose tissue and a few rudimentary ducts beneath the nipple. Histologically, three forms of gynecomastia are noted: (a) florid, which usually occurs over a short duration and is seen to have an increase in the ducts with proliferation of the epithelium, edema, and an increase in the stroma and fat; (b) fibrotic, which is more chronic and seen in elderly men who have dilated ducts without an increase in stroma or edema; and (c) intermediate (3).

The most common mammographic appearance of gynecomastia (54%) in a series by Chandrakant and Pareck (3) was that of mild prominence of the subareolar ducts. Dershaw (4) found the most common presentation of gynecomastia as a triangular or flame-shaped density symmetrically situated behind the nipple. The appearance, however, may range to diffuse ductal enlargement or even to a homogeneously dense breast having the appearance of that of a young woman. The condition may be unilateral or bilateral. Of importance in suggesting the diagnosis of gynecomastia on mammography is that the increased density or prominent ductal pattern be situated directly beneath the subareolar area and radiate out in a fan shape, as would be expected for the distribution of the ducts (Figs. 10.1–10.4).

Benign masses that have been described in the male breast include: cysts, abscesses, hematomas, enlarged lymph nodes (3), intraductal papillomas, and fibroadenomas (2) (Fig. 10.5). The mammographic manifestations of these masses are similar to those found in the female breast.

Carcinoma of the male breast accounts for about 0.9% of all breast cancers (5). The disease is more common in men over 60 years but has been seen rarely in young men. Most patients present clinically with a palpable breast lump (6). Factors that increase the risk of male breast cancer include: altered estrogen metabolism, exogenous estrogens, infectious orchitis, Klinefelter's syndrome, and radiation to the chest (7).

On mammography, male breast cancer usually presents as a spiculated mass, like scirrhous cancer of the female breast (Figs. 10.6 and 10.7). Calcifications may occur, but they are usually larger and fewer in number than are found in cancers of the female breast (3). Male breast carcinoma is distinguished from gynecomastia by its eccentric location, spiculation, microcalcifications, and secondary features, such as skin or nipple retraction (8). If, however, gynecomastia presents in an eccentric location (4), it may not be readily distinguished from carcinoma, and biopsy is warranted.

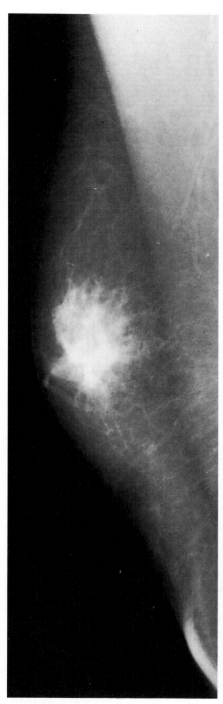

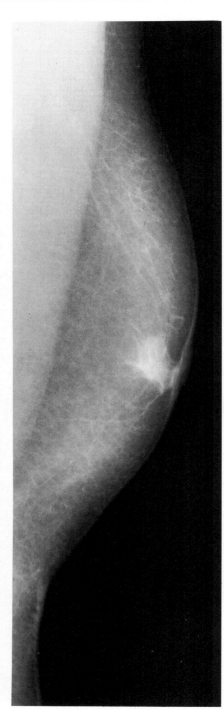

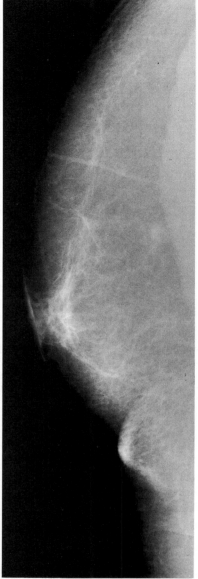

A-1

Figure 10.1.

Clinical: 45-year-old man with a history of recurrent Hodgkin's lymphoma, presenting with a tender left breast mass beneath the nipple.

Mammogram: Bilateral oblique views. The breasts are enlarged and fatty. In the right subareolar area, there is slight prominence of the ducts. On the left, there is an irregular area of increased density beneath the nipple. No secondary signs of malignancy are associated with this mass. The finding is nonspecific, and although gynecomastia with ductal enlargement was considered most likely, aspiration was performed to exclude a malignancy.

Cytology: Benign ductal cells consistent with gynecomastia.

Figure 10.2.

Clinical: 53-year-old obese man with tenderness and enlargement of the right breast.

Mammogram: Bilateral mediolateral (**A-1** and **A-2**) and craniocaudal (**B-1** and **B-2**) views. Both breasts are enlarged. The left breast is fatty, related to the generalized obesity of the patient. The right breast contains prominent glandular tissue diffusely.

Impression: Right gynecomastia.

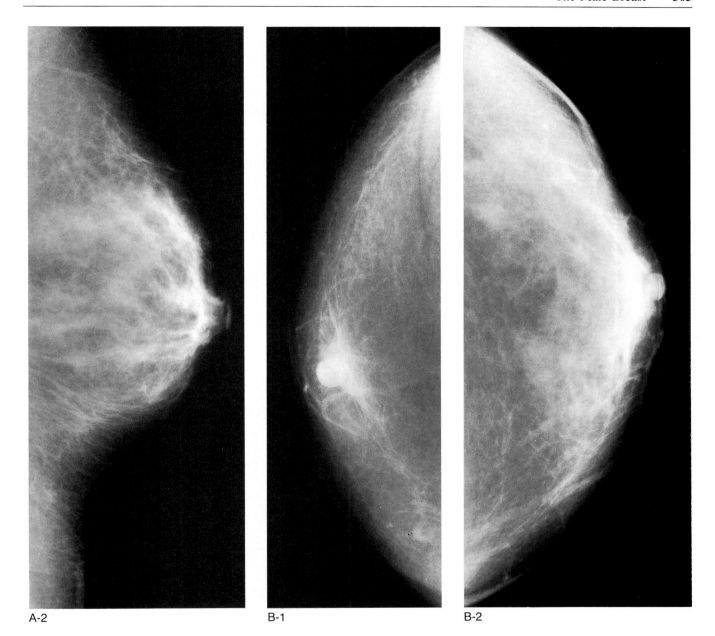

A-2   B-1   B-2

Figure 10.3.

Clinical: 63-year-old man with a 3-cm tender lump beneath the left nipple.

Mammogram: Bilateral oblique views. Marked asymmetry in the appearance of the breasts is present. The right breast is fatty except for some rudimentary ducts beneath the nipple. There is prominent glandular tissue in the left breast, which has the appearance of a female breast. This finding represents unilateral gynecomastia.

Impression: Unilateral gynecomastia.

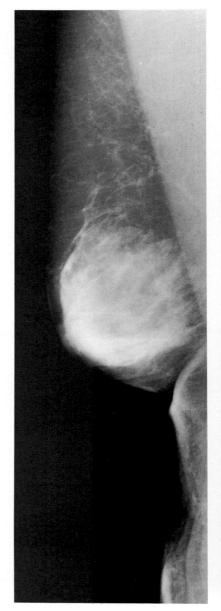
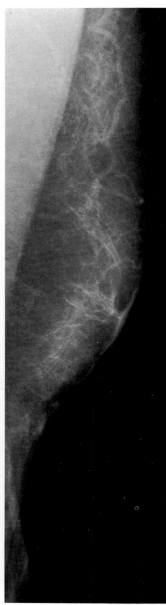

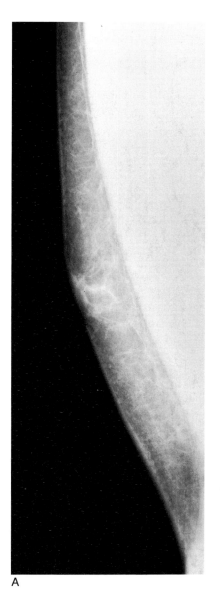
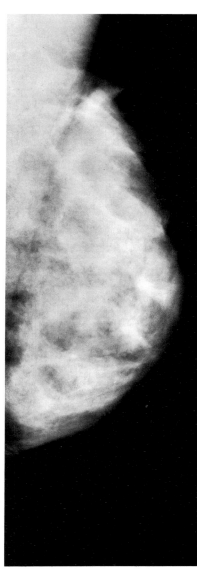

A

Figure 10.4.

Clinical: 21-year-old man who presented with unilateral breast enlargement. He stated that he had sustained blunt trauma to the right chest 2 weeks earlier; no bruising, mass, or tenderness was found on physical examination.

Mammogram: Bilateral oblique views (**A**) and ultrasound (**B**). There is striking asymmetry in the appearance of the breasts. (**A**). The left breast has a normal appearance for a male, with minimal fat and rudimentary ductal structures noted. The right breast is strikingly enlarged and is dense and glandular, having the appearance of an adult female breast. Sonography (**B**) of the right breast showed ductal and glandular tissue without solid or cystic masses being noted.

Impression: Unilateral gynecomastia.

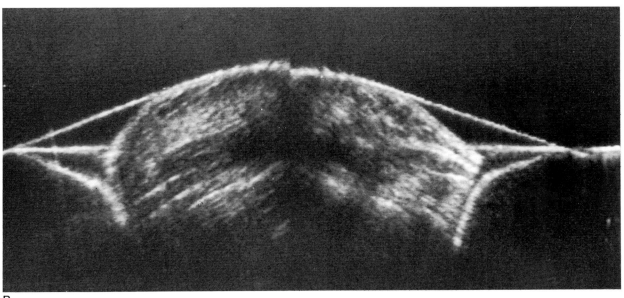

B

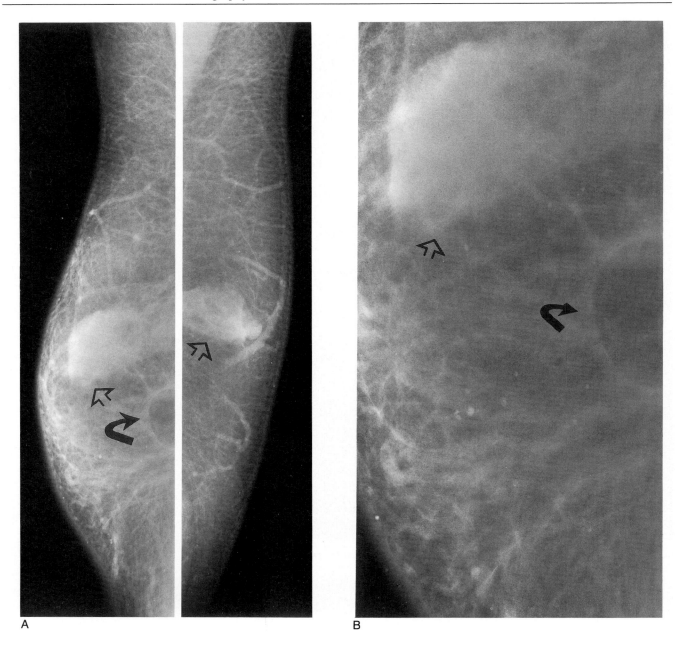

A

B

Figure 10.5.

Clinical: 41-year-old man who had been bitten by a horse on the left breast 6 months earlier, presenting with a firm mass in the upper inner quadrant.

Mammogram: Bilateral oblique (**A**) and enlarged (2×) left craniocaudal (**B**) views and ultrasound (**C**). There is some prominent ductal tissue in both subareolar areas *(open arrows)* (**A** and **B**), consistent with a mild degree of gynecomastia. On the left, near the chest wall, there is a radiolucent circumscribed encapsulated mass *(curved arrows)* (**A** and

B) having the characteristic appearance of an oil cyst. Sonography (**C**) shows this mass to be relatively anechoic, with good through-transmission of sound and a well-defined back wall. These findings corresponded to the area of palpable abnormality. Incidentally noted also are extensive skin calcifications.

Impression: Large oil cyst secondary to previous trauma.

Histopathology: Fibrous walled cyst, fat necrosis.

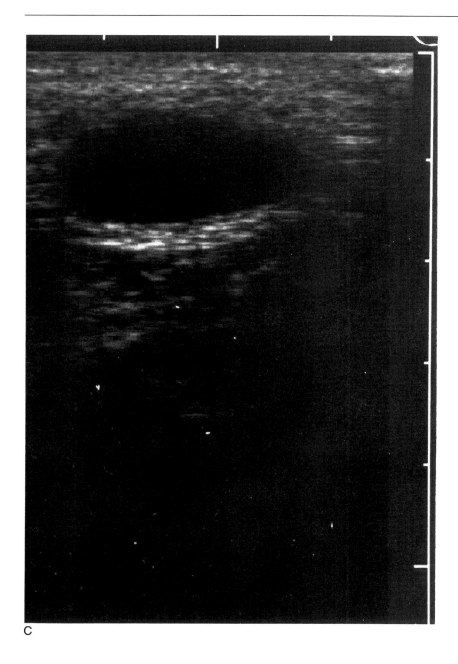

C

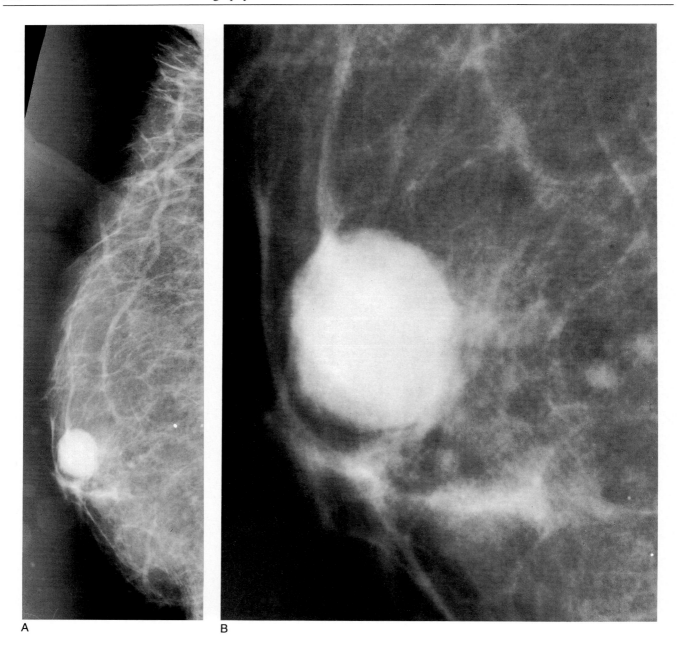

A

B

Figure 10.6.

Clinical: 80-year-old man with a firm mass beneath the left nipple.

Mammogram: Left mediolateral view (**A**) and magnified image (**B**). The breast is somewhat enlarged but fatty and not containing prominent ductal tissue, as would be found in gynecomastia. In the subareolar area, there is a well-defined high-density mass with slight nodularity of the margins, suggesting a suspicious nature.

Impression: Mass in the left breast, highly suspicious for carcinoma.

Histopathology: Medullary carcinoma.

Note: The scalloping of the edges of this lesion (**B**) and the high density are the features suggestive of malignancy. (Case courtesy of Dr. Luisa Marsteller, Norfolk, VA.)

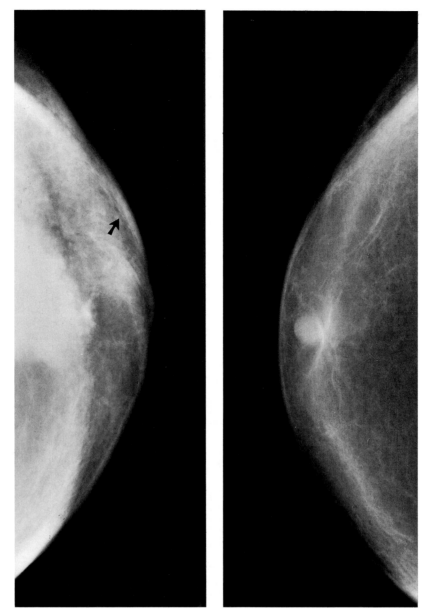

Figure 10.7.

Clinical: 80-year-old man with a fixed mass in the right breast.

Mammogram: Bilateral craniocaudal views. There is a large, very irregular nodular mass of high density in the outer portion of the right breast. Associated skin thickening *(arrow)* is present. The features are characteristic of malignancy.

Impression: Carcinoma.

Cytology: Carcinoma.

References

1. Cole-Beuglet C, Schwartz GF, et al. Ultrasound mammography for male breast enlargement. J Ultrasound Med 1982;1:301–305.
2. Jackson VP, Gilmor RL. Male breast carcinoma and gynecomastia: comparison of mammography with sonography. Radiology 1983;149:533–536.
3. Chandrakant CK, Pareck NJ. The male breast. Radiol Clin North Am 1983;21:137–148.
4. Dershaw DD. Male mammography. AJR 1986;146:127–131.
5. Yap HY, Tashima CK, Blimensheim GR, et al. Male breast cancer: a natural history study. Cancer 1979;44:748–754.
6. Hultborn R, Friberg S, Hultborn KA. Male breast carcinoma. Acta Oncol 1987;26:241–256.
7. Meyskins FL, Tormey DC, Neifeld JP. Male breast cancer: a review. Cancer Treat Rev 1976;3:83–93.
8. Michels LG, Gold RH, Arndt RD. Radiography of gynecomastia and other disorders of the male breast. Radiology 1977;122:117–122.

CHAPTER
11

INTERVENTIONAL PROCEDURES

Several interventional procedures are now performed regularly in conjunction with mammography. These procedures enable the radiologist to make a more accurate or specific diagnosis and to conduct a more comprehensive evaluation of the patient. The techniques for performing these procedures are described in this chapter.

Needle Localization of Nonpalpable Abnormalities

Preoperative localization of a nonpalpable mammographic abnormality is necessary before surgical removal. With preoperative localization a smaller amount of tissue can be excised than without radiographic guidance. This is important not only from the patient's standpoint, because of a lesser degree of postoperative deformity, but also from the pathologist's standpoint, because the ease and accuracy of identifying a tiny focus of carcinoma in situ are improved when the amount of tissue to be sectioned is less.

The techniques for localization are varied, including triangulation and needle placement (1), needle localization with dye injection (2, 3), and needle localization with wire placement. There are a number of wires available, most of which have a type of hook (4) or J configuration (5) when released from the needle. Many of the newer dedicated mammographic units are equipped with a localization device. Two basic designs are available: a rectangular aperture or multiple 1-cm-round perforations (6) in a plastic compression plate.

Prior to the localization, a 90° lateral (mediolateral) view is obtained if only craniocaudal and oblique projections are available. From these films the closest skin surface to the abnormality is determined—superior, medial, or lateral. The localization plate is placed over the surface determined, and a film is made (Fig. 11.1). While the patient remains in position, compressed, the coordinates of the aperture overlying the lesion are determined. A localization needle is placed into the breast, parallel to the chest wall at the indicated location; the depth of placement is estimated only, because the breast is compressed by the localization device. A film is made with the needle in place to determine if the placement is accurate (Fig. 11.2). The localization plate is then carefully removed, leaving the needle in place, and the orthogonal view is made. If the needle is too deep, it is with-

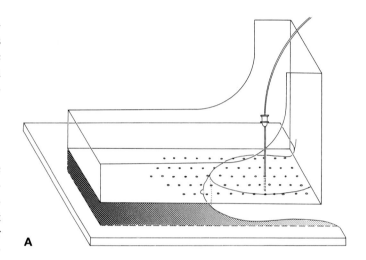

A

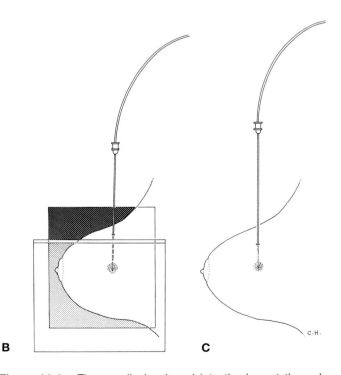

B   C

Figure 11.1. The needle is placed into the breast through the appropriate aperture (**A**), the opposite view is made to determine the depth of the needle (**B**), and the wire is ejected (**C**).

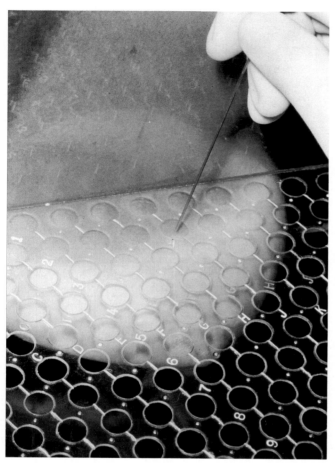

Figure 11.2. A localization grid with 1-cm-round perforations is in place.

for the localization of a lesion in a breast augmented with a prosthesis to avoid puncture of the prosthesis, particularly if it contains silicone. Robertson et al. (13) described wire localization in 8 patients with implants, with placement of the needle using the Eklund technique (14) of displacement of the implant. Another option in these patients is to place the localization grid over the breast and mark the lesion with skin markers only, giving instructions of the depth from the skin surfaces.

Most series report a true positive rate in needle localization series of 10–35% (15–29). The vast majority of benign lesions biopsied represent some form of fibrocystic disease, although proliferative lesions, which increase the risk of the patient to develop breast cancer by 1.9 (without atypia) to 5.3 (with atypia) times, account for a significant number of nonpalpable lesions biopsied (26). Without meticulous techniques and attention to subtle signs of malignancy, early breast cancers will be missed. Rosenberg et al. (25) found that in a series of 927 needle-guided breast biopsies, 29% were malignant and 30% of the patients with invasive lesions had axillary nodal metastases. Hermann et al. (29) retrospectively reviewed the mammograms of 220 women who underwent needle localization biopsy procedures and classified the lesions as ''probably benign'' or ''probably malignant.'' The radiologic diagnosis was correct in 68% of cases; 27 of the cancers were retrospectively interpreted as ''probably benign'' and would have been missed had there not been an aggressive approach to indeterminate lesions. A high-quality screening program coupled with needle localization biopsy procedures for suspicious or indeterminate lesions will yield increasing numbers of early breast cancers at biopsy.

drawn until the tip is within the lesion, and then the wire is ejected. The needle is removed, the wire is taped to the skin, and two final films, craniocaudal and mediolateral views, are made to show the position of the hook relative to the lesion. Specimen films (7) are necessary to confirm that the lesion has been removed, particularly for calcifications or nodules (8) (Figs. 11.3 and 11.4). Particularly for noncalcified lesions, specimen radiography in two projections may be needed to confirm removal of the abnormality (9).

If care is used in needle placement, the risks of the procedure are minimal. Although a pneumothorax could occur, attention to placement of a localization wire parallel to the chest wall should avoid this problem. Hematomas are infrequent and, if significant, are usually related to a vascular puncture (10). Migration of a lost wire at surgery has been described (11); to avoid a lost wire, it is important that a wire be used of sufficient length to allow at least 10 cm to protrude from the breast at the end of the procedure. In patients treated for breast cancer that was diagnosed by a needle localization biopsy procedure, there has been no documented increase in local recurrence rate to suggest seeding of tumor cells along the wire tract (12). Care must be taken

Pneumocystography

The evaluation of a patient with a well-defined breast mass on mammography may include ultrasonography, needle aspiration, and pneumocystography. Pneumocystography can be performed if breast ultrasound is not available or if the sonographic findings are equivocal. Some studies (30) have shown a therapeutic value from breast cyst puncture and pneumocystography. With pneumocystography, or air injection into the cyst cavity, an intracystic tumor can be identified. The incidence of intracystic carcinoma ranges from 0.2% (31) to 1.3% (32). Tabar et al. (30) identified 13 benign and 13 malignant tumors on a series of 434 pneumocystograms. The fluid aspirated from 5 of 13 cancers was not bloody, as is generally thought to be indicative of malignancy, and cytology performed in 11 of the cases was negative in 8 (30). In a 1-year follow-up of 130 simple cysts diagnosed at pneumocystography, 88% did not refill after initial puncture, and 97% were definitively treated with pneumocystography after a repeat puncture. The presence of air within the cyst cavity may induce collapse and sclerosis of the wall (33).

Pneumocystography is a simple technique to perform and produces minimal discomfort to the patient (Fig. 11.5). The aspiration of the cyst can be performed by palpating it, under ultrasound guidance (34), or under mammographic guidance. Palpable and nonpalpable cysts can be aspirated easily under mammographic guidance because the lesion can be more easily fixed for puncture by compressing the breast. This technique is described as follows.

On viewing the initial mammogram, one determines the shortest distance from the lesion to the skin surface—medial, superior, or lateral. The localization compression plate is placed over the breast at the determined location, and a film is made. The patient remains in position with the breast compressed while the film is developed; the coordinates of the lesion are determined. A 20-gauge needle attached to a syringe is placed into the breast and is slowly withdrawn while mild suction on the syringe is applied. When liquid is aspirated, the needle is held in place until aspiration is complete; the syringe is removed and replaced with a syringe containing slightly less room air, and the air is injected into the cyst cavity. If the fluid aspirated is bloody, it is sent for cytologic examination.

In mediolateral and craniocaudal projections, films are made immediately after injection of air. The walls of the cyst cavity should be thin and smooth (Fig. 11.6). Any intraluminal filling defect or focal irregularity of the wall is regarded with suspicion for an intracystic tumor. Benign intracystic papillomas and papillary carcinomas can be visualized in this way. If an intracystic abnormality is identified, excision of the lesion is indicated.

Fine-Needle Aspiration

Fine-needle aspiration biopsies (FNABs) for palpable breast masses have been performed with success in lieu of open biopsy (35, 36). Fine-needle aspiration of a solid breast mass can also be performed in a similar fashion to the previously described method for cyst aspiration. For a questionably palpable lesion that cannot be satisfactorily aspirated by palpation only or for a nonpalpable lesion, fine-needle aspiration can be done under mammographic or sonographic guidance. Critical for fine-needle aspiration of nonpalpable lesions to be of value are the following: extremely accurate needle placement, good techniques of aspiration and preparation of the smear, experienced cytologists for interpretation of the sample, and accurate and consistent results for cytologic determination of benign and malignant lesions (37). The experience of the person performing the aspiration is reflected in the percentage of aspirates that have sufficient material for analysis (35, 38).

The technique for needle placement for fine-needle aspiration is identical with the technique for needle localization of nonpalpable masses. Once a 22-gauge needle has been placed into the lesion, suction is applied and the needle is moved back and forth within the lesion; the suction is released, the needle is withdrawn, and the aspirate is ejected from the needle onto slides and is smeared and fixed. Multiple passes will increase the yield of cells for cytologic analysis. If an aspirate of a suspicious mammographic lesion is negative, open biopsy is necessary for accurate diagnosis.

The advent of stereotaxis for mammography has greatly impacted on the ease of accurate needle placement into small nonpalpable lesions and has allowed for a nonsurgical approach. Stereotactically guided fine-needle aspirations for biopsy or cyst puncture can be performed for nodules as small as 3–5 mm. Stereotaxis can also be used for needle localizations and is particularly advantageous for the localization of a lesion seen clearly on only one view and superimposed over dense tissue on the orthogonal view.

The basic principle of stereotaxis is based on movement of the x-ray tube relative to the breast at angles of a fixed degree of obliquity. The technique described here is based on the Siemen's Mammomat 2 stereotactic unit. The breast is compressed and is not moved during the entire procedure. Two 16° oblique spot views of the lesions are made. The radiologist identifies the lesion on each film and places the film onto the computer viewbox. The coordinates on the computer are zeroed, and then the coordinates are moved over the center of the lesion on each oblique view. From this information the computer calculates the X, Y, and Z coordinates of the lesion. The length of needle is chosen and entered into the computer. The stereotactic attachment is then zeroed, thereby moving the needle guides into position. The needle is placed through the guides to the hub, and in this position the tip is within the lesion. Repeat spot oblique views are made to confirm accurate needle placement. For aspiration procedures a coaxial system can be used in order to avoid multiple needle punctures. An outer cannula of 19 or 20 gauge can be placed at the proximal edge of the lesion, and 22-gauge needles are passed through the cannula for aspiration (Fig. 11.7).

Stereotactically guided fine-needle aspiration is of help for small well-defined nodules that are new in comparison with prior examinations and that are not definitely identified as cystic on ultrasound. Fluid can be aspirated from these cysts under stereotactic guidance. Either pneumocystography or follow-up mediolateral and craniocaudal views should be performed to confirm the disappearance of the nodule (Fig. 11.8). Cytology of cysts usually shows apocrine metaplasia.

Needle localizations can be performed rapidly under stereotactic guidance. For localization of a lesion seen well on one view only, stereotaxis is of particular advantage. The oblique views are made with the breast in the position in which the abnormality is seen. During the procedure, radiation exposure to the breast other than the region of the lesion is limited by the spot views. For wire localizations it is important that the wire not be advanced into the needle for final placement. With the breast compressed a slight advancement of the wire can cause the hook to be located deep to the lesion. Once the needle tip is confirmed to be in the lesion, the needle is withdrawn over the wire (Fig. 11.9).

Fine-needle aspiration biopsy (FNAB) under stereotactic guidance is becoming an option for the evaluation of non-palpable solid lesions (39–49). Although most reported series have described the technique as a fine-needle aspiration procedure, there are also reports (50) of stereotactic core biopsies being performed for nonpalpable lesions. Variable results from studies comparing cytology and histology for nonpalpable lesions have demonstrated a relatively high sensitivity and specificity for this procedure. For FNAB to be of value and to be cost effective, it is necessary that lesions that are called ''malignant'' be malignant and that there be no false positives. Otherwise, histologic confirmation would be necessary prior to definitive treatment (Figs. 11.10–11.12). Because of the small size of these lesions, the mixed nature of the aspirate (49), the necessity for highly accurate needle placement, and the technique for aspiration, the numbers of ''insufficient for cytologic analysis'' specimens during FNAB have ranged from 0% (42) to 36% (44), with most series reporting on insufficient sampling in approximately 20% of cases. Stereotactic systems have allowed for improved sampling in comparison with the standard mammographic localization grid system (49). It is important that a comparative analysis of FNAB with histologic analysis be conducted in one's own institution prior to eliminating open biopsies for mammographically identified lesions.

The greatest advantages of FNAB is in the elimination of some open biopsies, but for this advantage to be present, it is critical that the radiologist and cytologist be highly experienced in the procedure. If there should be any false positive diagnoses, then histologic confirmation prior to definitive therapy for ''malignant'' lesions would be necessary. Certainly, FNAB has a definite role in the evaluation of some benign lesions. Small equivocal nodules that are cysts can be aspirated with a high degree of accuracy and need not be subjected to open biopsy. Similarly, an option for lesions that are of low suspicion on mammography, such as ''probable fibroadenomas,'' can be confirmed with cytologic analysis and followed mammographically rather than be resected.

Galactography

Nipple discharge in a nonlactating breast can be produced by a variety of conditions including duct ectasia, fibrocystic disease, inflammation, intraductal papilloma, and intraductal carcinoma. The most common cause of a bloody or serosanguineous discharge at all ages is, however, intraductal papilloma (31). Ductography or galactography can be useful in the evaluation of a spontaneous nipple discharge, particularly when there are no mammographic or physical find-

ings to account specifically for the etiology of the leakage. Although nipple discharge from the nonlactating breast may be white, creamy, clear, greenish, serosanguineous, or bloody, the most significant discharges are those that come from one orifice and are serous, serosanguineous, or bloody. Discharges that are not spontaneous and are expressible only are usually of benign origin and related to fibrocystic disease (51). Galactography is the only method to determine preoperatively the nature, location, and extent of the lesion producing the discharge, and it allows for more precise and limited surgical excision of the area of abnormality.

Galactography is relatively simple to perform. The patient may be seated or supine. A small amount of discharge is expressed from the breast, and the orifice of the duct is identified. The nipple is cleansed with an antiseptic solution, and the breast is draped. A blunt needle, such as a 27-gauge pediatric sialography cannula, is filled with water-soluble radiographic contrast, the duct is cannulated, and the solution is injected. The most difficult step is cannulation of the duct, particularly if it is not dilated. Very gentle placement of the cannula is necessary to avoid penetration of the duct wall and extravasation of contrast. The cannula is taped with Steri-Strips to the nipple. The amount of contrast needed ranges from 0.1 to 3.0 ml and varies with the number of secondary ducts draining into the main lactiferous duct and the degree of dilatation.

While contrast is being injected, the patient is asked to state if she feels the contrast being injected and when she feels tightness or pressure. When she says she feels the tightness or pressure, the injection is terminated, the cannula is left in place, and films are made with mild compression. Should the patient experience pain, indicating possible extravasation of contrast, injection should be terminated. The mammograms are taken in two projections: craniocaudal and mediolateral; magnification views may be of help in the demonstration of intraductal filling defects (52).

The normal ducts converge toward the nipple into dilated ampullae that are then drained by thin (2–3 mm in diameter (51)) distal ductal segments. As the ducts arborize back into the breast, the caliber gradually decreases. The walls of the lumens are smooth, and no beading, angulation, or abrupt narrowing should be present (51).

In duct ectasia or secretory disease, the ducts are dilated, may be tortuous, and may contain filling defects from inspissated secretions (53). The ducts may be up to 8 mm in diameter, and there may be some beading present (51). In simple fibrocystic disease, the ducts may be irregular in diameter, and there may be filling of multiple tiny or even large cysts (53) (Fig. 11.13). In intraductal hyperplasia, multiple small filling defects are seen within the ductal lumen (Fig. 11.14).

Intraductal filling defects may be single or multiple. The etiology of a solitary defect is most often an intraductal papilloma, and these more commonly occur near the nipple-areolar complex (51). It is, therefore, important that the most terminal portion of the duct be filled during galactography to avoid bypassing a small papilloma in the nipple with the cannula. The borders of the papilloma are usually rounded or lobulated, and if the lesion is large, it may completely obstruct the duct (Figs. 11.15 and 11.16). Papillomatosis, like intraductal hyperplasia, produces multiple defects and may appear as irregularity of the luminal wall of the affected duct (53) (Fig. 11.17).

The appearance of intraductal carcinoma on ductography may be a solitary irregular mass, multiple intraluminal fill-ing defects, encasement and abrupt areas of narrowing and dilatation of the duct, distortion of the arborization, and obstruction of the duct lumen (51). In particular, encasement and distortion of irregular ducts are features quite suspicious for malignancy (Figs. 11.18–11.20).

In general, however, one cannot differentiate with certainty benign papillomas or papillomatosis from intraductal malignancy with the finding of a solitary defect or of multiple intraluminal defects. Galactography is important, however, in identifying an intraluminal defect and its exact location for surgical removal.

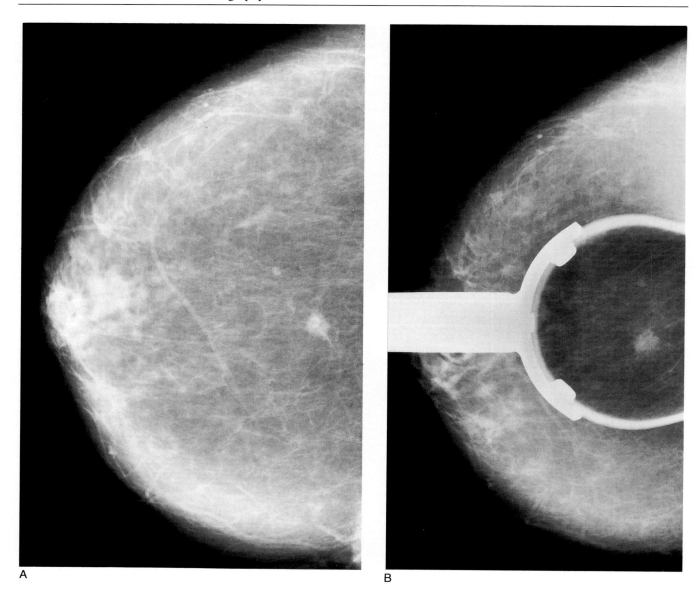

A   B

Figure 11.3.

Clinical: 70-year-old woman for screening mammography.

Mammogram: Left craniocaudal (**A**), spot magnification (**B**), and needle localization (**C–G**) views. There is a high-density spiculated nodule in the upper middle aspect of the left breast (**A** and **B**). The localization grid was placed on the superior aspect of the breast (**C**), and the hole overlying the nodule was identified. A Kopan's needle was placed parallel to the chest into the nodule (**D**). The mediolateral view (**E**) shows the depth of the needle tip relative to the nodule. After removal of the needle, the localization wire is identified in relationship to the nodule (**F** and **G**).

Histopathology: Infiltrating ductal carcinoma.

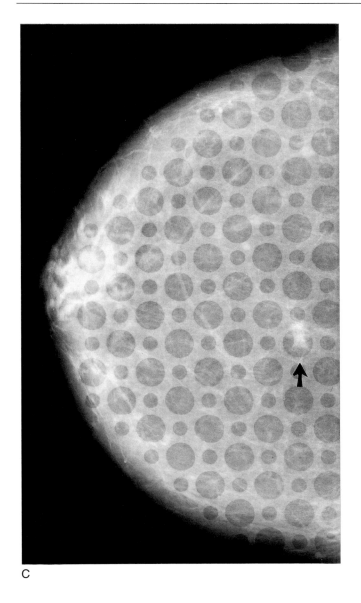

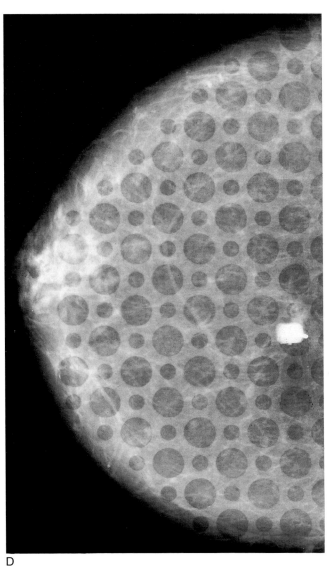

C

D

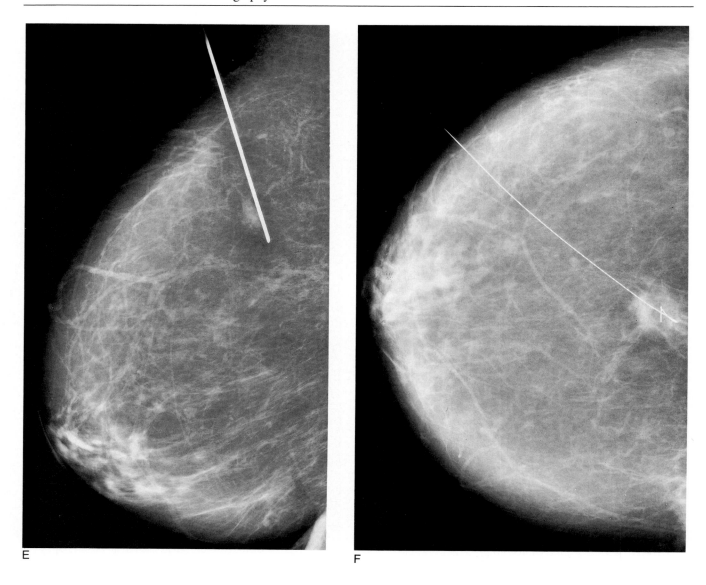

E

F

Figure 11.3. *Continued*

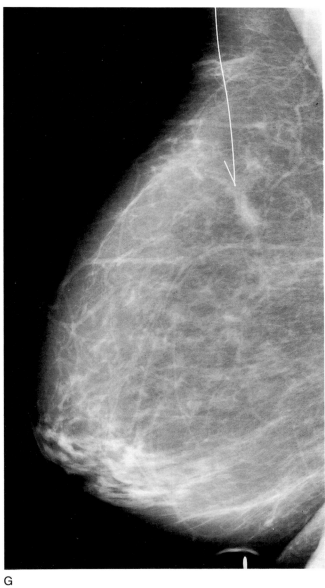

G

Figure 11.4.

Clinical: 56-year-old woman for screening mammography.

Mammogram: Left oblique view (**A**) and specimen film (**B**). A high-density spiculated lesion is present deep in the breast *(curved arrow),* and there are two other areas of nodularity located more superficially *(straight arrows)* (**A**). Between these nodules are extensive ductal-type microcalcifications. These findings are highly suspicious for extensive malignancy, and it is important that the extent of disease be demonstrated. In approaching this patient, it is best to place two wires for needle localization, with one marking the anterior extent of the process, and the other, the more posterior extent of the process (**B**).

Impression: Two needle localization wires placed to mark extensive area of microcalcifications and nodularity, consistent with breast carcinoma.

Histopathology: Infiltrating ductal and extensive intraductal carcinoma.

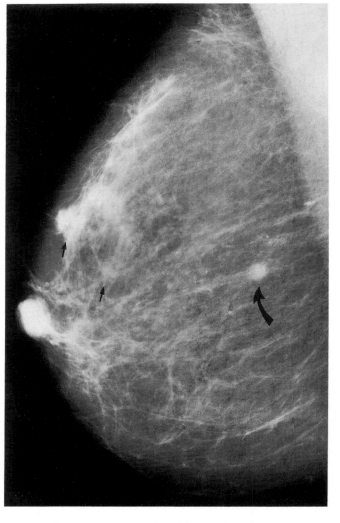

A

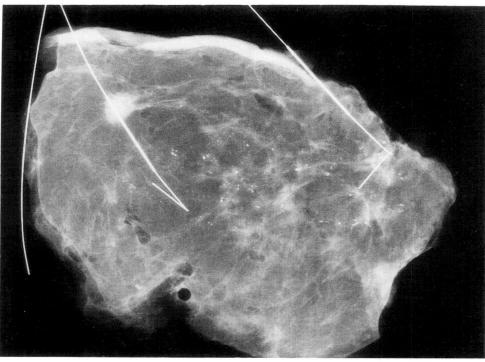

B

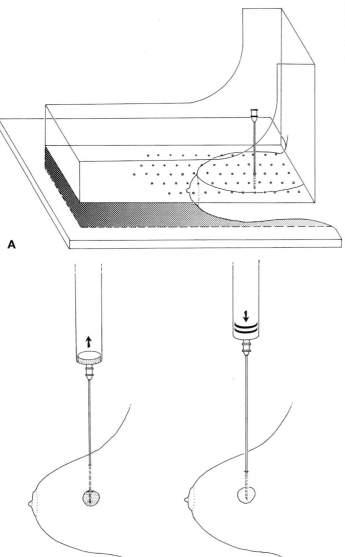

A

B

C

C.H.

Figure 11.5. For pneumocystography, the needle is placed into the breast overlying the lesion to be aspirated (**A**). The needle is slowly withdrawn into the lesion while aspiration is being performed (**B**), and after aspiration is complete, air is injected (**C**).

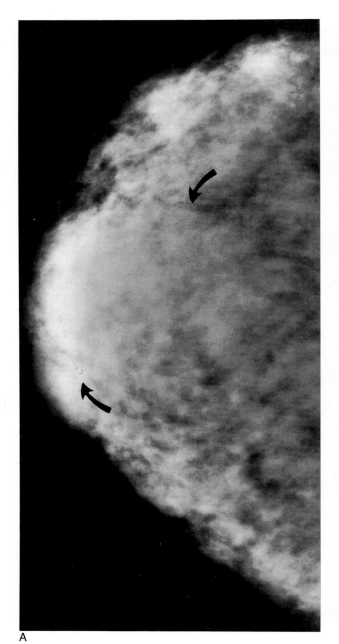
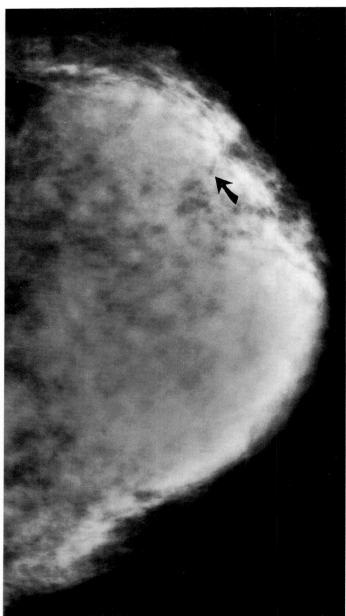

A

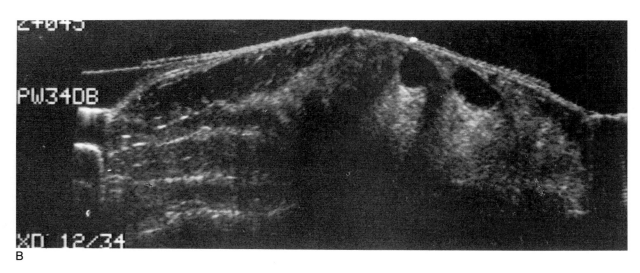

B

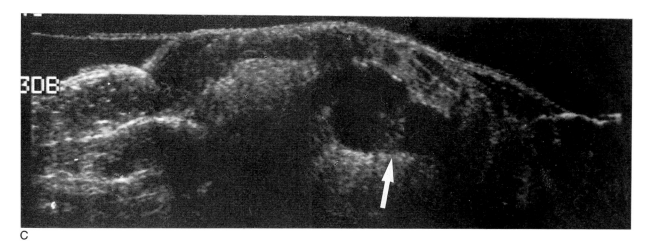

C

Figure 11.6.

Clinical: 39-year-old G0 woman with a nonpainful 5-cm mass in the left breast.

Mammogram: Bilateral craniocaudal views (**A**), ultrasound (**B** and **C**), and left pneumocystogram (**D**). The breasts are very dense and diffusely nodular. There are also areas that are more dense and rounded with halo signs in both breasts *(arrows),* suggesting well-defined masses. Sonography reveals multiple cysts in both breasts (**B**). In the left outer quadrant the palpable mass appears cystic, but there is some irregularity *(arrow)* on the posterior wall (**C**). Because of this finding, cyst aspiration was performed, yielding 45 ml of clear yellowish fluid. Pneumocystography demonstrates loculated areas within the cyst and no intracystic mass (**D**).

Impression: Multilocular cyst, diffuse fibrocystic disease.

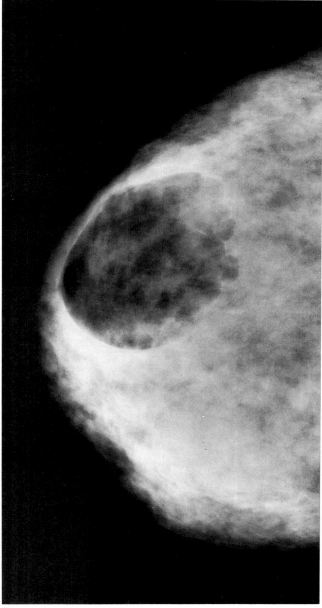

D

Figure 11.7. The patient is in position for a stereotactically guided procedure, and the tube is tilted at a 16° angle relative to the breast (**A**). The oblique spot film is on the computer viewbox, and the coordinates are in the zero position *(arrows)* (**B**). With the film in the same position, the coordinates are placed over the nodule *(arrows)* (**C**). The needle guides are moved into position over the lesion according to the computed X, Y, and Z coordinates (**D**). The needle is placed through the needle guides into the breast, and fine-needle aspiration is performed (**E**).

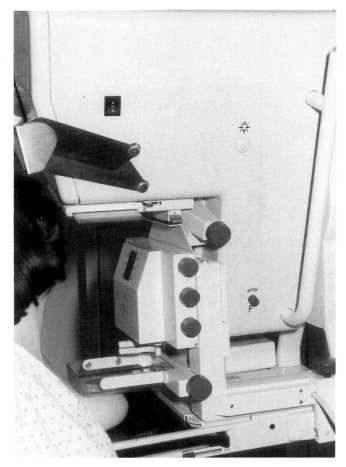

A

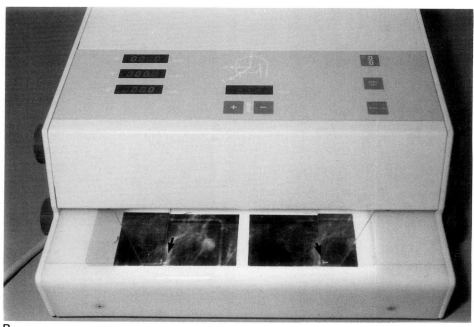

B

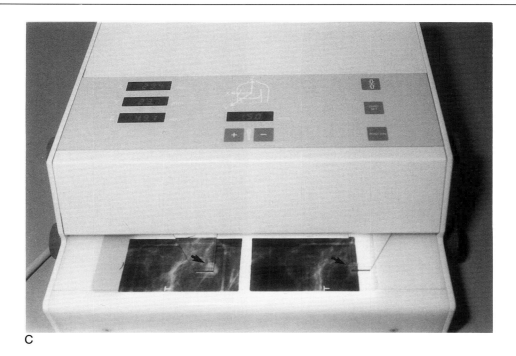

C

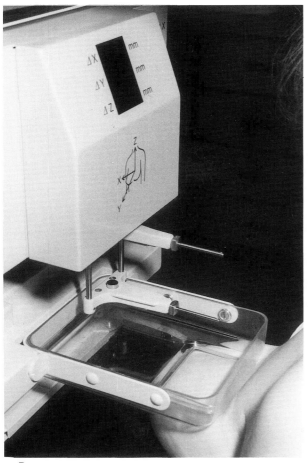

D

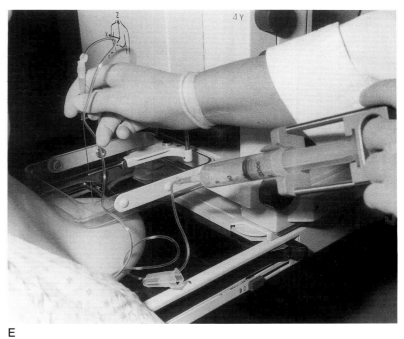

E

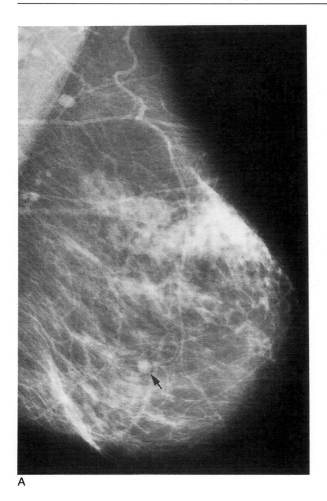

A

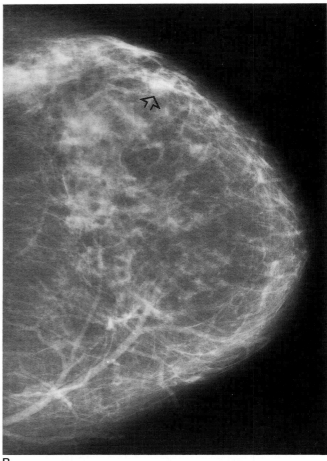

B

Figure 11.8.

Clinical: 64-year-old G3, P2 woman with a positive family history of breast cancer, for screening.

Mammogram: Right oblique (**A**) and craniocaudal (**B**) preliminary views, spot oblique views (**C** and **D**), spot oblique views with needle placement (**E** and **F**) for a stereotactically guided aspiration, and postaspiration oblique (**G**) and craniocaudal (**H**) views. There is a relatively well circumscribed 9-mm medium-density nodule (**A** and **B**) in the right lower outer quadrant *(arrow)*. This nodule had developed since the previous study 3 years earlier. Ultrasound was performed and showed the nodule to contain some internal echoes, and for this reason, stereotactically guided aspiration was performed. Preliminary spot oblique views (**C** and **D**) demonstrate the nodule in the field and a dot marking the nodule *(arrow)* for setting the coordinates of the lesion. Oblique spot views with the needle in place (**E** and **F**) show the needle within the nodule. Aspiration yielded 0.2 ml of clear fluid. Postaspiration films (**G** and **H**) demonstrate complete resolution of the nodule.

Impression: Simple cyst confirmed by stereotactically guided aspiration.

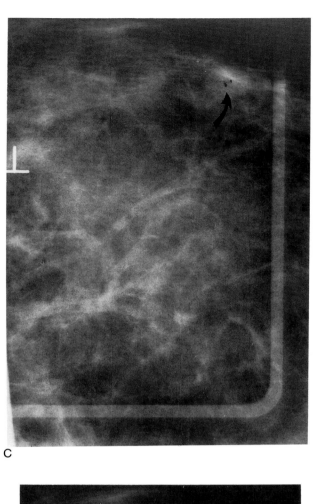

C

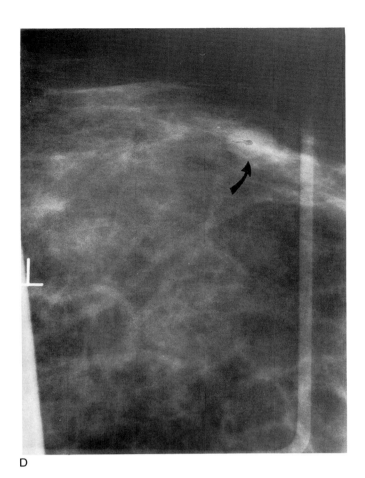

D

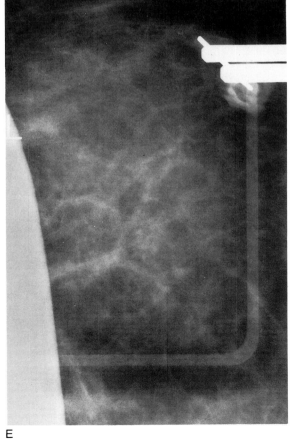

E

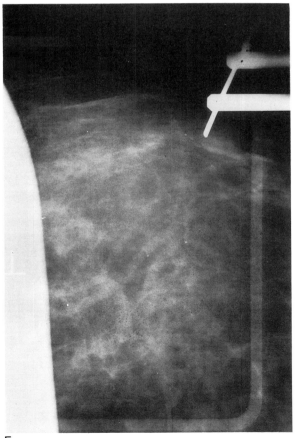

F

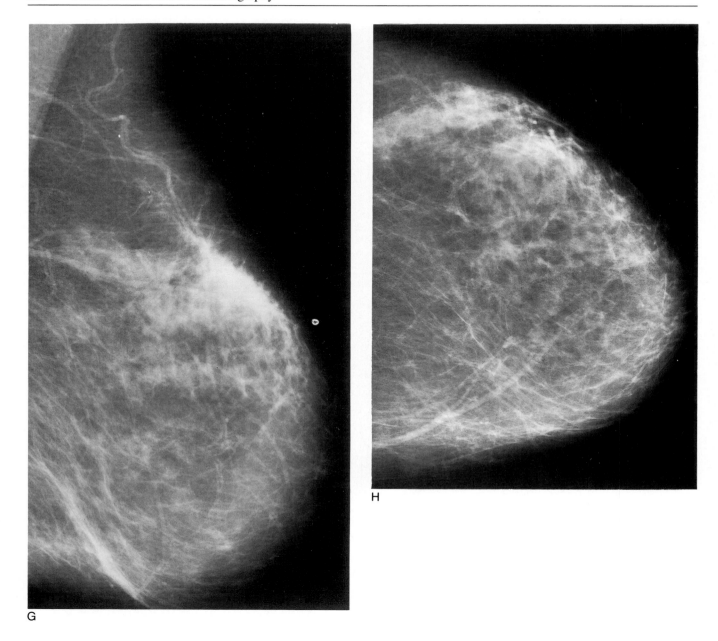

Figure 11.8. *Continued*

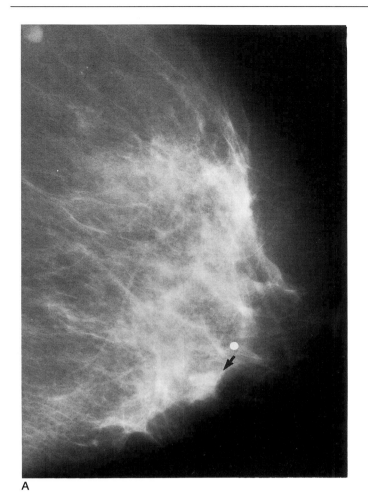

A

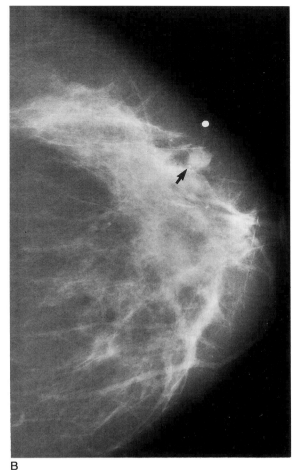

B

Figure 11.9.

Clinical: 44-year-old G3, P3 woman with a family history of breast cancer who had contralateral breast cancer 1 year earlier.

Mammogram: Right oblique (**A**) and craniocaudal (**B**) views, preliminary spot stereotactic view (**C**), oblique stereotactic spot views (**D** and **E**), oblique stereotactic spot views with needle in place (**F** and **G**), and final mediolateral (**H**) and craniocaudal (**I**) views with hookwire in place. On the preliminary films (**A** and **B**) a well-circumscribed nodule *(arrow)* is noted in the lower outer quadrant of the right breast; this nodule had developed since the previous examination. A BB marks a skin lesion near the parenchymal nodule. The lesion was considered suspicious, and a needle localization under stereotactic guidance was performed. The preliminary spot craniocaudal stereotactic view (**C**) shows the nodule *(arrow)* within the field. The two 16° oblique views (**D** and **E**) are made and are used to indicate to the computer the position of the nodule *(straight arrow)* relative to the zero marker *(curved arrow)*. Two 16° oblique views (**F** and **G**) after placement of a localization needle show the needle tip with the nodule *(arrow)*. The final films (**H** and **I**) show accurate hookwire placement within the nodule *(arrow)*.

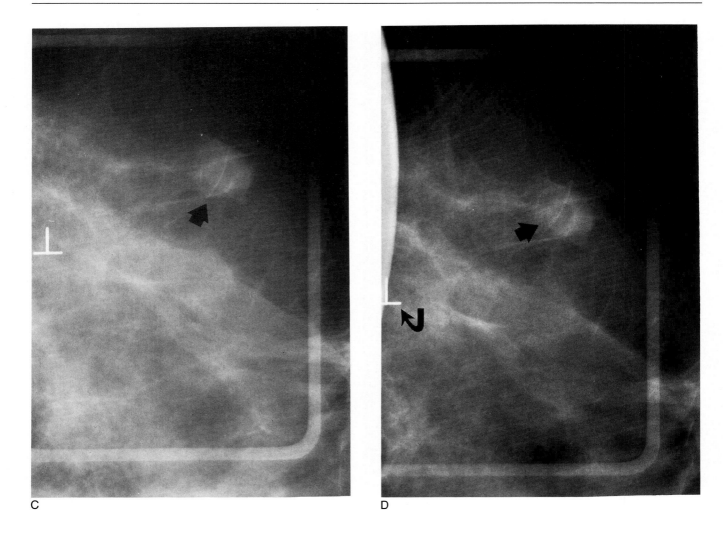

C

D

Figure 11.9. *Continued*

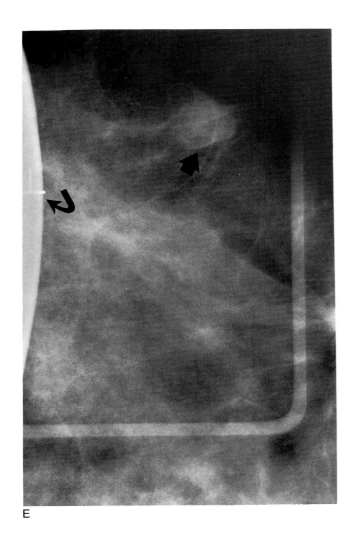

E

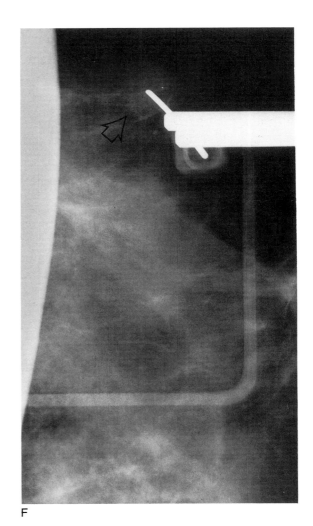

F

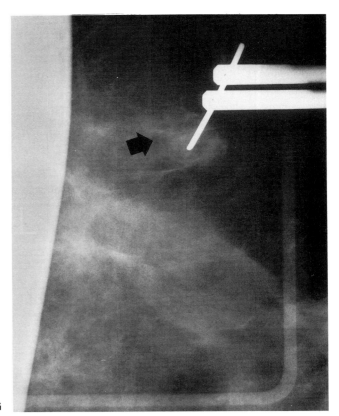

G

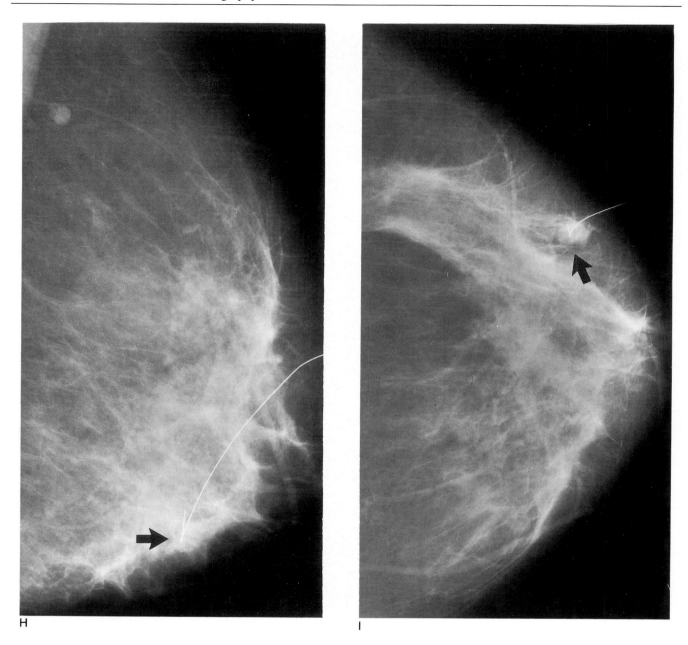

H

I

Figure 11.9. *Continued*

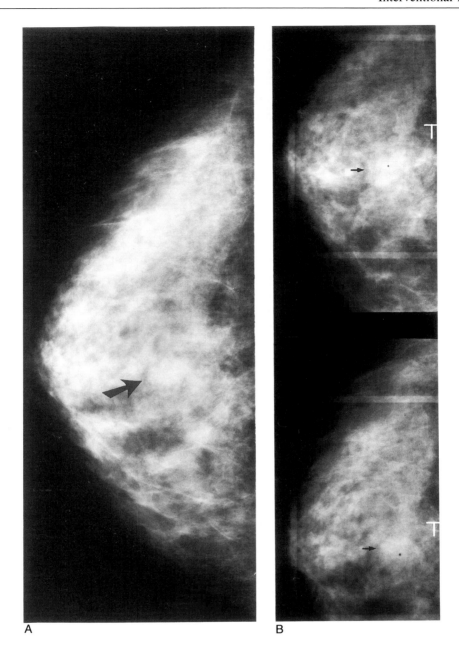

A   B

Figure 11.10.

Clinical: 45-year-old G0 patient for screening; no palpable findings were present on physical examination.

Mammogram: Left craniocaudal view (**A**) and spot oblique views (**B**) from a stereotactically guided fine-needle aspiration. There is a well-circumscribed lobulated nodule *(arrow)* in the central aspect of the left breast that was confirmed to be solid on ultrasound. The mammographic appearance suggests that this is most likely a fibroadenoma. Under ster-

eotactic guidance, fine-needle aspiration of the nodule *(arrows)* was performed (**B**).

Cytology: Benign ductal cells consistent with a fibroadeoma.

Note: Because of the mammographic appearance and the cytology, the lesion was considered to be a fibroadenoma. It was later excised because of the patient's concerns, and histopathology revealed a fibroadenoma.

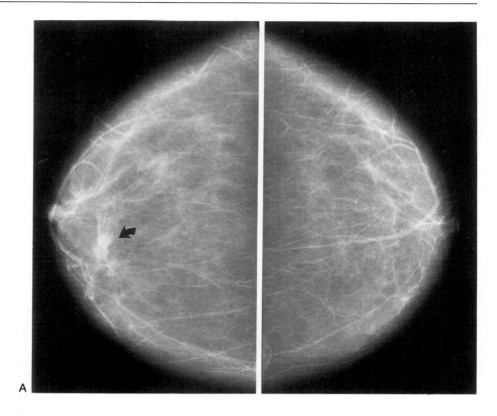

A

Figure 11.11.

Clinical: 67-year-old G0 woman for screening.

Mammogram: Bilateral craniocaudal (**A**), left oblique (**B**), and spot compression (**C**) and stereotactic spot oblique (**D** and **E**) views. In breasts showing otherwise fatty replacement, an irregular nodular density *(arrows)* is noted in the left subareolar area (**A** and **B**). The spot compression view (**C**) dissipates some of the glandular tissue in this area, but a medium- to high-density nodule persists. It is moderately suspicious for malignancy. Fine-needle aspiration of the area was performed under stereotactic guidance. The 16° oblique stereotactic views (**D** and **E**) show the needle tip within the lesion *(arrows)*.

Cytology: Positive for carcinoma.

Note: Lumpectomy was performed, and histologic examination showed intraductal carcinoma and a focus of infiltrating ductal carcinoma. The patient was further treated with radiotherapy.

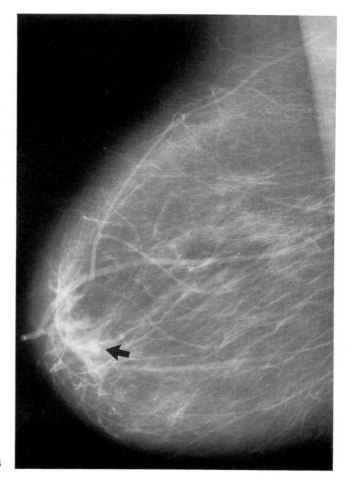

B

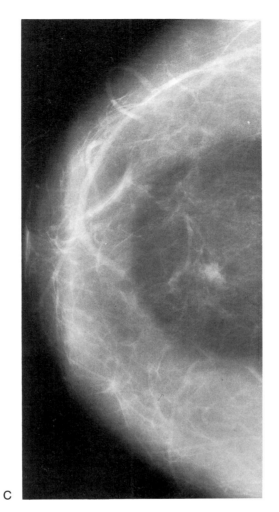

C

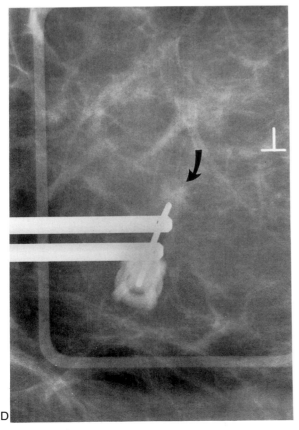

D

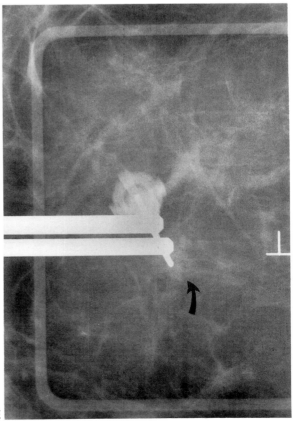

E

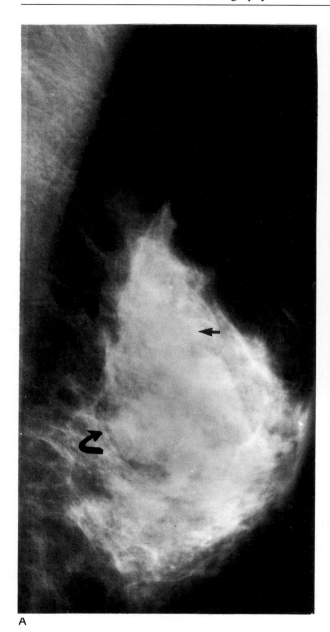

A

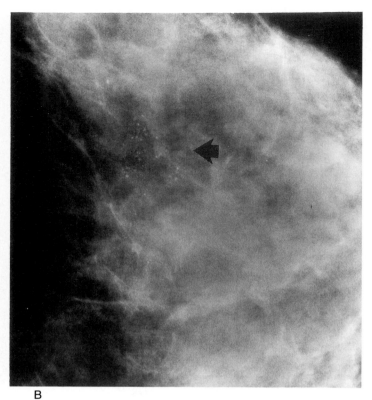

B

Figure 11.12.

Clinical: 47-year-old woman referred because of an abnormal mammogram and a vague palpable thickening in the right breast superiorly.

Mammogram: Right oblique (**A**) and magnification (2×) craniocaudal (**B**) views. The background parenchymal pattern is dense for the patient's age. There are clustered microcalcifications in the superior aspect of the breast (**A**) *(arrow)* that on magnification (**B**) are quite irregular and of mixed size and shape. The mammographic appearance is highly suspicious for carcinoma. Incidental note (**A**) is made of a circumscribed medium-density mass *(curved arrow)* inferior to the calcifications, which was shown on ultrasound to be a simple cyst. The calcifications were approached by mammographically guided fine-needle aspiration. Cytology was suspicious for carcinoma. Needle localization was performed prior to excision for confirmation of the diagnosis.

Histopathology: Comedocarcinoma.

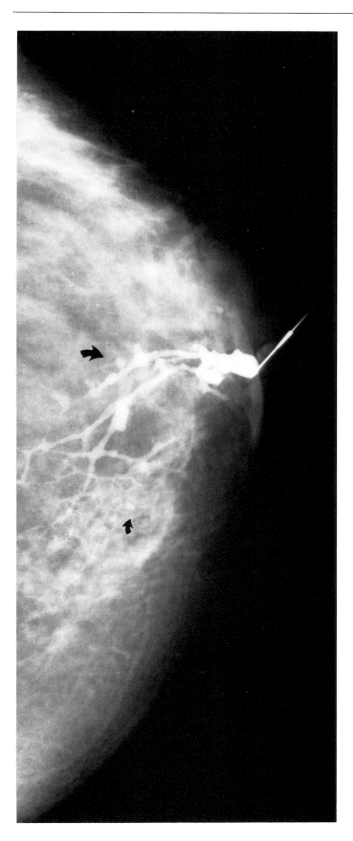

Figure 11.13.

Clinical: 41-year-old G2 woman with a history of fibrocystic disease and cysts, presenting with a clear right nipple discharge.

Mammogram: Right craniocaudal galactogram. There is normal arborization of the ducts from the orifice cannulated. There is moderate duct ectasia of the major ducts, where normally the caliber is much finer. There is also filling of some microcysts *(arrows)*. No intraluminal masses are seen.

Impression: Mild ductal dilatation with microcysts.

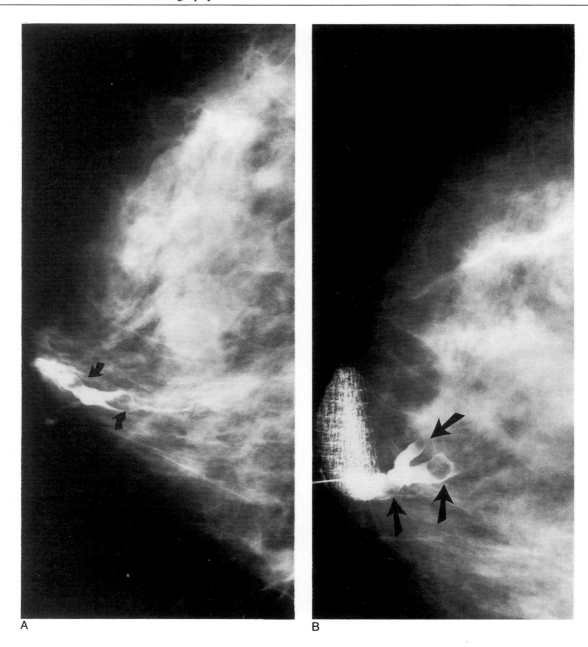

A

B

Figure 11.14.

Clinical: 72-year-old G3, P3 woman with a bloody left nipple discharge.

Mammogram: Left galactogram mediolateral (**A**) and magnification (2×) (**B**) views. The left breast is very dense for the patient's age. No abnormalities were noted on routine mammography. Galactography was performed because of the nipple discharge; however, only a small amount of contrast could be injected without retrograde flow. On galactography, there are at least three intraductal filling defects *(arrows)* that persisted. There was incomplete filling of the duct system drained by this major duct. The filling defects are rather smooth, and there is no encasement present, suggesting more likely a benign etiology. However, the termination of the duct lumen is of some concern. The differential diagnosis includes papillomas, papillomatosis, duct hyperplasia, and intraductal carcinoma.

Impression: Intraluminal filling defects of uncertain nature, favoring a benign process.

Histopathology: Atypical ductal hyperplasia.

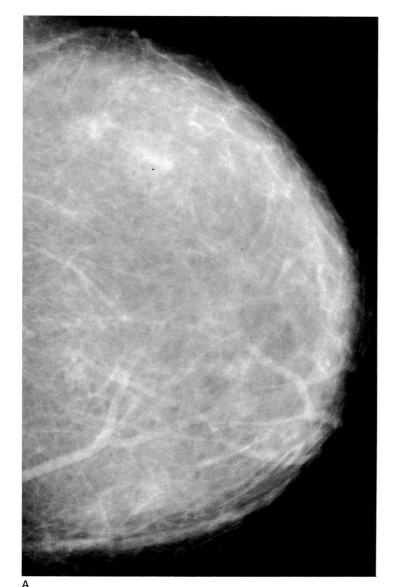

A

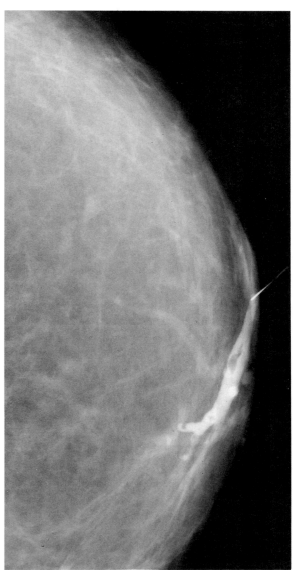

B

Figure 11.15.

Clinical: 46-year-old premenopausal woman with a serosanguineous right nipple discharge.

Mammogram: Right craniocaudal view (**A**) and galactogram (**B** and **C**). No abnormalities are seen on mammography. On the galactogram (**B** and **C**), a persistent irregular polypoid intraluminal filling defect is present in a main lactiferous duct. Intraductal papilloma is most likely, but also included in the differential diagnosis are clot, inspissated lactiferous material, and intraductal papillary carcinoma.

Impression: Filling defect, probable intraductal papilloma.

Histopathology: Intraductal papilloma.

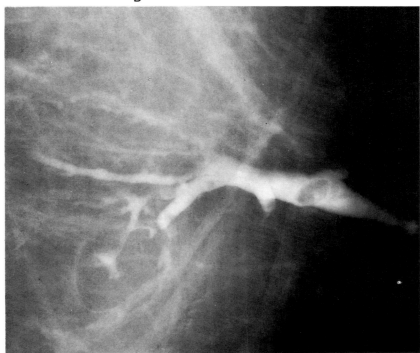

C

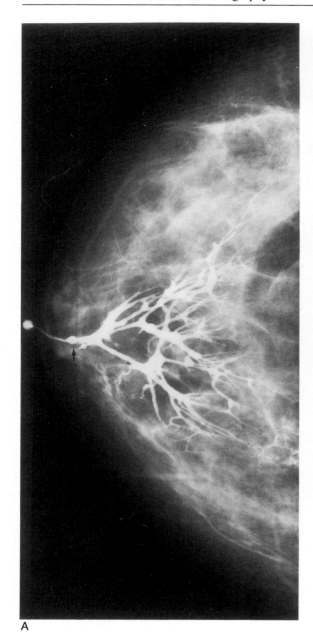

A

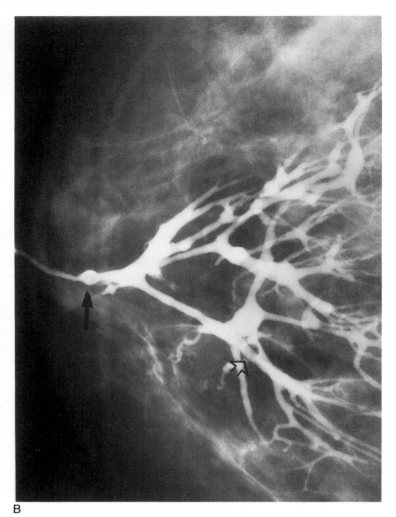

B

Figure 11.16.

Clinical: 38-year-old woman with a bloody left nipple discharge.

Mammogram: Left craniocaudal view from galactography (**A**) and enlarged (2×) craniocaudal view (**B**). The cannulated duct arborizes into mildly dilated lactiferous ducts. There is a solitary filling defect approximately 1 cm deep to the nipple *(closed arrow)*. This defect expands the duct and is well circumscribed and persistent. A second well-circumscribed defect is seen more peripherally in the medial aspect of the breast *(open arrow)* (**B**), and this was found to represent an air bubble. The subareolar lesion is consistent with an intraductal lesion. The differential diagnosis includes an intraductal papilloma, hyperplasia, or carcinoma (less likely).

Histopathology: Intraductal papilloma.

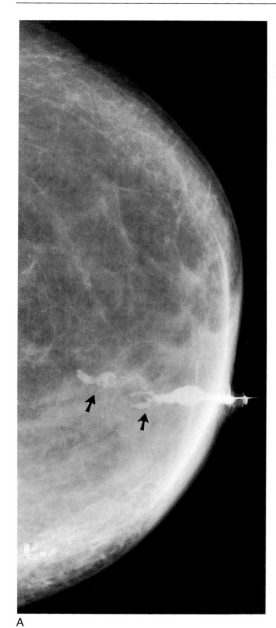

A

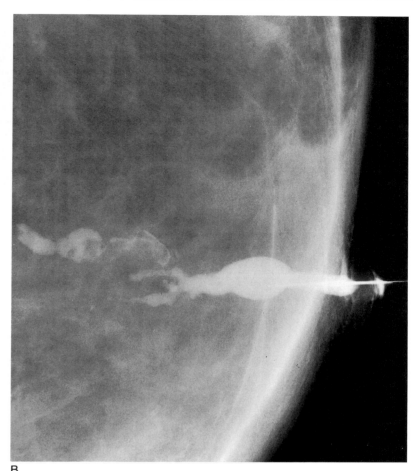

B

Figure 11.17.

Clinical: 58-year-old woman with chronic renal failure who developed a spontaneous bloody left nipple discharge.

Mammogram: Left galactogram (**A**) and magnified image (**B**). The breast is edematous related to the renal failure. The cannulated duct is dilated, and there is an irregular filling defect *(arrows)* extending over a 1.5-cm segment of duct with distal dilatation of the duct. The finding most likely represents a large papilloma or papillomatosis, but intraductal carcinoma cannot be excluded.

Impression: Intraluminal filling defect, favoring papilloma.

Histopathology: Marked intraductal hyperplasia and papillomatosis.

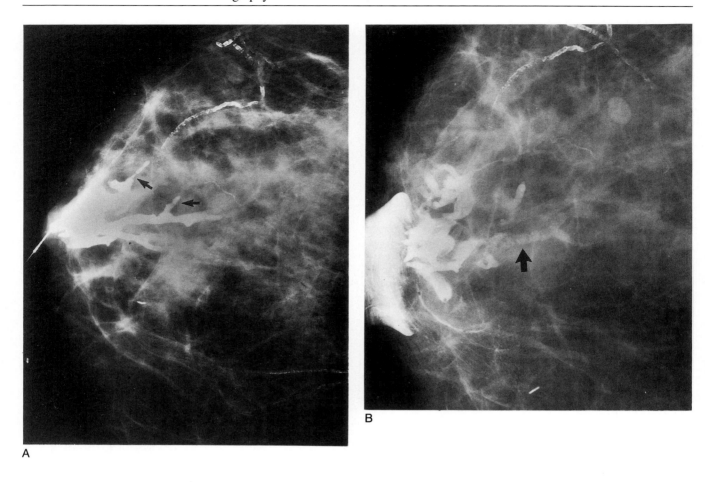

A

B

Figure 11.18.

Clinical: 78-year-old G4, P4 woman with a bloody discharge from the left nipple.

Mammogram: Left craniocaudal (**A**) and magnification (2×) craniocaudal (**B**) views from a galactogram. The cannulated duct and its branches are dilated in the subareolar area. There are multiple areas of encasement *(arrows)* with narrowing and changes in caliber (**A**), as well as irregular filling defects *(ar-*

row) (**B**) and areas of abrupt termination of the lactiferous ducts. These findings are highly suggestive of intraductal carcinoma.

Impression: Extensive intraductal carcinoma.

Histopathology: Intraductal carcinoma, solid and cribriform varieties.

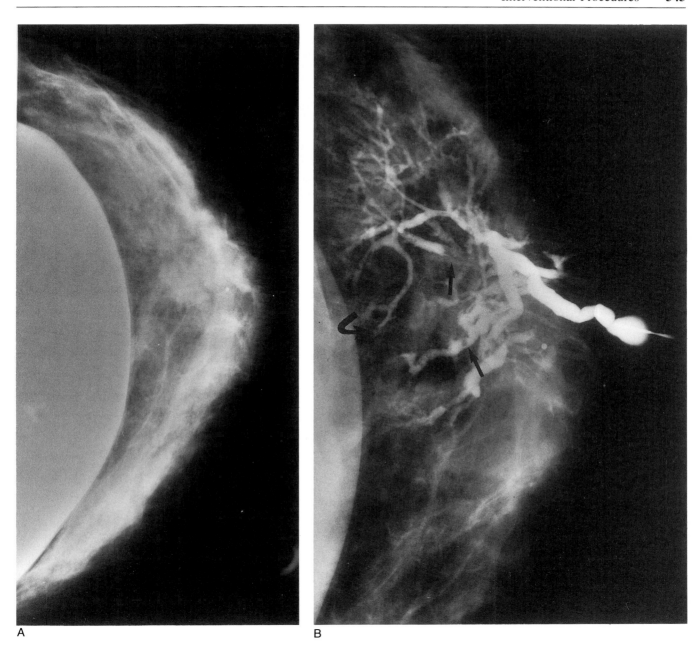

A   B

Figure 11.19.

Clinical: 39-year-old G3, P4 woman with a bloody right nipple discharge.

Mammogram: Right craniocaudal (**A**) and magnification (1.5×) craniocaudal (**B**) views from a galactogram. On the initial film (**A**) a breast implant is noted, and there is a moderate amount of overlying glandular tissue without focal suspicious findings. On the galactogram (**B**) the injected ducts are mildly dilated. There are multiple irregular filling defects *(straight arrows)* and some areas of abrupt termination *(curved arrow)* of the ductal lumen. The filling defects could represent papillomatosis, hyperplasia, or carcinoma, but the finding of the abrupt terminations is more suspicious for intraductal carcinoma.

Impression: Multiple filling defects suspicious for intraductal carcinoma.

Histopathology: Intraductal carcinoma.

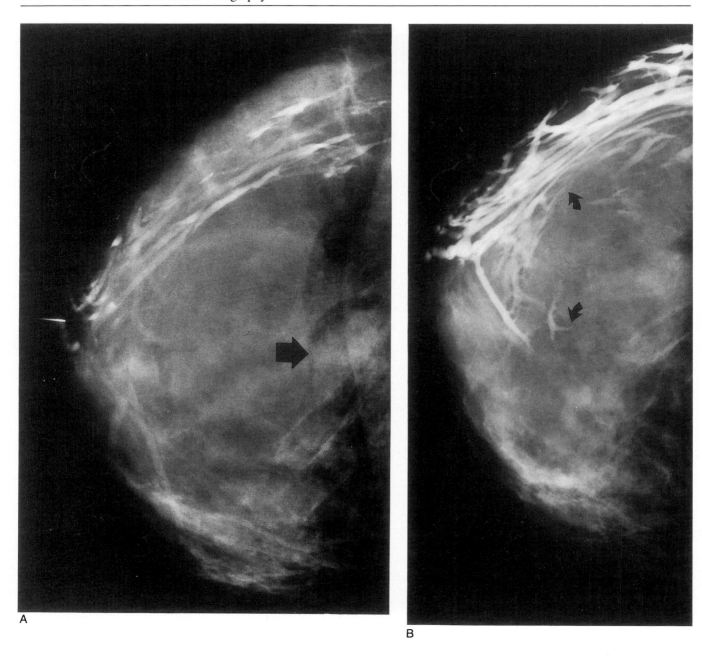

A

B

Figure 11.20.

Clinical: 33-year-old woman with a 2-cm palpable mass at the 6 o'clock position in the left breast and bloody left nipple discharge.

Mammogram: Left craniocaudal views with early filling (**A**) and with late filling (**B**) during galactography. On the initial film (**A**) the breast is very dense, consistent with the patient's age. There is a multinodular mass *(arrow)* deep in the breast, corresponding to the palpable lesion and suspicious for carcinoma. It is important to evaluate the patient via galactography, because the lesion lies very deep in the breast and

the nipple discharge suggests the possibility of intraductal extension. On the galactogram (**B**), there is a straightening of the ducts, with multiple areas of narrowing and abrupt termination *(arrows)* suspicious for intraductal extension of tumor.

Impression: Probable carcinoma with extensive intraductal extension.

Histopathology: Infiltrating ductal carcinoma, extensive intraductal carcinoma, and comedocarcinoma.

References

1. Kalisher L. An improved needle for localization of nonpalpable breast lesions. Radiology 1978;128:815–817.
2. Edeiken S, Suer WD, Vitale SF, et al. Needle localization of nonpalpable breast lesions using methylene blue. Breast Dis 1990;3:75–80.
3. Raininko R, Linna MI, Rasanen O. Preoperative localization of nonpalpable breast tumours. Acta Chir Scand 1976;142:575–578.
4. Kopans DB, DeLuca S. A modified needle-hookwire technique to simplify preoperative localization of occult breast lesions. Radiology 1980;134:781.
5. Homer MJ. Nonpalpable breast lesions localization using a curved-end retractable wire. Radiology 1985;157:259–260.
6. Goldberg RP, Hall FM, Simon M. Preoperative localization of nonpalpable breast lesions using a wire marker and perforated mammographic grid. Radiology 1983;146:833–835.
7. Snyder RE. Specimen radiography and preoperative localization of nonpalpable breast cancer. Cancer 1980;46:950–956.
8. Stomper PC, Davis SP, Sonnenfeld MR, et al. Efficacy of specimen radiography of clinically occult noncalcified breast lesions. AJR 1988;151:43–47.
9. Rebner M, Pennes DR, Baker DE, et al. Two view specimen radiography in surgical biopsy of nonpalpable breast masses. AJR 1987;149:283–285.
10. Sistrom C, Abbitt PL, Shaw de Paredes E. Hematoma of the breast: a complication of needle localization. Va Med 1988;115(2):78–79.
11. Davis PS, Wechsler RJ, Feig SA, March DE. Migration of breast biopsy localization wire. AJR 1988;150:787–788.
12. Kopans DB, Gallagher WJ, Swann CA, et al. Does preoperative needle localization lead to an increase in local breast cancer recurrence? Radiology 1988;167:667–668.
13. Robertson CL, Kopans DB, McCarthy KA, Hart NE. Nonpalpable lesions in the augmented breast: preoperative localization. Radiology 1989;173:873–874.
14. Eklund GW, Busby RC, Miller SH, Job JS. Improved imaging of the augmented breast. AJR 1988;151:469–473.
15. Libshitz HI, Feig SA, Fetouh S. Needle localization of nonpalpable breast lesions. Radiology 1976;121:557–560.
16. Hall FM, Frank HA. Preoperative localization of nonpalpable breast lesions. AJR 1979;132:101–105.
17. Peyster RG, Kalisher L. Needle localization of nonpalpable lesions of the breast. Surg Gynecol Obstet 1979;148:703–706.
18. Gisvold JJ, Martin JK Jr. Prebiopsy localization of nonpalpable breast lesions. AJR 1984;143:477–481.
19. Oppedal BR, Drevvatne T. Radiographic diagnosis of nonpalpable breast lesions: correlation to pathology. Acta Radiol (Diagn) 1983;24:259–265.
20. Meyer JE, Kopans DB, Stomper PC, Lindfors KK. Occult breast abnormalities: percutaneous preoperative needle localization. Radiology 1984;150:335–337.
21. Hoehn JL, Hardacre JM, Swanson MK, Williams GH. Localization of occult breast lesions. Cancer 1982;49:1142–1144.
22. Yankaskas BC, Knelson MH, Abernathy ML, et al. Needle localization biopsy of occult lesions of the breast: experience in 199 cases. Invest Radiol 1988;23:729–733.
23. Hall FM, Storella JM, Silverstone DZ, Wyshak G. Nonpalpable breast lesions: recommendations for biopsy based on suspicion of carcinoma at mammography. Radiology 1988;167:353–358.
24. Ciatto S, Cataliotti L, Distante V. Nonpalpable breast lesions detected with mammography: review of 512 consecutive cases. Radiology 1987;165:99–102.
25. Rosenberg AL, Schwartz GF, Feig SA, Patchefsky AS. Clinically occult breast lesions: localization and significance. Radiology 1987;162:167–170.
26. Rubin E, Visscher DW, Alexander RW, et al. Proliferative disease and atypia in biopsies performed for nonpalpable lesions detected mammographically. Cancer 1988;161:2077–2082.
27. Hallgrimsson P, Karesen R, Artun K, Skjennald A. Nonpalpable breast lesions: diagnostic criteria and preoperative localization. Acta Radiol 1988;29:285–288.
28. Meyer JE, Sonnenfeld MR, Greene RA, Stomper PC. Preoperative localization of clinically occult breast lesions: experience at a referral hospital. Radiology 1988;169:627–628.
29. Hermann G, Janus C, Schwartz IS, et al. Nonpalpable breast lesions: accuracy of prebiopsy mammographic diagnosis. Radiology 1987;165:323–326.
30. Tabar L, Pentek Z, Dean PB. The diagnostic and therapeutic value of breast cyst puncture and pneumocystography. Radiology 1981;141:659–663.
31. Haagenson CD. Disease of the breast. Philadelphia: WB Saunders, 1971.
32. Gatchell FG, Dockerty MB, Clagett OT. Intracystic carcinoma of the breast. Surg Gynecol Obstet 1958;106:347–352.
33. Hoeffken W, Hintzen C. Die Diagnostik der Mammazysten durch Mammographie and Pneumozystographie. ROFO 1970;112:9–18.
34. Fornage BD, Faroux MJ, Simatos A. Breast masses: ultrasound-guided fine-needle aspiration biopsy. Radiology 1987;162:409–414.
35. Wanebo HJ, Feldman PS, Wilhelm MC, et al. Fine needle aspiration cytology in lieu of open biopsy in management of primary breast cancer. Ann Surg 1984;199:569–579.
36. Palombini L, Fulciniti F, Vetrani A, et al. Fine needle aspiration biopsy of breast masses. Cancer 1988;61:2273–2277.
37. Kopans DB. Fine-needle aspiration of clinically occult breast lesions. Radiology 1989;170:313–314.
38. Lee KR, Foster RS, Papillo JL. Fine needle aspiration of the breast: importance of aspirator. Acta Cytol 1987;31:281–84.
39. Ciatto S, Del Turco MR, Bravetti P. Nonpalpable breast lesions: stereotaxic fine-needle aspiration cytology. Radiology 1989;173:57–59.
40. Dowlatshahi K, Gent HJ, Schmidt R, et al. Nonpalpable breast tumors: diagnosis with stereotaxic localization and fine-needle aspiration. Radiology 1989;170:427–433.
41. Masood S, Frykberg ER, McLellan GL, et al. Prospective evaluation of radiologically directed fine-needle aspiration biopsy of nonpalpable breast lesions. Cancer 1990;66:1480–1487.
42. Fajardo LL, Davis JR, Wiens JJ, Trego DC. Mammography-guided stereotactic fine-needle aspiration cytology of nonpal-

pable breast lesions: prospective comparison with surgical biopsy results. AJR 1990;155:977–981.

43. Azavedo E, Svane G, Auer G. Stereotactic fine-needle biopsy in 2594 mammographically detected non-palpable lesions. Lancet 1989;1:1033–1035.

44. Lofgren M, Andersson I, Bondeson L, Lindholm K. X-ray guided fine-needle aspiration for the cytologic diagnosis of nonpalpable breast lesions. Cancer 1988;61:1032–1037.

45. Dent DM, Kirkpatrick AE, McGoogan E, et al. Stereotaxic localization and aspiration cytology of impalpable breast lesions. Clin Radiol 1989;40:380–382.

46. Evans WP, Cade SH. Needle localization and fine-needle aspiration biopsy of nonpalpable breast lesions with use of standard and stereotactic equipment. Radiology 1989;173:53–56.

47. Hann L, Ducatman BS, Wang HH, et al. Nonpalpable breast lesions: evaluation by means of fine-needle aspiration cytology. Radiology 1989;171:373–376.

48. Bibbo M, Scheiber M, Cajulis R, et al. Stereotaxic fine needle aspiration cytology of clinically occult malignant and premalignant breast lesions. Acta Cytol 1988;32:193–201.

49. Lofgren M, Andersson I, Lindholm K. Stereotactic fine-needle aspiration for cytologic diagnosis of nonpalpable breast lesions. AJR 1990;154:1191–1195.

50. Lovin JD, Parker SH, Jobe WE. Stereotactic percutaneous core biopsy: technical adaption and initial experience. Breast Dis 1990;3:135–143.

51. Threatt B. Ductography. In: Bassett LW, Gold RH, eds. Mammography, thermography and ultrasound in breast cancer detection. New York: Grune & Stratton, 1982.

52. Tabar L, Dean PB, Pentek Z. Galactography: the diagnostic procedure of choice for nipple discharge. Radiology 1983; 149:31–38.

53. Diner WC. Galactography: mammary duct contrast examination. AJR 1981;137:853–856.

THE POSTSURGICAL BREAST

A wide variety of mammographic findings are seen after surgical procedures on the breast. Surgical procedures including fine-needle aspirations, excisional breast biopsy, wide excision or segmental mastectomy, subcutaneous or modified radical mastectomy with reconstruction, augmentation, or reduction mammoplasty, and lumpectomy with radiation therapy produce a spectrum of classical and unusual findings. Critical to an accurate analysis of a mammogram and to determination that findings are of postsurgical origin is knowledge of the history and clinical examination of the patient.

It is of help to place a wire or BB marker on the skin to avoid repeating films because of uncertainty about positions of scars. If this is not done, then it is absolutely necessary that the technologist be responsible for clearly marking the location and orientation of any scars on a drawing of the breast. Additionally, it is equally important to document the location and size of any palpable masses and particularly their relationship to the surgical scar (Fig. 12.1).

In interpreting a mammogram of a postsurgical breast it is important for the radiologist to compare present studies with previous studies regarding the location and appearance of the mammographic abnormalities biopsied and the confirmation of mammographic abnormalities on the specimen film.

Postbiopsy Changes

After a fine-needle aspiration of a breast lesion, there may be irregular increased density at the site from edema and hematoma formation. Unless there is significant bleeding during the aspiration, the changes are subtle; nonetheless, it is best to perform imaging prior to any interventional procedures. If there is a puncture of a vessel during an aspiration, a large hematoma may form. If the hematoma dissects through the tissue, an amorphous ill-defined density is seen. If it is more loculated, then the appearance is that of a relatively circumscribed mass.

The mammographic findings associated with excisional biopsy are localized to the area of the biopsy site. It is, therefore, important to correlate the position of the scar to the mammographic findings and to be aware of the temporal changes that are expected postsurgically. In a study of 1049

breast biopsies, Sickles and Herzog (1) found mammographic abnormalities attributed to postsurgical changes in 474 (45%). Normal postsurgical changes include: localized skin thickening or retraction, an asymmetric glandular defect, architectural distortion, contour deformity of the breast, hematoma and fat necrosis formation, parenchymal scarring, calcifications of fibrosis, fat necrosis and sutures, and opaque foreign bodies (1, 2).

Skin thickening is localized to the biopsy site unless there is superimposed infection, in which case a more generalized thickening is present. A contour deformity may be associated with the skin thickening. Skin thickening is maximum on mammography during the first 6 months after biopsy and gradually diminishes.

A hematoma may be seen at the biopsy site on a mammogram performed soon after biopsy. Postoperative hematomas or seromas are seen more commonly if a drain has not been placed and may actually be related to an improved cosmetic result with a lesser degree of contour deformity (3). On mammography, fluid collections are usually relatively circumscribed medium- to high-density masses and may range from 2 to 10 cm in diameter (Fig. 12.2). In a series of postlumpectomy patients who were referred for radiotherapy, Mendelson (3) found postoperative fluid collections in 47%. On ultrasound, hematomas are relatively smooth and anechoic but may contain some internal echoes or debris, depending on the degree of organization. Because these may contain debris if they are not infected, the clinical findings are of more help to suggest the presence of superimposed infection.

Areas of architectural disturbance are a common finding after surgery and include asymmetric decrease in glandular tissue from resection, which does not change over time (1), architectural distortion, and focal increased density or parenchymal scar and fat necrosis. On resolution of a hematoma it is usual to see some residual irregular increased density and/or distortion (Figs. 12.3–12.5). Architectural distortion was the second most common postsurgical finding after skin thickening by Sickles and Herzog (1) in the evaluation of 474 postoperative breasts. The changes of increased density and architectural distortion are maximum at 0–6 months after surgery and gradually diminish over time (1). When one is interpreting a stellate density as a postsurgical change, it is important to review the mammogram prior to biopsy to confirm that the lesion removed was in fact in the area of concern and, if nonpalpable, was present in the specimen (Fig. 12.6). The most helpful factor that can aid one in making the diagnosis of "postsurgical change" is a mammogram at 3–6 months after biopsy (1). This is particularly important when the biopsy demonstrated an atypical lesion.

Calcifications of fat necrosis form at a variable time after biopsy but usually later than 6 months. These calcifications are typically ringlike, with lucent centers, and may be small (liponecrosis microcystica calcificans) or larger oil cysts— radiolucent masses with calcified rims (Figs. 12.7–12.9). Occasionally, fat necrosis may be associated with clumps of irregular but rather coarse microcalcifications. Other forms of calcification that occur postoperatively include ringlike dermal calcifications in the scar and calcified sutures, which are in linear or knot shapes (Fig. 12.10) (2, 4).

Foreign bodies left in the breast inadvertently include surgical clips (Fig. 12.11), often used for marking a tumor bed for location of a boost dose of radiotherapy and sutures that may calcify. Inadvertent transection of a needle localization wire and lack of its retrieval will result in the observation of a small segment of wire in the breast (Fig. 12.12). Another cause of an iatrogenic foreign body in the breast is the inadvertent severing of the tip or cuff of a central venous catheter for chemotherapy, which may be embedded in the upper inner aspect of the breast (5) (Fig. 12.13).

The Augmented Breast

Approximately 150,000 women in the United States undergo an augmentation mammoplasty annually. The augmented breast presents a challenge to the radiologist to image the residual parenchyma adequately and to detect any abnormalities. Fortunately, most women in the United States who have had augmentation mammoplasty have undergone placement of implants rather than direct silicone or paraffin injection. Augmentation may be performed for cosmetic reasons—to increase the size of both breasts or, unilaterally, for an asymmetric hypoplastic breast or after mastectomy for reconstruction. Augmentation procedures have included direct injection of silicone or paraffin into the breast, placement of a variety of types of implants in either a subpectoral or retroglandular location, and the use of several types of myocutaneous flaps for reconstruction.

Many patients seen in the United States with augmentation by direct injection have had the procedure performed in the Orient or Mexico (6). Because of the intense response to the foreign material, management of the patient is quite difficult. Clinically, the breasts are quite hard or lumpy, and the exclusion of a tumor by palpation is impossible (6). Par-

sons and Thering (6) found that mastodynia was the most common presenting symptom in 28 patients with silicone-injected breasts. Another problem these patients face is the tendency for the silicone to migrate far outside the breasts (7). Histologically, the silicone incites areas of fat necrosis, infiltration with fibrocytes, and cystlike spaces lined by fibrous tissue (7). There may be hyaline degeneration with calcification of the inner surface of the fibrous capsule of the siliconoma (8). The calcification may represent deposition of calcium and phosphates near necrotic tissue (8).

Mammography is markedly limited in these patients because the breasts are thick and hard and therefore difficult to compress well (Fig. 12.14). The injected substance and the fibrous response create a very dense appearance requiring a long exposure. Technically, by increasing the kVp to 30 or 32, one is sometimes able to penetrate the breasts adequately.

Koide and Katayama (8) found differences in the mammographic findings in breasts augmented by injection, depending on the substance used for injection. In patients who had paraffin injections, radiolucent masses were seen; 75% of these patients developed extensive small annular calcifications, and lymphadenopathy was common. In patients who received silicone injections, the mammographic nodules were of high density, and 29% of these women were found to have large localized eggshell calcifications in the breasts. Others (9, 10) have found, in patients with silicone injections, calcifications in patterns varying from irregular to small ringlike, to eggshell shaped.

Implants used for augmentation have included saline filled, silicone gel, inflatable double lumen, and polyurethane coated (11, 12). Implants may be placed beneath the pectoralis major muscle or may be located anteriorly, in the retroglandular area (Figs. 12.15 and 12.16). The imaging of a patient with implants is limited, in that on routine mammography the devices may obscure large areas of glandular tissue. The use of manual techniques (13) rather than phototiming is usually of help in imaging these patients. Eklund et al. (14) have described a modified positioning technique in which the implant is displaced posteriorly and the breast tissue is pulled anteriorly as compression is applied. This technique allows for improved compression and visualization of the parenchyma (Figs. 12.17–12.19). This technique is more easily performed on patients with a moderate amount of native tissue over the implant or in patients with subpectoral implants. The description of Eklund et al. (14) for imaging the augmented breast includes *(a)* standard lateral oblique and craniocaudal views using normal positioning techniques and *(b)* modified oblique and craniocaudal views with phototiming. In those patients who have encapsulated implants or in whom the Eklund technique is not successful, a third view, the lateromedial oblique, can prove useful in imaging the upper inner and lower outer quadrants that are obscured on the routine views. Ultrasound (15) is also of help in evaluating complications of the implant and the overlying parenchyma.

Complications associated with implants include infection, hematoma, encapsulation, leakage or rupture, and collapse. In the 2–3 weeks after an implant has been inserted, a fibrous capsule is deposited around it (11). This capsule may become fibrotic and contract, which is the most commonly associated complication with implants (16); encapsulation may occur in as many as 10–40% of patients (16, 17). Retromuscular implants are much less likely to develop contractures (11). On mammography, the finding of a crenulated or irregular contour of the implant may suggest capsular contraction (12) (Figs. 12.20–12.22). Irregularity of the implant contour may be palpated as a mass (10, 12, 18), but the irregular contour as opposed to a parenchymal mass can be differentiated with mammography.

Palpable irregularity may also be associated with rupture of the implant with silicone extravasation. Mammography can identify the dense globules of silicone that may be calcified outside the contour of the implant, indicating rupture (12) (Figs. 12.23 and 12.24). The leaking silicone not only can form calcified nodules but also can present as intraductal casts of silicone (19) (Fig. 12.25). Calcifications that are coarse and ringlike may also develop in the capsule of the implant and are indicative of an inflammatory reaction to the prosthesis (12) but not leakage of silicone.

Parenchymal abnormalities can be demonstrated with imaging, but it is important to maximize information obtained by tailoring the examination to the patient. Benign and malignant lesions may be demonstrated (Figs. 12.26–12.28). Masses may be less readily detected than microcalcifications (12) on mammography, but ultrasound may be of help in the evaluation of dense parenchyma over the prostheses and of palpable masses (15).

Patients who have undergone subcutaneous mastectomy and reconstruction with an implant may have residual ductal tissue (Figs. 12.29 and 12.30). If a patient is known to have had a subcutaneous mastectomy or if she has her native nipple, then it is important that the augmented breast be imaged.

In most cases, patients who have had a total or modified radical mastectomy and reconstruction are not imaged. The reconstruction may be performed by placement of an expandable implant or by a plastic repair with a myocutaneous flap (Fig. 12.31). Several types of myocutaneous flaps have been used for breast reconstruction. One complication of this procedure, which is related to maintaining an adequate blood supply, is fat necrosis of the flap (19). The patient presents with a firm mass (20, 21), and the differential diagnosis includes recurrent carcinoma or fat necrosis (Fig. 12.32). Mammography may be used in this circumstance and may demonstrate changes of fat necrosis ranging from an irregular increased density, to lucent cystic lesions, to ringlike calcifications characteristic of a benign process.

Reduction Mammoplasty

Breast reduction is performed for cosmetic reasons—to treat macromastia—or to achieve symmetry of the contralateral breast after the patient has undergone mastectomy with reconstruction. The surgical procedure involves elevation of the nipple, resection of glandular tissue, and skin removal (22). If there is a nipple transposition procedure, the nipple-areolar complex remains attached to the lactiferous ducts, and the whole complex is transposed upward. In a transplantation procedure, the nipple-areolar complex is severed from the ducts and is transplanted upward (22).

Mammographic findings vary with the type of procedure performed. In patients with a transposition, the subareolar ducts are in a normal relationship with the nipple-areolar complex, but there is a disruption of this orientation after transplantation procedures. Miller et al. (22) found parenchymal redistribution, with most of the fibroglandular tissue below the level of the nipple, as the most common finding in 24 patients who had undergone reduction mammoplasties. Elevation of the nipple was also a common finding, along with thickening of the skin of the lower aspect of the breast and the areola (22). There may be disorientation of the normal parenchymal pattern, with swirled patterns of tissue distribution (23) (Fig. 12.33).

Calcifications are a common finding in patients who have had reductions (3) (Figs. 12.34–12.37). Dermal calcifications, which are smooth and round, may occur in the areola (22) or in scars. Areas of fat necrosis are more common in patients who have undergone reduction than those who have had routine biopsies. Calcifications may be eggshell shaped in typical oil cysts or may be irregular (24) or even lacy in appearance. Often these calcifications are oriented in the direction of the scars. Even sutural calcification may be identified after reduction procedures (23) (Fig. 12.38). Again, with reduction mammoplasties it is important to correlate the location of surgical scars to the mammographic findings.

Lumpectomy and Radiation Therapy

During the past 10 years, there has been a striking increase in breast conservation procedures for treatment of carcinomas. Several studies (25, 26) have shown that the long-term survival of women treated for grade I and II breast cancer with lumpectomy and radiation therapy is similar to that of those treated with mastectomy. Patients who have the option for breast conservation therapy are usually those who have tumor confined to the breast and ipsilateral nodes, a tumor size of <4 cm without fixation, and a size or location of tumor that, after treatment, will yield satisfactory cosmetic results (3, 25). Multicentric carcinoma (27) is also considered by many radiotherapists as a contraindication to breast conservation therapy.

In patients who are treated with lumpectomy and radiation therapy, the rate of local recurrence is in the range of 6–10% (28–30) and is at a rate of 2% per year (3). There is a significant salvage rate (58% at 5 years, 50% at 10 years) in patients who develop local recurrences after lumpectomy and radiation (31). A majority of local recurrences occur in the same quadrant as the initial primary (30). Because of this, not only whole-breast irradiation but also a boost dose to the tumor bed may be given (32). Careful clinical and mammographic follow-up is necessary in order to detect these recurrences when they are early enough for the patient to be salvaged.

Normal mammographic and clinical changes that may be expected after breast conservation therapy include (a) local changes at the tumor bed related to surgery and (b) diffuse changes related to irradiation. Mammography is necessary for accurate monitoring of the postirradiation changes as well as the possible development of recurrent carcinoma (33).

An initial postlumpectomy, preradiotherapy mammogram is recommended to serve as a baseline for follow-up studies and to evaluate the breast for residual carcinoma (3, 33–36). This study should be performed at least 10 days after surgery, allowing time for the incision to heal. Comparison must be made with the preoperative mammogram to determine the exact location of the tumor and its appearance. Particularly if the tumor contained microcalcifications, the postoperative study can provide valuable information about the presence of residual calcification (28, 34) (Figs. 12.39–12.41).

On this baseline, a normal expected finding is skin thickening at the lumpectomy site, architectural distortion, and oftentimes a fluid collection. Postoperative hematomas are of maximum size on this initial baseline study and gradually diminish in size, becoming more irregular in contour. When a patient is found to have irregular density on a 6-month posttreatment mammogram, it is extremely useful to have a baseline postoperative study that showed a larger hematoma at the site (Fig. 12.42).

At 6–12 months the maximum changes of increased interstitial markings and skin thickening are seen. These diffuse findings are secondary to the edema from irradiation of the breast. These edematous changes will stabilize and then diminish, usually at 2 years or later (3). The skin thickness may increase to as much as 1 cm. Dershaw et al. (37) found that in 160 women treated with lumpectomy and radiation therapy, 96% had skin thickening which stabilized by 1 year. At 3 years, 50% of women had persistent edema and skin thickening (Figs. 12.43–12.45).

The latent normal changes after radiation are the development of calcifications of fat necrosis, developing usually after 1 year (Fig. 12.46). Libshitz et al. (38) found that benign calcifications developed in treated breasts from 2 to 44 months after irradiation. These calcifications have the same mammographic appearance of liponecrosis microcystica secondary to trauma or biopsy, and they may occur at the lumpectomy site or elsewhere in the treated breast.

The findings of recurrent carcinoma include the development of new microcalcifications, increased skin thickening after stabilization, increased density, particularly at the tumor bed, after stabilization, and the development of a new mass (Fig. 12.47). Because of the difficulty in differentiating benign from malignant microcalcifications with certainty, biopsy is indicated unless the calcification are those of fat necrosis. New spiculated masses and irregular ductal-type malignant microcalcifications are highly suspicious for recurrence. Stomper et al. (39) found that 65% of recurrences in 23 women occurred at the primary site, 22% recurred in different sites, and 13% were multifocal. The positive rates for recurrent tumor on biopsies for mammographic or clinical abnormalities in treated breasts range from 20% to 58% (35, 40–42). A combination of clinical findings and mammographic findings is highly suspicious for recurrence (35). To detect the changes indicative of recurrence, careful attention to and comparison with all previous studies, not just the most recent, are necessary.

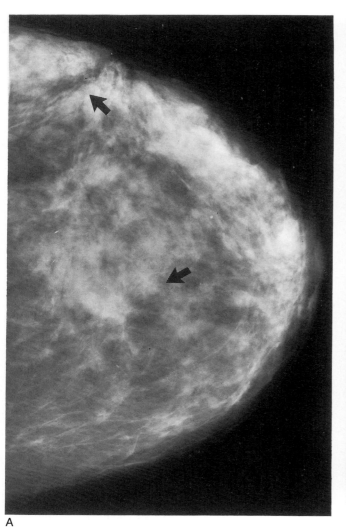

A

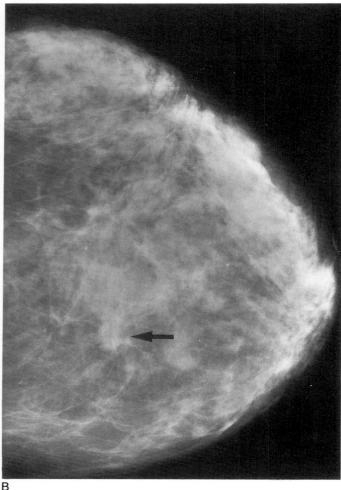

B

Figure 12.1.

Clinical: 50-year-old G9, P2, Ab7 woman who has a positive family history of breast cancer and a personal history of multiple breast biopsies showing fibroadenomas and fibrocystic changes. She presents for routine follow-up; comparison is made with her mammogram from 3 years earlier.

Mammogram: Right craniocaudal view from 1987 (**A**), and right craniocaudal (**B**) and oblique (**C**) views and specimen film (**D**) from 1990. The breast is moderately dense, with an adenosis pattern. There are areas of architectural distortion (**A**) related to surgical scarring *(arrows)*. On the subsequent mammogram (**B** and **C**), a new spiculated nodule *(arrows)* is present medial to the scar. Although initially a scar could have this appearance, over time it should become less dense and spiculated, not more so. The lesion is highly suspicious for malignancy. It was biopsied after needle localization, and the specimen film (**D**) shows it to be of high density and with spicules surrounding its entire margin, characteristic of carcinoma.

Impression: Developing density highly suspicious for carcinoma.

Histopathology: Infiltrating ductal carcinoma.

Note: If there is any question as to the location of a density in the breast relative to the position of a scar, skin markers should be placed over the scar, and the film should be repeated.

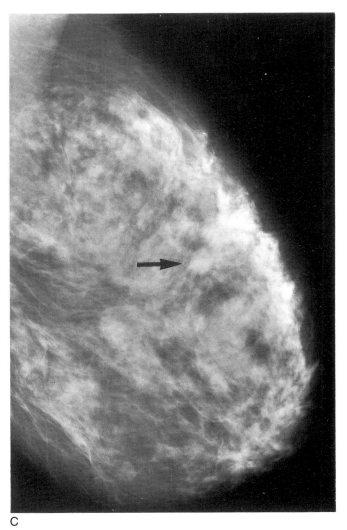

C

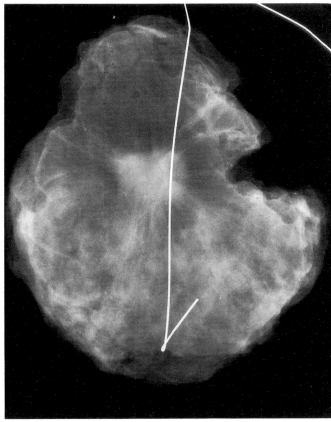

D

Figure 12.2.

Clinical: 48-year-old G2, P2 woman 6 months after left breast biopsy, presenting with no new palpable findings.

Mammogram: Left craniocaudal view from a needle localization (**A**) and left craniocaudal view (**B**) and ultrasound (**C**) 6 months after biopsy. On the initial film (**A**), a needle localization wire is marking a cluster of microcalcifications *(arrow)* for biopsy. The histopathology was benign. On the subsequent study (**B**), there is a large high-density, partially circumscribed mass at the biopsy site. On ultrasound (**C**), the mass is complex, appearing circumscribed with some acoustic enhancement. The features are typical of a postoperative hematoma or seroma, and a lesion of this size may not be palpable. The patient was followed without aspiration of the lesion.

Impression: Large postoperative hematoma or seroma.

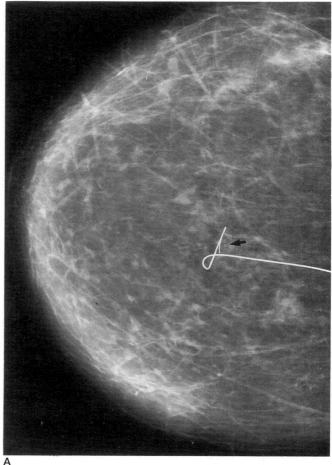

A

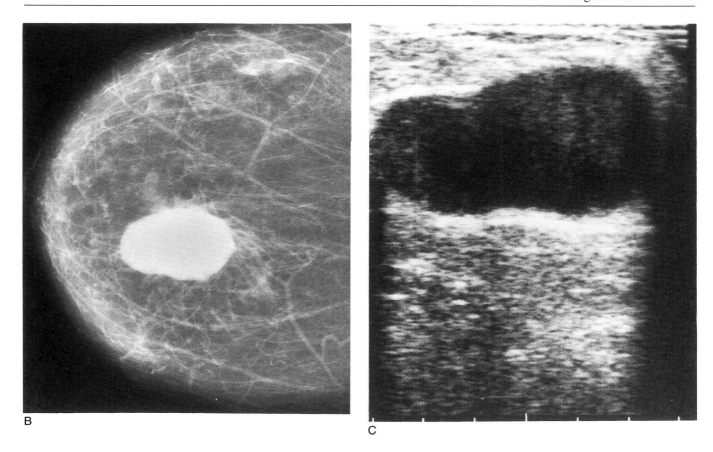

B

C

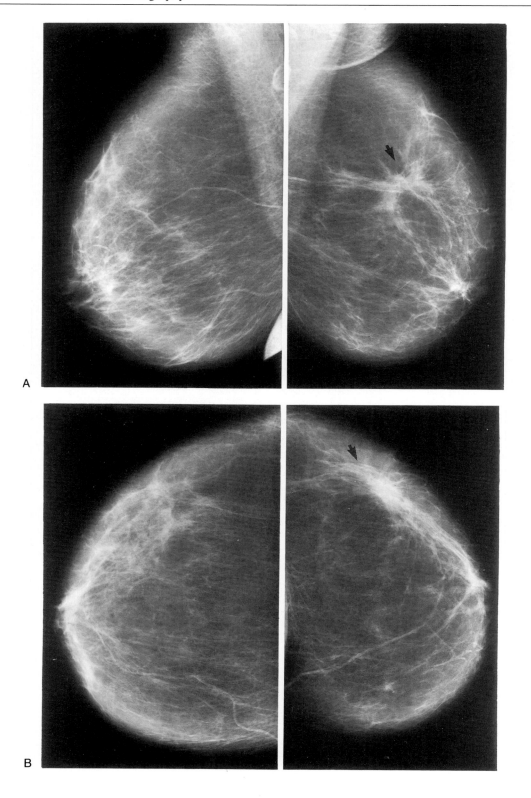

Figure 12.3.

Clinical: 72-year-old G2, P2 woman for follow-up 1 year after a right breast biopsy that showed fibrocystic change.

Mammogram: Bilateral oblique (**A**) and craniocaudal (**B**) views. There is an irregular density in the right upper outer quadrant *(arrows)*. On the oblique view (**A**) the lesion appears less dense and spiculated than on the craniocaudal view (**B**). The difference in shape of such a density suggests more likely a benign rather than a malignant etiology. This density was confirmed to be in the location of the scar from the previous biopsy.

Impression: Irregular density consistent with fat necrosis after excisional biopsy.

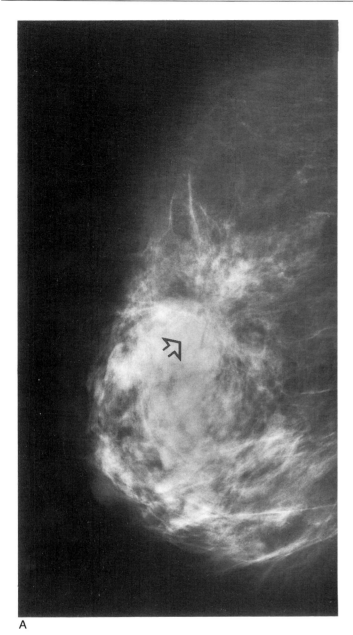

A

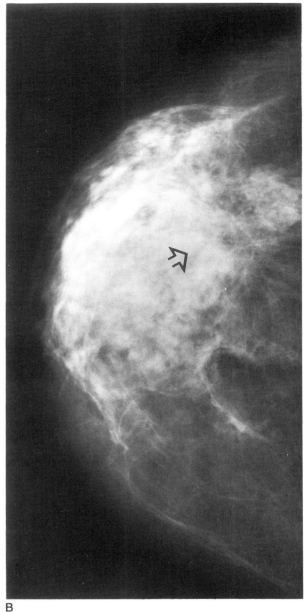

B

Figure 12.4.

Clinical: 71-year-old woman 1 year after left breast biopsy for a palpable nodule that was found on histopathologic examination to be fibrosis.

Mammogram: Left oblique (**A**) and craniocaudal (**B**) views. There is dense glandular tissue present throughout the left breast. In the upper outer quadrant, there is a prominent area of architectural distortion *(arrows)*. Although the area appears somewhat spiculated, it does not have a high-density center, and it appears somewhat less prominent on the craniocaudal view (**B**), features suggesting more likely a benign nature. The area corresponded to the surgical scar from recent biopsy and was, therefore, considered to be most likely fat necrosis. It was followed and gradually decreased in size.

Impression: Fat necrosis, surgical scar.

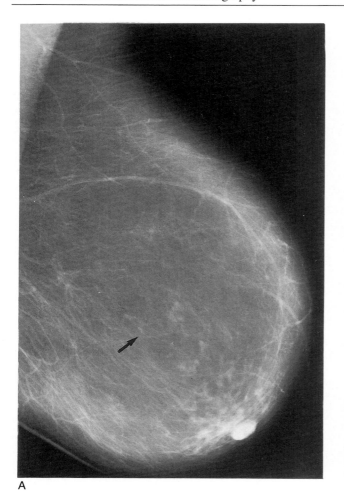

A

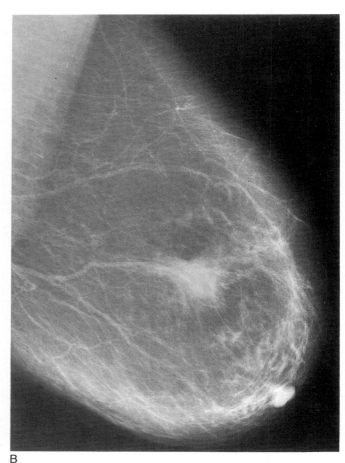

B

Figure 12.5.

Clinical: 55-year-old G0 woman for follow-up mammography after a benign biopsy in the right breast.

Mammogram: Right oblique film (preoperative) (**A**), right oblique (**B**) and craniocaudal (**C**) views 6 months after biopsy, and right oblique (**D**) and craniocaudal (**E**) views 12 months after biopsy. The preoperative film (**A**) demonstrates a small cluster *(arrow)* of microcalcifications that were biopsied and found to be benign. On the initial postoperative study

(**B** and **C**), there is a 3-cm ill-defined area of increased density in the right middle outer quadrant. On the craniocaudal view (**C**), the area is of lower density than would be expected for a neoplastic process. Because the location of the biopsy was in this area, the density is most consistent with fat necrosis. Six months later (**D** and **E**), the area of fat necrosis has decreased in size as would be expected.

Impression: Postoperative fat necrosis decreasing in size.

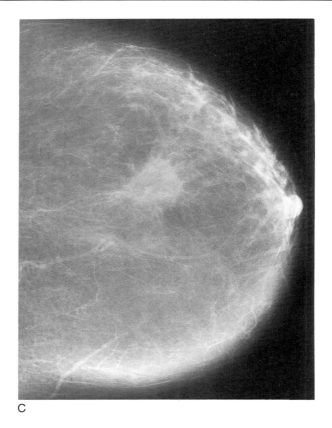

C

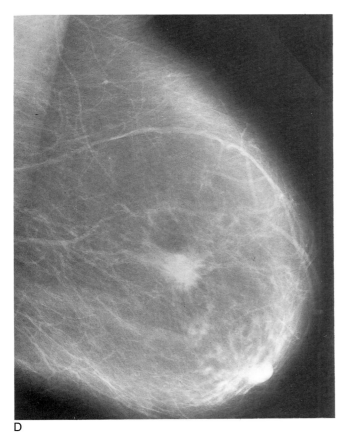

D

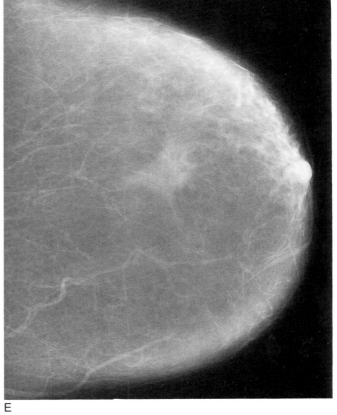

E

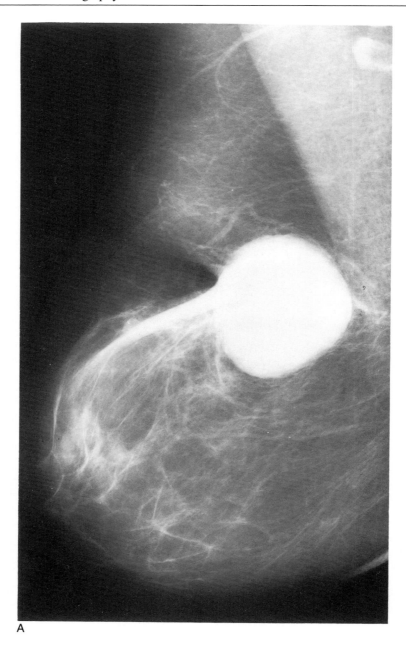

A

Figure 12.6.

Clinical: 64-year-old G2, P2 woman with a history of carcinoid tumor and a left breast biopsy 1 year ago. The biopsy was performed for a nonpalpable nodule that was confirmed on specimen radiography and found to represent sclerosing adenosis.

Mammogram: Left oblique (**A**) and craniocaudal (**B**) views. There is a large very high density, relatively well circumscribed mass in the upper inner quadrant, producing marked skin retraction. (This mass was in the region of previous biopsy.) Ultrasound showed the lesion to be solid. Because of the history of biopsy for a benign lesion, the favored diagnosis is hematoma with fat necrosis; however, neoplasia is a definite consideration because of the skin changes and high density of the mass.

Impression: Large mass, favoring postoperative changes, fat necrosis.

Histopathology: Fibromatosis.

Note: Fibromatosis is a benign lesion that occurs in the area of fascia and may be related to trauma. Although rare, when it does occur in the breast, it is more often an ill-defined lesion. In this case, the mass was found to be completely attached to the deep fascia at the time of resection.

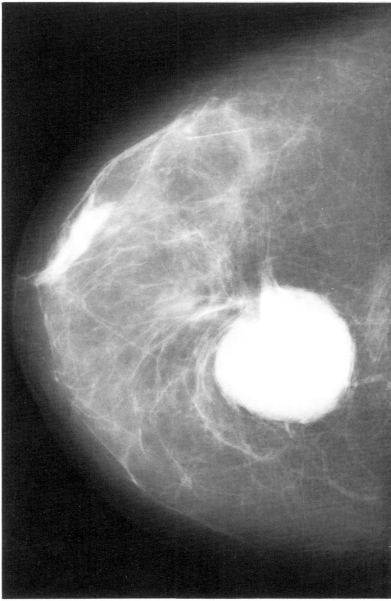

B

Figure 12.7.

Clinical: 32-year-old G0 woman who had had breast reduction 3 years ago, presenting with a firm irregular nodule in the right lower inner quadrant.

Mammogram: Bilateral oblique (**A**), craniocaudal (**B**), and enlarged (2×) right craniocaudal (**C**) views. The breasts show fatty replacement. In the right lower inner quadrant, there is an irregular area of increased density associated with a radiolucent nodule containing ringlike calcification in the wall *(curved arrow)*. A radiolucent lesion is typical of an oil cyst and is most consistent with posttraumatic changes from reduction mammoplasty. The area was biopsied because of clinical concern about the palpable findings. Incidental note is also made of a small degenerating fibroadenoma in the left middle inner quadrant *(arrow)*.

Impression: Fat necrosis, oil cyst.

Histopathology: Fat necrosis.

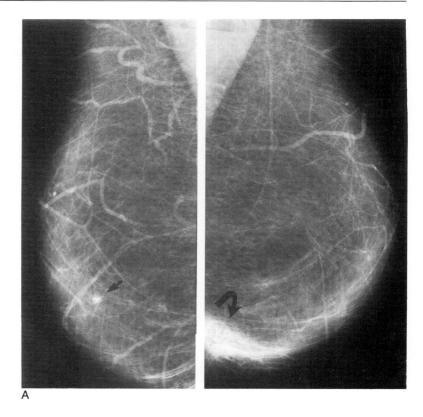

A

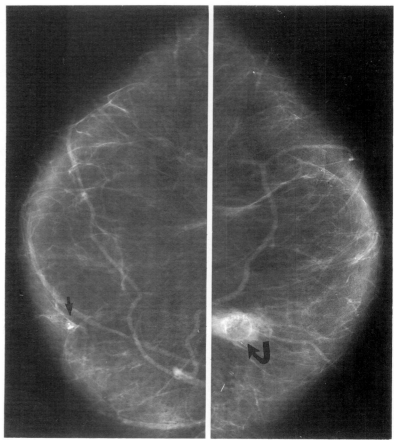

B

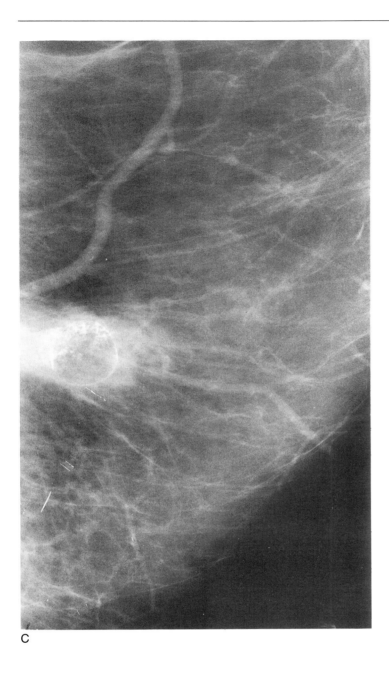

C

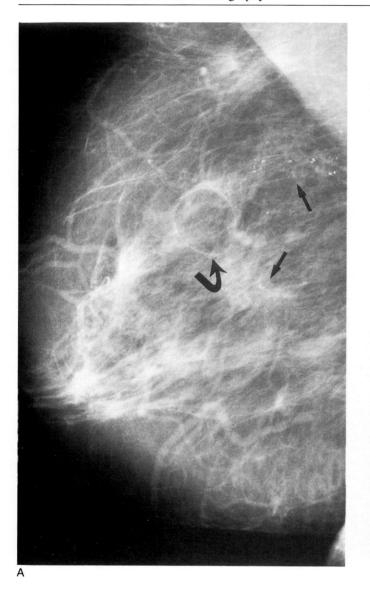

A

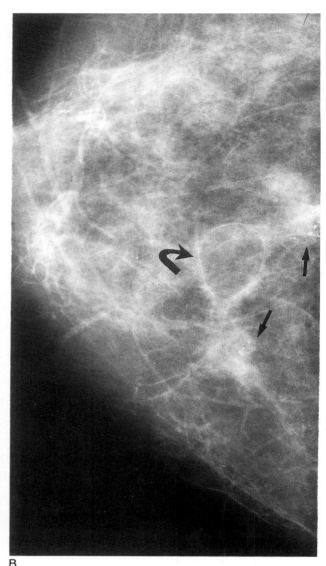

B

Figure 12.8.

Clinical: 58-year-old G6, P6 woman with a history of right breast cancer and of reduction mammoplasty on the left.

Mammogram: Left oblique (**A**) and enlarged (1.5×) craniocaudal (**B**) views. The breast is moderately dense. In the left upper inner quadrant, there is a radiolucent well-circumscribed lesion *(curved arrow)* with early calcification in the rim, consistent with an oil cyst. Adjacent to the oil cyst are two clusters of coarse irregular microcalcifications *(arrows)* that had developed since the prior mammogram. Because of

their morphology and their association with the nearby oil cyst, these microcalcifications were thought to represent most likely fat necrosis and fibrosis. However, because of the risk status of the patient and the interval change, the area was biopsied.

Impression: Probable fat necrosis.

Histopathology: Changes compatible with old biopsy, fat necrosis.

Figure 12.9.

Clinical: 78-year-old G2, P2 woman after right breast biopsy for microcalcifications that were found to be epithelial hyperplasia, presenting for routine follow-up.

Mammogram: Right enlarged (2×) craniocaudal view (**A**) 6 months postoperatively and right oblique (**B**) and enlarged craniocaudal (**C**) views 12 months postoperatively. On the initial study (**A**), there is an irregular area *(arrow)* of increased density in the outer aspect of the breast. This corresponded in location to the scar and was presumed to represent fat necrosis. Six months later (**B** and **C**), the density has resolved and has been replaced with a lucent nodule with a calcifying rim *(arrow)* (**B**), consistent with an oil cyst.

Impression: Postoperative fat necrosis evolving into an oil cyst.

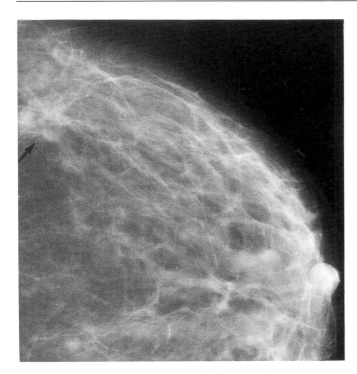

A

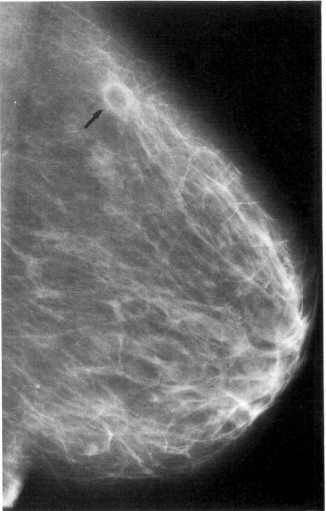

B

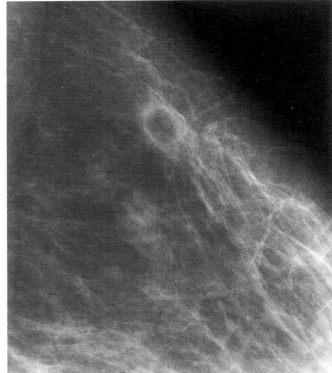

C

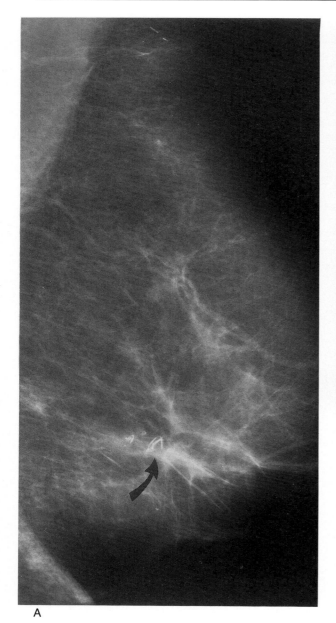

A

B

Figure 12.10.

Clinical: 68-year-old G6, P4 woman for follow-up after lumpectomy and radiation therapy on the right for infiltrating lobular carcinoma. She had also undergone a reexcision at the tumor bed for new microcalcifications found to be atypical epithelial hyperplasia.

Mammogram: Right oblique (**A**) and magnification (2×) (**B**) views at the tumor bed 2 years after treatment. There is irregular increased density at the lumpectomy site, consistent with postsurgical changes. There are curvilinear coarse calcifications at the biopsy site *(curved arrow)* (**A**) seen better on the magnification view (**B**). Behind the curvilinear calcifications is a group of calcifications in a knotted shape (**A** and **B**). The smooth curvilinear shape of the calcifications is typical of sutural calcification. (These have been followed for 3 years and are stable.)

Impression: Sutural calcifications.

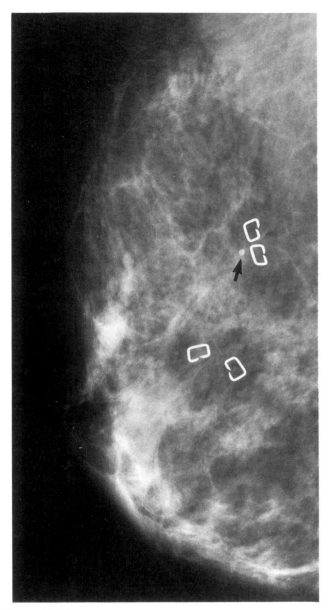

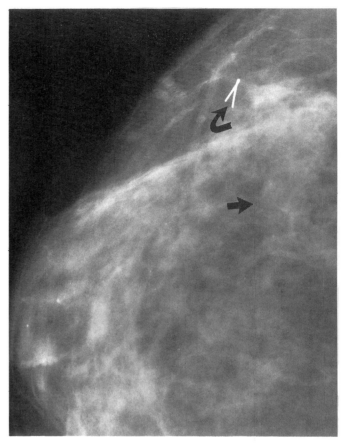

Figure 12.11.

Clinical: 52-year-old woman 5 years after treatment for intraductal carcinoma of the left breast with lumpectomy and radiation therapy.

Mammogram: Left oblique view. The breast is moderately dense. Surgical clips have been placed at the lumpectomy site to outline the tumor bed for radiation therapy planning. A single calcification of fat necrosis *(arrow)* is noted at the tumor bed.

Impression: Foreign bodies: surgical clips marking tumor bed.

Figure 12.12.

Clinical: 46-year-old woman who has been treated for carcinoma of the right breast and who has had a biopsy of the left upper outer quadrant for microcalcifications, which showed lobular carcinoma in situ.

Mammogram: Magnified (2×) left craniocaudal view. A metallic foreign body is present *(curved arrow)* and represents the end of a needle localization hookwire severed during surgery. Residual microcalcifications *(straight arrow)* are also present and have a rounded morphology, suggesting a lobular origin. Because of the prior histopathology in this region, reexcision was recommended; lobular carcinoma in situ was found on the reexcision biopsy.

Impression: Foreign body—retained localization wire.

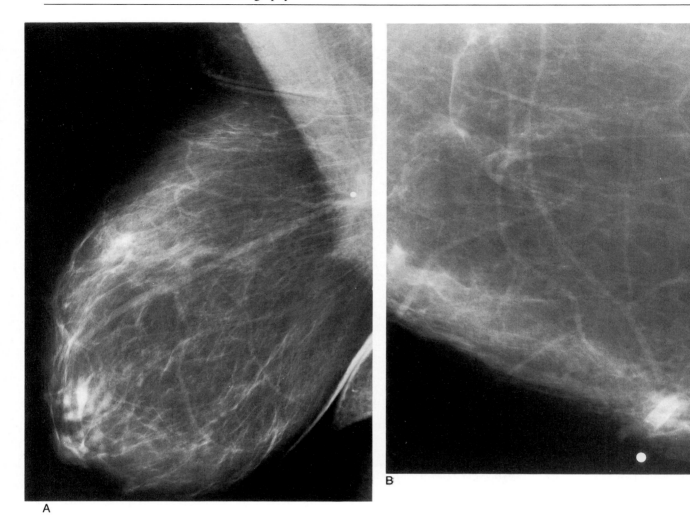

A

B

Figure 12.13.

Clinical: 24-year-old woman with acute leukemia and neutropenia, presenting with a 2 × 2-cm tender mass in the left upper inner quadrant. (A BB was placed over the palpable lesion for mammography.)

Mammogram: Left oblique view (**A**), left enlarged (2×) craniocaudal view (**B**), and ultrasound (**C**). The breast is mildly glandular. Far posteriorly in the upper inner quadrant in the area of the palpable mass is a tubular intraparenchymal artifact. Some surrounding increased density is present (**A** and

B). On ultrasound the structure is producing a dense shadow (**C**) but no surrounding fluid collection to suggest an abscess is seen. This tubular structure is the tip of a catheter for chemotherapy, which had been removed several months earlier. The tip was severed and remained in the breast and had not been clinically evident until the surrounding inflammation occurred.

Impression: Catheter tip with surrounding inflammatory changes.

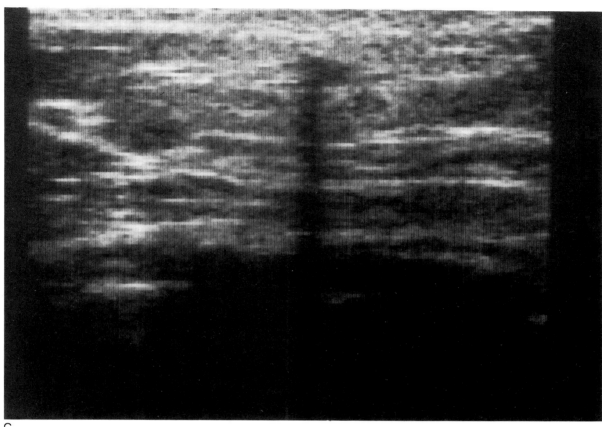

C

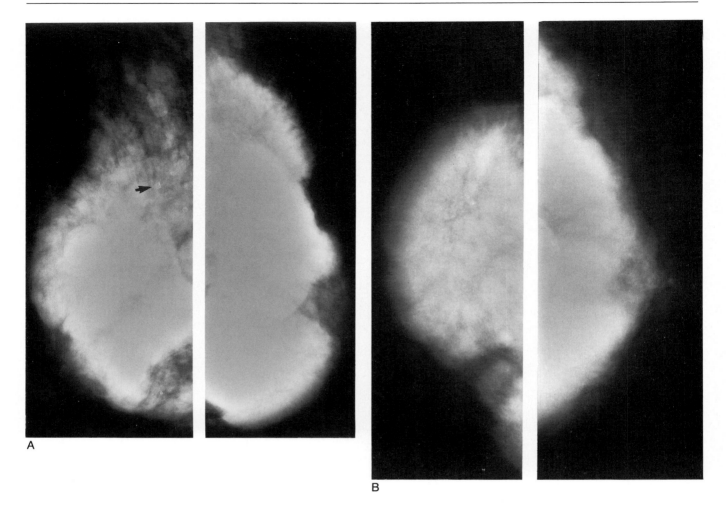

A

B

Figure 12.14.

Clinical: 41-year-old woman after augmentation mammoplasty with silicone injections, presenting with numerous hard masses and distortion of the contour of the breasts bilaterally.

Mammogram: Bilateral oblique (**A**), craniocaudal (**B**), and enlarged right mediolateral (**C**) views. Technically, the examination is limited by the extreme density of the breasts and the inability to compress them adequately. The study was performed at 32 kVp with a tungsten target and rhodium filtration to attempt to penetrate the tissue. The breasts are extremely dense, with multiple soft tissue masses bilaterally. There are also innumerable circular calcifications *(arrows)* bilaterally that represent dystrophic and granulomatous reaction to the silicone injections. Ultrasound was not of help because of diffuse shadowing from this process.

Impression: Extensive dystrophic changes secondary to silicone injection for augmentation mammoplasty.

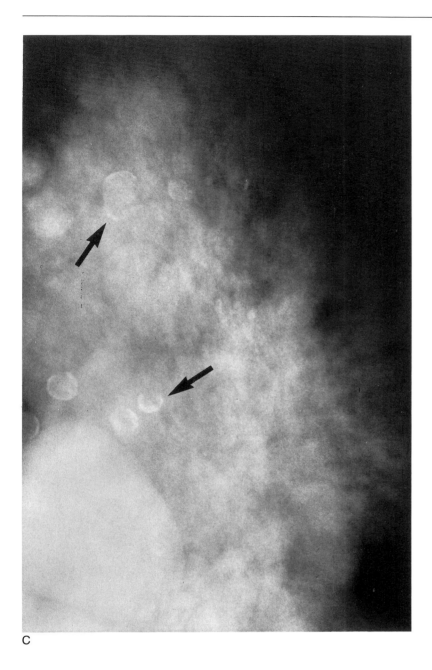

C

Figure 12.15.

Clinical: 38-year-old G2, P2 woman for routine follow-up mammography.

Mammogram: Bilateral oblique (**A**) and craniocaudal (**B**) views. Bilateral suprapectoral saline implants are present. Saline implants are more radiolucent than those filled with silicone, and in this case the valves in the implant are evident. There is a focal nonpalpable area of asymmetric glandular tissue in the right upper outer quadrant *(arrow)* (**A**), which had been identified on a prior study and has remained unchanged.

Impression: Bilateral suprapectoral saline implants.

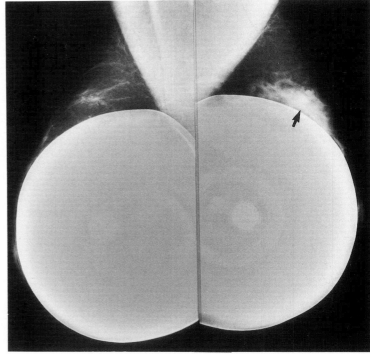

A

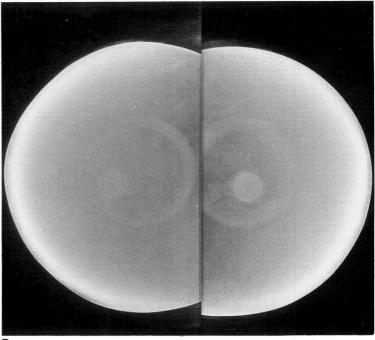

B

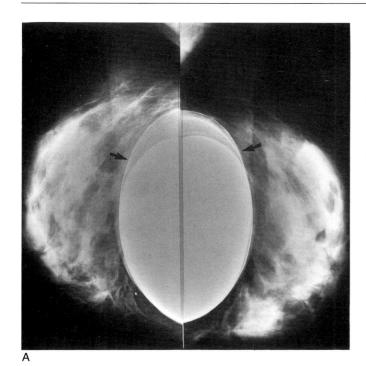

A

Figure 12.16.

Clinical: 42-year-old G3, P2, Ab1 woman for routine follow-up after augmentation mammoplasty.

Mammogram: Bilateral oblique (**A**), medial oblique (**B**), and craniocaudal (**C**) views. The patient has had bilateral augmentation mammoplasty. Subpectoral *(arrows)* (**A**) silicone double-chamber implants are present, and dense fibroglandular tissue overlies the prostheses. The medial oblique view is an optional position that can be used to demonstrate areas that may be obscured by the implants on the standard oblique and craniocaudal views.

Impression: Status of woman after augmentation mammoplasty with subpectoral implants.

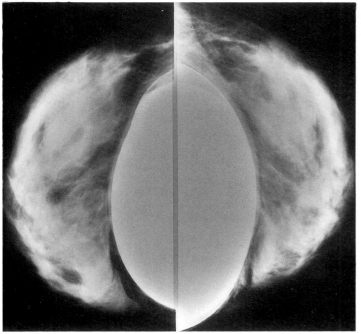

B

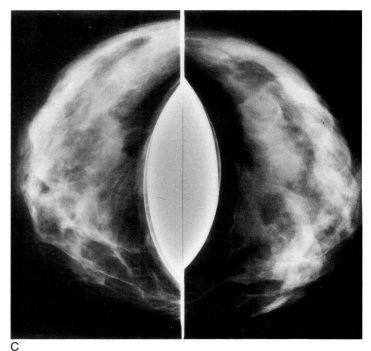

C

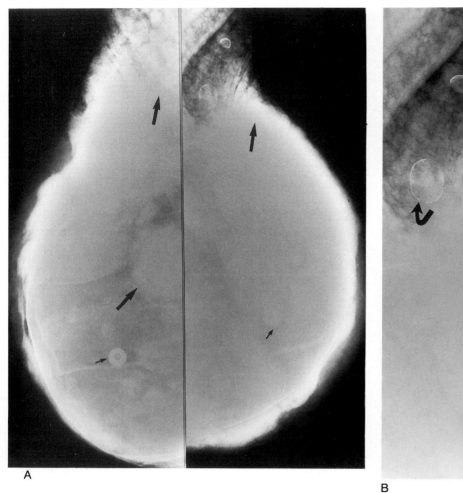

A

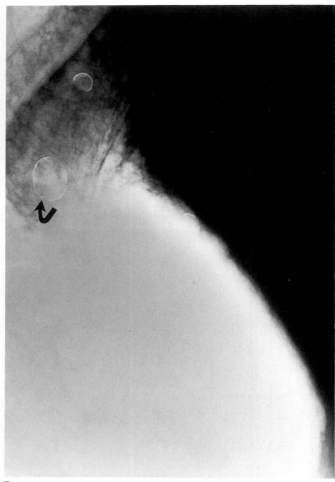

B

Figure 12.17.

Clinical: 40-year-old woman after augmentation mammoplasty with both silicone injections and saline implants. On clinical examination the breasts were filled with hard nodules, particularly in the upper outer quadrants.

Mammogram: Bilateral oblique (**A**) and right enlarged (2×) oblique (**B**) views. The breasts are very difficult to image because of the postsurgical changes. Saline implants are present bilaterally, and the valves of these prostheses are seen *(small arrows)* (**A**). There are also extremely dense nodules bilaterally *(large arrows)* (**A**) that are related to the silicone injections. On the enlarged view (**B**) these very dense nodules are seen, and some areas of fat necrosis (ringlike lucent nodules) are also identified *(curved arrow)* (**B**). The nodules are granulomas that have formed secondary to the silicone injections.

Impression: Postoperative changes of augmentation mammoplasty with both implants and direct silicone injections. (Case courtesy of Dr. Cherie Scheer, Richmond, VA.)

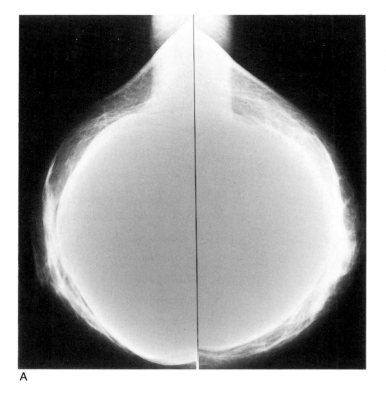

A

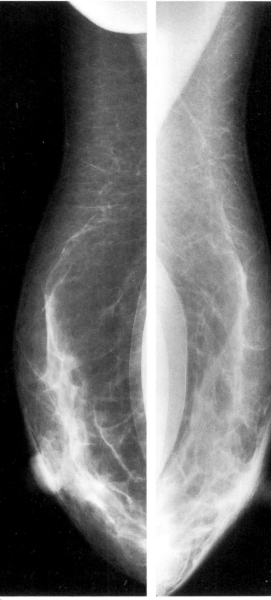

B

Figure 12.18.

Clinical: 44-year-old woman for routine mammography after augmentation mammoplasty.

Mammogram: Bilateral standard oblique (**A**) and bilateral Eklund oblique (**B**) views. The subpectoral implants are present bilaterally and obscure much of the overlying parenchyma with standard views (**A**). Using the Eklund technique (**B**), the implants are displaced posteriorly, and the moderately dense anterior parenchyma is well visualized.

Impression: Bilateral augmentation mammoplasty imaged with standard and Eklund techniques. (Case courtesy of Dr. Cherie Scheer, Richmond, VA.)

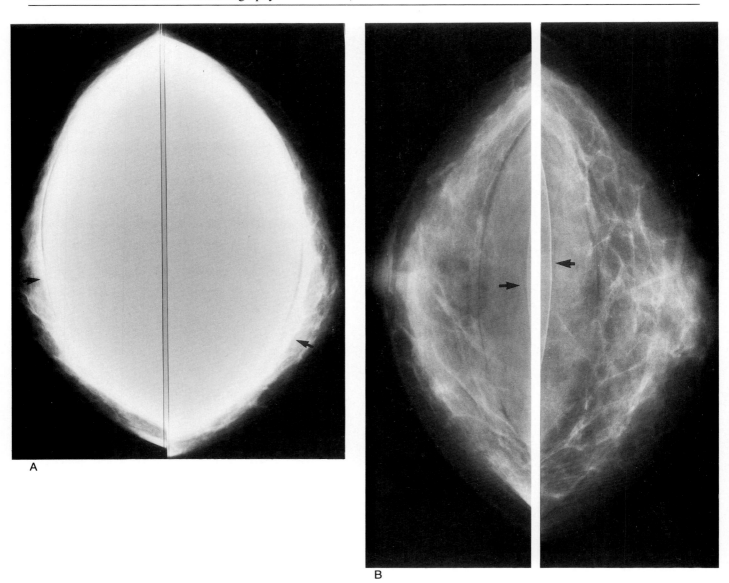

A

B

Figure 12.19.

Clinical: 45-year-old patient for routine mammography after augmentation mammoplasty.

Mammogram: Bilateral craniocaudal (**A**) views and bilateral craniocaudal views (**B**) with the Eklund technique. On the standard view (**A**), bilateral subpectoral implants are present, obscuring much of the parenchyma. The thin stripe of pectoralis muscle *(arrows)* is seen covering the implants. With

the Eklund technique (**B**), the implants have been displaced posteriorly, with only the anterior edge of each implant *(arrows)* being visualized.

Impression: Eklund technique demonstrating better visualization of parenchyma over subpectoral implants. (Case courtesy of Dr. Cherie Scheer, Richmond, VA.)

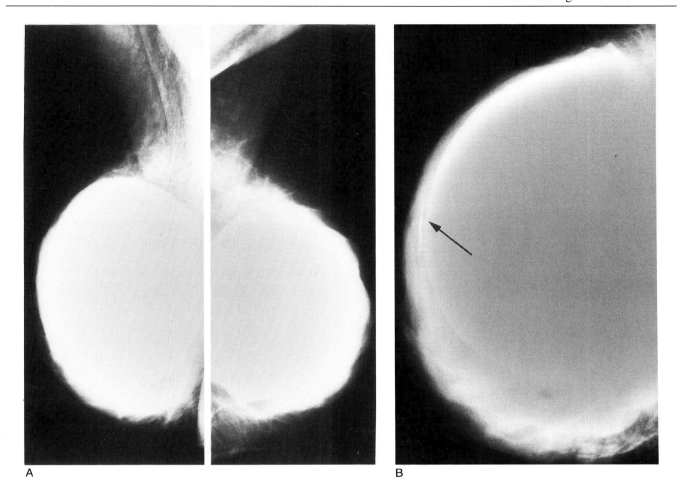

A   B

Figure 12.20.

Clinical: 46-year-old G3, P3 woman after bilateral augmentation mammoplasty, for screening; her implants were clinically considered to be encapsulated.

Mammogram: Bilateral oblique (**A**) and left craniocaudal (**B**) views. Implants anterior to the pectoralis major muscle are present, and there is a moderate amount of irregular dense tissue surrounding the prostheses (**A**). On the left (**B**), there is a dense circumlinear calcification *(arrow)* around the margin of the implant. The calcification is dystrophic in origin and may be related in part to encapsulation of the implant.

Impression: Bilateral implants with dystrophic calcification in the capsule on the left, suggesting encapsulation.

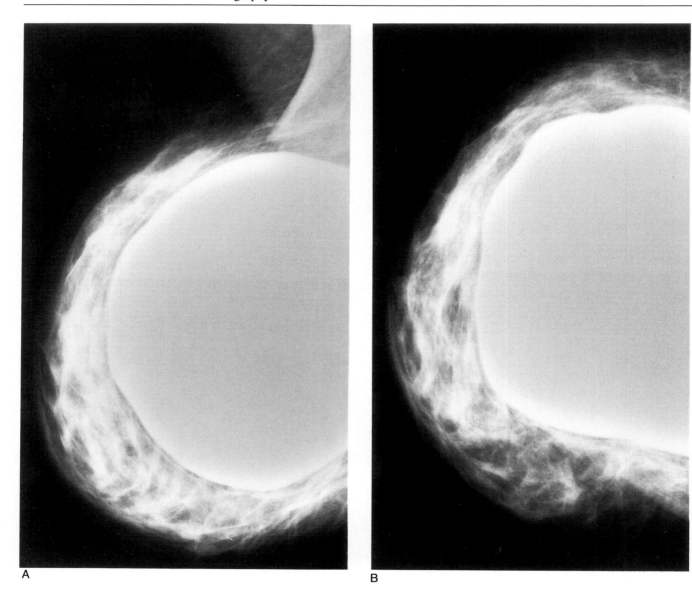

A

B

Figure 12.21.

Clinical: 45-year-old G2, P2, Ab1 woman after bilateral augmentation mammoplasty, with a smooth nodule in the left breast.

Mammogram: Left oblique (**A**), medial oblique (**B**), and craniocaudal (**C**) views. There is a suprapectoral silicone implant in place with moderate overlying glandularity. There is

irregularity to the contour of the implant, particularly medially *(arrow)* (**C**), and this irregularity corresponds to the palpable finding for which the patient was referred. Such irregularity may indicate encapsulation of the implant.

Impression: Irregularity of the left implant; possible encapsulation.

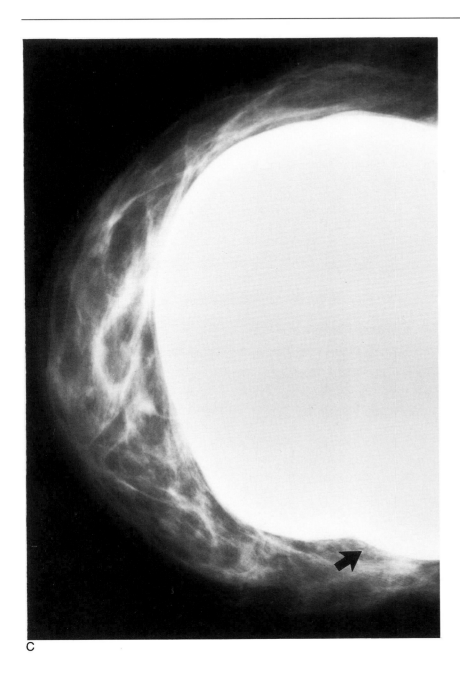

C

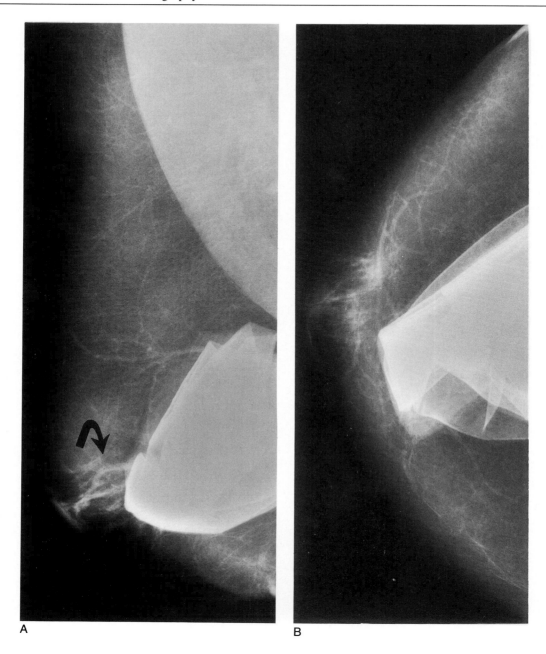

A   B

Figure 12.22.

Clinical: 56-year-old G4, P4 woman with a positive family history and personal history of breast cancer, treated with bilateral subcutaneous mastectomies and placement of prostheses.

Mammogram: Left oblique (**A**), left craniocaudal (**B**), right oblique (**C**), and right craniocaudal (**D**) views. Bilateral subpectoral implants are present. There has been collapse of the left implant (**A** and **B**) and partial collapse of the right

implant (**C** and **D**). Also noted on the right (**D**) is dystrophic calcification along the edge of the implant *(straight arrow),* probably related to encapsulation. Residual ductal tissue *(curved arrows)* is present in both subareolar areas (**A** and **C**), even though the patient had undergone subcutaneous mastectomies.

Impression: Collapsed subpectoral implants bilaterally, minimal residual ductal tissue.

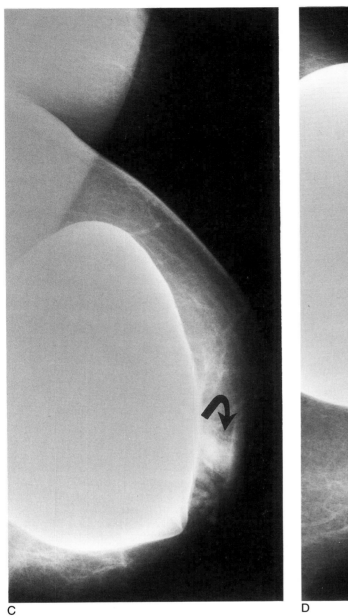

C

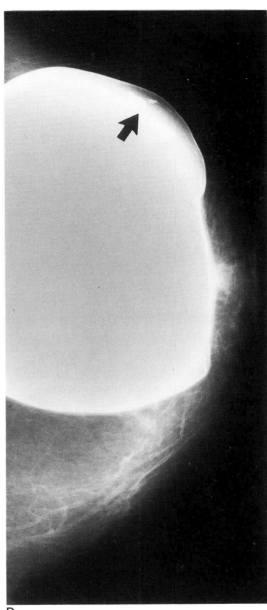

D

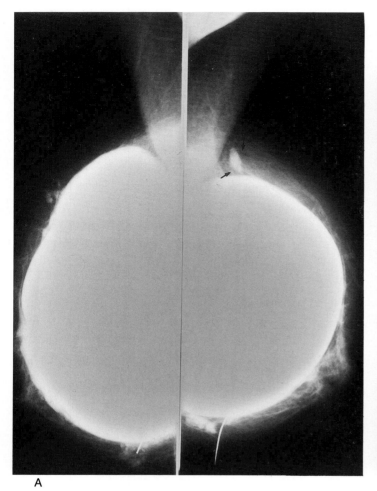

A

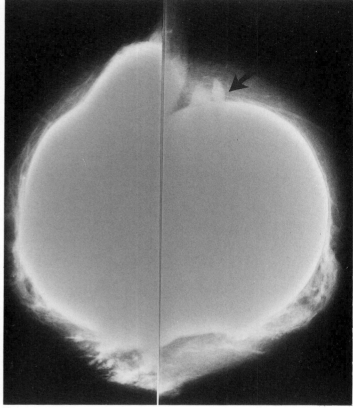

B

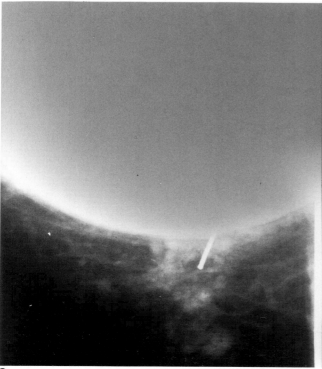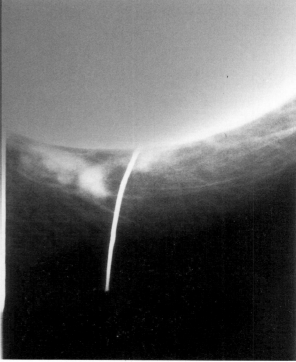

C

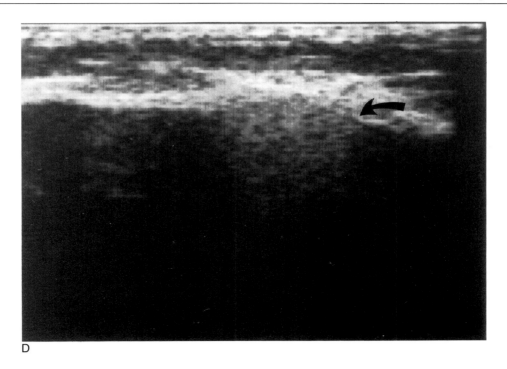

D

Figure 12.23.

Clinical: 42-year-old woman after bilateral augmentation mammoplasty, presenting with bilateral palpable nodularity at the inferior aspects of the implants.

Mammogram: Bilateral oblique view (**A**), craniocaudal view (**B**), coned-down oblique view (**C**), and ultrasound (**D** and **E**). Bilateral retroglandular silicone-filled implants are present. There is some deformity of the contour of both implants, which may be associated with encapsulation. There are also multiple areas *(arrows)* of high-density nodularity near the border of the implants, both inferiorly and superiorly. On the enlargement (**C**) these nodules contain densities that appear to be calcific. Ultrasound (**D**) in the region of the palpable nodularity showed disruption of the border of the implant and a hyperechoic region *(arrow)* with vague glandularity in the capsule at the point of disruption. This contrasts with other areas (**E**) where the implant is intact and the overlying parenchyma is normal.

Impression: Bilateral leakage of silicone implants.

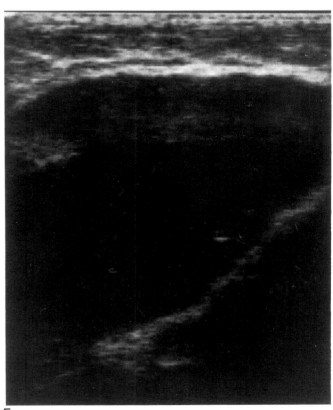

E

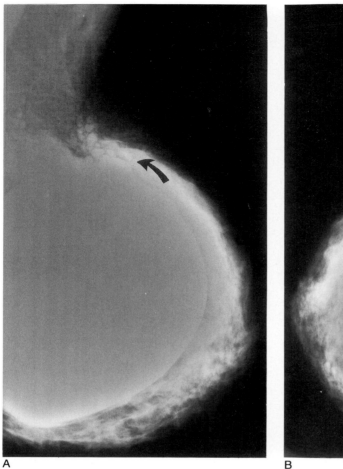

A

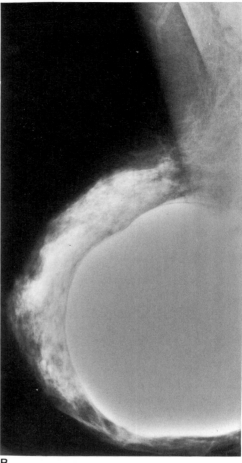

B

Figure 12.24.

Clinical: 38-year-old woman after bilateral augmentation mammoplasty who had sustained a blunt trauma to the right breast in a car accident 4 months ago. She now presents with palpable nodularity in the right axillary tail.

Mammogram: Right oblique (**A**), left oblique (**B**), and enlarged (2×) right oblique (**C**) views. Bilateral suprapectoral silicone implants are present. A moderate amount of glandular tissue overlies the implants. Slight irregularity of the superior margin of the right implant is present (**A** and **C**), and just above this, in the parenchyma, there are multiple high-density circumscribed nodules *(arrows)*. This finding is typical of silicone leakage into the parenchyma and may be related to the trauma.

Impression: Silicone leakage from ruptured implant.

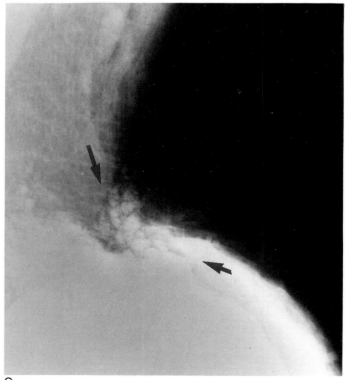

C

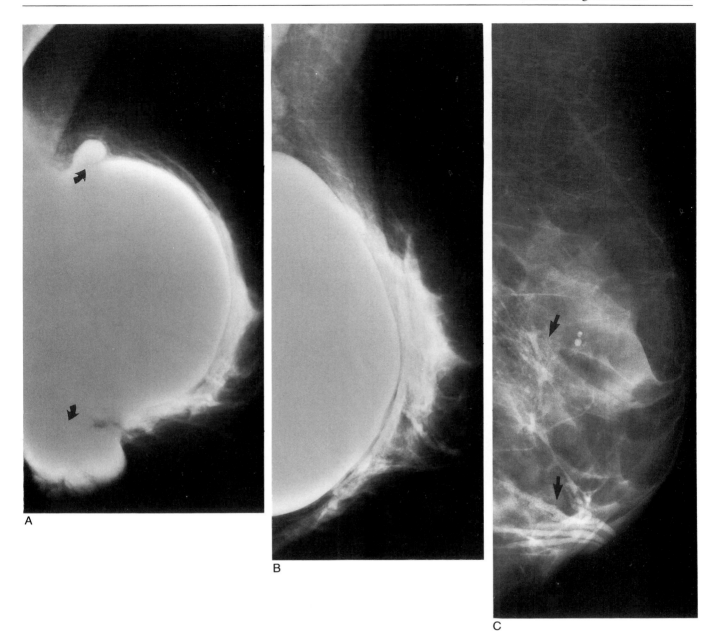

Figure 12.25.

Clinical: 44-year-old woman after bilateral augmentation mammoplasties who presents with a firm nodule in the inferior aspect of the right breast.

Mammogram: Right oblique view (**A**) and right oblique (**B**) and Eklund oblique (**C**) views 1 year later. On the initial study a suprapectoral silicone implant is present. There are globules of free silicone beneath and above the implant in the surrounding parenchyma *(arrows)* (**A**). This silicone was leaking from a rupture in the implant and was removed at the same time as a replacement of the implant. On the subsequent mammogram (**B** and **C**) the silicone globules have been removed. There is, however, a dense cast of the ductal system *(arrows)* (**C**), consistent with silicone in the lactiferous ducts.

Impression: Rupture of implant treated surgically, with the development of silicone casts of lactiferous ducts. (Case courtesy of Dr. Cherie Scheer, Richmond, VA.)

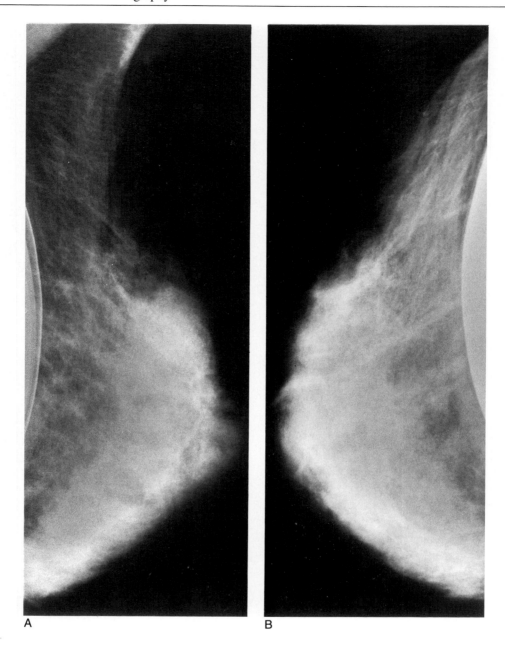

A

B

Figure 12.26.

Clinical: 35-year-old G0 woman with a positive family history of breast cancer, for routine screening after augmentation mammoplasty.

Mammogram: Right oblique view (**A**), left oblique view (**B**), right craniocaudal view (**C**), and ultrasound (**D**). The implants are small and subpectoral and do not obscure much of the overlying breast tissue. The parenchyma is dense, but no focal masses are identified. Ultrasound demonstrates a somewhat irregular hypoechoic lesion located in the 9 o'clock position of the right breast. The lesion was localized under

sonographic guidance by placement of skin markers. Sonography can be of help in the evaluation of the patient who has had augmentation with implants. The presence of the implants can make clinical evaluation of the breasts more difficult and can obscure overlying parenchyma.

Impression: Status after augmentation mammoplasty: solid nodule on the right of moderate suspicion for malignancy. Differential diagnosis included primarily fibroadenoma, fibrocystic change, and carcinoma.

Histopathology: Focal fibrosis.

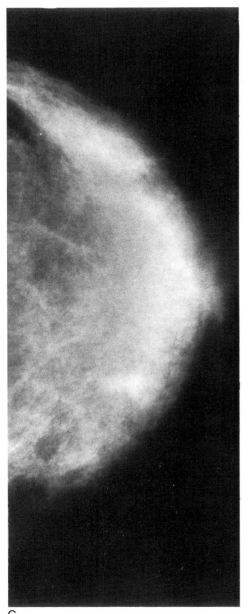

C

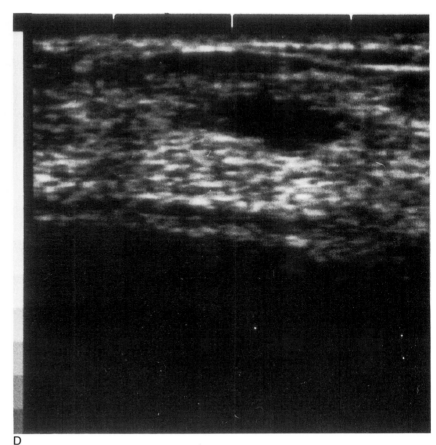

D

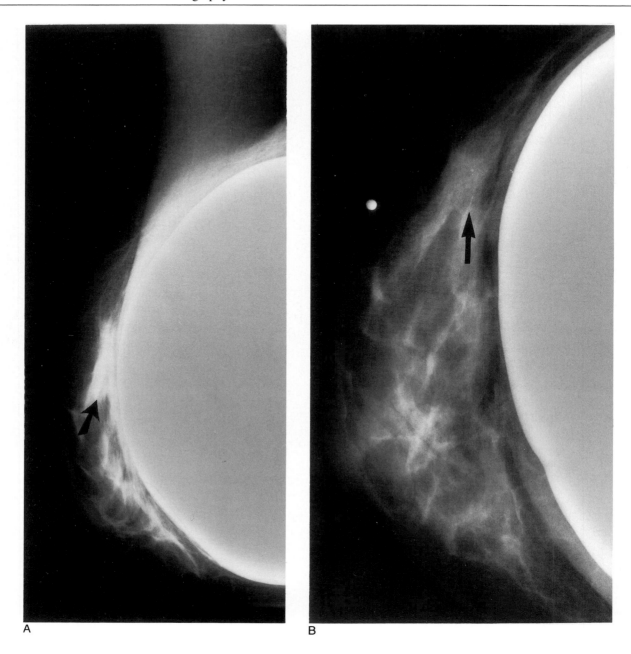

A

B

Figure 12.27.

Clinical: 40-year-old G6, P2 woman with bilateral breast implants, for screening.

Mammogram: Left oblique (**A**), craniocaudal (**B**), enlarged (2×) craniocaudal (**C**), and specimen (**D**) views. A subpectoral implant is present, and moderately dense glandular tissue overlies the prosthesis. In the left upper outer quadrant (**A–C**), there is a focal area of increased density associated with fine, granular microcalcifications *(arrows)*. The area was considered suspicious for malignancy and was localized under mammographic guidance by placement of a skin marker rather than a needle over the lesion. The specimen film (**D**) confirms removal of the suspicious area.

Impression: Irregular density with microcalcifications anterior to the implant, moderately suspicious for carcinoma.

Histopathology: Infiltrating ductal carcinoma.

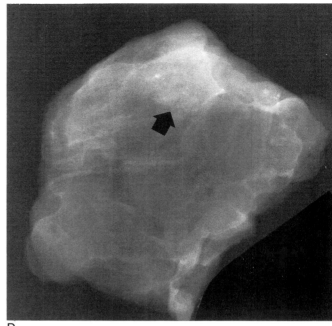

D

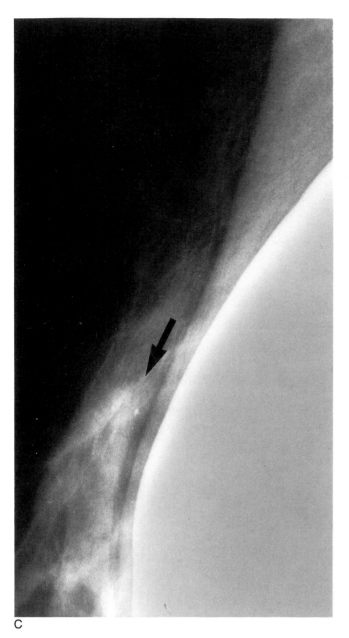

C

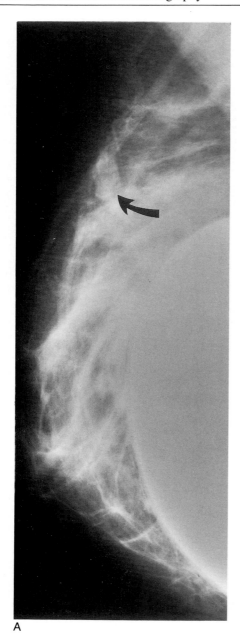

A

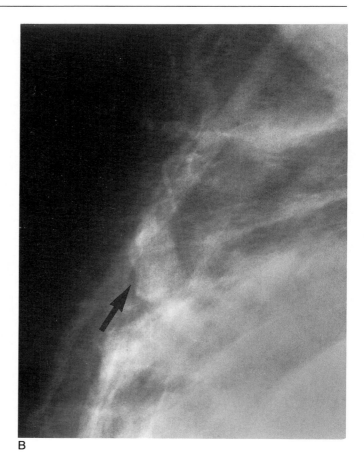

B

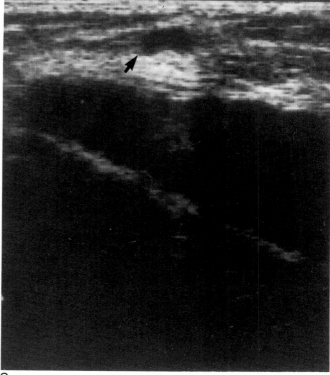

C

Figure 12.28.

Clinical: 38-year-old woman with bilateral breast implants and a palpable nodule in the left axillary tail.

Mammogram: Left oblique view (**A**), coned-down oblique view (**B**), and ultrasound (**C**). A retroglandular implant and a moderate amount of overlying glandular tissue are present. There is a well-circumscribed lobulated nodule *(arrow)* in the upper outer quadrant of the left breast (**A** and **B**). Ultrasound (**C**) demonstrates the nodule to be a cyst *(arrow),* and this corresponded to the palpable nodule.

Impression: Simple cyst anterior to the retroglandular implant.

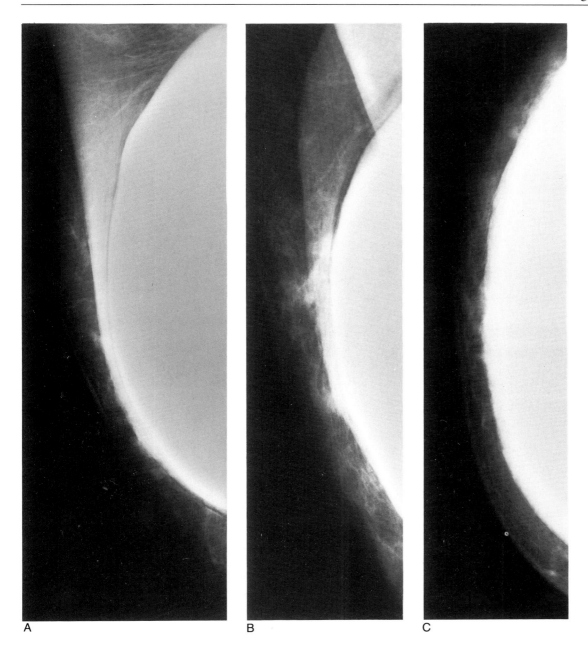

A   B   C

Figure 12.29.

Clinical: 51-year-old G1, P1 woman with a history of bilateral breast carcinomas treated with a right modified radical mastectomy and a left subcutaneous mastectomy.

Mammogram: Left oblique (**A**), medial oblique (**B**), and craniocaudal (**C**) views. A subpectoral implant has been placed for reconstruction of the breast treated with subcutaneous mastectomy. Although no definite ducts are identified, there are patchy densities in the subcutaneous fat, seen best on the medial oblique view (**B**). These densities can be residual fibroglandular tissue or areas of fat necrosis. These areas were followed and were stable in comparison with prior studies.

Impression: Normal appearance of a reconstructed breast with a prosthesis, after subcutaneous mastectomy.

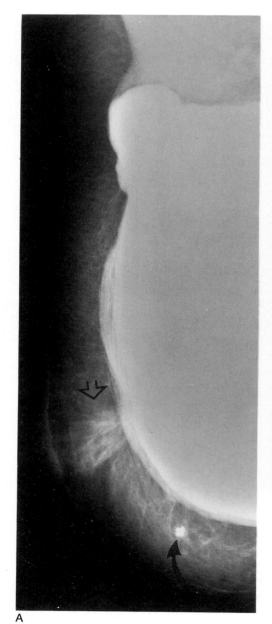

A

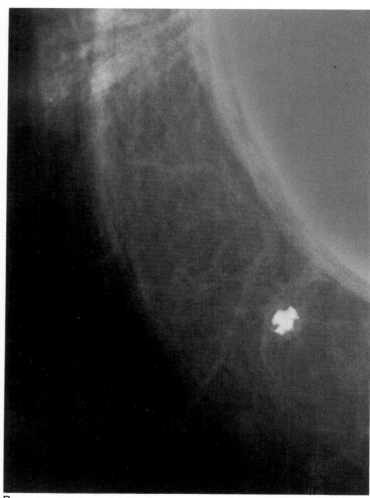

B

Figure 12.30.   70-year-old G4, P3 woman after bilateral subcutaneous mastectomies for benign disease, presenting with a palpable nodule in the left upper outer quadrant.

Mammogram: Left oblique (**A**) and coned-down (**B**) views. There is a subpectoral silicone implant in place. Irregularity of the superior margin of the implant is present, and this corresponded to the palpable nodularity. Even though the patient has undergone a subcutaneous mastectomy, there is residual ductal tissue *(open arrow)* in the subareolar area and a calcified fibroadenoma *(curved arrow)* in the lower aspect of the breast. This emphasizes the importance of imaging patients who have undergone a subcutaneous mastectomy or in which the native nipple is present.

Impression: Residual glandular tissue, irregularity of superior margin of implant; fibroadenoma present after subcutaneous mastectomy and reconstruction.

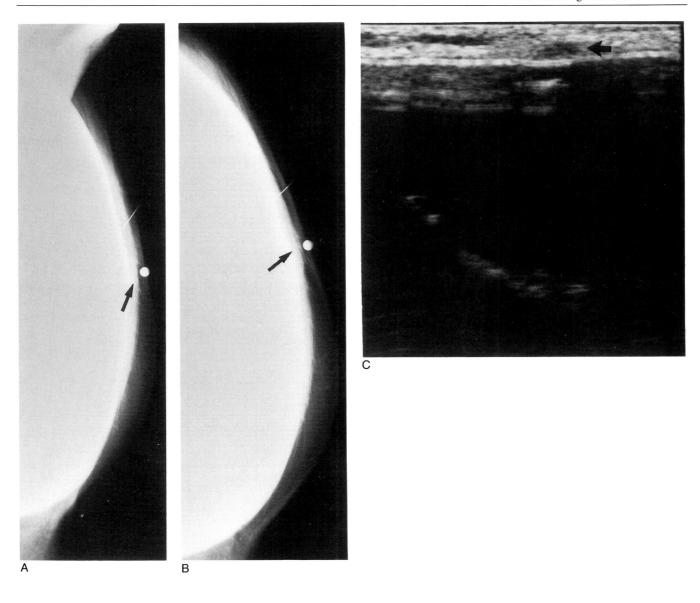

A   B   C

Figure 12.31.

Clinical: 51-year-old woman 6 years after right mastectomy and reconstruction with an expandable implant. She presents with palpable thickening of questionable duration, inferior to the mastectomy scar.

Mammogram: Right oblique view (**A**), right medial oblique view (**B**), and ultrasound (**C**). A wire is present over the scar, and a BB overlies the palpable nodule. A small focal area of irregular tissue *(arrow)* is present beneath the BB (**A** and **B**). The ultrasound (**C**) clearly demonstrates the hypoechoic nodule *(arrow)* in the subcutaneous area.

Impression: Recurrent carcinoma.

Cytology: Positive for malignancy.

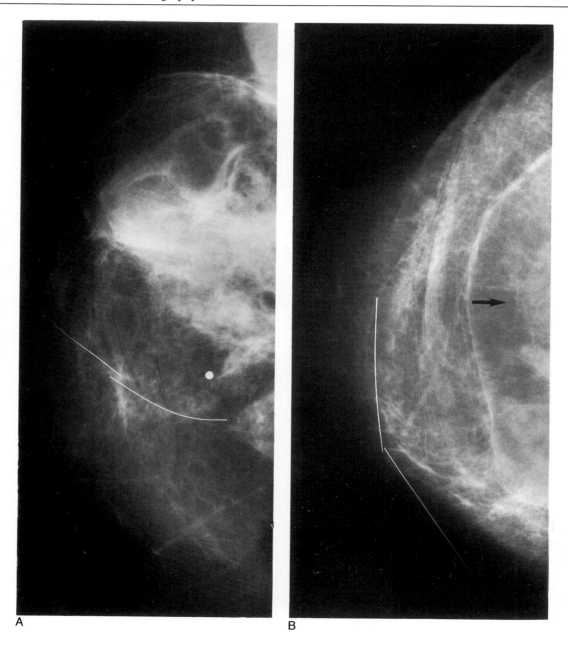

A   B

Figure 12.32.

Clinical: 51-year-old woman after left breast cancer treated with a modified radical mastectomy and reconstruction with a myocutaneous flap. She presents with a palpable mass in the upper aspect of the reconstructed breast.

Mammogram: Left oblique (**A**) and craniocaudal (**B**) views and ultrasound (**C** and **D**). The wires mark the surgical scars, and the BB marks the palpable nodule. There is no ductal tissue present; instead, the reconstructed breast is composed of bandlike densities of muscle, fascia, and fatty tissue (**A** and **B**). In the upper central aspect, there is an irregular mass *(arrow)* (**B**). On ultrasound, the superior aspect of

the density is complex, containing fluid and echogenic components (**C**), most consistent with an organizing hematoma. Adjacent to the hematoma is a focal area of shadowing *(arrow)* (**D**), which could represent fat necrosis, fibrosis, or tumor. This shadowing corresponded to the palpable nodule and was biopsied.

Impression: Reconstructed left breast with a probable hematoma and a solid shadowing area representing either fat necrosis or recurrent tumor.

Histopathology: Fat necrosis, lipogranuloma, foreign body giant cell reaction.

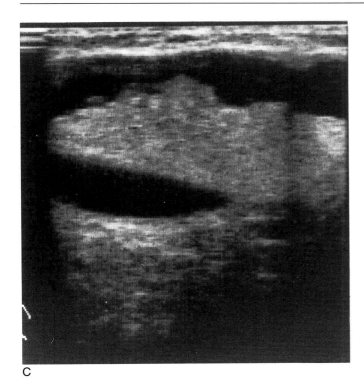

C

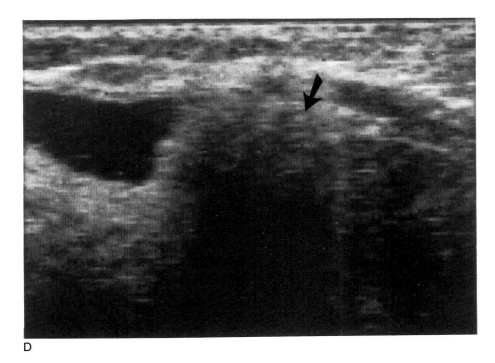

D

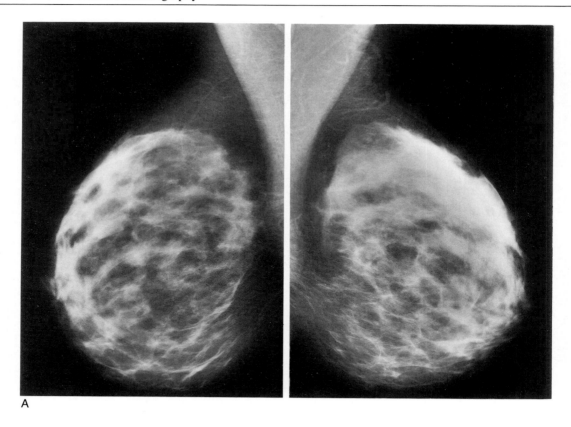

A

Figure 12.33.

Clinical: 36-year-old woman who underwent reduction mammoplasties, for routine follow-up.

Mammogram: Baseline preoperative bilateral oblique views (**A**), oblique (**B**) and craniocaudal (**C**) views 1 year postoperatively, and enlarged (2×) right oblique view (**D**) 2 years postoperatively. On the baseline mammogram (**A**), the breasts are composed of dense symmetrical fibroglandular tissue. After reduction (**B** and **C**), a large amount of fibroglandular tissue has been removed, and there is disorientation of the remaining tissue and elevation of the nipples consistent with normal changes after this procedure. This pattern should suggest to one the findings of a reduction procedure, even without knowledge of the clinical history. One year later (**D**), there has been interval development of multiple oil cysts *(arrow)* and some smaller coarse calcifications of fat necrosis in the upper outer quadrant.

Impression: Postreduction changes, with development of fat necrosis. (Case courtesy of Dr. Cherie Scheer, Richmond, VA.)

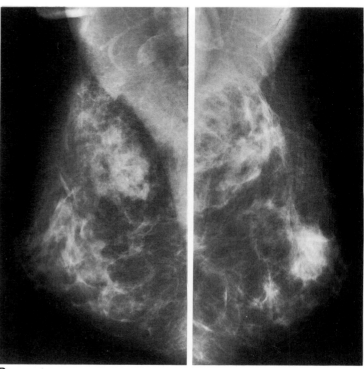

B

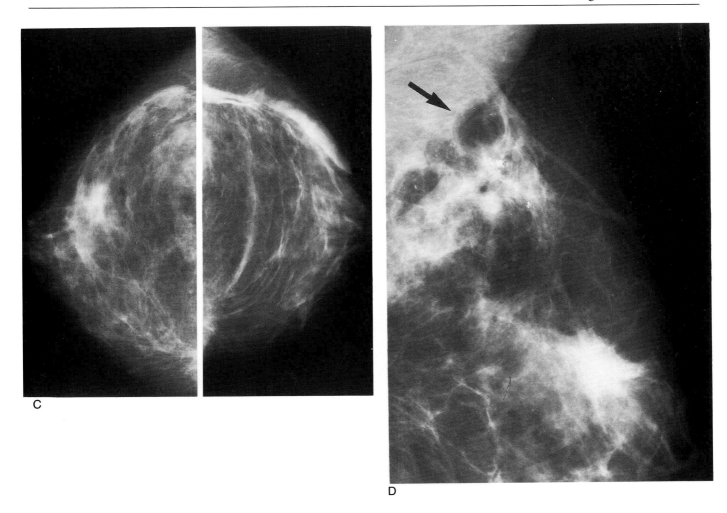

C

D

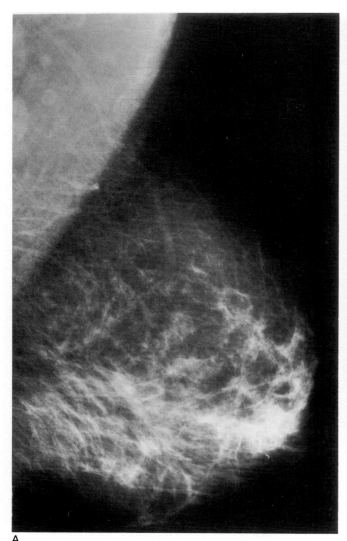

A

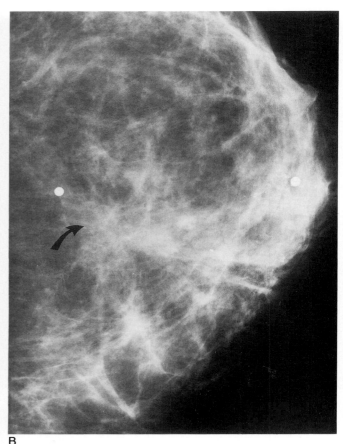

B

Figure 12.34.

Clinical: 44-year-old G3, P3 woman after left mastectomy and reduction mammoplasty on the right.

Mammogram: Right oblique (**A**) and craniocaudal (**B**) views. There is distortion of normal architecture with disturbance of the normal orientation of the ducts toward the nipple. In the lower central aspect of the right breast, there is focal irregu-

lar increased density *(arrow)* (**B**) along the direction of the reduction scar (marked by BBs). This finding is typical of the fat necrosis and scarring that is seen after reduction mammoplasty.

Impression: Postoperative changes after reduction mammoplasty.

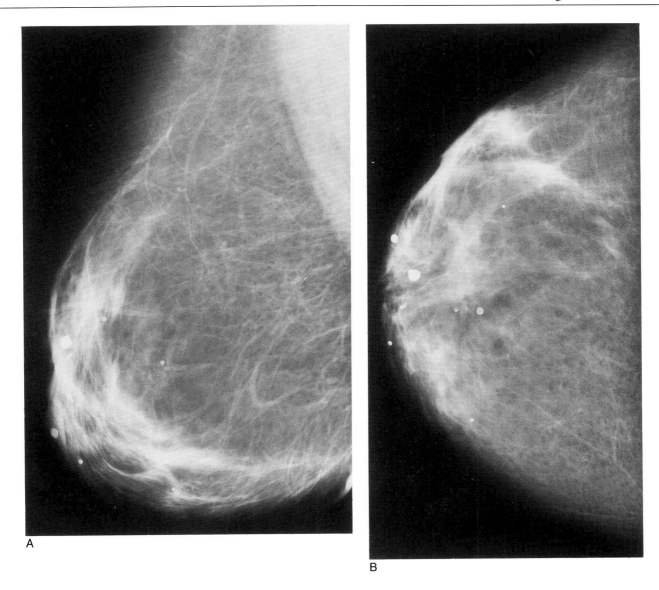

A

B

Figure 12.35.

Clinical: 55-year-old G2, P2 woman after breast reduction, for routine screening.

Mammogram: Left oblique (**A**) and craniocaudal (**B**) views. The breast is mildly glandular. Elevation of the nipple is seen, and there is some disorientation of the parenchymal pattern, consistent with postreduction changes. Multicentric ringlike calcifications are present in the region of the scars, consistent with calcified cysts and fat necrosis.

Impression: Manifestation of fat necrosis, after reduction mammoplasty.

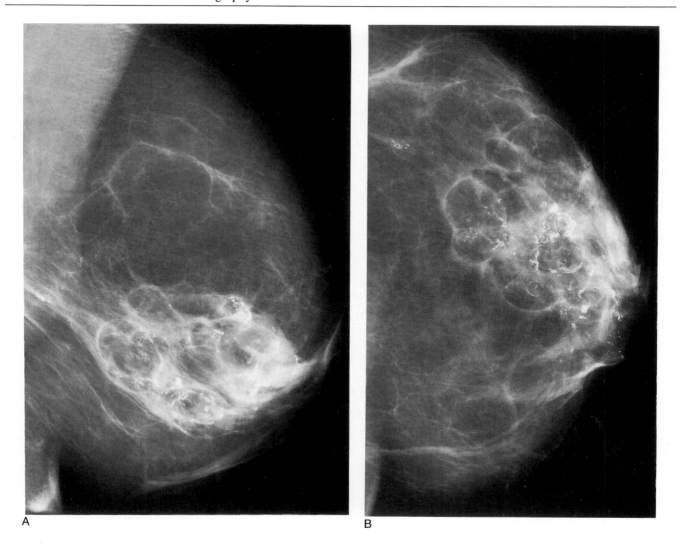

A

B

Figure 12.36.

Clinical: 45-year-old woman after bilateral reduction mammoplasties, with firm nodularity in both subareolar areas.

Mammogram: Right oblique (**A**) and craniocaudal (**B**) views and left oblique (**C**) and craniocaudal (**D**) views. The breasts show primarily fatty replacement. There are extensive areas of calcification in both breasts, more prominent on the right than on the left. Many of the calcifications are thin ringlike areas of liponecrosis macrocystica (fat necrosis). On the right (**A** and **B**), there is a mixture of the large oil cysts with coarse irregular calcifications. The findings represent dystrophic changes of fat necrosis secondary to reduction mammoplasty. Generally, this extent of fat necrosis is not seen after biopsy or lumpectomy and, instead, represents a more significant trauma such as a reduction procedure or severe nonsurgical breast trauma.

Impression: Extensive changes of fat necrosis secondary to reduction mammoplasty. (Case courtesy of Dr. M. C. Wilhelm, Charlottesville, VA.)

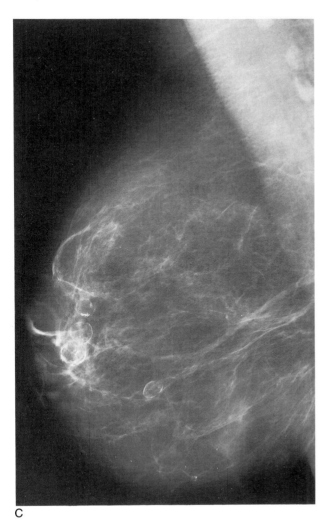

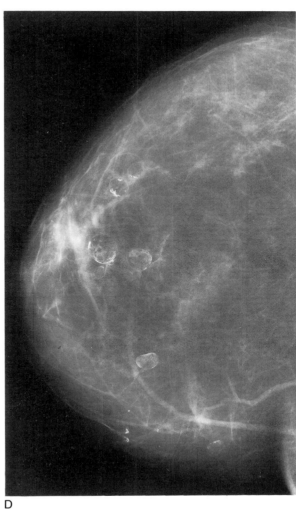

C

D

Figure 12.37.

Clinical: 50-year-old woman after bilateral reduction mammoplasties, for routine mammogram.

Mammogram: Bilateral oblique (**A**), left craniocaudal (**B**), and right craniocaudal (**C**) views. There is disorientation of the parenchymal pattern, without the normal flow of ducts toward the nipples (**A**). This disorientation of parenchyma is a typical postreduction finding. On the craniocaudal views (**B** and **C**), there are circular, round and lacy, coarse calcifications associated with the dense areas of parenchymal scarring. These findings are seen after reduction mammoplasty and represent dystrophic changes of fat necrosis.

Impression: Fat necrosis secondary to reduction mammoplasty.

Note: The patient has been followed for 18 months, and the calcifications are stable.

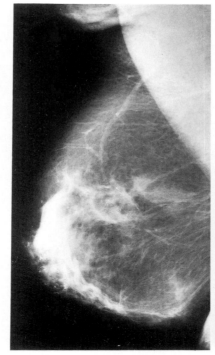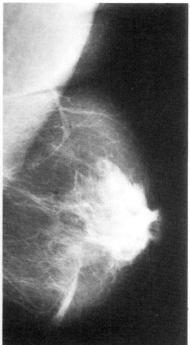

A

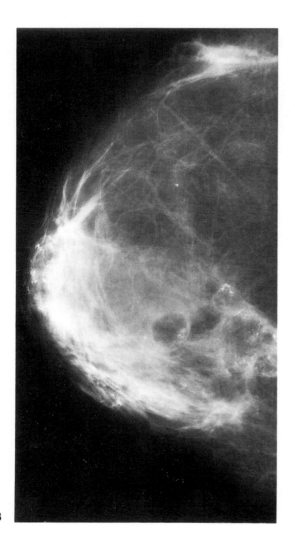

B

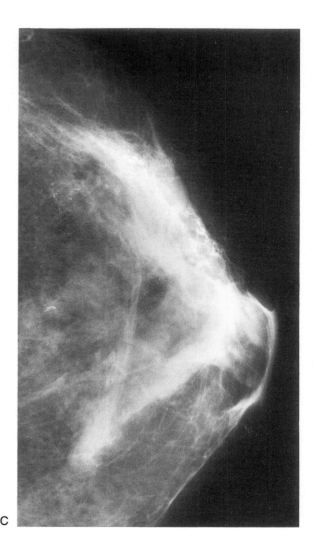

C

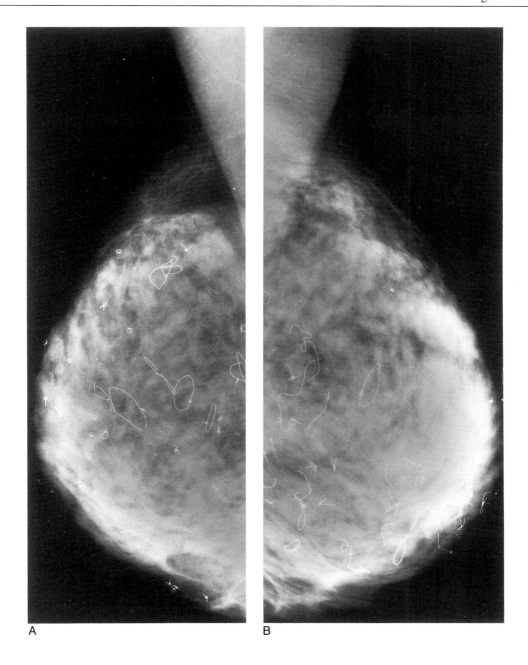

A   B

Figure 12.38.
Clinical: 35-year-old woman after reduction mammoplasty, for routine screening.

Mammogram: Left oblique (**A**) and right oblique (**B**) views. The breasts are very dense and glandular, with an adenosis pattern. Multiple calcified and radiopaque sutures are present bilaterally, corresponding to the scars involved with the reduction procedure.

Impression: Calcified sutures.

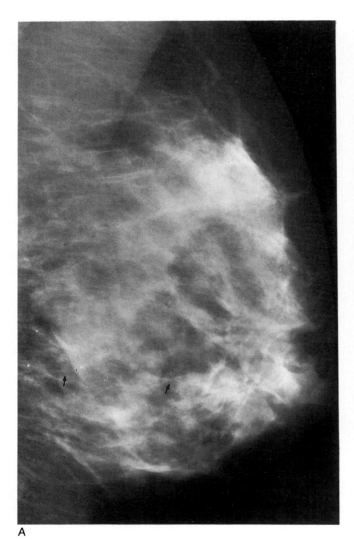

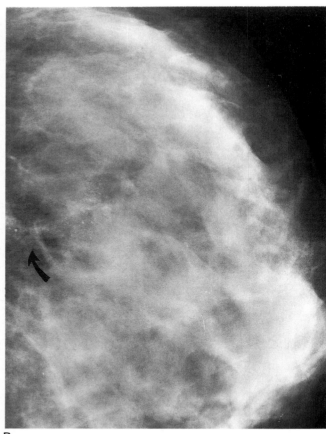

Figure 12.39.

Clinical: 60-year-old woman referred for radiotherapy after having had a lumpectomy elsewhere for comedocarcinoma.

Mammogram: Right oblique (**A**) and craniocaudal (**B**) views prior to lumpectomy; postlumpectomy bilateral oblique (**C**), right breast ultrasound (**D**), right magnification (2×) craniocaudal (**E**), and left magnification (2×) craniocaudal (**F**) views. On the initial prebiopsy films (**A** and **B**) the right breast is dense. There are extensive irregular, mixed-morphology microcalcifications *(arrows)* extending from the retroareolar area to the deep central aspect of the breast. These microcalcifications, which are of malignant morphology, were biopsied and revealed intraductal carcinoma. Because of the extensive nature of calcification the patient would not have been a good candidate for radiotherapy. On her postlumpectomy, preradiotherapy mammogram (**C**) a large medium-density circumscribed mass occupies the central aspect of the right breast *(arrows)*. On ultrasound (**D**) the mass was hypoechoic

and circumscribed and is consistent with an organizing post-operative hematoma. On magnification (**E**) of the tumor bed a few residual microcalcifications are seen anteriorly *(arrows)* and are highly suspicious for residual carcinoma. Incidental note on evaluation of the left breast (**F**) demonstrated two clusters of microcalcifications *(arrows)* best seen on magnification and of nonspecific nature. Some variation in size was seen, and because of their clustered nature and the high-risk status of the patient, biopsy was recommended.

Impression: Right microcalcifications highly suspicious for residual carcinoma, left microcalcifications moderately suspicious for contralateral carcinoma.

Histopathology: Intraductal carcinoma, right breast; multicentric intraductal carcinoma, left breast.

Note: The patient was treated with bilateral mastectomies rather than radiotherapy.

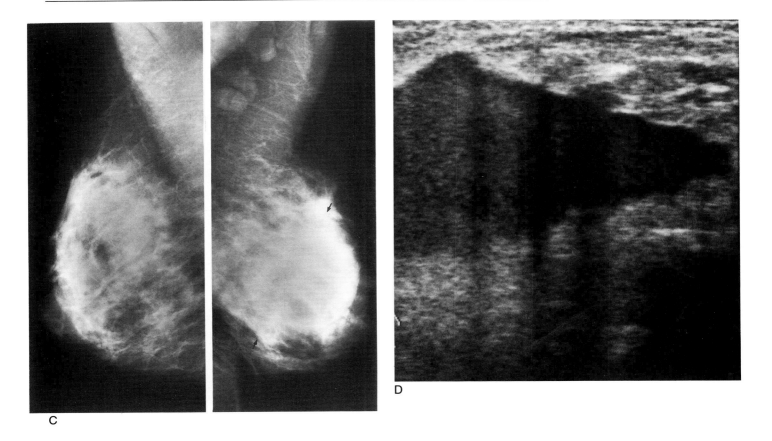

C

D

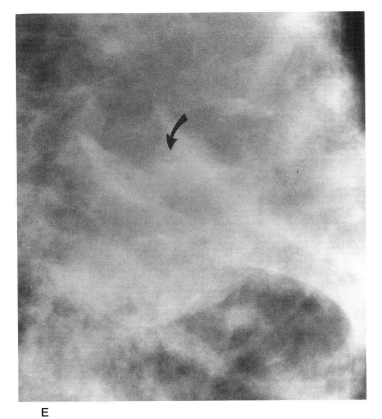

E

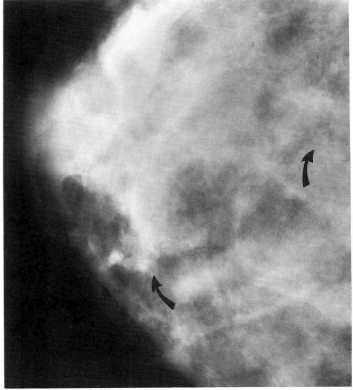

F

Figure 12.40.

Clinical: 31-year-old woman who had a lumpectomy for a palpable carcinoma in the left axillary tail 3 weeks earlier. She was referred for radiation therapy, and a postoperative baseline mammogram was obtained.

Mammogram: Left oblique (**A**), right oblique (**B**), and left oblique craniocaudal (**C**) views. The scar from the recent lumpectomy is evident as a flat irregular density in the upper outer quadrant *(curved arrow)* (**A** and **C**) of the left breast. There is also a subtle area of asymmetry (**A**) in the left supra-areolar area *(arrow)* in comparison with the right breast (**B**). A focal area of increased density is present, and on the craniocaudal view (**C**) it appears finely spiculated *(arrow)*. This supra-areolar lesion is suspicious for residual multicentric nonpalpable carcinoma.

Impression: Highly suspicious for residual carcinoma, separate focus, left breast.

Histopathology: Infiltrating ductal carcinoma.

Note: This case demonstrates the importance of obtaining a mammogram, even in a young patient, prior to definitive therapy to confirm the absence of residual carcinoma.

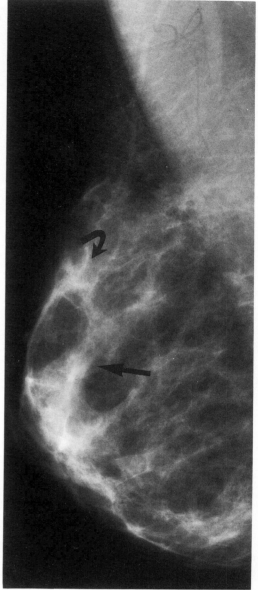

A

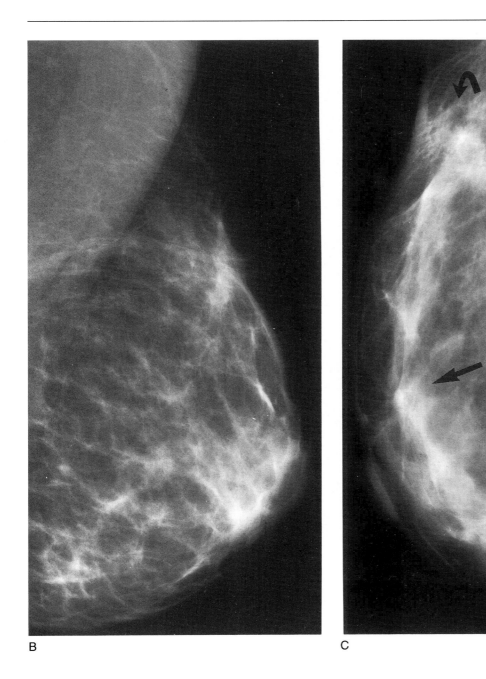

B   C

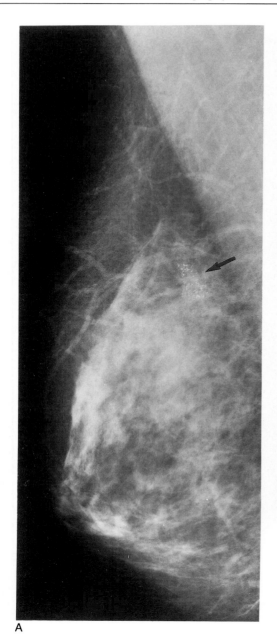

A

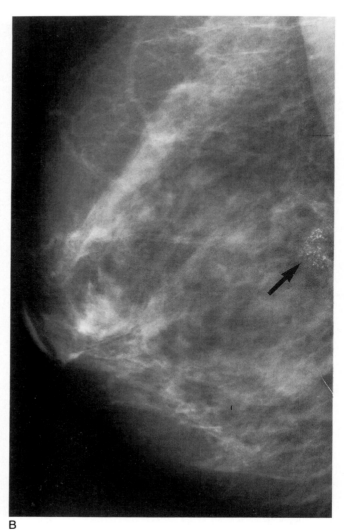

B

Figure 12.41.

Clinical: 66-year-old G2, P2 woman with a family history of breast cancer, for screening.

Mammogram: Left oblique (**A**) and enlarged lateral oblique craniocaudal (**B**) views, specimen radiograph (**C**), and enlarged left mediolateral (**D**) and craniocaudal (**E**) views after biopsy. On the initial mammogram a cluster of innumerable, irregular malignant calcifications *(arrows)* is seen (**A** and **B**). The specimen radiograph (**C**) demonstrates the calcifications, which were noted to extend to the edge of the tissue. Histopathology demonstrated intraductal carcinoma of the comedo type, extending close to the surgical margin. The patient wished to have breast conservation therapy. The postbiopsy, preradiotherapy baseline mammogram (**D** and **E**) demonstrates residual malignant-appearing calcifications at the lumpectomy site *(arrows)*. The spiculated soft tissue density *(curved arrow)* represents hematoma and fat necrosis. Reexcision was performed prior to radiotherapy, and residual intraductal carcinoma was found.

Impression: Preradiotherapy baseline mammogram demonstrating residual carcinoma.

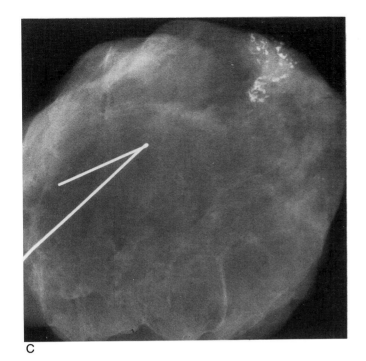

C

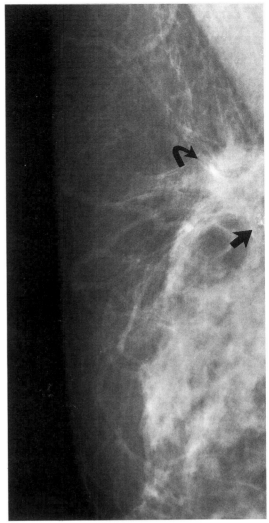

D

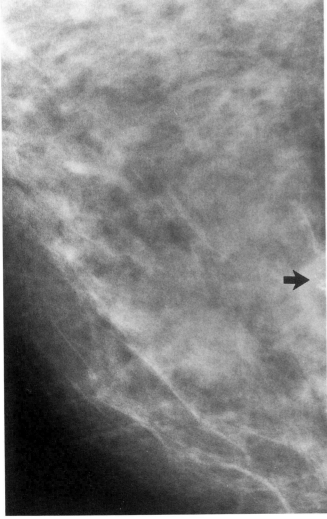

E

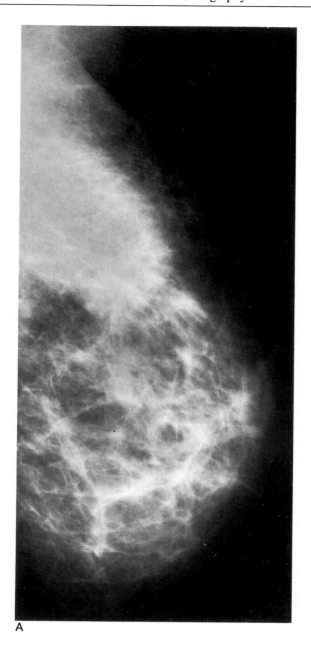

A

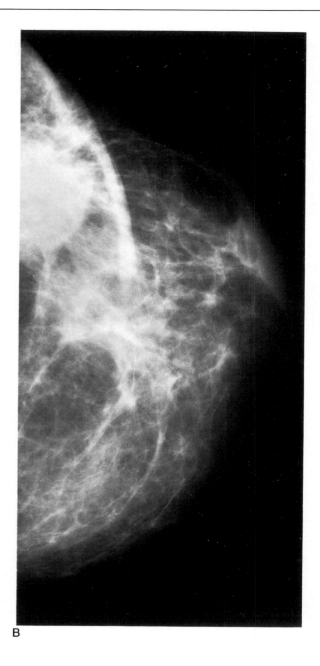

B

Figure 12.42.

Clinical: 50-year-old G4, P4 woman after lumpectomy for a carcinoma in the right upper outer quadrant and referred for radiation therapy. A preliminary mammogram, after lumpectomy and before radiotherapy, was obtained.

Mammogram: Right oblique (**A**) and craniocaudal (**B**) views 1 month after lumpectomy, and right oblique (**C**) and craniocaudal (**D**) views 6 months later. On the postlumpectomy films (**A** and **B**) a large, medium-density, partially circumscribed mass is present at the surgical site and is consistent with a postoperative hematoma. Six months after therapy (**C** and **D**), the hematoma has resolved, and there is a small

residual area of increased density, consistent with scar and fat necrosis *(arrows)*. There is also a mild increase in the overall density of the interstitium and an increase in skin thickness that are normal postradiation changes.

Impression: Normal evolution of postlumpectomy and radiation changes in the acute-subacute phase.

Note: It is not unusual to see a hematoma on the baseline postlumpectomy study. The mammogram can usually be performed with adequate compression of the breast no sooner than 10 days after lumpectomy.

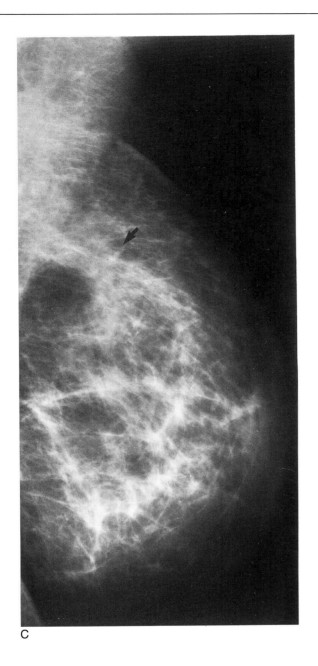

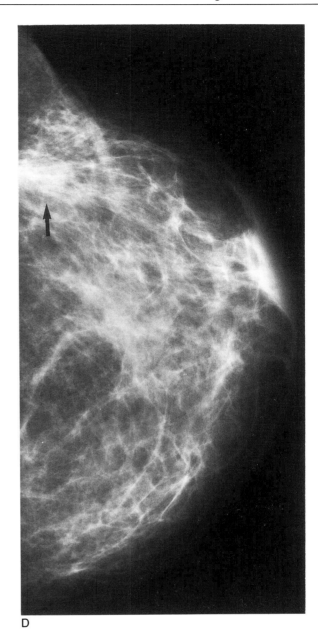

C

D

Figure 12.43.

Clinical: 66-year-old G3, P3 woman who was referred for radiation therapy after a lumpectomy and axillary dissection in the left upper outer quadrant.

Mammogram: Left oblique view 3 weeks after lumpectomy (**A**), and left oblique views 6 months (**B**) and 12 months (**C**) later. On the initial postoperative film (**A**), there is architectural distortion associated with irregular areas of increased density in the left upper outer quadrant and in the axilla *(arrows)*. This density represents hematoma and postsurgical change, and the examination will serve as a baseline for follow-up after radiotherapy. Six months after treatment (**B**), the distortion from the scar persists, but the hematoma and surrounding density have significantly decreased in size. Very minimal increase in interstitial markings is seen, an effect of radiotherapy. On the study 1 year after treatment (**C**), further diminution in the density is seen as would be expected, and there are no new findings to suggest recurrence.

Impression: Postlumpectomy scarring showing resolution.

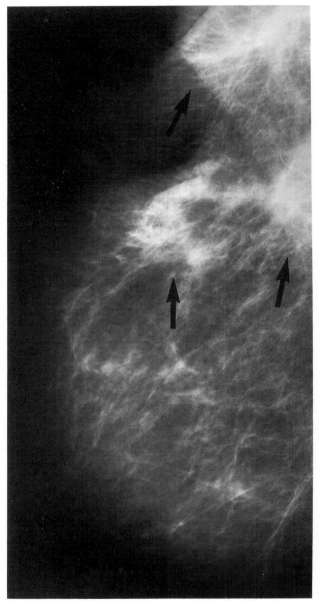

A

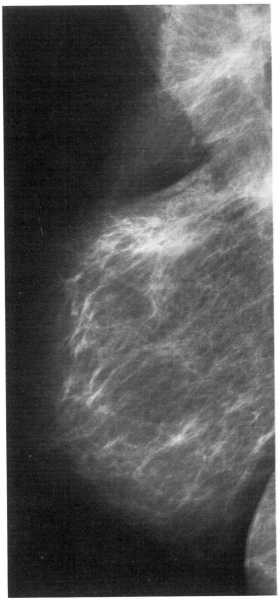

B

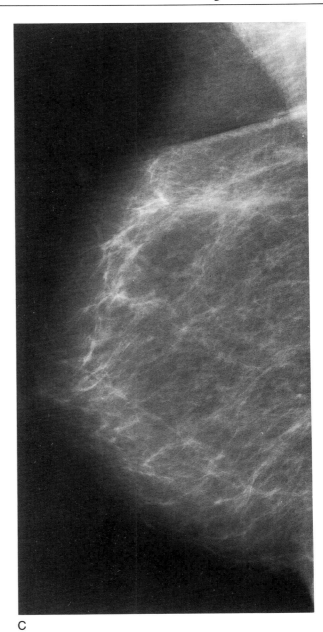

C

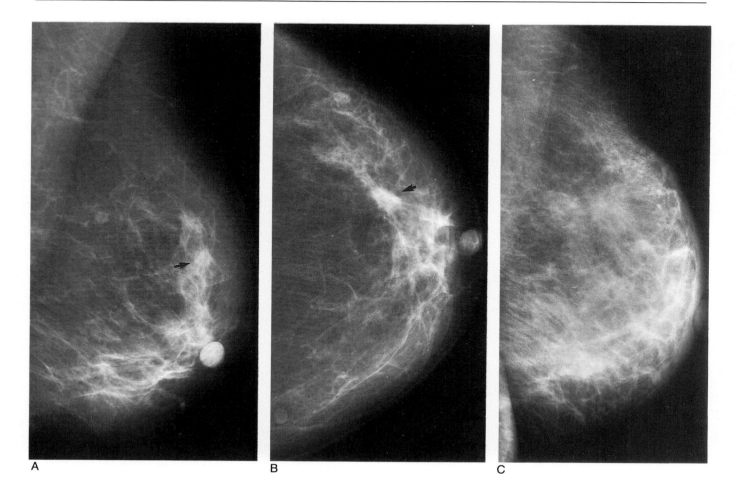

A   B   C

Figure 12.44.

Clinical: 67-year-old G6, P5 woman with a positive family history of breast cancer, for routine screening.

Mammogram: Right oblique (**A**) and craniocaudal (**B**) views from April 1988, right oblique (**C**) and craniocaudal (**D**) views from April 1989, and right oblique (**E**) and craniocaudal (**F**) views from October 1989. On the initial screening examination (**A** and **B**), there is a high-density spiculated mass in the upper outer quadrant (arrows). The lesion was considered highly suspicious and was biopsied after needle localization. The histopathology demonstrated infiltrating ductal carcinoma, and the patient was treated with lumpectomy and ra-

diation therapy. One year later (**C** and **D**), the breast is diffusely edematous, with prominent interstitial markings, increased density, and skin thickening. These are normal changes in the first year after radiation therapy. At 18 months after diagnosis (**E** and **F**), the edema pattern secondary to radiation is decreasing. There also has been a decrease in skin thickening. The scar in the upper outer quadrant is evident (arrow), but there are no changes to suggest recurrence.

Impression: Normal evolution of postradiation changes after treatment of primary breast carcinoma.

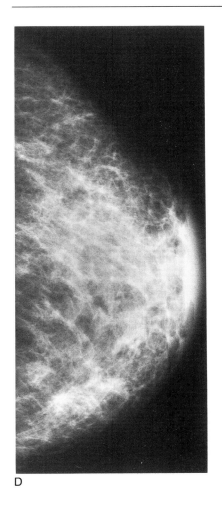

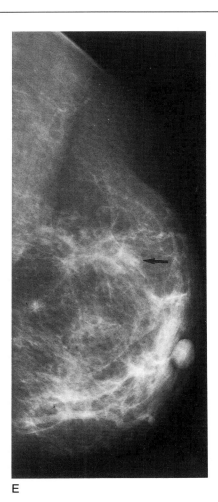

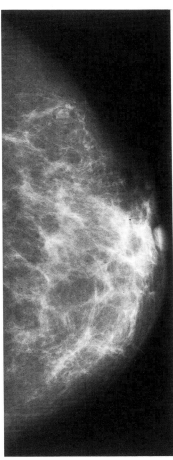

D

E

F

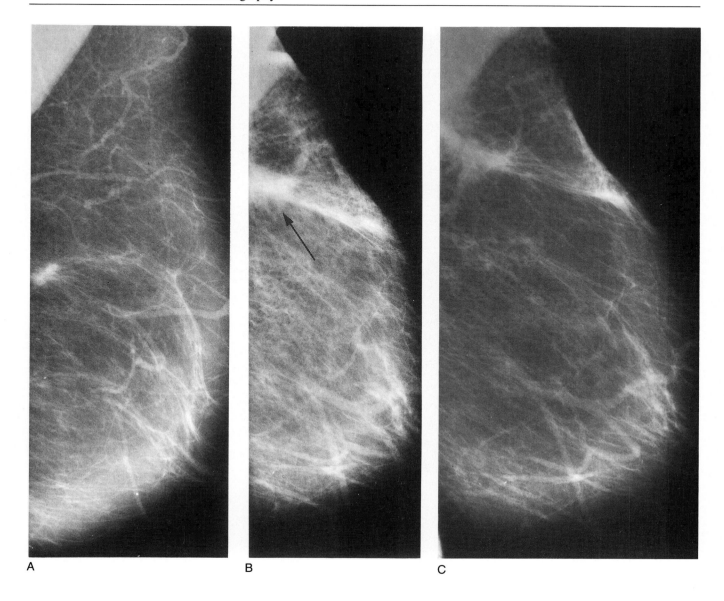

A   B   C

Figure 12.45.

Clinical: 65-year-old woman after lumpectomy and radiation therapy for infiltrating ductal carcinoma of the right breast.

Mammogram: Prebiopsy right oblique view (**A**) and post-treatment right oblique views at 6 months (**B**) and at 12 months (**C**). On the initial study (**A**), there is a high-density spiculated mass deep in the right breast, consistent with carcinoma. This was biopsied after a needle localization, and histopathology revealed infiltrating ductal carcinoma. On the next examination (**B**) 6 months after lumpectomy and radiation therapy, the breast is diffusely more dense and does not compress as well. There is a focal irregular density (arrow) at the lumpectomy site that is most consistent with fat necrosis. Subsequently, at 12 months posttreatment (**C**), there has been a decrease in the edema of the breast as well as a decrease in the size and density of the scar and fat necrosis.

Impression: Normal evolution of postoperative and radiation changes.

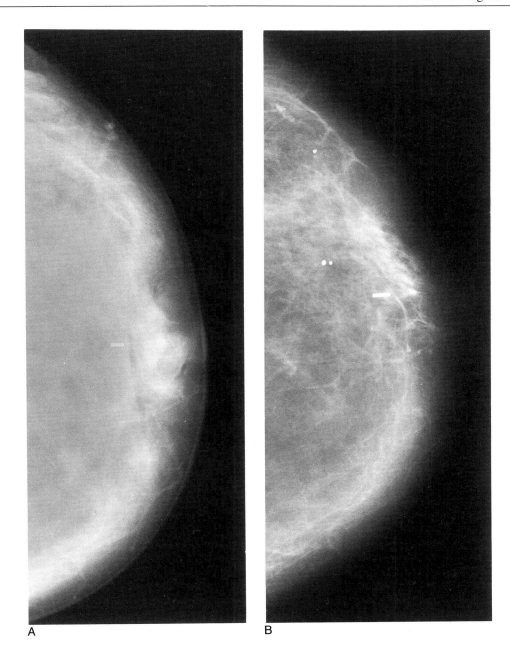

A

B

Figure 12.46.

Clinical: 57-year-old G2, P2 woman after breast conservation therapy on the right, for routine follow-up.

Mammogram: Right craniocaudal view in June 1983 (**A**) and right craniocaudal view in April 1989 (**B**). On the initial study that was postlumpectomy and preradiotherapy, the breast is dense, and there is minimal skin thickening present. A surgical clip is noted in the subareolar area. Six years later, there

has been interval development of coarse dystrophic calcifications of fat necrosis, both at the lumpectomy site near the clip and laterally in the breast. Such calcifications may develop as a normal change after breast conservation therapy.

Impression: Dystrophic calcifications secondary to breast conservation therapy.

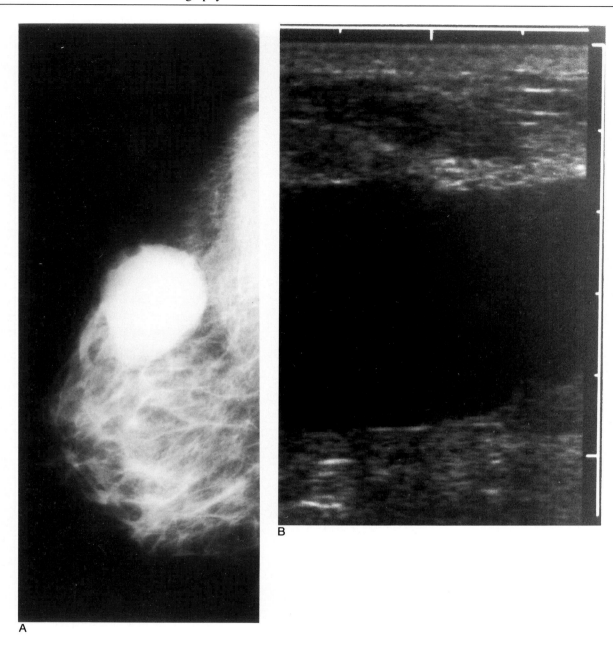

A

B

Figure 12.47.

Clinical: 39-year-old G1, P1 woman 20 months after treatment for stage I breast carcinoma with lumpectomy and radiation therapy. She became pregnant and delivered a child approximately 12 months after radiation therapy was completed.

Mammogram: Left oblique view (**A**) and ultrasound (**B**) 4 weeks after lumpectomy, left oblique view (**C**) 14 months after lumpectomy and radiotherapy, and left oblique (**D**) and craniocaudal (**E**) views 18 months after lumpectomy. On the initial postlumpectomy mammogram (**A**), there is a large high-density, relatively circumscribed mass at the biopsy site. On ultrasound (**B**) this mass is relatively anechoic, consistent with a postoperative hematoma. The mammogram 1 year later, when the patient was postpartum (**C**), demonstrates an irreg-

ular medium-density area at the lumpectomy site. This had decreased in size considerably from the postoperative mammogram and was thought to represent most likely postoperative scarring. However, because of the lack of sequential mammograms a repeat study in 3 months was recommended. On the final films (**D** and **E**) 4 months later, there is a high-density spiculated lesion at the lumpectomy site. (Clinical examination revealed increased induration in this area.) The findings are highly consistent with recurrent carcinoma in the treated breast.

Impression: Sequence of changes demonstrating a recurrent carcinoma in the treated breast.

Cytology: Carcinoma.

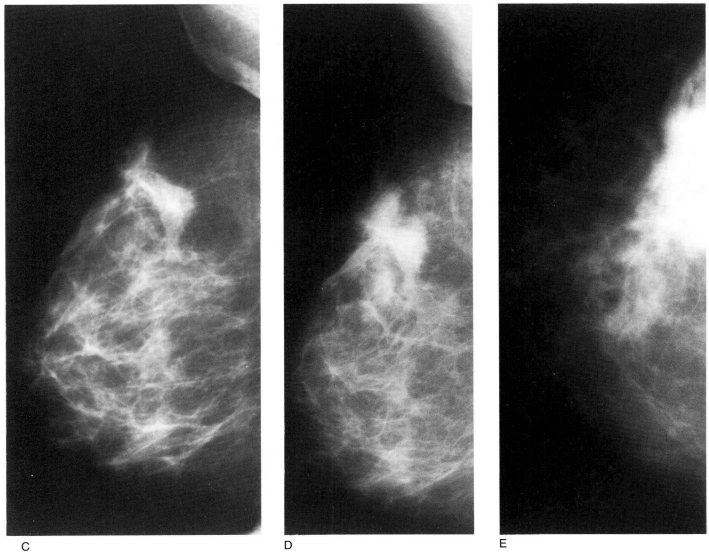

C   D   E

References

1. Sickles EA, Herzog KA. Mammography of the postsurgical breast. AJR 1987;136:585–588.
2. Stigers KB, King JK, Davey DD, Stelling CB. Abnormalities of the breast caused by biopsy: spectrum of mammographic findings. AJR 1991;156:287–291.
3. Mendelson EB. Imaging the post-surgical breast. Semin Ultrasound CT MR 1989;10(2):154–170.
4. Davis SP, Stomper PC, Weidner N, Meyer JE. Suture calcification mimicking recurrence in the irradiated breast: a potential pitfall in mammographic evaluation. Radiology 1989;172:247–248.
5. Beyer GA, Thorsen MK, Shaffer KA, Walker AP. Mammographic appearance of the retained Dacron cuff of a Hickman catheter. AJR 1990;155:1203–1204.
6. Parsons RW, Thering HR. Management of the silicone-injected breast. Plast Reconstr Surg 1977;60(4):534–538.
7. Delage C, Shane JJ, Johnson FB. Mammary silicone granuloma. Arch Dermatol 1973;108:104–107.
8. Koide T, Katayama H. Calcification in augmentation mammoplasty. Radiology 1979;130:337–340.
9. Jenson SR, Mackey JK. Xeromammography after augmentation mammoplasty. AJR 1985;144:629–633.
10. Segel MC, Schnitt EL, Binns JH. Carcinoma of the breast associated with silicone paraffin injections. Breast Dis 1988;1:225–229.
11. McGrath MH, Burkhardt BR. The safety and efficacy of breast implants for augmentation mammoplasty. Plast Reconstr Surg 1984;74(4):550–560.
12. Dershaw DD, Chaglassion TA. Mammography after prosthesis placement for augmentation or reconstructive mammoplasty. Radiology 1989;170:69–74.
13. Mitnick JS, Harris MN, Roses DF. Mammographic detection of carcinoma of the breast in patients with augmentation prostheses. Surg Gynecol Obstet 1989;168:30–32.
14. Eklund GW, Busby RC, Miller SH, Job JS. Improved imaging of the augmented breast. AJR 1988;151:469–473.
15. Cole-Reuglet C, Schwartz G, Kurtz AB, et al. Ultrasound mammography for the augmented breast. Radiology 1983;146:737–742.
16. Biggs TM, Cukier J, Worthing LF. Augmentation mammoplasty: a review of 18 years. Plast Reconstr Surg 1982;69(3):445–449.
17. McKinney P, Tresley G. Longterm comparison of patients with gel and saline mammary implants. Plast Reconstr Surg 1983;72:27–29.
18. Grant EG, Cigtay OS, Mascatello VJ. Irregularity of Silastic brest implants mimicking a soft tissue mass. AJR 1978;130:461–462.
19. Shermis RB, Adler DD, Smith DJ, Hall JD. Intraductal silicone secondary to breast implant rupture. An unusual mammographic presentation. Breast Dis 1990;3:17–20.
20. Rebner M, Stevenson TR. Fat necrosis of bilateral musculocutaneous flap breast reconstruction. Breast Dis 1988;1:199–203.
21. Holmes FA, Singletary ES, Kroll S, et al. Fat necrosis in an autogenously reconstructed breast mimicking recurrent carcinoma at mammography. Breast Dis 1988;1:211–218.
22. Miller CL, Feig SA, Fox JW. Mammography changes after reduction mammoplasty. AJR 1987;149:35–38.
23. Swann CA, Kopans DB, White G, et al. Observations on the postreduction mammoplasty mammogram. Breast Dis 1989;1:261–267.
24. Baber CE, Libshitz HI. Bilateral fat necrosis of the breast following reduction mammoplasties. AJR 1977;128:508–509.
25. Fisher B, Redmond C, Poisson R, et al. Eight-year results of a randomized clinical trial of comparing total mastectomy and lumpectomy with or without irradiation in the treatment of breast cancer. N Engl J Med 1989;320:822–828.
26. Veronesi U, Zucali R, Luini A. Local control and survival in early breast cancer: the Milan trial. Int J Radiat Oncol Biol Phys 1986;12:717–720.
27. Peters ME, Fagerholm MI, Scanlan KA, et al. Mammographic evaluation of the postsurgical and irradiated breast. RadioGraphics 1988;8(5):873–899.
28. Romsdahl MM, Montague ED, Ames FC, et al. Conservative surgery and irradiation as treatment for early breast cancer. Arch Surg 1983;118:521–528.
29. Stehlin JS, de Ipolyi PD, Greeff PJ, et al. A ten year study of partial mastectomy for carcinoma of the breast. Surg Gynecol Obstet 1987;165:191–198.
30. Fisher ER, Sass R, Fisher B, et al. Pathologic findings for the National Surgical Adjuvant Breast Project. Relation of local breast recurrence to multicentricity. Cancer 1986;57:1717–1724.
31. Harris JR, Recht A, Amalric R, et al. Time course and prognosis of local recurrence following primary radiation therapy for early breast cancer. J Clin Oncol 1984;2(1):37–41.
32. Krishnan I, Krishnan EC, Mansfield C, et al. Treatment options in early breast cancer. RadioGraphics 1989;9(6)1067–1079.
33. Paulus DD. Conservative treatment of breast cancer: mammography in patient selection and follow-up. AJR 1984;143:483–487.
34. Homer MJ, Schmidt-Ullrich R, Safaii H, et al. Residual breast carcinoma after biopsy. Role of mammography in evaluation. Radiology 1989;170:75–77.
35. Spaulding C, Shaw de Paredes E, Anne P, et al. Detection of recurrence after breast conservation treatment with radiotherapy. Breast Dis in press.
36. Gefter WB, Friedman AK, Goodman RL. The role of mammography in evaluating patients with early carcinoma of the breast for tylectomy and radiation therapy. Radiology 1982;142:77–80.
37. Dershaw DD, Shank B, Reisinger S. Mammographic findings after breast cancer treatment with local excision and definitive irradiation. Radiology 1987;164:455–461.
38. Libshitz HI, Montague ED, Paulus DD. Calcifications and the therapeutically irradiated breast. AJR 1977;128:1021–1025.

39. Stomper PC, Recht A, Berenberg AL, et al. Mammographic detection of recurrent cancer in the irradiated breast. AJR 1987;148:39–43.

40. Dershaw DD, McCormick B, Cox L, Osborne MP. Differentiation of benign and malignant local tumor recurrence after lumpectomy. AJR 1990;155:35–38.

41. Rebner M, Pennes DR, Adler DD, et al. Breast microcalcifications after lumpectomy and radiation therapy. Radiology 1989;170:691–693.

42. Solin LJ, Fowble BL, Troupin RH, Goodman RL. Biopsy results of new calcifications in the post irradiated breast. Cancer 1989;63:1956–1961.

INDEX